CONTRIBUTORS

The authors thank the following colleagues for their contributions and expertise in preparing questions for this student study guide.

Amy Deutschendorf, MS, RN, AOCN
Senior Director, Care Management, Practice and Education
Johns Hopkins Bayview Medical Center
Principal, Clinical Resource Consultants, LLC
Faculty Associate, Johns Hopkins University School of Nursing
Baltimore, Maryland
Chapter 12: Interventions for Clients with Fluid Imbalances
Chapter 15: Acid-Base Balance
Chapter 16: Interventions for Clients with Acid-Base Imbalances

Susan Anne Frosbrook, MS, RN
Medical-Surgical Nurse Clinician and Educator
Annapolis, Maryland
Chapter 65: Interventions for Clients with Diabetes Mellitus

J. Penny Gonella, MPH, RN, CIC
Infection Control Nurse
Augusta, Georgia
Unit 9: Problems of Mobility, Sensation, and Cognition: Management of Clients with Problems of the Nervous System

Maureen D. Holtzman, MN, RN, C
Assistant Professor, Nursing Department
Anne Arundel Community College
Arnold, Maryland
Chapter 6: Cultural Aspects of Health

Jodi Hudgins, MSN, RNC, CLC
Education Services Coordinator
Enterprise Communities/Healthy Start Initiative Project
Medical College of Georgia
Clinical Instructor, School of Nursing
Augusta State University
Augusta, Georgia
Unit 4: Management of Perioperative Clients

Melissa T. Williams, MSN, RN, PCS
Assistant Professor, School of Nursing
Augusta State University
Augusta, Georgia
Unit 16: Problems of Reproduction: Management of Clients with Problems of the Reproductive System

PREFACE

Critical Thinking Study Guide is a companion publication for *Medical-Surgical Nursing: Critical Thinking for Collaborative Care*, fourth edition, by Ignatavicius and Workman. This study guide is designed and written by experts in the fields of adult medical-surgical nursing and nursing education. It is primarily written to enable the nursing student to understand the textbook content and learn about collaborative practice in the care of the adult medical-surgical client.

The format and learning exercises have undergone extensive revision and redesign from the previous edition. The overall goal was to provide a study guide with a format that is logically structured, understandable, and user-friendly, with practical, thought-provoking critical thinking questions related to clinical practice, and learning exercises that offer comprehensive coverage of adult medical-surgical content. Because of the format and structure of the learning exercises, this study guide is a useful tool to prepare for classroom examinations and standardized tests, as well as a review for clinical practice.

The overall organization of the *Critical Thinking Study Guide* directly corresponds to the unit/chapter name and number in the textbook so that the student or faculty member can readily select the corresponding learning exercises in the study guide. Each unit is divided into the following parts, which the student completes with each chapter assignment:

a) *Core Concepts Grid*. These grids highlight the key concepts that are covered in the text and study guide for that unit. Students should read these grids and familiarize themselves with these concepts.

b) *Learning Plan*. This plan maps out an approach and structure for the student to maximize the learning for each chapter. Learning Plans are divided into *Learning Outcomes*, *Learning Activities*, and *Supplemental Resources*.

- *Learning Outcomes* correspond directly to the Learning Objectives listed in the text. They represent the essential learning outcomes that students should achieve for each chapter.
- *Learning Activities* provide a three-step approach for completing the Learning Plan. First, key prerequisites are provided for review as needed by the student. Next, the student has the opportunity to review critical terms and their definitions that are highlighted in each chapter. These first two steps maximize the impact and benefit of the final step: the Learning Exercises that are provided for each chapter. These Learning Exercises are designed to encourage prioritizing, critical thinking, and application of the steps of the nursing process.
- *Supplemental Resources*. In addition to the textbook, a wide variety of resources have been provided to support all three steps in the Learning Activities. For all of the interventions chapters, the related assessment chapter for that unit is first on this list. The assessment chapter is specifically listed for students in order to highlight the importance of assessment data in the care of clients; we recommend that the assessment chapters be considered required reading to serve as the foundation for the interventions chapters that address health care problems. The assessment chapter name and number are listed as a quick reference. All other resources listed are suggestions for additional information.

The answers, with some rationales and references to the text, are given at the end of the *Critical Thinking Study Guide* for each corresponding Learning Exercise. Answer Guidelines for Case Studies are provided on the companion SIMON Web site at http://www.wbsaunders.com/SIMON/Iggy/.

This unique format, including Core Concept Grids and complete Learning Plans, should facilitate student learning and foster critical thinking that can be applied in any clinical setting.

Critical Thinking Study Guide for
Ignatavicius & Workman

Medical-Surgical Nursing: Critical Thinking for Collaborative Care
4th edition

Carol Gamer Dignon, MSN, RN, OCN
Independent Education Consultant
Education Specialist, NIH R-25 Grant, University of Maryland, Baltimore, Maryland
Formerly, Visiting Assistant Professor, Towson University, Towson, Maryland
Instructor, Christ Hospital School of Nursing, Cincinnati, Ohio
Adjunct Faculty, Medical College of Georgia, Augusta, Georgia

Sheryl R. Alba, MSN, RN
Clinical Nurse Specialist, Center for Senior Health
Clinical Instructor, Department of Community Nursing, Medical College of Georgia, Augusta, Georgia
Formerly, Assistant Professor, Learning Resource Coordinator, School of Nursing, Augusta State University,
    Augusta, Georgia

Rosemarie Helen Delya, MSN, RN
Illinois-Certified Train the Trainer
Assistant Professor and BSN Coordinator, Lakeview College of Nursing, Danville, Illinois
Adjunct Faculty, South Suburban College, South Holland, Illinois

Nancy C. Scarlett, MS, RNC
Assistant Professor, Lakeview College of Nursing, Danville, Illinois

With contributions by Donna D. Ignatavicius, MS, RN, Cm

W.B. Saunders Company
Philadelphia   London   Montreal   Sydney   Tokyo   Toronto

W.B. Saunders Company

Vice President and Publishing Director: Sally Schrefer
Executive Editor: Robin Carter
Managing Editor: Lee Henderson
Senior Developmental Editor: Kristin Geen
Project Manager: Gayle Morris
Production Editor: Stephanie M. Hebenstreit
Designer: Teresa Breckwoldt

W.B. Saunders Company
The Curtis Center
Independence Square West
Philadelphia, Pennsylvania 19106-3399

International Standard Book Number: 0-7216-8975-2

Printed in the United States of America

01 02 03 04 05 FG/EB 9 8 7 6 5 4 3 2 1

CONTENTS

UNIT 1 HEALTH PROMOTION AND ILLNESS ■ Core Concepts Grid

Critical Thinking in the Role of the Medical/Surgical Nurse	Community-Based Care	Introduction to Managed Care and Case Management	Introduction to Complementary and Alternative Therapies	Health Care of Older Adults

• **Definitions of health**
• **Health promotion and protection**
• **Roles**
• **Teaching/learning process**
• **Concept of caring**
• **Practice settings**
• **Nursing process**
	• **Ambulatory care**
	• **Home care**
	• **Nursing home care**
	• **Subacute care**
	• **Rehabilitative care**
		• **Purpose**
		  Types
		• **Role of the nurse**
		• **Focus on outcomes**
		• **Case management**
		• **Role of case manager**
		• **Clinical pathways**
			• **Spirituality and religion**
			• **Relaxation**
			• **Imagery**
			• **Music**
			• **Touch**
			• **Laughter/humor**
			• **Herbalism**
			• **Progressive muscle relaxation**
			• **Aromatherapy**
				• **Subgroups of older adults**
				• **Health issues**
				  Health promotion
				  Nutritional needs
				  Accidents
				  Drug use/misuse
				  Mental health
				  Neglect/abuse
				• **Economic issues**
				  Income
				  Housing
				  Other resources
				• **Role of gerontologic nurse**

Unit 1 (Chapters 1-5)

Health Promotion and Illness

Learning Plan

Chapter 1: *Critical Thinking in the Role of the Medical-Surgical Nurse*

Learning Outcomes

1. Compare and contrast common definitions of health.
2. Explain why some populations are more likely to experience health problems than others.
3. Differentiate the three levels of illness prevention and provide at least one example of each level.
4. Explain the purpose of Healthy People 2010.
5. Identify the major roles of the medical-surgical nurse.
6. Explain the relationship between critical thinking and evidence-based practice.
7. Describe best practice interventions for client education.
8. Describe typical health care settings in which medical-surgical nursing is practiced.
9. Identify the key components of a nursing assessment.
10. Describe the difference between a nursing diagnosis and a collaborative problem.
11. Formulate expected outcomes based on data analysis.
12. Identify best practice interventions for clinical documentation.

Learning Activities

1. Prior to completing the study guide exercises for this chapter, it is recommended to review the following:
   - Concepts of health and health promotion
   - Consumer education and awareness
   - Teaching-learning process
   - North American Nursing Diagnosis Association (NANDA) current nursing diagnoses

2. Review the **boldfaced** words and their definitions in Chapter 1 to enhance your understanding of the content.

3. Go to Study Guide Number 1.1 on the following pages and complete the learning exercises for this chapter.

Supplemental Resources

1. Textbook—Chapter 1
2. Other resources:
   - Hamer, S. & Collinson, G. (1999). *Achieving evidence based practice: A handbook for practitioners.* Edinburgh: Balliere Tindall.
   - U.S. Department of Health and Human Services, Public Health Service. (2000). *Healthy People 2010: National promotion and disease prevention objectives.* Washington, DC: U.S. Government Printing Office.

Chapter 2: *Community-Based Care*

Learning Outcomes

1. Explain the primary purpose of ambulatory care.
2. Discuss the growth of home care in the United States.
3. Describe the role of the nurse in home care.
4. Identify examples of interventions for which Medicare pays in home care.
5. Compare and contrast the common types of nursing homes.
6. Describe the term *subacute care.*

Learning Activities

1. Prior to completing the study guide exercises for this chapter, it is recommended to review the concept of home care, long-term care, and acute care facilities as health providers.

2. Review the **boldfaced** words and their definitions in Chapter 2 to enhance your understanding of the content.

3. Go to Study Guide Number 1.2 on the following pages and complete the learning exercises for this chapter.

Supplemental Resources

1. Textbook—Chapter 2
2. Other resources:
   - Invite a nursing home director to discuss regulated residency, the nursing home as a health care setting, and special provisions for confused clients.
   - Spillman, B.C., & Lubitz, J. (2000). The effect of longevity on spending for acute and long-term care. *New England Journal of Medicine, 342*(19), 1409-1415.
   - Stahl, D.A. (1994). Subacute care: The future of health care. *Nursing Management, 25*(10), 34-40.

- Visit an acute care unit at a local nursing home and determine the type, length of stay, and acuity of the clients residing there.

Chapter 3: *Introduction to Managed Care and Case Management*

Learning Outcomes

1. Explain the primary purpose of managed health care.
2. Contrast the fee-for-service and capitated reimbursement systems.
3. Describe the process of case management.
4. Identify at least three certifications for case managers.

Learning Activities

1. Prior to completing the study guide exercises for this chapter, it is recommended to review the following:
   - Concepts of health and health promotion
   - Consumer education and awareness

2. Review the **boldfaced** words and their definitions in Chapter 3 to enhance your understanding of the content.

3. Go to Study Guide Number 1.3 on the following pages and complete the learning exercises for this chapter.

Supplemental Resources

1. Textbook—Chapter 3
2. Other resources:
   - Contact a local hospital and visit with a practicing case manager and management of difficult and long-term clients.
   - Forbes, M. (1999). The practice of professional nurse case management. *Nurse Case Management, 4*(10), 28-33.
   - Locate an insurance company office in your area and discuss managed health care practices and reimbursement issues.

Chapter 4: *Introduction to Complementary and Alternative Therapies*

Learning Outcomes

1. Describe selected low-risk complementary and alternative therapies that nurses can use with their clients in a variety of health care settings.
2. Identify at least one purpose for each selected complementary and alternative therapy.
3. Discuss the implications of complementary and alternative therapies for health care professionals.

Learning Activities

1. Prior to completing the study guide exercises for this chapter, it is recommended to review the following:
   - Concepts of health and health promotion
   - Consumer education and awareness

2. Review the **boldfaced** words and their definitions in Chapter 4 to enhance your understanding of the content.

3. Go to Study Guide Number 1.4 on the following pages and complete the learning exercises for this chapter.

Supplemental Resources

1. Textbook—Chapter 4
2. Other resources:
   - Augustin, P. & Hains, A.A. (1996). Effect of music on ambulatory surgery patients' preoperative anxiety. *AORN Journal, 63,* 750,753-758.
   - Contact a massage therapist and/or music therapist and discuss benefits and applications of these therapies in practice.

Chapter 5: *Health Care of Older Adults*

Learning Outcomes	Learning Activities	Supplemental Resources
1. Identify four subgroups of older adults. 2. Describe nursing interventions for relocation stress syndrome. 3. Discuss common health issues that may concern older adults. 4. Explain why older adults are often at high risk for falls. 5. State common interventions for older clients at high risk for falls. 6. Describe the nursing care required for clients who are restrained. 7. Explain the effects of drugs on the older adult. 8. Compare and contrast delirium and dementia. 9. Interpret the signs and symptoms of elder neglect or abuse. 10. Discuss potential economic issues for older adults. 11. Describe government and community resources that are available for older adults.	1. Prior to completing the study guide exercises for this chapter, it is recommended to review the following: • Concepts of health and health promotion • Consumer education and awareness • Normal growth and development • Principles of sociology • Principles of developmental psychology 2. Review the **boldfaced** words and their definitions in Chapter 5 to enhance your understanding of the content. 3. Go to Study Guide Number 1.5 on the following pages and complete the learning exercises for this chapter.	1. Textbook—Chapter 5 2. Other resources: • Christmas, C. & Andersen, R. A. (2000). Exercise and older patients: Guidelines for the physician. *Journal of the American Geriatric Society, 48*(3), 318-324. • Contact the Center for Aging Organization in your area and find out what resources there are in your community for support of older adults.

STUDY GUIDE NUMBER 1.1

Critical Thinking in the Role of the Medical-Surgical Nurse

Study/Review Questions

1. The definition of health has been influenced by which factors?

    a. _____

    b. _____

    c. _____

Answer Questions 2 through 6 on a separate sheet of paper.

2. What is the holistic view of health? How does it differ from the sociologic perspective?

3. One concept related to health is homeostasis. Why is this concept losing popularity?

4. Health reflects a person's biologic, psychologic, and sociologic states. Define these terms.

    a. _____

    b. _____

    c. _____

5. The Healthy People 2010 campaign has an aggressive plan to improve the nation's health. What are the two overall national health goals?

6. Identify examples of practices that individuals can use to promote their health.

7. Match the following examples of preventive health behavior with their associated levels of intervention. *Answers may be used more than once.*

Prevention Health Behavior	Level of Intervention
___ a. Mammogram	1. Primary
___ b. Prevention of severe disability	2. Secondary
___ c. Flu vaccine	3. Tertiary
___ d. Seat belts	
___ e. Cardiac rehabilitation	
___ f. Purified protein derivative (PPD)	

8. Match the following role characteristics with their associated nursing roles. *Answers may be used more than once.*

Role Characteristics	Nursing Roles
___ a. Provides information	1. Caregiver
___ b. Arranges for home care	2. Care coordinator
___ c. Conducts team conferences	3. Community- based
___ d. Arranges for post- hospitalization equipment	care planner
___ e. Performs collaborative functions	4. Educator 5. Advocate
___ f. Works with legislators in effecting changes for better health care	6. Change agent
___ g. Administers medications	
___ h. Plans continued care	
___ i. Provides physical care	
___ j. Evaluates client's willingness to learn	
___ k. Works to improve conditions on unit for better client care	
___ l. Explains implications of decisions	

9. Explain the relationship between critical thinking and evidence-based practice.

10. Your client, a 60-year-old African-American woman, is a newly diagnosed diabetic and requires teaching by the interdisciplinary team. On a separate sheet of paper, list the important factors that could enhance or impede the teaching-learning process.

11. This client (see Question 10) is anxious about the major lifestyle change that having diabetes will require. Which approach may facilitate her learning?
    a. Providing most of the teaching in the evening when she can concentrate.
    b. Reviewing all the information and then repeating it later to ensure she has retained it.
    c. Providing written information for the client to reference along with a small group of other clients.
    d. Have her watch a videotape and complete a self-assessment.

Answer Questions 12 and 13 on a separate sheet of paper.

12. What cultural factors make this client (see questions 10 & 11) one of the most vulnerable of all populations?

13. Identify settings in which a medical-surgical nurse may practice.

14. What are the three general types of hospital nursing units?
    a. _____
    b. _____
    c. _____

15. You have been considering a nursing position at a hospital. You thrive in crisis situations and work well under high stress. Which would be a good choice for your skills?
    a. Urology specialty unit
    b. Rehabilitation or transitional unit
    c. Shock trauma unit
    d. Orthopedic unit

16. Identify the five steps of the nursing process.
    a. _____
    b. _____
    c. _____
    d. _____
    e. _____

17. An example of a medical diagnosis in contrast with a nursing diagnosis is which of the following?
    a. Fever of Unknown Origin
    b. Impaired Gas Exchange
    c. Risk for Infection
    d. Disturbed Sleep Pattern

18. On a separate sheet of paper, describe the difference between a nursing diagnosis and a collaborative problem.

19. Which of these activities would be included in a nursing assessment?
    a. Administering medications
    b. Determining client outcomes
    c. Analyzing client data
    d. Interviewing and taking a history

20. What is the end result of the data analysis step of the nursing process?
    a. Planning interventions based on problems
    b. Identifying actual or potential problems
    c. Determining data collection techniques for older adults
    d. Evaluating client response to plan

21. What are three critical functions of the planning step of the nursing process?
    a. _____
    b. _____
    c. _____

22. Expected client outcomes should have which of the following characteristics?
    a. Based on the Nursing Interventions Classification system
    b. Realistic for the client, measurable, and achievable
    c. Nurse- or health care provider–centered
    d. Focused on collaborative management activities

23. Match the following abbreviations to their definitions.

Abbreviations	Definitions
___ a. NANDA	1. Classification for nursing outcomes
___ b. NIC	2. Interdisciplinary document that outlines essential aspects of client care
___ c. NOC	
___ d. POC	3. Nursing diagnosis association
	4. Nursing classification system for interventions

24. Which of the following statements about the collaborative client plan of care is correct?
    a. It is a means of communicating the nursing problems regarding client's care.
    b. It is an interdisciplinary document that outlines essential aspects of client care.
    c. It identifies exclusively the nursing interventions for client problems.
    d. It requires few modifications regardless of client's length of hospital stay.

25. Identify the four possible outcomes for the evaluation phase and the implications for further nursing actions.

    a. _____

    b. _____

    c. _____

    d. _____

26. Identify six important guidelines for nursing documentation.

    a. _____

    b. _____

    c. _____

    d. _____

    e. _____

    f. _____

27. On a separate sheet of paper, write an outcome objective that would indicate a positive result for your client for each of the nursing diagnoses below.

    a. Imbalanced nutrition, less than body requirements, related to nausea

    b. Disturbed sleep pattern related to pain

    c. Risk for aspiration related to impaired swallowing

STUDY GUIDE NUMBER 1.2

Community-Based Care

Study/Review Questions

1. What is the primary purpose of ambulatory care?

2. Identify five ambulatory settings in which clients may receive care.

    a. _____

    b. _____

    c. _____

    d. _____

    e. _____

3. Identify three major roles of nurses working in the ambulatory care setting.

    a. _____

    b. _____

    c. _____

4. On a separate sheet of paper, discuss the factors that have contributed to the growth and acceptance of home care.

5. The major source of reimbursement for skilled home care services is which of the following?

    a. Private payment by the client

    b. Insurance companies

    c. Medicare

    d. Medicaid

6. On a separate sheet of paper, identify the differences between nursing in the home setting and nursing in an inpatient setting.

7. An older adult client has been discharged from the hospital after a stroke. The plan is to make a referral to a home care agency for physical therapy. Which home care agency would provide that service?

    a. A skilled home care service

    b. Home infusion therapy

    c. Private duty service

    d. Home medical equipment

8. An older adult client has dementia and the family wants a sitter to stay with her at night. Which home care agency would provide this service?

    a. A skilled home care service

    b. Home infusion therapy

    c. Private duty service

    d. Home medical equipment

9. Medicare will pay for home care services if which of the following qualifying conditions are met?

    a. The client needs assistance with ADLs.

    b. The client is confined to the home.

    c. The health care provider writes an order for home care.

    d. The client needs follow-up care.

10. Once client eligibility has been established, which of the following services would be reimbursed by Medicare?
    a. Teaching a family member to manage a colostomy
    b. Transporting a client to get batteries for a hearing aid
    c. Preparing meals for an older client
    d. Providing wound care
    e. Management of a urinary catheter
    f. Homemaker services

11. Identify three advantages to computerized documentation in home care.
    a. _____
    b. _____
    c. _____

12. In 1999, new regulations were instituted that require tracking outcome in Medicare-certified home care agencies by OASIS. Identify three benefits of this change.
    a. _____
    b. _____
    c. _____

13. On a separate sheet of paper, identify the cause of nursing homes accepting short-term residents for care.

14. For the client situations listed below, select the most appropriate placement from the following choices.
    a. Residential facility
    b. Nursing facility
    c. Chronic care facility
    d. Skilled nursing facility
    ___ A male client is retired and is doing well but needs minor assistance with his activities of daily living.
    ___ A female client has sustained a severe head injury and requires ventilator support.
    ___ A male client has severe dementia and requires ongoing supervision.
    ___ A female client has fractured her hip and needs short-term rehabilitative services.

15. Which of the following statements are true about nurses working in a nursing home?
    a. They are often in charge of a unit or shift.
    b. They require less training and fewer skills because the clients are always medically stable.
    c. They must be familiar with laws that protect the clients.
    d. They are less autonomous than nurses working in the acute care setting.
    e. They must document carefully to meet regulations.

STUDY GUIDE NUMBER 1.3

Introduction to Managed Care and Case Management

Study/Review Questions

1. The cost of health care in the United States has dramatically increased over the past 20 years and now accounts for ____ of the gross national product.
   a. 15%
   b. 5%
   c. 8%
   d. 10%

2. On a separate sheet of paper, discuss and contrast the fee-for-service arrangement and the capitated reimbursement system.

3. The primary purpose of managed care is to _____ _____.

4. In response to the managed care environment, nurses need to:
   a. Focus their care on the traditional disease-oriented approach.
   b. Learn to emphasize the curative process with client illnesses.
   c. Focus on empowering clients to stay well and care for themselves.
   d. Encourage long hospital stays to prepare clients for discharge.

5. Which statement about health maintenance organizations (HMOs) is true?
   a. They provide contractual arrangements with physicians, hospitals, and other providers who meet their criteria.
   b. HMOs are the oldest and most common type of managed care organization.
   c. Clients can choose any hospital for their acute care.
   d. There is usually no charge or copayment for services.

6. The Joint Commission of Accreditation of Health Care Organizations (JCAHO) mandates that all accredited agencies must provide:
   a. Cost-effective, focused client care.
   b. Collaborative, interdisciplinary care for clients.
   c. Comprehensive but purely nursing-directed care.
   d. Hospital-based comprehensive client care.

7. Identify three certifications for case managers.
   a. _____
   b. _____
   c. _____

8. The process of case management is similar to the steps of the nursing process. On a separate sheet of paper, give an example of best practice for each step of the process.

9. List three goals of case management identified by the American Nurses Association (ANA).
   a. _____
   b. _____
   c. _____

10. Internal case managers are focused on _____ care in a health care agency, whereas external case managers are focused on _____ of resources for insurance companies.

Answer the following two questions on a separate sheet of paper.

11. Case managers in the United States practice disease state management. What is the purpose of this approach?

12. Clinical pathways is a commonly used format for delineating the client's plan of care. There are two other names for this interdisciplinary guideline. What are they?

STUDY GUIDE NUMBER 1.4

Introduction to Complimentary and Alternative Therapies

Study/Review Questions

1. On a separate sheet of paper, explain the difference between traditional medicine (allopathic) and complementary and alternative therapies.

2. Match the commonly used complementary therapies listed below with their definitions.

Definition	Complementary Therapy
____ a. Use of needles to stimulate certain points on the body to treat health problems	1. Acupuncture
	2. Acupressure
	3. Aromatherapy
	4. Chiropractic
____ b. Use of manipulation to realign the spine and nervous system to promote healing	5. Homeopathy
	6. Hypnotherapy
	7. Imagery
	8. Massage therapy
____ c. Use of dilute forms of biologic materials to produce symptoms similar to those caused by disease	9. Naturopathy
	10. Osteopathy

____ d. A system of prevention, diagnosis, and management of health problems using natural medicines and therapies

____ e. Use of pressure to stimulate the energy points of the body

____ f. Use of hypnosis or other processes that prepare the client to be susceptible to suggestion or direction

____ g. Use of the medicinal properties of essential oils extracted from plants and herbs

____ h. Manipulation of muscles to relieve stress or muscle tension

____ i. Use of positioning and manipulative techniques to detect faulty body structure and function

____ j. Use of technique in which a client uses dreams and fantasies to relieve stress, decrease pain, and promote healing

3. On a separate sheet of paper, compare the terms spirituality and religion.

4. Which of the following are physiologic effects of relaxation?
   a. Decreased blood pressure
   b. Increased peripheral blood flow
   c. Increased heart rate
   d. Decreased epinephrine levels
   e. Increased oxygen consumption
   f. Decreased respiratory rate

5. Identify three relaxation techniques that do not require specialized training but would reduce your client's physical, mental, and emotional tension.
   a. _____
   b. _____
   c. _____

6. On a separate sheet of paper, explain what should affect your decision to use touch therapy with your client.

7. Which of the reactions listed below are benefits of laughter and humor therapy?
   a. Increased cortisol levels
   b. Increased salivary immunoglobulin A
   c. Increased circulation
   d. Stimulation of the left and right sides of the brain

Answer the following two questions on a separate sheet of paper.

8. Although herbs are not classified as drugs in the United States, why is it important for clients to inform you concerning which herbs they are taking?

9. Discuss the implications of complementary and alternative therapies for health professionals.

STUDY GUIDE NUMBER 1.5

Health Care of Older Adults

Study/Review Questions

1. Which of the statements below about the health of older adults in the United States are true?
   a. The fastest growing group is between 85 and 99 years of age.
   b. Only 5% of older adults are in nursing homes.
   c. Many older adults are mentally sound and competent.
   d. The highest rate of suicide is in the older adult population.

2. Identify four interventions to reduce relocation stress in the older hospitalized client.
   a. _____
   b. _____
   c. _____
   d. _____

3. Which of the following statements would be included in an educational program on wellness behaviors for the older adult?
   a. Allow at least 10 to 15 minutes of sun exposure 2 to 3 times weekly.
   b. Take one aspirin twice a day.
   c. Obtain a yearly pneumococcal vaccination.
   d. Create a hazard-free environment to prevent falls.
   e. Increase calcium intake to between 1000 and 1500 mg daily.
   f. Take time alone at home and relax.

4. Which statement regarding how nutrition is affected in older adults is true?
   a. Changes in smell and taste can result in a decrease in use of sugar.
   b. Older adults need increased calorie intake to maintain ideal body weight.
   c. Loneliness and boredom may impact the older adult's incentive to eat.
   d. Obesity is the most common nutritional problem in nursing homes.

5. Identify six benefits of exercise in promoting and maintaining a high level of functioning.
   a. _____
   b. _____
   c. _____
   d. _____
   e. _____
   f. _____

6. An older client's ability to maintain a positive self-concept and self-control can be impacted by which of the following?
   a. Loss of a loved one
   b. Ability to allow others to make decisions
   c. Retirement from work
   d. Loss of resources

7. Identify five factors that indicate a risk for falling in the older adult.
   a. _____
   b. _____
   c. _____
   d. _____
   e. _____

8. Common nursing interventions for hospitalized older clients at risk for falls include:
   a. Ensuring that the client is near the nursing station.
   b. Using bed and chair alarms.
   c. Toileting the incontinent client every 3 to 4 hours.
   d. Encouraging client to ambulate independently.

9. Nursing interventions for the client requiring restraints must include:
   a. Checking the client every 30 to 60 minutes.
   b. Releasing the restraint at least every 4 hours for repositioning and toileting.
   c. Using the most restrictive restraints and documenting interventions.
   d. Placing the client in an area where he or she can be observed carefully.

10. Which of the following types of psychoactive drugs is the most potent?
    a. Antidepressants
    b. Antipsychotics
    c. Antianxiety agents
    d. Sedative-hypnotics

11. Match the following physiologic changes affecting the drug use in older adults with their associated pharmacodynamic actions.

Physiologic Changes	Pharmacodynamics
___ a. Increased proportion of adipose tissue	1. Absorption
	2. Distribution
	3. Metabolism output
___ b. Reduced glomerular filtration	4. Excretion
___ c. Decreased cardiac	
___ d. Decreased liver enzyme	

12. Identify eight common adverse reactions that may occur in older adults.
    a. _____
    b. _____
    c. _____
    d. _____
    e. _____
    f. _____
    g. _____
    h. _____

13. Which of the following statements are true?
    a. Older adults have less reserve capacity in most organ systems.
    b. Severity of chronic disease may cause a more dramatic effect of drug reactions.
    c. When prescribing medications for older adults, a policy of generalized "start high but taper quickly" is essential for safety.
    d. All symptoms should be assessed for possible adverse reactions to medications in the older adult population.

14. Identify three common reasons why older adults may make mistakes when self-administering medications.
    a. _____
    b. _____
    c. _____

15. Which of these interventions is effective in helping to reorient a client suffering from delirium?
    a. Reorient the client frequently using a calm voice.
    b. Restrict visitors during periods of agitation.
    c. Remove personal items and store them safely.
    d. Apply wrist restraints to keep client from pulling at tubing.

16. Which of the following may be signs and symptoms of depression in older adults?
    a. Alcoholism
    b. Sense of helplessness and hopelessness
    c. Anger and aggressive behavior
    d. Increased pain

17. On a separate sheet of paper, differentiate dementia and depression in older adults.

18. Which of the following statements regarding elder abuse is true?
    a. The abuser is often a close family member.
    b. All older adults are vulnerable to being victims of elder abuse.
    c. Male adult children are usually the caregivers for their older family members.
    d. Approximately one half of all cases involve physical force.

19. Identify factors that impact economic self-reliance in older adults.
    a. _____
    b. _____
    c. _____
    d. _____
    e. _____

20. Match the funding programs below with the governmental resources that support older adults.

Funding Program	Governmental Resource
___ a. Older Americans Act of 1965	1. Rental assistance
	2. Health care
___ b. Social Security Act insurance	3. Transportation services
___ c. Housing program	4. Retirement income
___ d. Medicare and Medicaid	

Case Study: Medication Use in Older Adults

An 80-year-old client is brought to the emergency department after fainting at home. His serum digoxin level is 2.3 ng/mL. He is transferred to a medical nursing unit. The next day the nurse asks the client to tell her about his routine for taking his daily digoxin tablets. He states that he was told to check his pulse every morning before taking a pill. He does this in his kitchen because the clock on the wall has big numbers and he can see the second hand go around. The nurse asks him how long he measures his pulse. He replies, "I keep counting the beats until I get to 60. Sometimes it takes a long time. Then I take my heart pill."

Answer the following questions on a separate sheet of paper.

1. Identify factors that may affect the client's understanding of digoxin self-administration.

2. Devise a teaching-learning plan to re-teach this client about taking digoxin at home.

3. Discuss how the nurse can validate whether the teaching plan has been effective.

Concepts	Assessment	Assessment	Concepts
Culture	**Pain**	**Pain**	**Pain**
Definition	Site/location	Monitoring pain	Nonopioid drugs
Cultural competence	Intensity	Cutaneous stimulation	Opioid analgesics
Assessment	Quality/chronology	Distraction	Tricyclic antidepressants
Cultural care plan	Nonverbal indicators of pain	Acupuncture	Other adjunctive drugs
Religion	Vital signs	Imagery	**End-of-life care**
Folk medicine	Anxiety	Transcutaneous electrical nerve	Opioids in varying routes
Pain	Sweating	stimulation (TENS)	Diuretics
Ethics	Restlessness	Heat/cold	Bronchodilators
Pain	Confusion	Touch	Corticosteroids
Theories of pain	**Substance abuse**	**Substance abuse**	Antibiotics
Types of pain	Hallucinations	Health teaching	Anticholinergics
Addiction	Seizures	Avoidance	Sedatives
Dependence	Cardiac dysrhythmias	Rehabilitation	Antianxiety drugs
Tolerance	Dilated pupils	Symptom management	Barbiturates
Placebos	Vital sign changes	**End-of-life care**	**Rehabilitation**
Substance abuse	Tremors	Oxygen	Cholinergics
Stimulants	Nausea/vomiting	Oral hygiene	Rectal suppositories
Hallucinogens	Abdominal cramps	Alternative drug routes	
Depressants	Mental health disorders	Positioning	
Narcotics	Visual disturbances	Rest	
Inhalants	Euphoria	Energy conservation	
Steroids	Relaxation	Foley catheter	
End-of-life care	Sexual arousal	Enema	
Goals	Poor attention and memory	Physical support	
Hospice care	**End-of-life care**	Presence	
Death	Lethargy	Being realistic	
Postmortem care	Decreased level of consciousness	Promoting spirituality	
Euthanasia	(LOC)	Referral to bereavement services	
Rehabilitation	Discomfort or pain	Health teaching	
Settings	Dyspnea	**Rehabilitation**	
Team	Agitation	Transfers	
	Nausea/vomiting	Gait training	
	Dysphagia	Prevention of complications of	
	Rehabilitation	immobility	
	Body system assessment	Assistive/adaptive devices	
	Functional assessment	Energy conservation	
	Psychosocial assessment	Skin care	
	Vocational assessment	Bladder and bowel training	
		Community-based care	

Unit 2 (Chapters 6-10)

Biopsychosocial Concepts Related to Health Care

Learning Plan

Chapter 6: *Cultural Aspects of Health*

Learning Outcomes	Learning Activities	Supplemental Resources
1. Define cultural competence, culture, and subculture. 2. Explain the purpose of Healthy People 2010 as it relates to cultural groups. 3. Describe the three methods for assessing the culture of a client or group. 4. Identify two subcultures that have often been neglected. 5. Discuss specific cultural practices—religion, nutrition, and folk medicine—that the nurse should consider when assessing a client's culture.	1. Prior to completing the study guide exercises for this chapter, it is recommended to review the following: • Difference between religion and spirituality • Community health nursing • Concepts of communication 2. Review the **boldfaced** words and their definitions in Chapter 6 to enhance your understanding of the content. 3. Go to Study Guide Number 2.6 on the following pages and complete the learning exercises for this chapter.	1. Textbook—Chapter 6 2. Other resources: • Andrews, M.M. & Hanson, P.A. (1999). Religion, culture, and nursing. In M.M. Andrews & J.A. Boyle (Eds.). *Transcultural concepts in nursing care* (3rd ed.). Philadelphia: J.B. Lippincott. • Contact state government for statewide implication of "Healthy People 2010." • Leininger, M.M. (1995a). Overview of Leininger's culture care theory. In M.M. Leininger (Ed.), *Transcultural nursing: Concepts, theories, research, and practice* (2nd ed.). New York: McGraw-Hill. • Ludwig-Beymer, P. (1999b). Transcultural nursing's role in managed care setting. *Journal of Transcultural Nursing, 10*(4), 286-287. • Spector, R.E. (2000). *Cultural diversity in health and illness* (5th ed.). Upper Saddle River, NJ: Prentice-Hall Health. • See *Journal of Transcultural Nursing* for other articles that may interest you. • U.S. Department of Health and Human Services. (2000). Document "Healthy People 2010."

Chapter 7: *Pain: The Fifth Vital Sign*

Learning Outcomes	Learning Activities	Supplemental Resources
1. Define the concept of pain. 2. Describe briefly the gate control theory to explain the relationship between pain and emotion. 3. Explain the role of neuromodulators in the experience of pain.	1. Prior to completing the study guide exercises for this chapter, it is recommended to review the following: • Anatomy and physiology of the peripheral and central nervous system • Actions and side effects of opioid analgesics	1. Textbook—Chapter 7 2. Other resources: • American Pain Society: www.ampainsoc.org e-mail: info@ampainsoc.org

Chapter 7 (continued)

Learning Outcomes

4. Identify variables that influence a client's perception of pain.
5. Discuss the attitudes and knowledge of nurses, physicians, and clients regarding pain assessment and management.
6. Compare and contrast the characteristics of the major types of pain.
7. Describe the components of a comprehensive pain assessment.
8. Analyze assessment data to formulate nursing diagnoses for the client experiencing pain.
9. Plan nursing care for the client experiencing acute pain.
10. Differentiate commonly used drugs for acute pain and chronic pain.
11. Describe the nursing implications associated with drug therapy for clients with acute pain or chronic pain.
12. Identify special considerations for older adults related to pain assessment and management.
13. Discuss complementary and alternative therapies for clients experiencing pain.
14. Develop a teaching/learning plan for managing pain as part of community-based care for clients experiencing pain.

Learning Activities

- Central nervous system agents
2. Review the **boldfaced** words and their definitions in Chapter 7 to enhance your understanding of the content.
3. Go to Study Guide Number 2.7 on the following pages and complete the learning exercises for this chapter.

Supplemental Resources

- American Pain Society. (1999). *Principles of analgesic use in the treatment of acute pain and cancer pain.* (4th ed.) Glenview, IL: American Pain Society.
- Any pharmacology book
- Feldt, K.S. (2000). The checklist of nonverbal pain indictors. (CNPI). *Pain Management Nursing, 1*(1), 13-21.
- JCAHO standards for pain management http://www.jcaho.org/standard/pain_hap.htm *Journal of Pain and Symptom Management*
- Mayer, D.M., et al. (2001). Speaking the language of pain. *American Journal of Nursing, 101*(2), 44-50.
- McCaffery, M. (1998). *Pain: A clinical manual for nursing practice.* (2nd ed). St. Louis: Mosby.
- McCaffery, M. & Ferrell, B.R. (1999). Opioids and pain management—What do nurses know? *Nursing 99, 29*(3), 48-52.
- Partners Against Pain: www.partnersagainstpain.com
- Patient Bill of Rights

Chapter 8: *Substance Abuse*

Learning Outcomes

1. Discuss substance abuse as a major health problem in the United States.
2. Explain the effects of substance abuse on mental and physical health of individuals and society.
3. Describe the relationship of stress and substance abuse.
4. Identify assessment findings associated with the use of stimulants, hallucinogens, depressants, opioids, inhalants, and steroids.
5. Discuss priorities for care of clients who have or are experiencing substance abuse.
6. Identify signs and symptoms of alcohol withdrawal.

Learning Activities

1. Prior to completing the study guide exercises for this chapter, it is recommended to review the following:
   - Cultural competence
   - Stress and adaptation
   - Coping
   - DSM-IV criteria
2. Review the **boldfaced** words and their definitions in Chapter 8 to enhance your understanding of the content.

Supplemental Resources

1. Textbook—Chapter 8
2. Other resources:
   - Textbook Chapters 6 and 7
   - Acello, B. Controlling pain, facing fears about opioid addiction. *Nursing 2000, 30*(5), 72.
   - American Psychiatric Association. (1994). *Diagnostic and statistical manual of mental disorders* (4th ed.). Washington, DC: American Psychiatric Association.
   - Consultation with drug and rehabilitation unit staff
   - Gorman, M. (1998). Substance abuse. *AJN, 98*(7), 16.

Learning Activities	Supplemental Resources
3. Go to Study Guide Number 2.8 on the following pages and complete the learning exercises for this chapter.	• Keltner, N., Schwecke, L., & Bostrom, C. (1999). *Psychiatric nursing* (3rd ed.). St. Louis: Mosby. • National Institute of Drug Abuse (NIDA), National Institute of Health (NIH) U.S. Department of Health and Human Services. (2000). http://www.drugabuse.gov • Segatore, M., Adams, D., & Lange, S. Managing alcohol withdrawal in the acutely ill hospitalized adult. *Journal of Neuroscience Nursing, 31*(1), 129-141.

Chapter 9: *End-of-Life Care*

Learning Outcomes	Learning Activities	Supplemental Resources
1. Explain the goals of end-of-life care. 2. Describe the hospice concept. 3. Interpret the common physical and emotional signs of impending death. 4. Identify interventions for managing symptoms of distress at end of life. 5. Describe postmortem care. 6. Compare active euthanasia and passive euthanasia.	1. Prior to completing the study guide exercises for this chapter, it is recommended to review the following: 　• Concept of grief and loss 　• Death and dying 　• Concept of stress, coping, and adaptation 　• Pain management 　• Cultural diversity 　• Complementary and alternative therapies 2. Review the **boldfaced** words and their definitions in Chapter 9 to enhance your understanding of the content. 3. Go to Study Guide Number 2.9 on the following pages and complete the learning exercises for this chapter.	1. Textbook—Chapter 9 2. Other resources: 　• Textbook Chapters 4, 6, and 7 　• *American Journal of Hospice and Palliative Care* 　• Callanan, M. & Kelly, P. (1992). *Final gifts: Understanding the special awareness, needs and communications of the dying.* New York: Health Press. 　• Consultation with a palliative care clinical nurse specialist or a nurse practitioner 　• http://www.hospice-cares.com 　• Karnes, B. (1995). *Gone from my sight: The dying experience.* Stilwell: Barabara Karnes Books, Inc. 　• Levy, M. (1996). Pharmacologic treatment of cancer pain. *New England Journal of Medicine 335*, 1124-1132. 　• McCaffery, M. (1998). Pain: A clinical manual for nursing practice. (2nd ed.) St. Louis: Mosby. 　• McMillian, S.C. (1996). The quality of life of patients with cancer receiving hospice care. *Oncology Nursing Forum, 23*, 1221-1228. 　• Storey, P. (1994). *Primer of palliative care.* Gainsville, FL: The Academy of Hospice Physicians.

- Storey, P. & Knight, C. (1996). *Unipac four: Management of selected nonpain symptoms in the terminally ill.* Gainsville, FL: American Academy of Hospice and Palliative Medicine.
- Storey, P. & Knight, C. (1996). *Unipac three: Assessment and treatment of pain in the terminally ill.* Gainsville, FL: American Academy of Hospice and Palliative Medicine.

Supplemental Resources

1. Textbook—Chapter 10
2. Other resources:
   - Textbook Chapter 61
   - Any anatomy and physiology book
   - Any fundamentals of nursing book
   - Any psychology book and/or psychiatric mental health nursing book
   - Any techniques in nursing book
   - Hickey, J.V. *The clinical practice of neurological and neurosurgical nursing* (4th ed.). Philadelphia: J.B. Lippincott.
   - http://www.stroke.org/
   - Ignatavicius, D.D. (1998). *Introduction to long term care nursing.* Philadelphia: F.A. Davis.
   - Read nursing care protocols from a rehabilitation unit for clients with neurologic disabilities.
   - *Rehabilitation Nursing*
   - Visit a rehabilitation unit and observe the care of clients with disabilities.

Chapter 10: *Rehabilitation Concepts for Acute and Chronic Problems*

Learning Activities

1. Prior to completing the study guide exercises for this chapter, it is recommended to review the following:
   - Anatomy and physiology of the neurologic, muscular, cardiac, and respiratory systems
   - Techniques: urinary catheterization, bowel care, principles of bathing, transferring, range of motion exercises, and ambulation
   - Hazards of immobility
   - Concept of body image
   - Concept of self-esteem
   - Concept of loss and grieving
   - Concept of adult development
   - Concept of human sexuality
   - Concepts of nutrition
2. Review the **boldfaced** words and their definitions in Chapter 10 to enhance your understanding of the content.
3. Go to Study Guide Number 2.10 on the following pages and complete the learning exercises for this chapter.

Learning Outcomes

1. Differentiate between impairment, disability, and handicap.
2. Identify the roles of each member of the interdisciplinary rehabilitation team.
3. Interpret physical assessment findings for the client in a rehabilitation program.
4. Describe the major components of a functional assessment.
5. Prioritize nursing care needs for the client in a rehabilitation program.
6. Develop a teaching plan for the rehabilitation client at risk for complications of impaired physical mobility.
7. Assess client outcomes of the interdisciplinary rehabilitation program. Explain the primary concerns for clients being discharged to home after rehabilitation.

STUDY GUIDE NUMBER 2.6

Critical Thinking in the Role of the Medical-Surgical Nurse

Study/Review Questions

Match the following terms with the appropriate definitions.

a. Culture
b. Subculture
c. Culture care preservation
d. Culture competence
e. Culture care accommodation
f. Cultural assessment
g. Cultural restructuring
h. Transcultural nursing

_____ 1. A way to help people of a particular culture retain or preserve relevant care values so they can maintain and/or preserve their well-being, recover from illness, or face handicaps and/or death

_____ 2. The ability of health care providers and organizations to understand and respond effectively to the cultural and linguistic needs that clients bring to the health care setting

_____ 3. Learned beliefs, traditions, and guides for behaviors that are shared among members of a particular group

_____ 4. An area of study and practice that focuses on the care, health, and illness patterns of people with similarities and differences in their cultural beliefs, values, and practices

_____ 5. Data collected or research conducted to learn about the culture of clients

_____ 6. Interventions that help clients to reorder or greatly modify their life ways; providing a lifestyle more beneficial or healthier than that practiced before the changes were co-established with the clients

_____ 7. Part of a larger culture of the client

_____ 8. Professional actions and decisions that help people of a designated culture adapt to or negotiate with others for a beneficial or satisfying health outcome with professional care providers

9. Identify the three major methods for assessing the culture of a client and provide an example of each method.
   a. _____
   b. _____
   c. _____

10. Identify two ways a person can participate in a culture.
    a. _____
    b. _____

11. Identify two subcultures in our society that have been neglected often.
    a. _____
    b. _____

For Questions 12 through 19, read the statements and decide whether each is true or false. Write T for true and F for false in the blanks provided. **If the statement is false, correct the statement to make it true.**

_____ 12. Cultural practices that should be included as part of a cultural assessment include nutrition, family roles, pregnancy and childbirth, death rituals, and spirituality.

_____ 13. Transcultural nursing focuses on the care, health, and illness patterns of people with various cultural beliefs, values, and practices.

_____ 14. In the 2000 census, minorities accounted for 43.8% of the total population in the United States.

_____ 15. One goal of "Healthy People 2010" is to eliminate disparities in health status experienced by racial and ethnic minorities.

___ 16. All people within the same country will have the same health care needs.

___ 17. Garlic worn around the neck is thought to protect against cold and flu viruses in some cultures.

___ 18. The way pain is displayed is the same in all cultures.

___ 19. It is reasonable to expect that clients should always be on time for appointments.

20. The ability of health care providers to understand and respond effectively to the cultural and linguistic needs that clients bring to the health care setting is called:
    a. Cultural participation.
    b. Cultural competence.
    c. Cultural care preservation.
    d. Transcultural nursing.

21. Hypertension is referred to in some cultures as:
    a. High blood.
    b. Low blood.
    c. Sweet blood.
    d. Sour blood.

22. Which of the following is *not* likely to ensure good communication with someone who does not speak English?
    a. Learn his or her language
    b. Use an interpreter
    c. Use pictures with common phrases
    d. Look him or her directly in the eye

23. One way for organizations to achieve _____ _____ is to ensure that staff members are trained to work respectfully and effectively with clients in culturally diverse health care environments.

24. Give at least one example of a way to provide cultural care for deaf clients.

SiMON. *Case Study: Assessment of a Culture*

The hospital where you are a nurse manager is opening an outreach clinic and has asked you to help set it up. The clinic is located in a community with many recent immigrants from Guatemala.

Answer the following questions on a separate sheet of paper.

1. What do you need to know to be prepared to provide culturally appropriate care for your clients?

2. How will you find that information?

3. How will you use that information?

Pain: The Fifth Vital Sign

Study/Review Questions

1. Read the following statements and decide if each is true or false. *Write T for true or F for false in the blanks provided. If the statement is false, correct the statement to make it true.*

   ___ a. Pain is the number one symptom or complaint that causes people to seek health care.

   ___ b. Pain alters the quality of life more than any other single health-related problem.

   ___ c. Over the years, there have been major advances in how pain is managed.

   ___ d. Unrelieved and untreated pain is a major public health problem in the United States.

   ___ e. The amount of pain a person feels and the response to it is a universal experience.

2. Match the following definitions/descriptions of pain with the correct authorship. *Answers may be used more than once.*

   Description

   ___ a. Stimulus indicating tissue damage

   ___ b. Exists whenever the individual says it does

   ___ c. Personal sensation of hurt

   ___ d. Unpleasant sensory or emotional experience

   ___ e. Definable only by the individual

   ___ f. Whatever the individual says it is

   ___ g. Response that protects from harm

   ___ h. Described in terms of tissue damage

   Authorship

   1. International Association on Pain
   2. McCaffery
   3. Sternbach

3. Which of the following is not related to the Gate Control theory?

   a. It is an explanation of the relationship between pain and emotion.

   b. Perception of pain is influenced by physical and psychologic variables.

   c. Perception of pain occurs by way of the stimulus being transmitted directly to the gate in the brain.

   d. Interventions for pain management have been based on this theory.

4. The free nerve endings or receptors in the various body tissues that become activated by thermal, mechanical, or chemical stimuli to initiate the client's response to pain are called _____.

5. Identify the three anatomic structures from which painful stimuli can originate.

   a. _____

   b. _____

   c. _____

6. On a separate sheet of paper, briefly describe the following four categories relating to the location of pain:

   a. Localized pain
   b. Projected pain
   c. Radiating pain
   d. Referred pain

7. On a separate sheet of paper, briefly describe neuropathic pain.

8. Compare and contrast the two types of periphery nerve fibers that are responsible for transmitting pain stimuli by completing the following chart on a separate sheet of paper.

Fiber	**Structure**	**Function**
a. A delta fibers		
b. C fibers		

9. On a separate sheet of paper, trace the route of pain from the peripheral stimulus to the cerebral cortex.

10. On a separate sheet of paper, differentiate neurotransmitters and neuromodulators that inhibit or facilitate the pain sensory input to the spinal cord.

11. Match the following definitions of concepts related to the pain experience with their correct terms.

Definition	Term
___ a. Ability of a person to endure the intensity of pain	1. Pain perception
	2. Pain threshold
___ b. Point at which a person feels pain and reports it as such	3. Pain tolerance
___ c. Awareness of the painful sensation or feeling	
___ d. Affects the perception of pain even if there is no detectable cause	

12. On a separate sheet of paper, identify three barriers to good pain management and examples of each.

13. Age can be a factor that influences how pain is perceived and how it is assessed. On a separate sheet of paper, briefly summarize how this statement relates to pain and pain management in the older adult.

14. In the chart below, for each of the psychosocial variables that can affect an individual's perception of and response to pain, identify at least one example of the variable and the impact it can have on the treatment of pain. Use a separate sheet of paper for your answers.

Psychosocial Variables	Example	Impact on Treatment
Age		
Gender		
Cultural considerations		
Personality, affect/mood states		

15. Identify the sources of the following three types of pain:
    a. Somatic pain
    b. Visceral pain
    c. Neuropathic pain

16. A client complains of a deep, localized cramping type of pain. These assessment findings indicate which type of pain?
    a. Somatic
    b. Psychosomatic
    c. Neuropathic
    d. Visceral

17. A client complains of a constant "achy" type of pain after abdominal surgery. This is an indication of which type of pain?
    a. Somatic
    b. Visceral
    c. Neuropathic
    d. Psychosomatic

18. Compare acute and chronic pain by completing the following chart on a separate sheet of paper.

	Acute pain	Chronic pain
Purpose		
Etiology		
Onset		
Duration		
Intensity		
Localization		
Characteristics		
Emotional response/ assessment findings		
Physiologic response/ assessment findings		
Treatment		

Answer the following three questions on a separate sheet of paper:

19. Identify essential subjective data relevant to a pain assessment.

20. Identify objective client data relevant to pain.

21. Only the client can determine location, character, quality, pattern, and intensity of pain. Compare the advantages and disadvantages of using self-rating scales to measure pain.

22. The best type of pain scale to use for clients who have language problems or reading problems or for children is:
    a. 0-10 numeric rating scale.
    b. FACES (smile to frown).
    c. Verbal description scales.
    d. No type of scale.

23. Identify possible nursing diagnoses of clients with pain other than acute pain or chronic pain.

24. What are the expected outcomes for clients experiencing (a) acute pain, (b) nonmalignant chronic pain, or (c) cancer-related pain?
    a. _____
    b. _____
    c. _____

25. Identify the common classes of pharmacologic agents used to control pain. Give an example of each and a reason for use.

  a. _____
  b. _____
  c. _____

26. A nurse would monitor for gastric irritation, antiplatelet activity of bleeding, and bruising as side effects of which pain medication? *Check all that apply.*

  ___ a. Nonopioid analgesics such as aspirin
  ___ b. Nonopioid analgesics such as Tylenol
  ___ c. Nonsteroidal anti-inflammatory drugs (NSAIDs)
  ___ d. Opioid analgesics

27. A client with chronic bone pain as a result of osteo-arthritis or rheumatoid arthritis may be prescribed which of the following agents? *Check all that apply.*

  a. Aspirin
  b. COX 2 inhibitor such as Celebrex
  c. Opioid such as morphine
  d. Tylenol
  e. NSAID such as Motrin

Answer the following three questions on a separate sheet of paper:

28. Discuss the pitfalls of intermittent or prn (as needed) scheduling of pain medication.

29. What is the rationale for using a nonopioid agent with an opioid agent in the treatment of pain?

30. Identify all the routes of administration for opioid analgesics.

31. The drug that can cause life-threatening seizures, particularly in the older adult, because of an accumulation of toxic metabolites is:

  a. Motrin.
  b. Morphine.
  c. Demerol.
  d. Tylenol.

32. On a separate sheet of paper, identify the nursing interventions that should be performed when caring for a client receiving opioid analgesics.

33. Which of the following statements are true regarding the side effects of respiratory depression as a result of administering an opioid analgesic?

  ___ a. Respiratory depression is not very common in opioid-dependent clients.
  ___ b. Monitor for respiratory depression in clients receiving opioids by IV administration, especially monitor opioid-naive adults.
  ___ c. The pain, stress, and anxiety experienced by the client are potent respiratory stimulants that may override or negate the respiratory depression resulting from the drugs.
  ___ d. Respiratory depression is less of a problem in the older adult.
  ___ e. When the respiratory rate falls to 10 or below, the first action of the nurse is to attempt to rouse the client.
  ___ f. The drug used to reverse the respiratory depression is known as naloxone (Narcan).
  ___ g. A one-time dose of Narcan is all that is needed to reverse the effects of the opioid.

34. Which of the following statements about the adverse side effects of opioids is true?

  a. Bolus administration is less likely to produce central nervous system changes.
  b. Respiration may decrease with relaxation and pain relief.
  c. Opioid antagonists produce more respiratory depression than opioid agonists.
  d. Peripheral effects include vasoconstriction and elevated blood pressure.

35. On a separate sheet of paper, identify factors that may influence a nurse's ability to manage a client's pain episodes successfully.

36. Read the following statements and decide whether each is true or false. *Write T for true or F for false in the blanks provided. If the statement is false, correct the statement to make it true.*

  ___ a. Physical dependency means the same as addiction.
  ___ b. Clients who are prescribed opioids for pain rarely become addicted.

37. Match the following definitions of physiologic sequelae associated with opioid use with their correct terms. *Answers may be used more than once, and more than one term may apply to each sequela.*

    Physiologic Sequelae

    ____ a. Persistent drug craving

    ____ b. Withdrawal symptoms upon abrupt cessation

    ____ c. Amount of drug needed for normal tissue function

    ____ d. Gradual resistance to effect of the opioid

    ____ e. Abuse for recreational purposes

    ____ f. Adjustment of body to drug's adverse effects

    ____ g. Higher doses needed to achieve pain relief

    ____ h. A common fear in clients and health professionals

    ____ i. Physiologic adaptation

    ____ j. A psychologic, not physical, phenomenon

    ____ k. Problem with amount of medication given to a client with substance abuse

    Term

    1. Physical dependency
    2. Drug tolerance
    3. Addiction

38. Which of the following statements are true regarding the use of epidural catheters for pain management? *Check all that apply.*

    ____ a. It is an external catheter located in the lumbar or thoracic region near the spinal cord.

    ____ b. It is used for hospitalized clients in acute and chronic pain, especially postoperative pain.

    ____ c. Morphine, Dilaudid, and Fentanyl are common drugs used for pain with a local anesthetic such as Bupivacaine.

    ____ d. The nurse monitors for nausea and vomiting, pruritus, and infection at the site.

    ____ e. Nurses should read the hospital policy and procedures before caring for a client with an epidural catheter.

    ____ f. Catheters are usually in place for about 48 to 72 hours; then the oral route is used.

    ____ g. An epidural catheter affects sensory and motor nerves; therefore urinary retention and weakness in the legs can occur.

    ____ h. Nurses do not need to perform a complete pain assessment because this is an effective measure of pain control for all types of pain.

39. On a separate sheet of paper, define patient-controlled analgesia (PCA), when it is used, and the advantages of its use. Identify nursing care of clients with a PCA.

40. True or false? Cutaneous stimulation controls pain by stimulating the fibers in the skin and subcutaneous tissue, which then blocks the transmission of painful stimuli to the spinal cord.

41. Identify the various modalities of cutaneous stimulation that can be prescribed to control a client's acute or chronic pain.

    a. _____

    b. _____

    c. _____

    d. _____

    e. _____

    f. _____

    Answer Questions 42 through 45 on a separate sheet of paper.

42. What are the limitations of cutaneous stimulation as an effective measure to control a client's pain?

43. True or false? Clients with a history of substance abuse should not receive opioids to treat their pain. (Give a rationale for your answer.)

44. In your role as a nurse, practice performing a complete pain assessment by using a pain assessment tool and a pain scale of your choice. As a result of your assessment, identify the type of pain the client is having and work collaboratively with other health care providers to determine a plan of care for the client to help relieve the pain.

45. Briefly describe the use of a TENS unit to control pain.

46. Which of the following statements about the strategy of distraction is true?

    a. Distraction is effective for acute and chronic pain relief.

    b. Distraction influences the cause of pain directly.

    c. Distraction may be used instead of other pain control measures.

    d. Distraction alters the perception of pain.

47. True or false? NSAIDs cause renal toxicity; therefore renal function blood tests should be routinely monitored with long-term therapy, especially in the older adult.

48. A client complains of stabbing, burning nerve pain. Which of the following medications are not used to treat this type of pain.
   a. Tricyclic antidepressants (e.g., Elavil)
   b. Gabapentin (Neurontin)
   c. Anticonvulsants (e.g., Dilantin, Tegretol)
   d. NSAIDs

49. True or false? *Write T for true or F for false in the blanks provided. If the statement is false, correct the statement to make it true.*
   ___ a. Antianxiety medications such as Xanax and Ativan act directly on the pain pathway to relieve the pain.
   ___ b. Side effects of antianxiety drugs are confusion, drowsiness, and hypotension.

50. Identify two purposes of acupuncture.
   a. _____
   b. _____

51. On a separate sheet of paper, briefly discuss the surgical procedure of a rhizotomy for the treatment of chronic pain.

52. The drug category of choice for the treatment of mild-to-moderate bone pain is:
   a. NSAIDs.
   b. Opioids.
   c. Anticonvulsants.
   d. Antianxiety agents.

53. Match the following descriptions with their associated strategies for coping with pain. *Answers may be used more than once.*

Description	Associated Strategies
___ a. Massage to decrease muscle tension	1. Imagery
___ b. Physiologic responses monitored	2. Relaxation
___ c. Mental experience of sensations or events	3. Hypnosis
___ d. Altered state of consciousness	4. Biofeedback
___ e. Form of distraction	
___ f. Responses regulated using a variety of techniques	
___ g. More effective when combined with other techniques	
___ h. Overall sense of reality lost	

54. On a separate sheet of paper, define what is meant by the term equianalgesic. What would the equianalgesic dose of Dilaudid be for a client receiving 90 mg of morphine orally?

55. True or false? The best method for discontinuing opioids for a client who has become physically dependent is to abruptly stop the drug.

Answer Questions 56 and 57 on a separate sheet of paper.

56. Identify the best method for controlling pain of a hospice client who is unable to take oral medication. Identify the drug most commonly used by this route. Identify nursing responsibilities related to this method of administration.
   a. Intravenously
   b. Continuous subcutaneous infusion
   c. Sublingual
   d. Transdermal

57. Identify the two routes used to administer opioids via intraspinal medication for intractable pain. What is the purpose of using intraspinal medications? What are the methods for administration?

58. Read the following statements regarding Duragesic patches and decide whether each is true or false. *Write T for true or F for false in the blanks provided. If the statement is false, correct the statement to make it true.*
   ___ a. Duragesic is available in patch doses of 25 mcg/hr, 50 mcg/hr, 75 mcg/hr, and 100 mcg/hr.
   ___ b. It is reserved for those clients with continuous and relatively stable pain.
   ___ c. It is supplemented by intermittent doses of pain medication for episodic or breakthrough pain.
   ___ d. It is an easy-to-use method for anyone in chronic pain because it is easily titrated to control the pain.
   ___ e. When the patch is initially applied, it may take up to 24 hours before pain relief begins, so short-acting pain medication must be administered until the medication takes effect.
   ___ f. The patch is effective for 1 week; then a new patch is applied.
   ___ g. The client's body temperature has no affect on absorption of the medication.
   ___ h. Once the patch is totally discontinued, the effects can last up to 24 hours.

59. A temporary pain relief measure that involves localizing the nerve root by an anesthetic is called a

    _____.

60. On a separate sheet of paper, identify the five expected outcomes for any client in pain.

61. In recent years, more emphasis has been placed on good pain management in hospitals and other health care facilities. As a nurse, familiarize yourself with the quality improvement program in your place of employment/clinical sites regarding the implementation of pain strategies and the evaluation of pain care. Learn about the pain outcomes that serve as indicators of how well pain is managed. Continue to learn more about pain management and be a client advocate for achieving good pain management.

STUDY GUIDE NUMBER 2.8

Substance Abuse

Study/Review Questions

1. In caring for a hospitalized client, the nurse recognizes that the client has a history of substance abuse. On a separate sheet of paper, answer the following questions.
   a. In your own words, described the terms *substance abuse* and *addiction*, and then compare your answers with the textbook definitions.
   b. In the table below, identify the six categories of substances most commonly abused, describe the action and effect on the body, and give examples of the abused substance for each category.

Categories	Action of Drug and Overall Effects on the Body	Examples

   c. Briefly discuss the impact of substance abuse on society and the health care professional in the United States.
   d. As stated in the text, "The nurse must have a firm awareness of self to avoid reactive behaviors to the client's beliefs or absence of personal convictions." Spend a little time now to think about your own viewpoints regarding substance abuse.

2. Read the following statements about substance abuse and decide whether each is true or false. *Write* T *for true or* F *for false in the blanks provided. If the statement is false, correct the statement to make it true.*
   ____ a. NIDA is a component of the National Institutes of Health and an excellent resource on substance abuse in the United States.
   ____ b. Approximately 1 out 10 persons in the United States has a friend or family member with substance abuse problems.
   ____ c. A plan of care for a client with substance abuse should be based only on the type of chemical used.
   ____ d. Substance abuse only includes illicit or illegal drugs.
   ____ e. Substance abuse is only related to teenagers and young adults.
   ____ f. Any socioeconomic group is prone to substance abuse.
   ____ g. Knowledge of the client's religious preference will influence the treatment modality.
   ____ h. Older women are at risk for substance abuse because of normal body changes related to the aging process.
   ____ i. Women are generally prone to substance abuse because of biologic predisposition and stressors in the environment.

3. Which of the following statements regarding substance abuse, stress, and addiction are true?
   a. Stress is a contributing factor for substance abuse.
   b. Ingestion of substances causes the normal biologic stress response that originates from the hypothalamus.
   c. Stress responses that are frequently triggered can result in a more sensitive response to the substance.
   d. As a client responds to stress from substances, the more the client becomes conditioned to attain the same level of satisfaction.

The following questions are related to the category of stimulants.

4. Identify the two stimulants that are prescribed therapeutically for attention deficit disorders, obesity, and narcolepsy.
   a. _____
   b. _____

5. What assessment finding would indicate to the nurse that the client is a chronic user of cocaine, particularly crack/cocaine?

6. Cardiac arrest can occur with the first use of which stimulant?

7. A client withdrawing from stimulants should be assessed for which of the following?
   a. Insomnia
   b. Violence
   c. Seizures
   d. Lethargy

8. On a separate sheet of paper, identify the signs and symptoms of use and adverse and toxic effects of the following stimulants.
   a. Amphetamines
   b. Methamphetamine
   c. Cocaine
   d. Nicotine

9. As stress rises, additional stimulant of this substance is needed because the stress hormone corticosterone reduces its effect.
   a. Cocaine
   b. Nicotine
   c. Methamphetamine
   d. Amphetamine

10. Identify the stimulant that has both stimulant and sedative properties. Explain how this drug affects the body.

The following questions are related to the category of hallucinogens and related compounds.

11. True or false? *Write T for true or F for false in the blanks provided.*
    ___ a. Flashbacks are a common phenomenon when psychedelic drugs are used.
    ___ b. There are no therapeutic uses for hallucinogens that are acceptable for medical treatment.
    ___ c. Withdrawal symptoms are unlikely to occur from any hallucinogen.

12. Which drug affects the serotonin-producing neurons in the brain?

13. Tolerance to what particular drug can develop so that an increased amount of the drug is needed to attain the same level of experience?

14. Critical thinking and memory can be affected by the long-term use of what drug?

15. On a separate sheet of paper, briefly explain why LSD is a dangerous health hazard with unpredictable results.

16. A client in the emergency room is suspected of using PCP. A key assessment finding that would indicate this diagnosis is which of the following?
    a. Violent behavior
    b. Totally unaware of one's surroundings
    c. Seizures
    d. Sedation

Answer the following three questions on a separate sheet of paper.

17. Briefly describe assessment findings in a client suspected of PCP abuse.

18. What drug is used experimentally to control cancer pain?

19. Briefly describe the effect marijuana has on the body.

The following questions are related to depressants.

20. The depressants that are medically used to treat anxiety and emotional disorders are _____ and _____.

21. On a separate sheet of paper, describe the actions of the drug and the desired results of each of the following drugs:
    a. Benzodiazepines
    b. Barbiturates
    c. Alcohol

22. True or false? *Write* T *for true or* F *for false in the blanks provided.*
    ___ a. Abuse is present when the client continues to use benzodiazepines after clinical signs have subsided.
    ___ b. Dependence on barbiturates takes a long time to occur.
    ___ c. When medically indicated, older adults can tolerate only small doses of the barbiturate group.
    ___ d. The safest method for withdrawing a client from depressants is to gradually reduce the dosage.
    ___ e. When assessing a client with alcohol abuse, it is important to determine when the client last had a drink.

23. Anxiety, restlessness, insomnia, irritability, and impaired attention are assessment findings for withdrawal from which drug?
    a. Barbiturates
    b. Benzodiazepines
    c. Opioids
    d. Alcohol

24. An assessment of a postoperative client with a history of substance abuse documents diaphoresis, nausea and vomiting, and tremors. These assessment findings are symptoms of:
    a. Benzodiazepine withdrawal.
    b. Barbiturate withdrawal.
    c. Alcohol withdrawal.
    d. Amphetamine withdrawal.

25. Alcohol withdrawal is evaluated by categories of severity. On a separate sheet of paper, briefly explain the assessment findings that would be monitored by the nurse for each of the following three alcohol withdrawal categories.
    a. Minor
    b. Major
    c. Life-threatening

26. A hospitalized client has a history of alcoholism. How soon after the client's last drink should the nurse monitor the client for withdrawal symptoms?
    a. Several hours later
    b. 1 day
    c. More than 3 days afterwards
    d. 2 to 3 days

27. Seizures can occur as a result of alcohol withdrawal within what time frame?
    a. 6 to 12 hours
    b. 12 to 48 hours
    c. 48 to 72 hours
    d. After 72 hours

The following questions are related to narcotics: opioids and morphine derivatives.

28. Opioids and morphine are drugs of addiction because of the:
    a. Analgesic and euphoric effects.
    b. General anesthetic effect.
    c. Stimulation and increase in body activity effect.
    d. Medical indication in the treatment of anxiety.

29. The opioid derivative that has no medical use is called _____.

30. On a separate sheet of paper, briefly describe the effects heroin has on the body and why it is such a severe health hazard.

31. A client enters the emergency room and is diagnosed with opiate withdrawal Grade 2. The assessment findings of this client would include:
    a. Increased vital signs, abdominal cramps, diarrhea, vomiting, and weakness.
    b. Drug craving, anxiety, and drug-seeking behavior.
    c. Dilated pupils, muscle twitching, and anorexia.
    d. Sweating, lacrimation, yawning, and rhinorrhea.

32. A client is admitted to the hospital with a history of substance abuse and repeated episodes of infections and cellulitis. These findings can indicate a chronic use of which drug?
    a. Dilaudid
    b. Morphine
    c. Heroin
    d. Demerol

The following are questions related to inhalants and steroids.

33. The clients most likely to use inhalants are:
    a. Children
    b. Young adults
    c. Middle-aged adults
    d. Older adults

34. A young client states that solvents were inhaled. Examples of solvents are:
    a. Butane lighters, whipping cream aerosols, and spray paints.
    b. Cyclohexanol nitrite and amyl nitrite.
    c. Paint thinners, gasoline, glues, and paper correction fluid.
    d. Hair or deodorant sprays, ether, and chloroform.

35. True or false? *Write* T *for true or* F *for false in the blanks provided.*
    ____ a. A method to increase the effect of the inhalant is to dispense the substance from a paper bag to increase the concentration of the inhalant.
    ____ b. Young adults often are admitted to the hospital as a result of inhalants.

36. Reversible effects of inhalants include:
    a. Liver and kidney damage.
    b. Hearing loss.
    c. Limb spasms.
    d. Bone marrow suppression.

37. The clients most likely to abuse steroids are:
    a. Those diagnosed with depression.
    b. Athletes using them to increase strength and performance.
    c. Those with aggressive tendencies.
    d. Adults in extreme stress using them to relieve symptoms.

38. In the older adult, substance abuse can be a problem related to alcohol and which of the following?
    a. Stimulants
    b. Depressants
    c. Opioids
    d. Prescription and over-the-counter medications

STUDY GUIDE NUMBER 2.9

End-of-Life Care

Study/Review Questions

1. Match the following terms related to loss with their correct definitions.

Term	**Definition**
____ a. Death	1. Reaction to loss
____ b. Dying	2. Termination of life
____ c. Grieving	3. The state of being without something one once had
____ d. Loss	4. A process leading to the end of life

2. A terminally ill client has been referred to hospice. The nurse explains to the client and family that hospice care differs from the care for a client expected to recover from an illness in that it has the following goals:
   a. _____
   b. _____
   c. _____

3. Which of the following statements regarding the approach to hospice/end-of-life care is correct?
   a. Hospice programs only provide provisions of care in the home.
   b. Admission to hospice is involuntary and directed by a physician's order.
   c. The focus is on the provision for facilitating a quality of life just for the dying client.
   d. An interdisciplinary team approach is used for the care of the client and family.

4. A client receiving nursing care in a home hospice program can expect which of the following?
   a. The use of high technology equipment such as ventilators until time of death.
   b. To receive around-the-clock skilled direct nursing client care until time of death.

c. To be provided pain and symptom management that will achieve the best quality of life for the client and family.

d. To be given complete relief of only distressing physical symptoms.

5. To qualify for hospice benefits, a criterion for admission is that the client's prognosis needs to be:
   a. Limited to 2 weeks or less
   b. Limited to 3 months or less
   c. Limited to 6 months or less
   d. Limited to 1 year or less

6. Identify all of the following that apply when describing the concept of hospice:
   a. Unit of care is client and the family
   b. A special place
   c. Control of symptoms
   d. Ends with death
   e. Palliative care in multiple settings
   f. Available 24 hours/day, 7 days a week
   g. A philosophy of care
   h. Makes terminal illness pleasant
   i. Interdisciplinary team approach
   j. Nonfragmented care
   k. Support of family ends with client's death
   l. Supports active euthanasia
   m. Alleviates pain and suffering
   n. Does not hasten death
   o. Goal changes from curative to comfort
   p. Control of disease process

7. In teaching the client and family about the dying process, the nurse discusses the emotional signs of approaching death. Identify these four common emotional signs and related interventions.
   a. _____
   b. _____
   c. _____
   d. _____

8. When performing an assessment of a terminally ill client, which of the following interventions is correct?
   a. Assess only the client; do not include the family's perception of the client's symptoms.
   b. When the client is unable to communicate, there is no need to assess symptoms of distress any longer.
   c. Assess clients who are unable to communicate distress by teaching the family to observe for objective signs of discomfort.
   d. The nurse only assesses the client for pain, dyspnea, agitation, nausea, and vomiting.

9. Identify two examples of transcultural differences when dealing with the dying process.
   a. _____
   b. _____

10. On a separate sheet of paper, identify the physical signs of death.

11. Which of the following interventions is correct when performing postmortem care?
    a. Place the head of the bed at 30 degrees.
    b. Remove pillows from under the head.
    c. Leave a Foley (indwelling) catheter in place in the bladder.
    d. Place pads under the hips and around the perineum.

12. Which of the following interventions after the death of a client are correct? *Mark all that apply.*
    ____ a. Remove the body to the morgue or funeral home immediately after death.
    ____ b. Follow agency policies to remove all tubes and lines from the body, close eyes, and replace dentures.
    ____ c. A death certificate must accompany the body to the funeral home.
    ____ d. Provide privacy for the family and significant others with the deceased.
    ____ e. Allow family and significant other to perform religious and cultural customs.

13. Define the following terms:
    a. Euthanasia
    b. Active euthanasia
    c. Passive euthanasia

14. When a client makes known his or her wishes about treatment at the end of life, these are known as:
    a. Patient self-determination acts.
    b. Advance directives.
    c. Durable power of attorney.
    d. Euthanasia.

15. On a separate sheet of paper, briefly present your opinion about suicide. Include in the discussion your thoughts on whether this act is ever justifiable.

16. Give some thought to the following sentence: "Medical and scientific advances have contributed to the longevity of life, but they have also contributed to the longevity of dying." Share your thoughts with your clinical instructor and fellow students on how this impacts nursing care.

17. The priority outcome for the client at the end of life is to achieve physical and psychologic comfort until death. On a separate sheet of paper, identify the most common symptoms of distress of the terminally ill client.

18. Read the following statements regarding physically distressing symptoms of a terminally ill client and decide whether each is true or false. *Write* T *for true or* F *for false in the blanks provided. If the statement is false, correct the statement to make it true.*
    ___ a. Anorexia is normal; however, clients should be forced to eat small, frequent meals.
    ___ b. Cessation of food ingestion is a natural process and hydration with IV fluids can cause distressing respiratory symptoms.
    ___ c. A client's sense of hearing is intact even though the client is withdrawn from the external environment.
    ___ d. The most feared symptom of a terminally ill client is dyspnea.
    ___ e. Pain is a not a universal problem although it is common and has many causes.
    ___ f. The goals for a client with dyspnea are to relieve the primary cause and the psychologic distress and autonomic response.
    ___ g. Dyspnea is defined as the respiratory rate of less than 20 with observed labored breathing.
    ___ h. Dyspnea is common in about 50% to 70% of clients and is considered by health care providers to be the worst symptom of distress when a client is near death.
    ___ i. There are several causes of dyspnea, which therefore results in a variety of pathophysiologic conditions.
    ___ j. The cause of dyspnea is determined by diagnostic testing, a physical assessment, and knowledge of underlying condition.
    ___ k. Nausea and vomiting occur in about 40% of terminally ill clients in the last week of life.
    ___ l. There are a variety of causes of nausea and vomiting including constipation from opioid therapy.
    ___ m. Nausea and vomiting are prevalent only in individuals with certain types of cancer.
    ___ n. Agitation can result from either physical or spiritual causes.

19. The most common treatment of pain in a terminally ill client is administration of:
    a. Opioids.
    b. Steroids.
    c. Nonsteroidal anti-inflammatory agents.
    d. Radiation treatments.

20. A nursing diagnosis for a terminally ill client is Ineffective Breathing Pattern. On a separate sheet of paper, briefly discuss each of the following interventions for alleviating this distress.
    a. Opioids
    b. Diuretics
    c. Bronchodilators
    d. Anticholinergics
    e. Oxygen
    f. Sedatives
    g. Nonpharmacologic interventions

21. Assessment of a dying client and the family results in the nursing diagnosis of deficient knowledge related to dysphagia, pain, dyspnea, nausea and vomiting, agitation, and other common signs and symptoms. On a separate sheet of paper, develop a teaching plan for this client and family.

22. Adequate symptom management may result in what side effect that is not a treatment goal or an effort to hasten death?
    a. Aspiration
    b. Sedation
    c. Bowel obstruction
    d. Delirium

23. On a separate sheet of paper, develop a plan of care for a terminally ill client and the family for the nursing diagnoses of Risk for Ineffective Coping and Risk for Compromised Family Coping to incorporate the following points.
    a. Offering physical and emotional support
    b. Being realistic
    c. Encouraging reminiscence
    d. Promoting spirituality
    e. Fostering hope
    f. Avoiding explanation of the loss

STUDY GUIDE NUMBER 2.10

Rehabilitation Concepts for Acute and Chronic Problems

Study/Review Questions

1. On a separate sheet of paper, differentiate the following terms related to rehabilitation by defining these concepts in your own words.
   a. Rehabilitation
   b. Impairment
   c. Disability
   d. Handicap
   e. Chronic illness
   f. Disability condition

2. As a result of a car accident, an adult client is unable to perform certain activities of daily living such as bathing without assistance. This is an example of which of the following terms? On a separate sheet of paper, explain why you chose your answer.
   a. Rehabilitation
   b. Impairment
   c. Disability
   d. Handicap

3. The leading cause of disabling conditions in young adults and the third leading cause of death in adults 45 to 54 years of age is:
   a. Strokes.
   b. Cancer.
   c. Arthritis.
   d. Accidents.

4. Identify the two primary goals of the rehabilitation team and give an example for each of those goals.
   a. _____
   b. _____

5. Interdisciplinary team meetings are held for planning client and family care. Match the interdisciplinary team member with the example of the type of work performed. *Answers can be used more than once.*

Type of Work Performed

____ a. Screens, tests, and recommends feeding techniques for dysphagia
____ b. Assists in job placement and seeking work-related training
____ c. Works with clients in learning to feed, bathe, dress themselves
____ d. Teaches clients cognition training and skills related to coordination such as picking up coins from a table
____ e. Directs client care and writes physician orders
____ f. Involved in client and family coping skills
____ g. Identifies community resources
____ h. Usually coordinates client care/case manager
____ i. Teaches client skills such as transferring in and out of bed, strength training, and exercises
____ j. Administers care such as bathing and feeding
____ k. Works directly with clients who have experienced head injuries and have difficulty with memory

Interdisciplinary Team Members

1. Physiatrist
2. Rehab nurse/ case manager
3. Physical therapist
4. Occupational therapist
5. Speech-language pathologist
6. Recreational/ activity therapist
7. Cognitive therapist
8. School worker
9. Psychologist
10. Vocational counselor
11. Aides and health care assistant
12. Client
13. Neuropsychologist

Exercise continued on next page.

___ l. Assists clients in learning new interests such as working crossword puzzles or swimming

___ m. Involved in all aspects of restoration and maintenance of optimal health

___ n. Teaches clients to pronounce words and express thoughts

___ o. Addresses the architectural features of the home to determine needs of the client

___ p. Performs assessment of the client's living habits and schedule to include items such as meals, sleep, sexuality patterns, exercise, and recreational activities

___ q. Performs comprehensive physical, psychosocial, and spiritual assessments

___ r. Discharge planning to determine adequacy of current situation and potential needs and how care will be provided to meet those needs

___ s. Retrains clients with language or hearing problems

___ t. Has final authority regarding teaching plan

6. Which of the following would not be considered a setting for rehabilitation after hospitalization?
   a. Rest home
   b. Vocational rehabilitation center
   c. Independent living center
   d. Outpatient hospital rehabilitation center

7. According to evidence-based practice, two predictors of being able to recover activities of daily living (ADL) independence in the older adult following a hospital discharge are:
   a. Ability to dress and feed self with minimal assistance.
   b. No prehospital ambulatory device and good score on Mini-Mental exam.
   c. Ability to transfer and toilet self with minimal assistance.
   d. Ability to bathe with minimal assistance and level of continence.

8. Which of the following are true statements regarding nursing care of the older adult in rehabilitation? *Check all that apply. If the statement is false, correct it to make it true.*
   ___ a. Turning the client every 2 hours is adequate for the skin type of the older adult.
   ___ b. Older adults are at increased risk for injury related to antihypertensive medications and orthostatic hypotension.
   ___ c. Diarrhea is a risk factor because of mobility and increased intestinal motility.

___ d. Clients are at risk for ineffective coping related to a lack of family and significant other support systems.

___ e. Assess for urinary problems present before illness or rehabilitation to determine effectiveness of a bladder training program.

___ f. Fatigue and physical complications often affect the length of time of a given workout session.

___ g. Encouraging ingestion of 2000 to 2500 mL of fluid per day is an important consideration in the prevention of complications from flaccid bladder and heart disease.

9. Identify the six categories of data that should be collected on all clients preparing for rehabilitation.
   a. _____
   b. _____
   c. _____
   d. _____
   e. _____
   f. _____

10. A client with Decreased Cardiac Output is entering a rehabilitation program. What should data collection include about the client?
    a. Has shortness of breath on activity.
    b. Has the ability to ambulate without angina.
    c. Feels rested upon awakening from sleep.
    d. Uses an antihistamine for pollen allergies.

11. Gastrointestinal system assessment of the paraplegic client who is entering a rehabilitation program should include which *priority* finding?
    a. Family and cultural background
    b. Baseline hemoglobin and hematocrit measurements
    c. Habits of bowel elimination before illness
    d. Manual dexterity, muscle control, and mobility

12. A client with a neurogenic bladder is to be taught how to perform intermittent self-catheterization. Which of the following is essential for the nurse to assess before beginning the teaching-learning sessions?
    a. Motor function of both upper extremities
    b. The type of neurogenic bladder the client has
    c. The client's gender
    d. The age of the client

13. To maintain skin integrity of a client in a rehabilitation unit, the nurse assesses which of the following items? *Check all that apply.*
    ___ a. Amount of water or other fluids in a day
    ___ b. Type and amount of food
    ___ c. Sensation to the skin
    ___ d. Circulation of oxygen and elimination of waste
    ___ e. Ability to move extremities
    ___ f. Ability to feel pain from pressure
    ___ g. Ability to change position as needed
    ___ h. Ability to perform self-care activities
    ___ i. Respiratory status and oxygenation

14. Read the following statements regarding the Katz Index of Activities of Daily Living and decide whether each is true or false. *Write* T *for true or* F *for false in the blanks provided. If the statement is false, correct the statement to make it true.*
    ___ a. Client is scored on 10 areas of activities of daily living.
    ___ b. Each area is scored as to the client being dependent or independent.
    ___ c. From total score, the client is given a grade of A through G.
    ___ d. Grade ranges from complete independence to dependence in all six areas.
    ___ e. Tool is only used as an initial assessment tool for determining client care.
    ___ f. Tool is only useful for chronic illnesses related to neurologic deficits.
    ___ g. It is the most widely used tool to assess activities of daily living.

15. Identify four assessment tools other than the Katz functional assessment index and provide a brief description of each tool.
    a. _____
    b. _____
    c. _____
    d. _____

16. Identify the six areas that are assessed on the Katz Functional Assessment Index. Discuss how these may vary from other assessment tools.
    a. _____
    b. _____
    c. _____
    d. _____
    e. _____
    f. _____

Answer the following three questions on a separate sheet of paper:

17. Identify types of data and examples of data that are included in a baseline assessment for a client entering a rehabilitation program.

18. Nurses use the major body systems approach when performing a physical assessment of a client. Identify data collected for each of the following areas as they relate to the functional abilities of a client in rehabilitation and chronic illness.
    a. Cardiovascular assessment
    b. Respiratory assessment
    c. Gastrointestinal and nutritional assessment
    d. Renal and urinary assessment
    e. Neurologic assessment (motor, sensation, cognitive)
    f. Musculoskeletal assessment
    g. Skin assessment (risk for breakdown and actual breakdown)

19. Identify the purpose of a vocational assessment for a client in rehabilitation.

20. The nurse reviews with the client the results of manual muscle testing performed by physical therapy. This procedure determines the client's:
    a. Body flexibility and muscle strength.
    b. ROM and degree of muscle strength.
    c. Muscle strength and amount of pain on movement.
    d. Voluntary versus involuntary muscle movement.

21. A client is preparing for discharge from a rehabilitation facility. On a separate sheet of paper, identify and briefly explain the two methods that can be used to assess the readiness of the client and the home for this discharge.

22. When assessing the family of a client with a chronic illness, data collected include the client's:
    a. Strengths as an individual.
    b. Relationships with peers.
    c. Role and role functions in the group.
    d. Ability to communicate with the health care team.

23. Identify the type of data that are included in an assessment of the family of a client with rehabilitation needs.

24. A 24-year-old paraplegic client, as a result of a motor vehicle accident, is admitted to a rehabilitation unit after 6 weeks of hospitalization. On a separate sheet of paper, identify potential outcome(s) for each of the following problem areas and submit your answers for review to your clinical instructor. Use the outcome(s) in the "Planning: expected outcomes" section of your text as a guide.
    a. Impaired physical mobility
    b. Self-care deficit
    c. Risk for impaired skin integrity
    d. Altered urinary elimination
    e. Constipation
    f. Ineffective individual coping
    g. Body image disturbance

25. When assisting a client with a hemiparesis to transfer or ambulate, the nurse instructs the client to:
    a. Lean the body weight backward.
    b. Use the weaker hand to assist.
    c. Lean the body weight toward the nurse.
    d. Use the strong hand to assist.

26. Which of the following items would be helpful to use when transferring a quadriplegic to a bed or chair?
    a. Gait belt
    b. Sliding board
    c. "Quad" cane
    d. Long-handled reacher

27. A client with Impaired Physical Mobility must be monitored for which of the following early potential complications?
    a. Pressure ulcers
    b. Renal calculi
    c. Osteoporosis
    d. Fractures

28. Which of the following clients is at greatest risk of developing a pressure ulcer?
    a. A 26-year-old woman who has had a tonsillectomy
    b. A 74-year-old woman who has had a bowel resection
    c. An 80-year-old man who has metastatic prostate cancer
    d. A 35-year-old man who is somnolent from a head injury

29. The best ways to prevent pressure ulcers resulting from immobility is to teach the client and significant other which of the following? *Check all that apply.*
    ___ a. Change position often to relieve pressure on all bony prominences.
    ___ b. Maintain good skin care by keeping the skin clean and dry.
    ___ c. Inspect the skin at least twice a day for problems such as reddened areas that do not fade readily.
    ___ d. Use pressure-relieving devices but not as a substitute for changing position.
    ___ e. Eat foods high in protein, carbohydrates, and vitamins for sufficient nutrition.

30. When assisting a client to perform range-of-motion (ROM) exercises, the nurse knows that ROM exercises should be performed:
    a. Only on the knees, hips, elbows, and shoulders.
    b. On each joint three times per session.
    c. To the point of inducing pain or stiffness in the joint.
    d. On each joint two times per day.

31. A client in a rehabilitation unit has a nursing diagnosis of Risk for Falls related to the effects of orthostatic hypotension. On a separate sheet of paper, identify nursing interventions to prevent falls and injuries.

32. When a client needs to increase musculoskeletal strength, which type of ROM exercise is indicated? Identify indications for the other types of exercises.
    a. Active
    b. Passive
    c. Assisted
    d. Resistive

33. Which of the following assistive-adaptive devices would be recommended to a client with a weak hand grasp?
    a. Gel pad
    b. Foam buildups
    c. Hook and loop fastener straps
    d. Buttonhook

34. When teaching a client with hemiplegia about energy conservation techniques, the nurse would include which of the following?
    a. Using a walker instead of a cane
    b. Scheduling physical therapy immediately prior to eating
    c. Using a bedside commode
    d. Scheduling recreational activities in afternoon or evening

35. Which of the following is true regarding the use of mechanical pressure-relieving devices?
    a. They effectively eliminate the need to turn clients.
    b. They still require repositioning clients regularly.
    c. They prevent pressure ulcers in debilitated clients.
    d. They have been shown to be ineffective against pressure ulcers.

36. A client has a lower motor neuron injury below T-12. This injury results in which of the following types of neurogenic bladder? *On a separate sheet of paper, briefly explain why the other answers are incorrect.*
    a. Reflex or spastic bladder
    b. Flaccid bladder
    c. Uninhibited bladder
    d. Inhibited bladder

37. A client with a flaccid bladder will have which of the following urinary elimination problems?
    a. Incontinence and inability to empty the bladder completely
    b. Incontinence caused by inability to wait until on a commode or bedpan
    c. Urinary retention and dribbling because of overflow of urine
    d. Incontinence due to loss of sensation

38. Match the bladder training intervention with the type of neurogenic bladder problem. *Answers may be used more than once.*

Bladder Training Interventions
____ a. Credé maneuver
____ b. Facilitating/ triggering
____ c. Intermittent catheterization
____ d. Medications
____ e. Consistent toileting schedule
____ f. Valsalva maneuvers
____ g. Regulation of fluid intake
____ h. Drinking fluids to promote an acidic urine

Neurogenic Bladder Problem
1. Reflex or spastic
2. Flaccid
3. Uninhibited

39. Which of the following are correct principles for performing an intermittent catheterization? *Check all that are true and correct the false answers.*
    ____ a. A catheter is inserted every 2 to 4 hours.
    ____ b. It is usually performed after the Valsalva or Credé maneuver.
    ____ c. A residual of less than 150 mL increases the interval between catheterization.
    ____ d. The maximum time interval between catheterizations is 6 hours.
    ____ e. The client uses sterile technique at home.

40. Which of the following medications would the client with a flaccid bladder most likely be given?
    a. Dantrolene sodium (Dantrium)
    b. Bethanechol chloride (Urecholine)
    c. Flavoxate hydrochloride (Urispas)
    d. Oxybutynin chloride (Ditropan)

41. A client with a flaccid bladder is to receive Urecholine. On a separate sheet of paper, describe what should be included in the teaching plan for this medication.

42. When instructing a client about beverages, the nurse tells the client that which of the following juices does not create an acidic urine?
    a. Citrus juices
    b. Prune juice
    c. Tomato juice
    d. Cranberry juice

43. A paraplegic client is experiencing muscle spasms. Identify two medications that would be prescribed and give the related nursing interventions to perform when teaching clients about these drugs.
    a. _____
    b. _____

44. Which of the following clients is most likely to have a flaccid bowel dysfunction?
    a. A 28-year-old client with a crushed pelvis
    b. A 54-year-old man with Guillain-Barré syndrome
    c. An 18-year-old woman with a displaced cervical fracture
    d. A 68-year-old woman who has had a cerebrovascular accident

45. Digital stimulation of the rectum as a method of re-establishing bowel control is most successful in the client who has had what problem?
    a. A myocardial infarction and is starting cardiac rehabilitation
    b. Chronic diarrhea resulting from radiation to the bowel
    c. Constipation resulting from medications taken for pain control
    d. A spinal cord injury resulting from a diving accident

46. What is the drug of choice for long-term management of bowel dysfunction?
    a. Milk of magnesia
    b. Senna concentrate (Senokot)
    c. Dulcolax or glycerin suppository
    d. Dulcolax tablets

47. An example of a food that should be part of breakfast for the client with bowel dysfunction is:
    a. Raisins.
    b. White bread.
    c. Cheddar cheese.
    d. Sausage links.

48. A client with lower motor neuron disease or injury results in which of following bowel dysfunctions? Why are the other answers incorrect?
    a. Flaccid bowel pattern
    b. Reflex (spastic) bowel pattern
    c. Uninhibited bowel pattern
    d. Inhibited bowel pattern

49. A client with an uninhibited bowel pattern dysfunction has difficulty with:
    a. Defecation occurring suddenly and without warning.
    b. Defecation occurring infrequently and in small amounts.
    c. Frequent defecation, urgency, and complaints of hard stool.
    d. Intermittent constipation and diarrhea.

50. Support systems for the client with a disability may include:
    a. Clergy member.
    b. Family member.
    c. Self-help groups.
    d. All of the above

UNIT 3 MANAGEMENT OF CLIENTS WITH FLUID, ELECTROLYTE, AND ACID-BASE IMBALANCES

■ Core Concepts Grid

Anatomy	Physiology	Pathophysiology	History	Physical Exam	Diagnostic Tests	Interventions	Pharmacology
• **Body fluid** Intercellular Extracellular Intravascular Interstitial • **Lungs** • **Heart/vessels** • **Kidney**	• **Filtration** • **Osmosis** • **Diffusion** • **Active transport** • **Hydrostatic pressure** • **Tonicity** Isotonic Hypotonic Hypertonic • **Third-space fluids** • **Transport medium** • **Protection** • **Metabolism** • **Regulatory mechanisms for fluid-electrolyte balance** • **Regulatory mechanisms for acid-base balance**	• **Overhydration** • **Dehydration** Isotonic Hypertonic Hypotonic • **Solute excess** • **Solute deficit** • **Metabolic acidosis/ alkalosis** • **Respiratory acidosis/ alkalosis**	• **Client history** Anorexia Fatigue Headache Nausea/ vomiting Diarrhea Weakness Cramping Thirst Fever	• **Skin** Color/moisture Turgor • **Weight** • **Urine output** • **Vital signs** • **Breath sounds** • **Muscle weakness** • **Central nervous system** Mental status Hyperreflexia Tetany Chvostek's sign Trousseau's sign • **Cardiovascular system** Dysrhythmias Decreased cardiac output	• **Serum levels** Sodium Potassium Calcium Phosphorus Magnesium • **Urine tests** pH Specific gravity • **Blood urea nitrogen** • **Arterial blood gases** pH Pao_2 $Paco_2$ HCO_3 • **Anion gap** • **Hemoglobin/ hematocrit**	• **Oral rehydration** • **Therapeutic diets** • **Blood gas interpretation** • **Semi-Fowler's position** • **Respiratory** Oxygen Turn, cough, deep breathe Incentive spirometry • **Oral hygiene** • **Rest** • **Infusion therapy** Peripheral intravenous therapy Central intravenous therapy • **Health teaching**	• **Diuretics** • **Crystalloid/ colloid fluid replacement** • **Electrolyte replacement** • **Bronchodilators** • **Anti-inflammatory drugs** • **Antibiotics** • **Antidiarrheals** • **Kayexelate**

Unit 3 (Chapters 11-16)

Management of Clients with Fluid, Electrolyte, and Acid-Base Imbalances

Learning Plan

Chapter 11: *Fluid and Electrolyte Balance*

Learning Outcomes	Learning Activities	Supplemental Resources

1. Explain why women and older adults have less total body water than do men and younger adults.
2. Interpret whether a client's serum electrolyte values are normal, elevated, or low.
3. Describe the expected blood volume and osmolarity responses when isotonic, hypertonic, or hypotonic intravenous fluids are infused.
4. Explain the relationships between antidiuretic hormone, urine output volume, and osmolarity.
5. Analyze a client's hydration status on the basis of physical assessment findings.
6. Evaluate a client's food choices for compliance with a low-sodium diet.
	1. Prior to completing the study guide exercises for this chapter, it is recommended to review the following:
	  • Normal A & P
	  • Fluid requirements of adults
	  • Adult nutrition
	  • Adult growth and development
	
	2. Review the **boldfaced** words and their definitions in Chapter 11 to enhance your understanding of the content.
	
	3. Go to Study Guide Number 3.11 on the following pages and complete the learning exercises for this chapter.
		1. Textbook—Chapter 11
		2. Other resources:
		  • Any fluid and electrolyte book for reference
		  • Any clinical laboratory guide to laboratory tests
		  • Consult the lab instructor at the nursing school for audiovisual material on the subject.
		  • Guyton, A. & Hall, J. (2001). *Textbook of medical physiology* (10th ed.). Philadelphia: W.B. Saunders.
		  • Horne, M.M. & Heitz, U.E. (1997). *Pocket guide to fluids and electrolytes* (3rd ed.). St. Louis: Mosby.
		  • Infusion Nurses Society (INS) http://www.ins1.org
		  • Lee, C.A.B., Barrett, C.A., Ignatavicius D.D. (1996). *Fluids and electrolytes: A practical approach.* (4th ed.). Philadelphia: Davis.
		  • Metheny, N.M. (2000) *Fluid and electrolyte balance nursing consideration.* (4th ed.). St. Louis: J.B. Lippincott.
		  • Pennington, J. (1998). *Bowe's and Church's food values of portions commonly used* (17th ed.). Philadelphia: J.B. Lippincott.
		  • Stark, J. (1998). A comprehensive analysis of the fluid and electrolytes system. *Critical care nursing clinics of North America, 10*(4), 471-475.
		  • Toto, K. (1998). Fluid balance assessment: The total perspective. *Critical Care Nursing Clinics of North America, 10*(4), 383-400.

Chapter 12: *Interventions for Clients with Fluid Imbalances*

Learning Outcomes	Learning Activities	Supplemental Resources
1. Identify clients at risk for fluid imbalances. 2. Use laboratory data and clinical manifestations to determine the presence of fluid imbalance.	1. Prior to completing the study guide exercises for this chapter, it is recommended to review the following: • Normal nutrition for adults	1. Textbook—Chapter 11 (Fluid and Electrolyte Balance) 2. Textbook—Chapter 12

Learning Outcomes	Learning Activities	Supplemental Resources
3. Apply appropriate nursing techniques to promote comfort and safety in the client with dehydration. 4. Prioritize nursing care needs for the client with fluid imbalance. 5. Develop a teaching plan to prevent dehydration in the older adult client at continuing risk for fluid loss. 6. Analyze changes in clinical manifestations to determine the effectiveness of therapy for the client with fluid imbalance.	• Fluid and electrolyte requirements for adults 2. Review the **boldfaced** words and their definitions in Chapter 12 to enhance your understanding of the content. 3. Go to Study Guide Number 3.12 on the following pages and complete the learning exercises for this chapter.	3. Other resources: • Any pathophysiology book • Cook, L. (1999). The value of lab values. *American Journal of Nursing 99*(5), 66-75. • Edwards, S. (1998). Hypovolemia: Pathophysiology and management options. *Nursing Critical Care, 3*(2), 73-82. • Fluid and electrolytes as presented in any anatomy and physiology book • Guyton, A. & Hall, J. (2001). *Textbook of medical physiology* (10th ed.). Philadelphia: W.B. Saunders. • Methany, N.M. (2000). *Fluid and electrolyte balance: Nursing considerations.* (4th ed.). St. Louis: J.B. Lippincott. • Provide nursing care for adult clients with medical-surgical diagnoses that are prone to fluid and electrolyte imbalances. • Read client lab values, assess and evaluate changes in the client's condition. • See a school lab instructor for audiovisual material on fluid and electrolytes. • Toto, K. (1998). Fluid balance assessment: The total perspective. *Critical Care Nursing Clinics of North America, 10*(4), 382-400.

Chapter 13: *Interventions for Clients with Electrolyte Imbalances*

Learning Outcomes	Learning Activities	Supplemental Resources
1. Identify clients at risk for imbalances of potassium. 2. Use laboratory data and clinical manifestations to determine the presence or absence of potassium imbalance. 3. Prioritize nursing care needs for the client with potassium imbalance. 4. Develop a teaching plan to prevent deficiencies or excesses of potassium in the older adult client at risk for potassium imbalance. 5. Analyze changes in clinical manifestations to determine the effectiveness of therapy for the client with potassium imbalance.	1. Prior to completing the study guide exercises for this chapter, it is recommended to review the following: • Fluids and electrolytes • Fluid requirements for adults • Dietary information in any nutrition reference for foods high in potassium and sodium • Normal nutrition requirements 2. Review the **boldfaced** words and their definitions in Chapter 13 to enhance your understanding of the content.	1. Textbook—Chapter 11 (Fluid and Electrolyte Balance) 2. Textbook—Chapter 13 3. Other resources: • Ahern-Gould, K. & Stark, J. (1998). Quick resource for electrolyte imbalance. *Critical Care Nursing Clinics of North America, 10*(4), 477-490. • Any pharmacology book • Castiglione, V. (2000). Emergency: Hyperkalemia. *American Journal of Nursing, 100*(1), 55-56. • Chmielewski, C. (1998). Hyperkalemic emergencies: Mechanisms, manifestations, and management. *Critical Care Clinics of North America, 10*(4), 449-457.

Learning Outcomes	Learning Activities	Supplemental Resources
6. Identify clients at risk for imbalances of sodium. 7. Use laboratory data and clinical manifestations to determine the presence or absence of sodium imbalance. 8. Prioritize nursing care for the client with sodium imbalance. 9. Develop a teaching plan to prevent deficiencies or excesses of sodium in the older adult client at risk for sodium imbalance. 10. Analyze changes in clinical manifestations to determine the effectiveness of therapy for the client with sodium imbalance. 11. Identify clients at risk for imbalances of calcium. 12. Use laboratory data and clinical manifestations to determine the presence or absence of calcium imbalance. 13. Prioritize nursing care needs for the client with calcium imbalance. 14. Develop a teaching plan to prevent deficiencies or excesses of calcium in the older adult client at risk for calcium imbalance. 15. Analyze changes in clinical manifestations to determine the effectiveness of therapy for the client with calcium imbalances.	3. Go to Study Guide Number 3.13 on the following pages and complete the learning exercises for this chapter.	• Consult with a dietitian for information on a low-sodium diet—one high in potassium and one low in potassium. • Fabius, D. (1998). How to recognize electrolyte imbalances on an ECG. *Nursing 98, 28*(2), 32hnl-32hn6. • Fabius, D.B. (1998). How to recognize electrolyte imbalances on an ECG. *Hospital Nursing 32*, 1. • Infusion Nurses Society (INS): http://www.ins1.org • Lee, C.A.B., Barrett, C.A., Ignatavicius, D.D. (1996). *Fluids and electrolytes: A practical approach* (4th ed.). Philadelphia: Davis. • Methany, N.M. (2000). *Fluid and electrolyte balance: Nursing considerations* (4th ed.). St. Louis: J.B. Lippincott. • Reber, P.M. & Heath, H. (1995). Hypocalcemia emergencies. *Medical Clinics of North America* 79, 93. • Review fluid and electrolytes in any anatomy and physiology book. • Review laboratory results to determine "hypo" and "hyper" levels of various electrolytes and provide appropriate interventions. • Review pathophysiology of electrolyte imbalances in any pathophysiology book. • Tasota, F.J. & Wesmiller, S.W. Balancing act: Keeping blood pH in equilibrium. *Nursing 28*:43.

Chapter 14: *Infusion Therapy*

Learning Outcomes	Learning Activities	Supplemental Resources
1. Explain the purpose of infusion filters. 2. Explain the primary advantage of needleless infusion systems. 3. Compare and contrast the use of controllers and pumps. 4. Identify important considerations when placing a venous access device (VAD). 5. Determine special needs of older adults who receive intravenous (IV) therapy. 6. Describe the major differences between nontunneled and tunneled central VADs.	1. Prior to completing the study guide exercises for this chapter, it is recommended to review the following: • Fluid and electrolyte balance • Anatomy and physiology of vascular system 2. Review the **boldfaced** words and their definitions in Chapter 14 to enhance your understanding of the content.	1. Textbook—Chapter 14 2. Other resources: • Assist with the insertion of a central line and monitor the line appropriately. • Contact the Infusion Nurses Society (INS), a professional nursing organization for infusion therapy nurses, for publications on standards of care regarding infusion therapy. • Lee, C.A.B., Barrett, C.A., Ignatavicius, D.D. (1996). *Fluids and electrolytes: A practical approach.* (4th ed.). Philadelphia: Davis.

7. Describe how a peripherally inserted central catheter differs from central lines.
8. Compare and contrast the major complications of peripheral and central IV therapy.
9. Identify the most common use for intra-arterial therapy.
10. Describe the nursing care of a client receiving hypodermoclysis.
11. Explain the indications for epidural and intrathecal therapy.

3. Go to Study Guide Number 3.14 on the following pages and complete the learning exercises for this chapter.

- Metheny, N.M. (2000). *Fluid and electrolyte balance: Nursing considerations.* (4th ed.). St. Louis: J.B. Lippincott.
- Provide nursing care for clients with central lines.
- Review policies and procedures of the employer to become familiar with the care and maintenance of all infusion therapies.
- Work with nurses on the IV team or with the infection control nurse.

Chapter 15: *Acid-Base Balance*

Learning Outcomes	Learning Activities	Supplemental Resources
1. Describe the relationship between hydrogen ion concentration and pH.	1. Prior to completing the study guide exercises for this chapter, it is recommended to review the following:	1. Textbook—Chapter 15
2. Explain the role of bicarbonate in the blood.	• Principles of acid and base solutions from basic chemistry	2. Other resources:
3. Explain the concept of compensation.	• Normal anatomy and physiology of the lungs and kidneys	• Demers, B. & Morfei, J. (1999). Role of bicarbonate ion concentration in acid-base balance. *Respiratory Care, 44*(8), 963-964.
4. Compare the role of a buffer in conditions of acidosis and alkalosis.		• Faris, S. (1997). Interpretation of arterial blood gases by nurses. *Journal of Vascular Nursing, 15*(4), 128-130.
5. Compare the roles of the respiratory system and the renal system in maintaining acid-base balance.	2. Review the **boldfaced** words and their definitions in Chapter 15 to enhance your understanding of the content.	• Guyton, A. & Hall, J. (2001). *Textbook of medical physiology* (10th ed.). Philadelphia: W.B. Saunders.
6. Describe the role of oxygen in maintaining acid-base balance.		• Horne, C. & Derrico, D. (1999). Mastering ABGs. *American Journal of Nursing, 99*(8), 26-32.
7. Interpret whether the client's arterial blood gas values are normal, elevated, or low.	3. Go to Study Guide Number 3.15 on the following pages and complete the learning exercises for this chapter.	• Lee CAB, Barrett CA, Ignatavicius DD. (1996). *Fluids and electrolytes: A practical approach.* (4th ed.). Philadelphia: Davis.
		• Metheny, N. (1996). *Fluid and electrolyte balance: Nursing considerations* (3rd ed.). Philadelphia: J.B. Lippincott.
		• Metheny, N.M. (2000). *Fluid and electrolyte balance: Nursing considerations.* (4th ed.). St. Louis: J.B. Lippincott.

Chapter 16: *Interventions for Clients with Acid-Base Imbalances*

Learning Outcomes	Learning Activities	Supplemental Resources

1. Identify clients at risk for acidosis.
2. Use laboratory data and clinical manifestations to determine the presence or absence of acidosis.
3. Analyze arterial blood gases to determine whether acidosis is respiratory or metabolic in origin.
4. Analyze arterial blood gases to determine whether respiratory acidosis is acute or chronic.
5. Prioritize nursing care for the client with acute acidosis.
6. Identify clients at risk for alkalosis.
7. Use laboratory data and clinical manifestations to determine the presence or absence of alkalosis.
8. Analyze arterial blood gases to determine whether alkalosis is respiratory or metabolic in origin.
9. Prioritize nursing care for the client with alkalosis.
	1. Prior to completing the study guide exercises for this chapter, it is recommended to review the following:
	  • Acid-base balance
	  • Anatomy and physiology of the lungs and kidneys
	2. Review the **boldfaced** words and their definitions in Chapter 16 to enhance your understanding of the content.
	3. Go to Study Guide Number 3.16 on the following pages and complete the learning exercises for this chapter.
		1. Textbook—Chapter 15 (Acid-Base Balance)
		2. Textbook—Chapter 16
		3. Other resources
		  • Any anatomy and physiology book
		  • Any fluid and electrolyte book
		  • Any pathophysiology book
		  • Cook, L. (1999). The value of lab values. *American Journal of Nursing, 99*(5), 66-75.
		  • Demers, B. & Morfei, J. (1999). Role of bicarbonate ion concentration in acid-base balance. *Respiratory Care, 44*(8), 963-964.
		  • Faria, S. (1997). Interpretation of arterial blood gases by nurses. *Journal of Vascular Nursing, 15*(4), 128-130.
		  • Guyton, A. & Hall, J. (2001). *Textbook of Medical physiology* (10th ed.). Philadelphia: W.B. Saunders.
		  • Horne, C. & Derrico, D. (1999). Mastering ABGs. *American Journal of Nursing, 99*(8), 26-32.
		  • Lee, C.A.B., Barrett, C.A., Ignatavicius, D.D. (1996). *Fluids and electrolytes: A practical approach* (4th ed.). Philadelphia: Davis.
		  • Markowitz, D. & Irwin, R. (1999). Evaluating acid-base disorders: Is venous blood gas testing sufficient? *Journal of Critical Illness, 14*(7), 403-406.
		  • Metheny, N.M. (2000). *Fluid and electrolyte balance: Nursing consideration* (4th ed.). St. Louis: J.B. Lippincott.
		  • Paulson, W. (1999). Quick take: Common causes of acid-base disorders. *Journal of Critical Care Illness, 14*(2), 110-111.
		  • Tasota, F. & Wesmiller, S. (1998). Balancing act: Keeping blood pH in equilibrium. *Nursing 98, 28*(12) 35-40.
		  • Wong, F. (1999). A new approach to ABG interpretation. *American Journal of Nursing, 99*(8), 34-35.

STUDY GUIDE NUMBER 3.11

Fluid and Electrolyte Balance

Study/Review Questions

1. What is homeostasis?
   a. The way the body attempts to keep itself in a balanced physiologic state.
   b. A balance of solvents and solutes for proper body functioning.
   c. A balance of fluid and electrolytes to maintain proper body function.
   d. The regulation of water and blood with other body substances.

2. Indicate which of the following statements regarding water is true. *Write* T *for true or* F *for false in the blanks provided.*
   ___ a. Water is the solvent that delivers substances such as glucose, sodium, and potassium to organs, tissues, and cells.
   ___ b. Water is a passive member of the homeostatic regulatory mechanism.
   ___ c. Fluids, especially water, make up approximately 55% to 60% of total adult body weight.
   ___ d. Water is the second largest component of body fluid next to blood.
   ___ e. When equilibrium occurs, filtration of water stops because there is no hydrostatic pressure gradient.
   ___ f. In osmosis, the physiologic activity is one of movement from a higher to a lower concentration of molecules.
   ___ g. Lean muscle tissue is higher in water content than is fat.
   ___ h. The amount of body fat and the gender and age of the client affect total body water content.

3. Match the physiologic influences on fluids and electrolytes in the body with their descriptions.

   Description
   ___ a. Hydrostatic pressure on both sides of a membrane that is the force behind the movement of water and substances from an area of high pressure to an area of low pressure.
   ___ b. The movement of electrolytes into or out of the cell.
   ___ c. The movement of water in or out of a compartment, depending on whether the solute concentration is highest inside or outside of the compartment.
   ___ d. The unit of measure in a liter of solution that reflects concentration of solutes.
   ___ e. Water creating a force against the walls of a given space.

   Physiologic Influences
   1. Filtration
   2. Diffusion
   3. Osmosis
   4. Osmolality
   5. Hydrostatic pressure

4. Describe the two major functions of body fluids.
   a. _____
   b. _____

5. A client requires blood work for serum electrolytes. Identify the six commonly reported lab values.
   a. _____
   b. _____
   c. _____
   d. _____
   e. _____
   f. _____

6. The major hypothalamic mechanism for stimulating fluid intake is _____.

7. On a separate sheet of paper, identify the four areas a nurse must consider when assessing serum electrolyte values for significance and follow-up interventions.

8. Identify three main goals and related nursing interventions for a client with Deficient Fluid Volume.

9. Match the type of osmolarity with its properties. *Types may be used more than once.*

Osmolarity Properties	Types of Osmolarity
___ a. 0.9% saline	1. Hypotonic
___ b. 45% saline	2. Isotonic
___ c. Dextrose 20%	3. Hypertonic
___ d. No effect on osmolarity of body fluids	
___ e. Osmolarity lower than body fluids	
___ f. Osmolarity higher than body fluids	
___ g. Causes movement of body fluids to increase blood volume	
___ h. Causes movement of body fluids to decrease blood volume	

10. The kidney is actively involved in which process of fluid balance?
   a. Osmosis
   b. Filtration
   c. Diffusion
   d. Active transport

11. Identify four factors that affect the process of filtration in the kidney.
   a. _____
   b. _____
   c. _____
   d. _____

12. Match each electrolyte with the corresponding lab value and description. *Answers can be used more than once.*

Normal Lab Values and Descriptions	Electrolytes
___ a. Normal plasma value is 3.5 to 5.0 mEq/L	1. Sodium
___ b. Major anion of extracellular fluid (ECF) and works with a cation to maintain osmotic pressure	2. Potassium
	3. Calcium
	4. Phosphorus
	5. Magnesium
	6. Chloride
___ c. Normal value is 90 to 110 mEq/L	
___ d. Main cation in ECF of the cell that maintains ECF osmolarity	

___ e. Works in balance with calcium
___ f. Normal plasma value is 136 to 145 mEq
___ g. Serum value must be kept in the narrow range
___ h. Major cation of intracellular fluid (ICF) in the cell that maintains the ICF osmolarity
___ i. Regulates glucose use and maintenance of electrical membrane excitability
___ j. Functions include contraction of skeletal, cardiac, and smooth muscle
___ k. Normal value is 3.0 to 4.5 mg/dL
___ l. Major intracellular mineral
___ m. Free form is physiologically active in the body
___ n. Normal value is 1.2 to 2.0 mg/dL
___ o. Absorbed from the GI tract
___ p. Mineral responsible for activating high energy substances (carbohydrate, protein, and lipid metabolism) and vitamin B.

13. Identify the three primary electrolytes that are involved in maintenance of acid-base balance.
   a. _____
   b. _____
   c. _____

14. Identify two factors that primarily control the electrolyte balance within the body.
   a. _____
   b. _____

15. Identify three sources of body fluid intake and give the average daily amount of each for an adult.
   a. _____
   b. _____
   c. _____

16. What is the total average amount of fluid intake for an adult in a 24-hour period?

17. Identify the factors that affect the renal tubules' ability to regulate fluid volume filtration.
   a. _____
   b. _____
   c. _____
   d. _____

18. Which of the following statements about fluid and electrolyte changes associated with aging is correct?
    a. Nearly 60% of the body weight of an older adult is water.
    b. Changes in the renal function increase the risk of electrolyte imbalance.
    c. Skin turgor is a reliable measure of body fluid levels.
    d. Thirst sensation is the best indicator of body fluid balance.

19. Which of the following statements regarding total body water in the older adult is correct?
    a. Decreased muscle mass results in decreased total body water.
    b. There is increased thirst and urination as a result of the aging process causing a loss of water.
    c. Loss of elasticity of the skin causes more evaporation of water from the skin.
    d. Older adults are prone to hypernatremia, which causes increased water retention.

20. When assessing for dehydration, what is the best location for assessing skin turgor on an older adult? How is this different than for other adults?
    a. Arms and sternum
    b. Sternum and forehead
    c. Back of hand and forehead
    d. Back of hand and thighs

21. The potassium laboratory value of a 65-year-old client was 5.0 mEq/L. This value can be interpreted as:
    a. High for the client's age.
    b. Low for the client's age.
    c. Normal for the client's age.
    d. It depends on the medical diagnosis.

22. Match the following cellular compartments with the descriptions. *Answers can be used more than once.*

Descriptions	**Cellular Compartments**
____ a. Contains the largest amount of body fluid	1. Extracellular compartment
____ b. Contains plasma	2. Intracellular compartment
____ c. Contains interstitial fluid	
____ d. High in sodium and chloride content	
____ e. High in potassium and phosphorous content	
____ f. High in magnesium content	

23. On a separate sheet of paper, identify and explain the four routes through which fluid is removed from the body.

24. The nurse assesses the urine specific gravity of 1.035 as an indication of:
    a. Overhydration.
    b. Dehydration.
    c. Normal value for an adult.
    d. Metabolic acidosis

25. On a separate sheet of paper, identify at least eight causes of fluid loss that may lead to a client's fluid imbalance.

26. A client is reviewing her dietary log with the nurse regarding maintenance of a low-sodium diet. Which of the following food items are high in sodium? *Check all that apply.*
    ____ a. Egg roll with soy sauce
    ____ b. Pork fried rice
    ____ c. Baked potato with butter
    ____ d. Salads with oil and vinegar dressing
    ____ e. Bacon and eggs each morning
    ____ f. Cottage cheese and tomato for lunch each day
    ____ g. Steak
    ____ h. Chicken breast
    ____ i. Canned tuna salad sandwich with pickles
    ____ j. Campbell's soup with saltine crackers
    ____ k. Canned vegetables

27. What is the nurse's response to a client when asked if a low-salt diet includes cooking with salt?

28. Which of the following substances increases osmotic pressure in the capillaries because of colloids?
    a. Salt
    b. Plasma
    c. Albumin
    d. Sugar

29. On a separate sheet of paper, identify common food sources for the following electrolytes:
    a. Magnesium
    b. Phosphorus
    c. Calcium
    d. Potassium
    e. Sodium

30. Match the following hormones with their corresponding effects on the body.

Hormone Effects on the Body	**Hormones**
___ a. Increases sodium and water loss in urine	1. Aldosterone
___ b. Stimulates release of aldosterone from the adrenal cortex	2. Angiotensin I
	3. Angiotensin II
___ c. Causes some vasoconstriction	4. Renin
___ d. Increases reabsorption of sodium in the distal convoluted tubule	

31. Which of the following best explains how antidiuretic hormone (ADH) affects urine output?
    a. It increases permeability to water in the tubules causing a decrease in urine output.
    b. It increases urine output as a result of water being absorbed by the tubules.
    c. Urine output is reduced as the posterior pituitary decreases ADH production.
    d. Increased urine output results from increased osmolarity and fluid in the extracellular space.

32. Identify three factors that affect the analysis of assessment findings in the older adult.
    a. _____
    b. _____
    c. _____

33. Which of the following best explains the difference between men and women in relationship to total body water?
    a. Women excrete more water than men and have less body water.
    b. Men have less body fat and therefore less body water.
    c. Men retain more body water because of more body fat.
    d. Men generally have less body fat than women do and more body water.

34. What effect does aldosterone have on the kidney and fluid balance?
    a. Water loss from the kidney increases.
    b. Potassium reabsorption in the tubules increases.
    c. Permeability to water increases in the tubules.
    d. Reabsorption of sodium and water occurs.

35. Which of the following clients would most likely have increased aldosterone secretion?
    a. Client who has excessive salt ingestion
    b. Client who drinks a lot of water
    c. Client who loses a lot of water and salt
    d. Client who loses potassium and water

36. Identify the two main hormones that regulate calcium absorption.
    a. _____
    b. _____

Answer the following questions on a separate sheet of paper:

37. Identify the subjective data relevant to fluid and electrolyte balance when performing a nursing assessment.

38. Identify the objective data relevant to fluid and electrolyte balance when performing a nursing assessment.

39. Briefly discuss why psychosocial factors are important to an accurate fluid and electrolyte status assessment.

Case Study: The Client with a Fluid Imbalance

Your client is a 45-year-old man who had GI surgery 4 days ago. He is NPO, has a nasogastric tube, and IV fluids of D5 ½ normal saline at 100 mL/hr. The nursing physical assessment includes the following: alert and oriented; fine crackles; capillary refill within normal limits (WNL); moving all extremities; complaining of abdominal pain, muscle aches, and dry mouth; moist mucous membranes; bowel sounds hypoactive, last BM was 4 days ago; skin turgor is poor; 200 mL of dark green substance has drained from NG tube in last 3 hours. Voiding dark amber urine without difficulty.

Intake for last 24 hours is 2500 mL. Output is 2000 mL including urine and NG drainage. Febrile and diaphoretic; BP 130/80; pulse 88; urine specific gravity is 1.035; serum potassium is 3.0 mEq/L; serum sodium 140 mEq/L; Cl 92 mEq/L; Mg 1.0 mg/dL.

Answer the following questions on a separate sheet of paper:

1. Analyze the data in the case study. Which of the assessment findings indicates a fluid volume deficit problem?

2. Evaluate this client's electrolyte values and give a rationale for the answer.

STUDY GUIDE NUMBER 3.12

Interventions for Clients with Fluid Imbalances

Study/Review Questions

1. Which of the following statements is true regarding dehydration in the adult?
   a. Dehydration may result from excessive sodium intake.
   b. Relative dehydration may be caused by fluid shifts.
   c. Persons over age 65 have increased thirst mechanisms.
   d. Water loss is the primary reason for dehydration.

2. Match the type of dehydration in column B with the corresponding pathophysiology in column A.
   Answers may be used more than once.

   Column A
   ___ a. Results from equal amounts of fluid and electrolyte loss
   ___ b. Results from decreased osmolality and fluid shifts
   ___ c. Results in cell shrinkage
   ___ d. Plasma osmolality remains normal
   ___ e. Fluid shifts without loss of total body water

   Column B
   1. Isotonic dehydration
   2. Hypertonic dehydration
   3. Relative dehydration
   4. Hypotonic dehydration

3. What serum laboratory values would you expect to see increased in hypertonic dehydration?
   a. _____
   b. _____
   c. _____
   d. _____

4. Which of the following compensatory mechanisms occurs as a result of hypertonic dehydration?
   a. Release of renin from the kidney
   b. Release of ADH from the pituitary gland
   c. Fluid shift from the ECF (extracellular fluid) to the ICF (intracellular fluid)
   d. Increased aldosterone release from the adrenal gland

5. Identify four clinical symptoms that you might observe in a client with circulatory volume overload as a result of renal failure.
   a. _____
   b. _____
   c. _____
   d. _____

6. Which of the following interventions would be effective for a client with fluid volume excess caused by congestive heart failure? *Identify all that apply.*
   a. Sodium and fluid restriction
   b. Slow infusion of hypotonic saline
   c. Administration of potassium
   d. Administration of loop diuretics
   e. Position in semi-Fowler's to high Fowler's position

7. State the change (increase or decrease) for the following parameters seen in hypotonic conditions.
   a. Serum sodium
   b. Urine osmolality
   c. Intracellular fluid
   d. Hematocrit

8. Match the following clinical conditions to the most likely type of resulting fluid imbalances. *Answers can be used more than once.*

Clinical Conditions	Resulting Fluid Imbalances
___ a. Vomiting	1. Hypertonic dehydration
___ b. Diabetes insipidus	2. Hypotonic dehydration
	3. Relative dehydration
___ c. Hemorrhage	4. Isotonic dehydration
___ d. Infusions of D5/0.2% NS	5. Hypotonic overhydration
	6. Hypertonic overhydration
___ e. Infusions of 0.9% NS	7. Isotonic overhydration
___ f. SIADH (syndrome of inappropriate antidiuretic hormone)	
___ g. Infusion of 3% NS	
___ h. Ascites	
___ i. End-stage renal disease	
___ j. Unconsciousness	
___ k. Congestive heart failure	

9. Explain why each of the following findings taken from a history from an older adult client are risk factors for dehydration. *Answer on a separate sheet of paper.*
   a. Age older than 70 years
   b. History of hypertension
   c. Weight loss of 4 pounds in 28 hours
   d. Feelings of lightheadedness
   e. Change in cognition

10. A client at risk for fluid volume excess should be taught to:
    a. Increase diuretic dose if swelling occurs.
    b. Limit the amount of free water in relation to sodium intake.
    c. Monitor his or her skin turgor.
    d. Weigh self each day on the same scale.

11. In which order would you provide the following interventions for an older adult client presenting to the emergency room with these symptoms: BP 80/60, pulse 120, temperature 105° F, headache, and flushed skin?
    a. Administration of oxygen
    b. Placement of ice packs at head, groin, and armpits
    c. Insertion of Foley catheter
    d. Insertion of IV catheter

ṢIMỌN. *Case Study: The Client with Overhydration*

A client is admitted to the hospital with a decreased serum osmolality and a serum sodium of 126 mEq/L. Dehydration or overhydration may accompany hypotonic conditions.

Answer the following questions in regard to this client:

1. In further assessing the client, which of the following assessments would indicate that the client has fluid volume excess?
   a. Distended hand and neck veins
   b. Decreased urine output
   c. Decreased capillary refill
   d. Increased rate and depth of respirations

2. Which of the following assessments would indicate that the client has fluid volume deficit?
   a. Increased, bounding pulse
   b. Jugular venous distension
   c. Presence of crackles
   d. Orthostatic hypotension

3. After determining by an in-depth clinical assessment that the client is not dehydrated, which of the following interventions would be appropriate to correct this hypotonic overhydration?
   a. Administration of 0.9% NS
   b. Restriction of free water
   c. Administration of antihypertensives
   d. Restriction of potassium

4. Which of the following would the nurse monitor for evidence of a worsening hypotonic condition?
   a. Mental status
   b. Urine output
   c. Skin changes
   d. Bowel sounds

ṢIMỌN. *Case Study: The Client with Dehydration*

A client with a history of voluminous diarrhea presents with a rapid pulse, orthostatic hypotension, urine output of 20 mL/hr, cool pale skin, and increased respiratory rate.

Answer the following questions in regard to this client.

1. In evaluating the client's laboratory values, you would expect to see which abnormality?
   a. Decreased urine specific gravity
   b. Increased serum sodium
   c. Decreased hematocrit
   d. Elevated BUN

2. The compensatory mechanism responsible for the client's rapid pulse is:
   a. Increased circulation of angiotensin.
   b. Increased sympathetic discharge.
   c. Increased aldosterone production.
   d. Increased renal reabsorption of sodium and water.

3. Immediate interventions to correct this client's fluid volume imbalance would include:
   a. Rapid hydration with 0.9% NS.
   b. Administration of a loop diuretic.
   c. Administration of an osmotic diuretic.
   d. Rapid hydration with D5/0.45% NS.

4. Which of the following would be most important to monitor to determine the client's response to corrective interventions?
   a. Respiratory rate and depth
   b. Skin turgor
   c. Urinary output
   d. Weight

5. Which of the following would indicate that the client has a negative response to fluid resuscitation?
   a. Increased blood pressure
   b. Urinary output of 40 mL/hr
   c. Presence of rales
   d. Widening of pulse pressure

STUDY GUIDE NUMBER 3.13

Interventions for Clients with Electrolyte Imbalances

Study/Review Questions

1. On a separate sheet of paper, briefly discuss the critical nature of the intracellular and extracellular effect potassium has on homeostasis.

2. The lab value that refers to hypokalemia is:
   a. Serum calcium level below 8.0 mg/dL.
   b. Serum potassium level below 5.0 mEq/L.
   c. Serum calcium level below 11.0 mg/dL.
   d. Serum potassium level below 3.5 mEq/L.

3. In addition to inadequate potassium intake, what type of clinical conditions would cause hypokalemia? Provide examples of the type of clients with these clinical conditions.

4. Which of the following clinical findings indicates the effect of hypokalemia on the body?
   a. Hypertension, bounding pulses, and bradycardia
   b. Moist crackles, tachypnea, and diminished breath sounds
   c. General skeletal muscle weakness, lethargy, and weak hand grasps
   d. Increased specific gravity and decreased urine output

5. Older adults are at increased risk for developing hypokalemia mainly because they:
   a. Often require medications that predispose them to hypokalemia.
   b. Avoid taking laxatives to promote bowel movements and relieve constipation.
   c. Have an increased capacity for the kidney to concentrate urine.
   d. Tend to consume large volumes of fluids leading to water intoxication.

6. A client is to receive potassium supplements for treatment of hypokalemia. Indicate the nursing interventions for safely administering oral and intravenous medications.

7. The complication of rapid infusion of intravenous potassium is:
   a. Pulmonary edema.
   b. Cardiac arrest.
   c. Postural hypotension.
   d. Renal failure.

8. Which of the following laboratory data are often found in association with hypokalemia?
   a. Decreased arterial blood P_{CO_2}
   b. Elevated blood glucose levels
   c. Inverted urine sodium/potassium ratio
   d. Increased urine potassium levels

9. Which of the following would *not* be included in discharge teaching regarding diet and medications for a client with hypokalemia?
   a. Reglan
   b. Nuts
   c. Metamucil
   d. Cheese

10. Which of the following statements indicates the client understands the treatment of hypokalemia?
    a. "My wife does all the cooking. She shops for food high in calcium."
    b. "When I take the liquid potassium in the evening, I'll eat a snack beforehand."
    c. "I usually have a bowl of corn flakes, a glass of cranberry juice, and a fried egg for breakfast."
    d. "I hate being stuck with needles all the time to monitor how much sugar I can eat."

11. On a separate sheet of paper, develop assessment criteria for a home care nurse with a cardiac client who was discharged from the hospital, is receiving loop diuretics, and is at risk for developing hypokalemia.

12. Which of the following lab values refers to hyperkalemia?
    a. Serum calcium level above 8.0 mg/dL
    b. Serum potassium level above 3.5 mEq/L
    c. Serum calcium level above 11.0 mg/dL
    d. Serum potassium level above 5.0 mEq/L

13. Which of the following statements explains the reason that hyperkalemia is uncommon?
    a. Symptoms do not develop until the serum electrolyte level is above 10 mEq/L.
    b. The kidney normally excretes any excess electrolytes at a fixed base rate.
    c. Few clients consume quantities of foods or liquids high in electrolytes.
    d. Hyperkalemic symptoms are indistinguishable from those of other conditions.

14. In the hospitalized client, which of the following is the most common cause of hyperkalemia?
    a. Overuse of potassium-sparing diuretics
    b. Failure to recognize acidosis in clients
    c. Too rapid administration of IV fluids with potassium
    d. Administering blood with an 18-gauge or larger needle

15. Laboratory findings associated with hyperkalemia include:
    a. Increased hematocrit and hemoglobin levels in renal failure.
    b. Elevated serum electrolyte levels in water intoxication.
    c. Increased urine potassium level in renal failure.
    d. Decreased urine potassium level in renal failure.

16. Which of the following interventions would be contraindicated in the emergency treatment of hyperkalemia?
    a. Cation exchange enemas (Kayexalate)
    b. Red blood cell/whole blood transfusion
    c. Hemodialysis or peritoneal dialysis
    d. IV glucose and insulin

17. Which of the following is *not* an assessment finding associated with hyperkalemia?
    a. Diminished breath sounds
    b. Numbness in hands, feet, and around the mouth
    c. Frequent, explosive diarrhea stools
    d. Irregular heart rate and hypotension

18. On a separate sheet of paper, identify nursing interventions that would be performed for clients with hyperkalemia.

19. Which of the following ECG changes reflect hyperkalemia? How is this different from hypokalemia?
    a. Tall tented T waves
    b. Narrow QRD complex
    c. Tail P waves
    d. Normal P-R interval

20. Which of the following clients are at risk for developing hyper- or hypokalemia? *Mark your answers with* hpr *for hyperkalemia or* hpo *for hypokalemia.*
    ___ a. Severely malnourished older adult man
    ___ b. COPD client on prednisone
    ___ c. Client with short bowel syndrome on TPN
    ___ d. Client with gout
    ___ e. Older adult receiving high-dose gentamicin
    ___ f. Client with hypertension receiving Aldactone
    ___ g. Client with CHF
    ___ h. Client with an ileostomy
    ___ i. Client in early stage of severe burns
    ___ j. Client with high CO_2 content in ABGs
    ___ k. Client with diabetic ketoacidosis receiving IV insulin
    ___ l. Oncology client receiving blood transfusions
    ___ m. Trauma client with crushed extremities
    ___ n. Client with congestive heart failure and taking loop diuretics

21. On a separate sheet of paper, compare and contrast subjective data for clients with hypokalemia and hyperkalemia in a nursing assessment.

22. On a separate sheet of paper, compare and contrast objective data for clients with hypokalemia and hyperkalemia in nursing assessment.

23. Match the following acid-balance imbalances with the associated conditions of hyperkalemia or hypokalemia.

Imbalance	Condition
___ a. Metabolic acidosis	1. Hyperkalemia
___ b. Metabolic alkalosis	2. Hypokalemia

24. The part of the body that is the most sensitive to the early effects of hyperkalemia and hypokalemia is which of the following? Indicate the potential complication that can result and give a rationale for your answer.
    a. Heart
    b. Skeletal muscles
    c. Gastrointestinal tract
    d. Kidney

25. Hyponatremia refers to which of the following lab values?
    a. Serum sodium level below 135 mEq/L
    b. Serum chloride level below 95 mEq/L
    c. Serum sodium level below 145 mEq/L
    d. Serum chloride level below 103 mEq/L

26. Which of the following statements is correct regarding the pathophysiology of hyponatremia?
    a. As the concentration of sodium falls in the ECF, it rises within the cell.
    b. Excitable membranes are more responsive during periods of hyponatremia.
    c. The nervous system tissues are the least affected by hyponatremia.
    d. Intracellular swelling may occur because of the shifts in osmotic pressure in the ECF.

27. Assessment findings of a client with hyponatremia include:
    a. Constipation and paralytic ileus.
    b. Watery explosive diarrhea with abdominal cramping.
    c. Muscle cramping and spasticity.
    d. Tachypnea and diminished breath sounds.

28. Which of the following clients is at risk of developing hyponatremia?
    a. Diabetic client with a blood glucose of 430 mg/dL
    b. Febrile client with copious diarrhea
    c. Client with diabetes insipidus
    d. COPD client on high doses of steroids

29. The nurse would monitor for which of the following complications that can occur with hyponatremia?
    a. Proteinuria/prerenal failure
    b. Change in mental status/increased intracranial pressure
    c. Pitting edema/circulatory failure
    d. Possible stool for occult blood/gastrointestinal bleeding

30. Laboratory findings associated with hyponatremia include:
    a. Decreased serum glucose.
    b. Increased total serum proteins.
    c. Decreased serum chloride levels.
    d. Normal hematocrit and hemoglobin.

31. Which of the following foods is contraindicated for the client who has hyponatremia?
    a. Cheese
    b. Stewed tomato
    c. Applesauce
    d. Whole milk

32. Which of the following clients are at risk for developing hyponatremia? *Check all that apply.*
    ____ a. A postoperative client who has been NPO for several hours
    ____ b. Client with prolonged diarrhea from food poisoning
    ____ c. Client with high blood cholesterol
    ____ d. Client with overactive adrenal glands
    ____ e. Client playing tennis in 100° F weather
    ____ f. Client with gastrointestinal fistula draining copious fluids
    ____ g. Client on high-salt diet
    ____ h. Diabetic client with blood glucose of 150 mg/dL
    ____ i. Client with excessive intake of 5% dextrose solution
    ____ j. No fluid intake for several days
    ____ k. Client with congestive heart failure
    ____ l. Febrile client with copious watery diarrhea
    ____ m. Client with massive systemic infection
    ____ n. Client with aldosterone deficiency
    ____ o. Client being given 0.9% normal saline at 100 mL/hr

33. When hyponatremia occurs with fluid deficit, the nurse can expect to administer:
    a. Saline infusions.
    b. 5% dextrose with saline.
    c. 10% dextrose with saline.
    d. Diuretics to promote excretion of water.

34. Hypernatremia refers to a:
    a. Serum chloride level above 95 mEq/L.
    b. Serum sodium level above 135 mEq/L.
    c. Serum chloride above 103 mEq/L.
    d. Serum sodium level above 145 mEq/L.

35. Which of the following systems is the most sensitive to changes in ECF sodium concentration? Give a rationale for your answer.
    a. Central nervous system/brain
    b. Skeletal muscles
    c. Cardiac tissue
    d. Sensory organs/hearing

36. Which two hormones are often used in the treatment of hypernatremia?
    a. Aldosterone and serotonin
    b. Antidiuretic hormone (ADH) and epinephrine
    c. Aldosterone and ADH
    d. ADH and oxytocin (Pitocin)

37. Match the clinical situations with the resulting effect leading to hypernatremia. *Answers may be used more than once.*

    Clinical Situations
    ___ a. Severe diarrhea
    ___ b. Presence of fever
    ___ c. Profound diaphoresis
    ___ d. Primary hyperaldosteronism
    ___ e. Kidney disease of the proximal tubule
    ___ f. Confused and disoriented
    ___ g. Multiple sodium bicarbonate injections
    ___ h. Severe vomiting
    ___ i. Restraints

    Resulting Effects Leading to Hypernatremia
    1. Inadequate water intake
    2. Excess fluid loss
    3. Excess sodium intake

38. The primary cause for hypernatremia relates to:
    a. Excessive sodium intake.
    b. Inadequate water intake.
    c. Excess fluid loss.
    d. Inadequate sodium intake.

39. The skin turgor assessment of a client with hypernatremia as a result of extracellular fluid loss would:
    a. Indicate a quick return to normal.
    b. Be unreliable to access.
    c. Be difficult to assess because of the edema.
    d. Last longer than 6 seconds.

40. Which of the following is the most common manifestation of a client with hypernatremia? Also provide specific assessment findings.
    a. Gastrointestinal disorders
    b. Altered urinary elimination
    c. Impaired skin integrity
    d. Altered cerebral functioning

41. The nurse identifies the client most at risk for developing hypernatremia as one who:
    a. Dislikes drinking milk and lacks calcium in the diet.
    b. Is receiving total parental nutrition related to GI surgery.
    c. Is being seen in the emergency department with excessive diarrhea and vomiting from food poisoning.
    d. Is an older adult client with decreased sensitivity to thirst.

42. The most effective way to treat mild hypernatremia as the result of water loss is to encourage clients to:
    a. Drink adequate amounts of water to prevent dehydration.
    b. Drink fluids such as those with caffeine and weigh themselves monthly.
    c. Maintain IV access of central line for fluid administration.
    d. Read the labels on canned foods to ensure plenty of sodium intake.

43. On a separate sheet of paper, compare and contrast subjective data for clients with hyponatremia and hypernatremia in a nursing assessment.

44. On a separate sheet of paper, compare and contrast objective data for clients with hyponatremia and hypernatremia in a nursing assessment.

45. As a result of hyponatremia or hypernatremia, a client is at Risk for Injury related to which of the following?
    a. Altered thought processes
    b. Spontaneous fractures
    c. Tetanic muscle contractions
    d. Painful paresthesia

46. Which of the following lab values indicates hypocalcemia?
    a. 1.5 mEq/L
    b. 2.0 mEq/L
    c. 4.5 mEq/L
    d. 9.0 mEq/L

47. Which of the following clinical conditions can result from hypocalcemia?
    a. Cardiac muscle contraction is stimulated.
    b. Intestinal and gastric motility are increased.
    c. Peripheral nerve excitability is decreased.
    d. Bone density is increased markedly.

48. Match the following clinical conditions that predispose a client to hypocalcemia with the etiologies. *Answers may be used more than once.*

Clinical Conditions	Etiologies
___ a. Alkalosis	1. Inhibited
___ b. Pancreatitis	calcium
___ c. Inadequate calcium intake	absorption
___ d. Lactase deficiencies	2. Decreased
___ e. Parathyroidectomy	ionized
___ f. Hyperphosphatemia	calcium
___ g. Decreased serum protein	3. Endocrine
___ h. Celiac disease	disorder
___ i. Orthopedic surgery	4. Other
___ j. Calcium-binding	etiology
medications	
___ k. Inadequate vitamin D intake	

49. Which of the following clients is at greatest risk of developing hypocalcemia?
    a. A 70-year-old African-American woman with long-standing celiac disease
    b. A 45-year-old Caucasian man with hypertension and diuretic therapy
    c. A 50-year-old Caucasian woman with a recent ileostomy
    d. A 70-year-old African-American man on long-term lithium therapy

50. Preventive measures for clients at risk for developing hypocalcemia include:
    a. Advising at-risk clients to increase the daily dietary calcium intake to 1000 mg.
    b. Administering calcium supplements once/day after the morning meal.
    c. Applying a sunblock and wearing protective clothing whenever outdoors.
    d. Administering calcium-containing IV fluids to clients receiving multiple blood transfusions.

51. Identify the laboratory finding that is often associated with hypocalcemia.
    a. Decreased level of serum phosphorus
    b. Increased total serum protein level
    c. Decreased arterial pH (below 7.35)
    d. Increased urinary level of potassium

52. A client is at risk for developing hypocalcemia as result of a deficiency in:
    a. Vitamin C
    b. Vitamin B_{12}
    c. Vitamin A
    d. Vitamin D

53. As a result of which of the following surgeries for an endocrine disorder is a client at risk for hypokalemia?
    a. Thyroidectomy
    b. Adrenalectomy
    c. Pancreatectomy
    d. Gastrectomy

54. A client with a parathyroidectomy is treated for hypocalcemia to prevent which of the following complications?
    a. Cardiac dysrhythmias
    b. Laryngeal spasms and respiratory arrest
    c. Esophageal reflux
    d. Renal failure

55. A typical nursing assessment finding of a client with hypocalcemia is:
    a. Paresthesias, tingling followed by numbness
    b. Shortened ST segment, tachycardia, and hypertension
    c. Constipation and hypoactive bowel sounds
    d. Severe muscle weakness

56. Which of the following medication orders should the nurse clarify before administering the medication to a client with hypocalcemia?
    a. Magnesium sulfate 1g intramuscularly (IM) every 6 hours for four doses
    b. Aluminum hydroxide (AlternaGEL) 15 mL tid PO
    c. Calcium carbonate 1000 mg pc tid ac
    d. Calcium gluconate 500 mg stat IM

57. The nurse would implement which of the following in treatment of a client with hypocalcemia?
    a. Encourage activity by the client as tolerated including weight-lifting
    b. Encourage socialization with friends and family to avoid social isolation
    c. Include a tracheostomy tray at the bedside for emergency use
    d. Provide adequate intake of vitamin D and calcium rich foods

58. Which of the following foods provides both calcium and vitamin D for the client who needs supplemental diet therapy for hypocalcemia?
    a. Eggs
    b. Cheese
    c. Milk
    d. Yogurt

59. Which of the following electrolyte imbalances is often associated with hypocalcemia as a result of chronic renal failure?
    a. Hypophosphatemia
    b. Hyperphosphatemia
    c. Hyperkalemia
    d. Hyponatremia

60. Hypercalcemia refers to a serum calcium level greater than:
    a. 4.5 mEq/L
    b. 5.5 mEq/L
    c. 8.0 mEq/L
    d. 11.0 mEq/L

61. Which of the following statements about the pathophysiology of hypercalcemia is true?
    a. Hypercalcemia has little effect on blood clotting.
    b. Hypercalcemia can lead to increased bone strength.
    c. Cardiac and nerve tissues are sensitive to various serum calcium levels.
    d. Excess ECF calcium ions increase the responses of excitable tissues.

62. Which of the following conditions can result in causing an increase in bone resorption of calcium?
    a. Dehydration
    b. Lung cancer
    c. Renal failure
    d. Excessive oral intake of vitamin D

63. What is the relationship between immobility and hypercalcemia?

64. What is the relationship between hypervitaminosis and hypercalcemia?

65. A preventive intervention for clients at risk for developing hypercalcemia is:
    a. Restricting dietary calcium by eliminating milk products.
    b. Discouraging weight-bearing activity such as walking.
    c. Monitoring the client for fluid volume excess.
    d. Administering multivitamin tablets twice per day.

66. Which of the following assessment findings is related to hypercalcemia? *Check all that apply.*
    ___ a. Bradycardia, late phase
    ___ b. Paresthesia
    ___ c. Leg cramping
    ___ d. Hyperactive bowel sounds
    ___ e. Ineffective respiratory movements
    ___ f. Decreased clotting time
    ___ g. Hypertension
    ___ h. Profound muscle weakness
    ___ i. Changes in mental status

67. Which of the following are examples of nursing interventions related to clients with hypercalcemia? *Check all that apply.*
    ___ a. Monitoring for a decreased urine output
    ___ b. Assessing the client for a positive Homan's sign
    ___ c. Measuring the abdominal girth
    ___ d. Neuromuscular assessment
    ___ e. Monitoring ECG changes for heart block
    ___ f. Assessing appetite, intake, and output
    ___ g. Monitoring for recurrence 1 to 3 days after cessation of treatment
    ___ h. During treatment, monitor for tetany

68. Treatment for hypercalcemia includes which of the following medications? *Check all that apply.*
    ___ a. Magnesium sulfate
    ___ b. Calcitonin
    ___ c. Indocin
    ___ d. Calcitriol
    ___ e. Calcium gluconate
    ___ f. Aluminum hydroxide

69. Hypercalcemia can potentiate which of the following drug toxicities?
    a. Tylenol
    b. Gentamycin
    c. Digoxin
    d. Anticonvulsants

70. A preventive intervention for the client at risk for fracture related to decreased bone density is:
    a. Encouraging independent ambulation about the room.
    b. Using a lift sheet for moving the client up in bed.
    c. Reminding the client to shift position in bed frequently.
    d. Providing an overhead trapeze to assist position changes.

71. On a separate sheet of paper, compare and contrast subjective data relating to hypocalcemia and hypercalcemia.

72. On a separate sheet of paper, compare and contrast objective data relating to hypocalcemia and hypercalcemia.

73. A positive Trousseau's or Chvostek's sign demonstrates neuromuscular irritation resulting from:
    a. Hypocalcemia.
    b. Hypercalcemia.
    c. Hyperkalemia.
    d. Hyperphosphatemia.

74. Match each of the following assessment findings for hypocalcemia with the technique and positive result for that finding.

Technique and Positive Results	Assessment Finding
___ a. Muscle twitching results when the facial nerve in front of the ear is tapped	1. Trousseau's sign 2. Chvostek's sign
___ b. Palmar flexion/contraction of the hand and fingers results upon inflation of a blood pressure cuff	

75. The immediate treatment of a client with a positive Trousseau's or Chvostek's sign is:
    a. Intravenous calcium.
    b. Calcitonin.
    c. Intravenous KCl.
    d. Large doses of oral calcium.

76. On a separate sheet of paper, discuss the responsibilities of the nurse when administering IV calcium therapy.

77. A client with congestive heart failure is receiving a loop diuretic. The nurse should monitor for which three electrolyte imbalances?
    a. _____
    b. _____
    c. _____

78. Which of the following clients would the nurse monitor for hypocalcemia, hypokalemia, and hyponatremia?
    a. Client with hypothyroidism
    b. Client with diabetes
    c. Client with chronic renal failure
    d. Client with adrenal insufficiency

79. The serum level of phosphorus exists in reciprocal balance to that of:
    a. Magnesium.
    b. Chloride.
    c. Potassium.
    d. Calcium.

80. For the parathyroid hormone to regulate phosphate metabolism, which vitamin is necessary in adequate levels?
    a. Vitamin B_{12}
    b. Vitamin C
    c. Vitamin D
    d. Vitamin K

81. Hypophosphatemia refers to which serum level of phosphorus below?
    a. 2.5 mg/dL
    b. 3.5 mg/dL
    c. 4.5 mg/dL
    d. 5.5 mg/dL

82. Match the following clinical conditions with their effects on serum phosphorus levels. *Answers are used more than once.*

Clinical Conditions	Serum Phosphorus Levels
___ a. Aggressive	1. Hyperphosphatemia
___ b. Malnutrition	2. Hypophosphatemia
___ c. Alcoholism	
___ d. Hypoparathyroidism	
___ e. Inadequate vitamin D intake	
___ f. Hypocalcemia	
___ g. Respiratory alkalosis	
___ h. Renal disease	
___ i. Hyperparathyroidism	

83. On a separate sheet of paper, indicate assessment findings for a client with hypophosphatemia.

84. Interventions for the client with hypophosphatemia include:
    a. Aggressive treatment with parenteral phosphorous.
    b. Administering oral vitamin D and phosphorus supplements.
    c. Concurrent administration of calcium supplements.
    d. Eliminating beef, pork, and legumes from the diet.

85. Which of the following clients are at risk for developing hyperphosphatemia?
    a. A client receiving radiation treatment for a large cancerous tumor
    b. A client with acute renal failure
    c. An older adult diagnosed with malnutrition
    d. A client with hyperglycemia

86. The nurse would monitor the client with hyperphosphatemia for which of the following accompanying electrolyte imbalances that potentially can cause life-threatening side effects?
    a. Hypercalcemia
    b. Hypocalcemia
    c. Hyponatremia
    d. Hyperkalemia

87. The normal range of serum magnesium levels is:
    a. 1.0 to 2.0 mEq/L.
    b. 1.5 to 2.5 mEq/L.
    c. 2.0 to 3.0 mEq/L.
    d. 2.5 to 3.5 mEq/L.

88. Indicate at least four clinical conditions that decrease intestinal absorption of magnesium causing hypomagnesemia.
    a. _____
    b. _____
    c. _____
    d. _____

89. Indicate five conditions that increase renal excretion of magnesium causing hypomagnesemia.
    a. _____
    b. _____
    c. _____
    d. _____
    e. _____

90. On a separate sheet of paper, indicate the objective data in a nursing assessment of a client with hypomagnesemia.

91. The most significant assessment finding in a client with hypomagnesemia that does *not* occur in clients with other electrolyte imbalances is:
    a. Muscle spasms in the legs.
    b. Paresthesia.
    c. Psychosis.
    d. Paralytic ileus.

92. Which of the following is *not* a clinical manifestation of hypomagnesemia that could also be an indication of hypocalcemia?
    a. Tetany
    b. Positive Trousseau's sign
    c. Positive Chvostek's sign
    d. Ventricular tachycardia

93. Which of the following is correct in treating clients with hypomagnesemia? Why are the other answers incorrect?
    a. Administer intramuscular $MgSO_4$.
    b. Encourage eating foods such as fruits.
    c. Administer oral preparations of $MgSO_4$.
    d. Discontinue diuretic therapy and administer IV $MgSO_4$.

94. The nurse monitors the effectiveness of $MgSO_4$ by hourly:
    a. Assessment of deep tendon reflexes.
    b. Assessment of vital signs.
    c. Assessment of serum lab values.
    d. Assessment of urine output.

95. On a separate sheet of paper, give the objective data that would be in the assessment of a client with hypermagnesemia.

96. A client predisposed to hypermagnesemia is taught to limit what types of foods and medications?

Case Study: The Client with a Potassium Imbalance

A male adult client is admitted for palpitations. His serum potassium level on admission is 5.3 mEq/L. Yesterday he ate two eggs, bacon, and toast for breakfast. For lunch he had a fresh fruit salad, and for dinner he ate baked halibut, baked potatoes, a salad, and green beans. He usually has a cola drink and salted peanuts for a snack. He uses a salt substitute regularly.

Answer the following questions on a separate sheet of paper:

1. Identify the foods in his diet that may be contributing to his hyperkalemia.

2. Which ECG changes would be typical for a client such as this?

3. Formulate relevant nursing diagnoses for this client based on the above data. This client states that he has had abdominal cramping and several very loose diarrhea stools since yesterday. The physician orders a sodium polystyrene sulfonate (Kayexalate) retention enema to be given stat.

4. Discuss the etiology of the client's symptoms.

5. Explain whether the nurse should clarify the physician's order before administering the enema.

6. The client is unable to retain the enema. What interventions should the nurse initiate to assist him in retaining the solution?

7. Eventually this client recovers and is scheduled for discharge. Develop a teaching-learning plan for him including information about his diet, self-monitoring of his pulse, and the need for regular follow-up care.

 ## Case Study: The Client with Sodium Imbalance

The nurse is caring for an 81-year-old man who is admitted after a 3-day period of weakness. A stroke is suspected because he has right-sided weakness and difficulty speaking. He appears dehydrated, with a skin turgor of 5 seconds and a urine specific gravity of 1.028.

Answer the following questions on a separate sheet of paper:

1. Discuss whether this client's serum sodium would be elevated, decreased, or normal.

2. Develop a specific assessment plan for this client.

3. The client is filling out his menu for the next day. Because he is somewhat confused, the nurse reviews his food choices. Which foods would not be advisable for the client? Which foods should be encouraged?

4. This client will be discharged to home care. Develop a teaching plan for him focusing on diet and safety.

STUDY GUIDE NUMBER 3.14

Infusion Therapy

Study/Review Questions

1. The following questions are related to filters on an infusion administration set. Write your answers on a separate sheet of paper.
   a. What is the purpose of a filter?
   b. Briefly discuss the types of filters, how to select the proper filter, and their uses.

2. Match each of the following definitions with the type of pump being described.
   ___ a. Volumetric or   1. Controller

   Definitions   **Types of Pumps**
   ___ a. A device with a   1. Ambulatory pump
         plunger that is used 2. Syringe pump
         for small volume   3. Cassette pump
         infusions   4. Implantable pump
   ___ b. Placed in a blood
         vessel to deliver
         medication directly
         into an organ
   ___ c. Used most often for home care clients,
         allowing them to return to their usual
         activities while receiving infusions
   ___ d. Uses a dedicated set that includes a
         pumping chamber of exact volume

3. Match the following characteristics with either a pump or a controller infusion device.

   Characteristic   **Device**
   ___ a. Volumetric or   1. Controller
         nonvolumetric   2. Pump
         device   3. Both controller
   ___ b. Pole-mounted only   and pump
   ___ c. Pole-mounted or
         implantable
   ___ d. Best for accurate infusion
   ___ e. Counts drops to regulate flow
   ___ f. Multiple types are available

4. On a separate sheet of paper, identify the main differences between volumetric and nonvolumetric pumps and controllers.

5. Which of the following central venous catheters requires a special needle for use?
   a. Broviac catheter
   b. Groshong catheter
   c. Hickman catheter
   d. MediPort vascular access device

6. Identify four reasons why clients receive intravenous (IV) therapy.
   a. _____
   b. _____
   c. _____
   d. _____

7. When initiating IV therapy for a client, which of the following items is *not* selected by the nurse?
   a. Tubing and filter
   b. Type of fluid
   c. Administration device
   d. Size and type of insertion device

8. On a separate sheet of paper, identify and describe the purpose of each component of an IV administration set.

9. When a client has an IV, what does a nurse assess to safely maintain the IV infusion?

10. Identify special considerations to follow when initiating or maintaining peripheral IV therapy for the older adult.

11. Match the name of each central intravenous catheter listed below with its type of catheter. *Answers can be used more than once.*

    Central Venous
    Catheter   **Type of Catheter**
    ___ a. Broviac   1. Tunneled catheter
    ___ b. Peripherally   2. Nontunneled
          inserted catheter
          central catheter
          (PICC)
    ___ c. Hickman
    ___ d. Groshong

12. On a separate sheet of paper, briefly explain the difference between an implanted port and a central venous catheter.

13. Which of the following is *not* a recommended nursing intervention when inserting a peripheral venous access device?
    a. Either an upper or lower extremity for the insertion site.
    b. Use the client's nondominant hand.
    c. Do not use the arm in which special procedures have been performed.
    d. Avoid placing an IV over a joint.

14. Which of the following clients could have an intra-arterial line? Explain why on a separate sheet of paper. *Check all that apply.*
    ___ a. A client receiving total parental nutrition
    ___ b. A client receiving blood and blood products
    ___ c. A client receiving chemotherapy
    ___ d. A client receiving medications for diagnostic tests

Answer Questions 15 through 23 on a separate sheet of paper.

15. Identify responsibilities the nurse has when caring for a client receiving intraarterial infusion.

16. What is the primary reason a client would receive intraperitoneal therapy?

17. Identify the complications of intraperitoneal therapy.

18. Identify the types of clients who might be candidates for continuous subcutaneous infusion.

19. A client who has cancer and is dying requires pain medication but is not able to swallow. Hypodermoclysis has been chosen as the infusion method to deliver the pain medication. Is this an appropriate method for this client? Explain why. Determine the responsibilities of the nurse caring for this client.

20. Answer the following questions concerning a client with a total knee replacement who is admitted to a general surgery floor with an epidural catheter for delivering pain medication.
    a. Briefly explain this method of pain medication delivery.
    b. What are the responsibilities of the nurse caring for a client with an epidural catheter?
    c. Identify medication-related complications for which the nurse assesses for clients receiving epidural pain medications.

21. Explain the difference between an epidural catheter and intrathecal therapy.

22. A client's IV site is very edematous, the pump continues to infuse fluids, and the client is complaining of burning at the site.
    a. Which of the following complications do these assessment findings indicate? Give a rationale for your answer.
       (1) Hematoma
       (2) Phlebitis
       (3) Infiltration
       (4) Infection
    b. Based on your conclusion as to the type of complication, what nursing intervention would be implemented?

23. A 65-year-old client has been receiving IV fluids at 150 mL/hr of D5 ½% NS for the past 3 days. Your assessment findings indicate crackles in both lower lobes with shortness of breath. Blood pressure is 150/96.
    a. What complication do these assessment findings indicate? Provide a rationale for your answer.
       (1) Infection in the blood
       (2) Anaphylactic shock
       (3) Speed shock
       (4) Circulatory overload
    b. Based on your conclusion as to the type of complication, what nursing interventions would be implemented?

24. A client having a central line inserted in the vena cava is at high risk for which of the following complications during this procedure?
    a. Pneumothorax
    b. Air embolism
    c. Circulatory overload
    d. Hydrothorax

25. The nurse is assisting a physician inserting a central line when the client develops chest pain and shortness of breath with decreased breath sounds and restlessness. The nurse would do which of the following?
    a. Tell the client to, "Relax, the procedure will soon be over."
    b. Administer pain medication to minimize the pain of insertion.
    c. Administer oxygen and assist with insertion of a chest tube.
    d. Monitor ongoing pulse oximetry and the client for respiratory changes.

26. Immediately after a triple lumen catheter central line is inserted, the nurse would:
    a. Start IV fluids but at a slower rate to prevent any fluid overload.
    b. Watch and wait for any complications before using the site.
    c. Get a portable chest x-ray as ordered and hold IV fluids until after results are obtained.
    d. Assess vital signs and perform a complete assessment and, if client is stable, start IV fluids.

27. After a tubing change to the central line, the line was later found to be disconnected from the catheter. The client develops chest pain, restlessness, HR 120, BP drops to 90/40, and pulse oximetry is 89%. The nurse performs which of the following interventions?
    a. Place client in Trendelenburg position on the left side, clamp the catheter, and notify the physician.
    b. Assess for patency of catheter and change the tubing and resume IV fluids.
    c. Notify physician, remove the central line, apply pressure, and place the client in a semi-Fowler's position.
    d. Notify physician and administer urokinase to declot the catheter.

28. Which of the following nursing interventions is key to preventing an infection in a client with a central line?
    a. Administer antibiotics for at least a week in a timely manner.
    b. Use aseptic technique during dressing changes, administering medications, and tubing changes.
    c. Change the catheter every 72 hours and tubing every 24 hours.
    d. Monitor the temperature for any elevation and give Tylenol as needed.

29. Review other complications of central and peripheral lines in Tables 14-3 and 14-4. Differentiate assessment findings and nursing interventions for each complication. Show your answer to your clinical instructor.

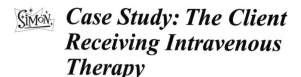

Case Study: The Client Receiving Intravenous Therapy

Your client is an older adult resident at a skilled nursing facility. She is receiving IV antibiotics and fluids for pneumonia via a peripheral site. She complains that her arm is hurting where she is receiving the IV, especially when the antibiotic is given.

Answer the following questions on a separate sheet of paper:

1. What would be the nurse's best action at this time?

2. What possible complications may explain her discomfort?

3. What interventions may prevent this problem in the future?

STUDY GUIDE NUMBER 3.15

Acid-Base Balance

Study/Review Questions

1. Which of the following statements regarding acid-base balance are true?
   a. Acid-base balance is mainly a function of cellular metabolism.
   b. pH is equal to the logarithm of hydrogen ion concentration.
   c. Arterial blood pH is slightly more acid than venous blood.
   d. Hydrogen ion reflects acid production and elimination.

2. Identify four ways that the hydrogen ion is produced by the body:
   a. _____
   b. _____
   c. _____
   d. _____

3. Match the following terms with their associated functions and substances.

   Associated Statements   **Terms**
   ___ a. Accepts hydrogen ion   1. Acid
   ___ b. Donates hydrogen ion   2. Base
   ___ c. Formed in the body as a   3. Buffer
          result of metabolism   4. pH
   ___ d. Regulates hydrogen ion
          and bicarbonate
   ___ e. Reflective of hydrogen ion concentration
   ___ f. $H_2CO_3^-$
   ___ g. Increases as the amount of base increases
   ___ h. HCO_3^-
   ___ i. Hemoglobin

4. A pH of 7.40 in the body reflects a ratio of bicarbonate to carbonic acid as:
   a. 50:50.
   b. 1:1.
   c. 1:20.
   d. 20:1.

5. Draw the direction of the carbonic anhydrase equation when excess carbon dioxide is produced.

6. Under the following conditions, what will happen to the plasma pH?
   a. Increase in CO_2
   b. Decrease in HCO_3^-
   c. Increase in lactic acid
   d. Increase in HCO_3^-
   e. Decrease in CO_2

7. Identify the sources of bicarbonate ions:
   a. _____
   b. _____
   c. _____
   d. _____

8. The immediate binding of excess $H^($ ions would primarily occur in the:
   a. Red blood cell.
   b. Renal tubule.
   c. Pulmonary capillary.
   d. Capillary micro-bed.

9. Match the buffer system with the statements.

   Statements   **Buffer Systems**
   ___ a. Chemoreceptor response   1. Chemical
          to increase in CO_2 2. Respiratory
   ___ b. Secretion of hydrogen   3. Renal
          ions to form H_2PO_4 4. Protein
   ___ c. Regenerates HCO_3^-
   ___ d. Binds H^+ with HCO_3^-
   ___ e. Binds H^+ with hemoglobin
   ___ f. Response occurs within minutes

10. Which of the following may occur as a result of acid-base imbalance?
    a. Paralytic ileus
    b. Hypertension
    c. Oliguria
    d. Cyanosis

11. Which buffer system will respond to acid-base imbalances most likely to occur from a metabolic origin?

12. Which of the following statements is true regarding compensation?
    a. The lungs compensate for acid-base imbalances of respiratory origin.
    b. Renal compensation is the most powerful and rapid.
    c. Compensation occurs as the body attempts to maintain a pH of 7.40.
    d. Compensation is the result of carbonic acid elimination.

13. Hypoxemia is most likely to result in:
    a. Ketoacidosis.
    b. Lactic acidosis.
    c. Hypochloremic metabolic alkalosis.
    d. Septicemia.

14. Determine whether the following values would indicate an acid or alkaline condition.
    a. CO_2 = 66 mm Hg   _____
    b. $HCO_3^{(}$ = 16 mEq/L   _____
    c. pH = 7.55   _____
    d. Lactate = 3.0 mmol/L _____

15. Identify the physiologic changes that occur in the lungs with aging that contribute to the older adult's risk for acid-base imbalances.
    a. _____
    b. _____
    c. _____

16. Identify the physiologic changes that occur in the kidneys with aging that contribute to the older adult's risk for acid-base imbalances.
    a. _____
    b. _____

17. Which of the following medications increases the older adult client's risk for acid-base imbalances?
    a. Carbamazepine (Tegretol)
    b. Conjugated estrogen (Premarin)
    c. Furosemide (Lasix)
    d. Metoclopramide (Reglan)

18. The serum pH value is:
    a. Directly related to the concentration of carbon dioxide.
    b. Directly related to the concentration of hydrogen ion.
    c. Inversely related to the concentration of hydrogen ion.
    d. Inversely related to the concentration of bicarbonate.

19. Which of the following is correct about pH?
    a. A solution with a pH of 6.5 is a weak base and has more hydrogen ions than a solution with a pH of 6.9.
    b. A solution with a pH of 7.0 is neutral and has fewer hydrogen ions than a solution with a pH of 6.8.
    c. A solution with a pH of 7.5 is a weak acid and has fewer hydrogen ions than a solution with a pH of 7.8.
    d. A solution with a pH of 8.7 is a strong base and has more hydrogen ions than a solution with a pH of 8.5.

20. Which of the following processes might be responsible for an increase in pH?
    a. Hypoventilation
    b. Ketoacidosis
    c. Nasogastric suction
    d. Diarrhea

21. Which of the following processes might be responsible for a decrease in HCO_3^-?
    a. Ketoacidosis
    b. Hypoventilation
    c. Vomiting
    d. Emphysema

22. A CO_2 of 55 mm Hg will most likely result in:
    a. A pH of 7.45.
    b. O_2 of 60 mm Hg.
    c. A pH of 7.55.
    d. HCO_3^- of 34 mEq/L.

23. Bicarbonate regeneration occurs primarily as a result of:
    a. Respiratory elimination of acid.
    b. Albumin binding with hydrogen ion.
    c. Renal reabsorption.
    d. Intracellular uptake of hydrogen ion.

24. In assessing a 75-year-old man, which of the following should alert the nurse to a potential acid condition?
    a. Twice daily furosemide use
    b. Jugular venous distension
    c. Serum creatinine of 3.4 mg/dL
    d. Bicarbonate of 26 mEq/L

25. Which of the following is a major extracellular fluid (ECF) buffer?
    a. Carbon dioxide
    b. Bicarbonate
    c. Ammonium
    d. Phosphate

26. The acid released by the lungs to regulate pH is:
    a. Bicarbonate.
    b. Phosphate.
    c. Hydrogen.
    d. Carbon dioxide.

27. Which of the following statements about the neural regulatory control of acid-base balance is correct?
    a. Baroreceptors in the ECF are sensitive to bicarbonate.
    b. Chemoreceptors in the ECF are sensitive to carbon dioxide.
    c. Chemoreceptors in the brain are sensitive to carbon dioxide.
    d. Baroreceptors in the brain are sensitive to bicarbonate.

28. When the respiratory rate slows, pH:
    a. Increases.
    b. Decreases.
    c. Is unchanged.
    d. Fluctuates.

29. The kidney regulates pH by controlling:
    a. Urea.
    b. Bicarbonate.
    c. Carbon dioxide.
    d. Hemoglobin.

30. Which of the following statements about the role of chemical buffers in regulating acid-base balance is correct?
    a. They are able to correct the imbalance permanently.
    b. They are present in the body fluids and act immediately.
    c. They constitute the largest store of buffers in the body.
    d. They can correct the underlying problems that lead to the imbalance.

31. Identify, in order of sequence, the three regulatory mechanisms that the body uses to control acid-base balance.
    a. _____
    b. _____
    c. _____

32. Ammonia, a normal by-product of protein metabolism, is converted to ammonium in the kidney by the addition of:
    a. Urea.
    b. Nitrogen.
    c. Hydrogen.
    d. Phosphate.

33. On a separate sheet of paper, describe a situation in which the renal system is used to compensate for acid-base imbalance.

34. On a separate sheet of paper, describe a situation in which the respiratory system is used to compensate for acid-base imbalances.

35. On a separate sheet of paper, briefly describe full compensation and partial compensation.

36. Identify four changes in the body that would occur if the pH was *not* closely regulated.
    a. _____
    b. _____
    c. _____
    d. _____

37. Which of the following blood pH values is within normal limits?
    a. 7.27
    b. 7.37
    c. 7.47
    d. 7.5

STUDY GUIDE NUMBER 3.16

Interventions for Clients with Acid-Base Imbalances

Study/Review Questions

1. Which of the following would cause acidosis resulting from excess production of hydrogen ion?
   a. Renal failure
   b. Emphysema
   c. Seizures
   d. Diarrhea

2. Which of the following statements regarding acidosis is true?
   a. Acidosis may result from a base deficit.
   b. Acidosis always occurs when excess hydrogen ion is produced.
   c. Acidosis is reflected by HCO_3^-.
   d. Acidosis results in an increased ratio of HCO_3^- to $H_2CO_3^-$.

3. Match the following etiologies of metabolic acidosis to the resulting state of pathophysiology.

Pathophysiology State	Etiology of Metabolic Acidosis
___ a. Anaerobic metabolism	1. ↑Hydrogen ion production
___ b. Renal failure	2. ↓Hydrogen ion elimination
___ c. Diarrhea	3. ↑Base elimination
___ d. Seizures	4. ↓Base production
___ e. Pancreatic insufficiency	

4. Respiratory acidosis occurs as a result of:
   a. Hyperventilation.
   b. Hypoventilation.
   c. Renal reabsorption of bicarbonate.
   d. Renal secretion of hydrogen ion.

5. Match the pathophysiologic causes of respiratory failure with the associated conditions.

Pathophysiology	Associated Conditions
___ a. Asthma	1. Respiratory depression
___ b. Guillain-Barré syndrome	2. Inadequate chest expansion
___ c. Morphine infusion	3. Airway obstruction
___ d. Pulmonary embolus	4. Altered alveolar capillary diffusion
___ e. Chronic bronchitis	
___ f. Ascites	
___ g. Cerebral vascular accident	
___ h. Flail chest	
___ i. Pneumothorax	
___ j. Hyperkalemia	
___ k. Pneumonia	

6. Which of the following laboratory values would indicate that a client was acidotic?
   a. Pa_{CO_2} = 55 mm Hg
   b. HCO_3^- = 25 mEq/L
   c. Lactate +2.5 mmol/L
   d. pH = 7.30

7. Identify four common medications that may be administered to decrease bronchial constriction.
   a. _____
   b. _____
   c. _____
   d. _____

8. Which of the following nursing assessment findings would indicate a worsening of the respiratory acidosis?
   a. Decreased respiratory rate
   b. Decreased blood pressure
   c. Use of accessory respiratory muscles
   d. Pale nail beds

9. State whether each of the following signs and symptoms would be seen in metabolic acidosis or respiratory acidosis.
   a. Kussmaul respirations
   b. Warm, flushed skin
   c. Hypertension
   d. Hypercapnia
   e. Decreased bicarbonate

10. Which of the following statements made by a client might indicate that he has an alkaline condition?
    a. "I am increasingly tired and can't concentrate."
    b. "I have tingling in my fingers and toes."
    c. "My feet and ankles are swollen."
    d. "I am short of breath all of the time."

11. The most important intervention for a client with ketoacidosis is to:
    a. Administer bicarbonate.
    b. Give furosemide.
    c. Administer insulin.
    d. Administer potassium.

12. Which of the following is likely to result in metabolic alkalosis as a result of base excess?
    a. Thiazide diuretics
    b. Nasogastric suction
    c. Vomiting
    d. Blood transfusions

13. Respiratory alkalosis is likely to occur as a result of:
    a. Lactic acidosis.
    b. Diarrhea.
    c. Hypoxemia.
    d. Antacid administration.

14. Metabolic alkalosis may result in which electrolyte imbalance?
    a. Hyperkalemia
    b. Hypophosphatemia
    c. Hyperchloremia
    d. Hypocalcemia

15. Tall peaked T waves on an ECG of a client who has metabolic acidosis is most likely the result of:
    a. An increase in ionized calcium.
    b. A shift of glucose from the ECF to the ICF.
    c. A shift of potassium from the ICF to the ECF.
    d. A decrease in serum magnesium.

16. A nursing intervention to correct metabolic alkalosis would include:
    a. Maintenance of fluid restriction.
    b. Administration of potassium.
    c. Administration of antiemetics.
    d. Oxygen administration.

17. Match each statement with its associated acid-base condition. *Answers may be used more than once.*

Statements	Acid-Base Condition
___ a. May occur as a result of anxiety	1. Respiratory acidosis
___ b. Results in hyperkalemia	2. Metabolis acidosis
___ c. Caused by hypoventilation	3. Respiratory alkalosis
___ d. May be a result of hypovolemia	4. Metabolic alkalosis
___ e. May be caused by diarrhea	
___ f. Associated with Kussmaul respiration	
___ g. Associated with ingestion of antacids	
___ h. Results in hypocalcemia	
___ i. Compensation occurs through renal reabsorption of bicarbonate	
___ j. Compensation occurs through hyperventilation	
___ k. Compensation occurs through hypoventilation	

18. Identify and describe two types of actions that lead to acid-base imbalances.
    a. _____
    b. _____

19. Describe the difference between acidosis and acidemia.

20. Describe the difference between alkalosis and alkalemia.

State whether the following arterial blood gases reflect metabolic acidosis, respiratory acidosis, metabolic alkalosis, or respiratory alkalosis. Determine which values indicate partial or complete compensation, and give a condition that may cause the abnormality.

21. pH 7.35, $Paco_2$ 66, HCO_3 38

22. pH 7.52, $Paco_2$ 45, HCO_3 36

23. pH 7.55, $Paco_2$ 24, HCO_3 20

24. pH 7.28, $Paco_2$ 24, HCO_3 15

25. pH 7.35, $Paco_2$ 24, HCO_3 15

26. pH 7.45, $Paco_2$ 50, HCO_3 42

27. Identify the three major causes of acidemia and alkalemia.

28. Which of the following electrolyte balances is likely to be disrupted in acidemia?
    a. Sodium
    b. Potassium
    c. Chloride
    d. Calcium

29. The cause of respiratory acidosis is:
    a. Overexcretion of hydrogen and bicarbonate ions from the kidney.
    b. Underelimination of carbon dioxide from the lungs.
    c. Overelimination of carbon dioxide from the lungs.
    d. Underelimination of metabolic waste products from the GI tract.

30. Inadequate chest expansion, which leads to respiratory acidosis, is most likely to be caused by:
    a. Lordosis.
    b. Emphysema.
    c. Prolonged bedrest.
    d. First-trimester pregnancy.

31. Interference with alveolar-capillary diffusion results in:
    a. Carbon dioxide retention and acidemia.
    b. Hydrogen ion elimination and acidemia.
    c. Hydrogen depletion from water vapor loss.
    d. Aerobic metabolism and lactic acid build-up.

32. One cause of metabolic acidosis is:
    a. Aspirin poisoning.
    b. Overuse of antacids.
    c. Prolonged diarrhea.
    d. Potassium-sparing diuretics.

33. Arterial Po_2:
    a. Decreases in respiratory acidosis and alkalosis.
    b. Increases in metabolic acidosis and alkalosis.
    c. Increases in respiratory and combined acidosis.
    d. Is unchanged in all conditions of alkalosis.

34. The hallmark of metabolic acidosis is:
    a. Increased bicarbonate and normal carbon dioxide levels.
    b. Decreased bicarbonate and normal carbon dioxide levels.
    c. Increased bicarbonate and carbon dioxide levels.
    d. Decreased bicarbonate and carbon dioxide levels.

35. The hallmark of chronic respiratory acidosis is:
    a. Elevated bicarbonate and increased arterial Pco_2 levels.
    b. Elevated bicarbonate and normal arterial Pco_2 levels.
    c. Decreased bicarbonate and normal arterial Pco_2 levels.
    d. Decreased bicarbonate and increased arterial Pco_2 levels.

36. The hallmark of metabolic alkalosis is:
    a. Increased bicarbonate and normal arterial Pco_2 levels.
    b. Increased bicarbonate and rising arterial Pco_2 levels.
    c. Increased bicarbonate and decreased arterial Pco_2 levels.
    d. Decreased bicarbonate and falling arterial Pco_2 levels.

37. The hallmark of respiratory alkalosis includes:
    a. Decreased bicarbonate and arterial Pco_2 levels.
    b. Increased bicarbonate and arterial Pco_2 levels.
    c. Decreased bicarbonate and normal arterial Pco_2 levels.
    d. Decreased bicarbonate and increased arterial $Paco_2$ levels.

38. The most effective way to administer oxygen to a client with chronic respiratory acidosis is by:
    a. High-volume intermittent positive pressure.
    b. Low-flow oxygen (2 L/min) via nasal cannula.
    c. High-flow 40% oxygen via face mask.
    d. Hyperbaric pressure chamber.

39. Which of the following assessments indicates that a client with chronic respiratory acidosis is responding favorably to treatment?
    a. Nail beds pale, extremities cool
    b. Respiratory stridor with inspiration
    c. Expectorating clear, stringy mucus
    d. Diffuse crackles auscultated bilaterally

40. The diet of a client with chronic respiratory acidosis should include:
    a. Milk products.
    b. Raw fruits and vegetables.
    c. Chicken noodle soup (low-sodium).
    d. Carbonated soft drinks and juices.

41. Discharge instructions for the client with chronic respiratory acidosis should include:
    a. Discussing how to plan for periods of increased activity.
    b. Teaching about low-protein, low-carbohydrate diet.
    c. Demonstrating exercises to increase vital capacity.
    d. Encouraging participation in activities such as jogging.

42. Interventions for the client with metabolic alkalosis include:
    a. IV infusion of lactated Ringer's solution.
    b. Administration of bolus IV calcium gluconate.
    c. Side rails padded and kept in the "up" position.
    d. Allowance for visitors after visiting hours.

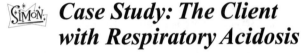

Case Study: The Client with Respiratory Acidosis

Your client is a 75-year-old man with a history of chronic bronchitis. He is admitted to the hospital with pneumonia.

Answer the following questions concerning this client:

1. Which of the following assessments would indicate that this client has impaired gas exchange?
    a. Decreased urine output
    b. Lethargy
    c. Decreased chest excursion
    d. Hypotension

2. Which of the following arterial blood gas values indicates that this client is a CO_2 retainer?
    a. $Paco_2 = 60$ mm Hg
    b. $HCO_3^- = 42$
    c. $Pao_2 = 60$ mm Hg
    d. pH $= 7.35$

3. The client's baseline arterial blood gases are: pH 7.36; $Paco_2$ 60 mm Hg, Pao_2 52 mm Hg, HCO_3^- 42 mEq/L. Which of the following would most likely indicate that he is having a negative response to the administration of oxygen?
    a. pH 7.35; $Paco_2$ 64, Pao_2 60, HCO_3^- 42 mEq/L
    b. pH 7.36, $Paco_2$ 60, Pao_2 60, HCO_3^- 42 mEq/L
    c. pH 7.36, $Paco_2$ 60, Pao_2 58, HCO_3^- 38 mEq/L
    d. pH 7.33, $Paco_2$ 66, Pao_2 66, HCO_3^- 42 mEq/L

Case Study: The Client with Metabolic Acidosis

A 65-year-old woman with a recent history of cellulitis is admitted to the hospital with fever, shortness of breath, and hypotension. Her ABG reveals a pH of 7.30, $Paco_2$ of 28, Pao_2 of 88, HCO_3^- of 18 mEq/L.

Answer the following questions concerning this client:

1. This client's symptoms are most likely a result of:
   a. Metabolic acidosis.
   b. Respiratory alkalosis.
   c. Metabolic alkalosis.
   d. Respiratory alkalosis.

2. The $Paco_2$ of 24 is the result of:
   a. Respiratory hypoventilation.
   b. Renal elimination of bicarbonate.
   c. Respiratory compensation.
   d. Renal reabsorption of hydrogen.

3. Which of the following symptoms would indicate a worsening acidotic condition?
   a. Increased blood pressure
   b. Anxiety
   c. Rising $Paco_2$
   d. Increased urinary output

4. Which of the following interventions would be critical in reversing this client's condition?
   a. Administration of antibiotics
   b. Administration of oxygen
   c. Administration of diuretics
   d. Administration of potassium

UNIT 4 MANAGEMENT OF PERIOPERATIVE CLIENTS ■ Core Concepts Grid

Anatomy	Physiology	Pathophysiology	History	Physical Exam	Diagnostic Tests	Interventions	Pharmacology
			• **Age** • **Previous medical history** • **Tobacco** • **Usual medications** • **Previous surgeries** • **Complications of surgeries** • **Autologous blood donation** • **Support** • **Advance directions**	• **Vital signs** • **Breath sounds** • **Nutritional status** • **Exposure to infection** • **Cardiovascular system** • **Renal/urinary system** • **Neurologic system** • **Musculoskeletal system**	• **Routine urinalysis** • **Complete blood count** • **Blood urea nitrogen** • **Creatinine** • **Coagulation studies** • **Electrolyte studies** • **Electrocardiogram**	• **Preoperative** Surgical consent Pulmonary toilet Excises to facilitate venous return Pain management Tubes Drains Dressings Intravenous fluids Skin preparation • **Intraoperative** Surgical team Nursing roles Holding area Positioning Anesthesia Complications Skin closures • **Postoperative** PACU assessment Return to unit Assessment Wound care Complications Infection Pulmonary embolism Deep vein thrombosis Paralytic ileus Dehiscence/Evisceration Fluid management Tubes/drains Dressings Respiratory care Pain management Health teaching	• **Anesthetic agents** Intravenous Inhaled Spinal Local or regional • **Adjunct drugs** Hypnotics Opioids Blocking agents

Unit 4 (Chapters 17-19)

Management of Perioperative Clients

Learning Plan

Chapter 17: *Interventions for Preoperative Clients*

Learning Outcomes	Learning Activities	Supplemental Resources
1. Assume the role of client advocate. **2.** Describe the legal implications and proper procedures for obtaining informed consent. **3.** Prioritize teaching needs for the client preparing for surgery. 4. Recognize client conditions or issues that need to be communicated to the surgical and postoperative teams.	1. Prior to completing the study guide exercises for this chapter, it is recommended to review the following: • Principles of teaching and learning in client care • Normal laboratory values • Normal ranges for vital sign measurements 2. Review the **boldfaced** words and their definitions in Chapter 17 to enhance your understanding of the content. 3. Go to Study Guide Number 4.17 on the following pages and complete the learning exercises for this chapter.	1. Textbook—Chapter 17 2. Other resources: • Baker, B., et al. (1999). Ambulatory surgical clinical pathway. *Journal of PeriAnesthesia Nursing, 14*(1), 2-11. • Visit a local hospital and discuss recommended practices with an operating room nurse. • Visit a surgical outpatient office and discuss patient outcomes and use of anesthesia in this setting.

Chapter 18: *Interventions for Intraoperative Clients*

Learning Outcomes	Learning Activities	Supplemental Resources
1. Discuss nursing interventions to reduce client and family anxiety. 2. Describe the roles and responsibilities of various intraoperative personnel. 3. Apply appropriate interventions to ensure the client's safety during an operative procedure. 4. Identify nursing responsibilities for management of clients receiving anesthesia. 5. Recognize the clinical manifestations of malignant hyperthermia. 6. Apply appropriate interventions for the client experiencing malignant hyperthermia. 7. Discuss the potential adverse reactions and complications of specific agents. 8. Assess clients for specific problems related to positioning during surgical procedures.	1. Prior to completing the study guide exercises for this chapter, it is recommended to review the following: • Principles of sterile technique • Principles of skin care • Normal ranges for vital sign measurements • Normal laboratory values 2. Review the **boldfaced** words and their definitions in Chapter 18 to enhance your understanding of the content.	1. Textbook—Chapter 18 2. Other resources: • Contact a nurse anesthetist and discuss this expanded nursing role in the operating room arena. • Gallo, S. (1999). Surgery in the twenty-first century. *Surgical Services Management, 5*(12), 18-21. • Visit a local hospital and discuss PACU units and evaluate how patients are monitored in this area.

3. Go to Study Guide Number 4.18 on the following pages and complete the learning exercises for this chapter.

Chapter 19: *Interventions for Postoperative Clients*

Learning Activities	Supplemental Resources
1. Prior to completing the study guide exercises for this chapter, it is recommended to review the following: • Assessment and care of the client having pain • The principles of fluid and balance • Principles of sterile technique • Principles of skin care • Normal ranges for vital sign measurements • Normal laboratory values • Principles of teaching and learning in client care 2. Review the **boldfaced** words and their definitions in Chapter 19 to enhance your understanding of the content. 3. Go to Study Guide Number 4.19 on the following pages and complete the learning exercises for this chapter.	1. Textbook—Chapter 19 2. Other resources: • Brenner, Z. (1999). Presenting postoperative complications: What's old what is new, what's tried and true. *Nursing 99, 29*(10), 34-40. • Contact a surgical center in your area and investigate types of surgeries performed, management of postoperative patients, and discharge practices for clients utilizing the center. • Jacobs, V. (2000). Informational needs of surgical patients following discharge. *Applied Nursing Research, 13*(1), 12-18. • Nazarko, L. (1999). Paying the price of early discharge. *Nursing Times, 95*(12), 51-52.

Learning Outcomes

1. Describe the ongoing head-to-toe assessment of the postoperative client.
2. Recognize wound complications in the postoperative period.
3. Prioritize common nursing interventions for the client recovering from surgery and anesthesia during the first 24 hours.
4. Prioritize nursing care for the client experiencing postoperative respiratory depression.
5. Discuss the criteria for determining readiness of the postoperative client to be discharged from the postanesthesia care unit.
6. Discuss teaching priorities for postoperative clients.

Interventions for Preoperative Clients

Study/Review Questions

1. Which of the following statements best describes the preoperative period?
   a. The preoperative period begins when the client makes the appointment with the surgeon to discuss the need for surgery.
   b. The preoperative period is the time during which the client receives education and testing related to the impending surgery.
   c. The preoperative period is a time during which the client's need for surgery is established.
   d. The preoperative period begins when the client is scheduled for surgery and ends at the time of transfer to the surgical suite.

2. Which of the following is *not* a category for surgical procedures?
   a. Reason for the surgery
   b. Hospital where the surgery is performed and the urgency of the procedure
   c. Degree of risk and extent of surgery required
   d. Anatomic location

3. The nurse screens the preoperative client for conditions that may increase the risk for complications during the perioperative period. Which of the following conditions are possible risk factors?
   a. The client is 70 years old and obese.
   b. The surgical procedure planned is a bunionectomy.
   c. The client is 5 feet tall and weighs 100 pounds.
   d. The surgery is planned as an ambulatory/same day surgery procedure.

4. Which of the following is *not* a correct rationale for asking specific questions about a client's history?
   a. The client's age must be known so that the risk of postoperative complications can be determined.
   b. The use of tobacco products is assessed because more anesthetic may be needed for clients who smoke.
   c. Medications or herbs routinely used are assessed because drug-drug interactions may occur.
   d. Previous surgeries are assessed because clients having had previous surgery will require very little preoperative teaching.

For Questions 5 to 10, read the following statements regarding preoperative care and decide whether each is true or false. Write T for true or F for false in the blanks provided. If the statement is false, correct the statement to make it true.

____ 5. The nurse functions as the client advocate by reporting to the physician and anesthesiology personnel any abnormalities found on the physical assessment.

____ 6. Throughout the physical assessment, the nurse focuses on the problem areas identified from the client's history that are limited to body systems affected directly by the surgical procedure.

____ 7. In the preoperative setting, the nurse is functioning as a client advocate when the client's home environment, self-care capabilities, and support systems are assessed and used in the discharge planning process.

____ 8. As a client advocate, the nurse can provide the client with educational materials appropriate to the client's ability to learn.

____ 9. The nurse has an awareness of factors that can influence coping and will use this knowledge when providing preoperative care.

____ 10. When the nurse evaluates preoperative laboratory test values, only abnormal values related to the surgery need to be reported to the physician and anesthesiology personnel.

11. When the nurse reports any abnormalities found on the physical assessment, this demonstrates the role of the client advocate and is exercising _____ _____.

12. The preoperative diagnostic assessment may include a variety of tests. On a separate sheet of paper, list the most common tests.

13. When a client has given consent for a surgical procedure, this indicates that:
    a. Information necessary to understand the nature of and reason for the surgery has been provided.
    b. Information about length of stay in the hospital has been preapproved by the managed care provider.
    c. Information about the surgeon's experience has been provided.
    d. The client has read all preoperative materials presented in the surgeon's office.

14. An informed consent is obtained by the nurse in the holding area after the preoperative nurse:
    a. Has explained the risks of the surgical procedure and its potential options.
    b. Has explained the risks associated with the administration of anesthesia.
    c. Has obtained the preoperative, diagnostic study results.
    d. None of the above

15. Which answer best describes the collaborative roles of the nurse and surgeon when obtaining the informed consent?
    a. The nurse is responsible for having the informed consent form on the chart for the physician to witness.
    b. The nurse may serve as a witness that the client has been informed by the physician before surgery is performed.
    c. The nurse may serve as witness to the client's signature after the physician has the consent form signed before preoperative sedation is given and before surgery is performed.
    d. The nurse has no duties regarding the consent form if the client has signed the informed consent form for the physician, even if the client then asks additional questions about the surgery.

Case Study: The Preoperative Client

Your client is a 42-year-old woman who is scheduled for a total hysterectomy under general anesthesia this morning. She is admitted to the preoperative area in the same-day surgery admitting area. During the admission assessment, the client mentions to the nurse that her last menses was 2 months ago and that the bleeding was heavier than usual, which she assumes is why her surgeon is recommending the surgery. When asking her about medications that she takes, the client denies taking any prescription medicines but does mention taking a baby aspirin a day and assorted herbal medicines for the bleeding.

Answer the following questions on a separate sheet of paper:

1. What assessment should the nurse make to determine this client's nutritional status and potential risk from the preoperative preparation and surgery?

2. What lab results of this client's should the nurse review? State the rationales for doing so.

3. Prioritize teaching needs for this client before surgery.

4. Develop a teaching-learning plan for this client's postoperative care.

5. Identify any client conditions or information that is to be shared with the surgeon or anesthesiologist.

6. The client states that she doesn't know whether her hysterectomy will be done vaginally or abdominally. Recognizing that the client is in need of more information, what would the nurse do?

7. The client asks if she will lose a lot of blood in surgery and, if so, can her daughter donate blood that she can receive if needed. What teaching would you give the client concerning blood donations?

8. Identify which category of surgery is related to each aspect of this client's impending surgery.
    a. Reason:
    b. Urgency:
    c. Degree of risk of surgery:
    d. Extent of surgery:

9. While this client is waiting in the preoperative area, she begins to cry and isn't sure what she wants to do about her surgery. The nurse observes her anxiety and suggests which of the following to help the client relax:
   a. Have a support person wait with her in the preoperative area if hospital policy allows.
   b. Encourage the client to take slow deep breaths to assist in relaxation.
   c. Ask the client about her previous surgical and/or hospital experiences.
   d. Ask the client about previous coping mechanisms she has used.

10. The client is about to be sent to the operating room. What items on a final checklist should be evaluated before leaving the preoperative area?

STUDY GUIDE NUMBER 4.18

Interventions for Intraoperative Clients

Study/Review Questions

1. Which of the following nursing interventions can reduce the preoperative client's anxiety?
   a. Provide a climate of privacy, comfort, and respect when caring for the client.
   b. Instruct the client that after the preoperative medication has taken affect the anxiety will go away.
   c. Avoid discussing the activities taking place around the client while in the holding area.
   d. Assist members of the surgical team readying the operating room suite.

2. Match the perioperative personnel with the descriptions of duties in the perioperative area.

Personnel
___ a. Surgeon
___ b. Holding area nurse
___ c. Anesthesiologist
___ d. Circulating nurse
___ e. Scrub nurse
___ f. Specialty nurse

Duties
1. Coordinates, oversees, and participates in the client's nursing care while he or she is in the operating room.
2. Assumes responsibility for the surgical procedure and any surgical judgments about the client.
3. Manages the client's care while he or she is in this area and initiates documentation on a perioperative nursing record.
4. Educated in a particular type of surgery and is responsible for intraoperative nursing care. specific to clients needing that type of surgery.
5. Sets up the sterile field, assists with the draping of the client, and hands sterile supplies, sterile equipment, and instruments to the surgeon.
6. Specializes in the administration of anesthetic agents.

3. During surgery, anesthesia personnel monitor, measure, and assess which of the following? *Check all that apply.*
   ___ a. Intake and output
   ___ b. Vital signs
   ___ c. Cardiopulmonary function
   ___ d. Level of anesthesia

Answer the following three questions on a separate sheet of paper.

4. How does the anesthesiologist monitor, assess, and measure the client's cardiopulmonary function?

5. Define the term *anesthesia.*

6. What is the purpose of anesthesia?

7. Match the following nursing interventions with the stage of general anesthesia.

Nursing Interventions	Stage of Anesthesia
___ a. Prepare for and assist in treatment of cardiovascular and/or pulmonary arrest. Document in record.	Stage 1 Stage 2 Stage 3 Stage 4
___ b. Shield client from extra noise and physical stimuli. Protect the client's extremities. Assist anesthesia personnel as needed. Stay with client.	Stage 5
___ c. Close operating room doors and control traffic in and out of room. Position client securely with safety belts. Maintain minimal discussion in operating room.	
___ d. Assist anesthesia personnel with intubation of client. Place the client in position for surgery. Prep the client's skin in area of operative site.	

8. What anesthetic agents are known most commonly to trigger a malignant hyperthermia (MH) crisis?

9. Which of the following clinical features are *not* found in an MH crisis?
   a. Rapid heart rate, supraventricular tachycardia
   b. Tightness and rigidity of the client's jaw area
   c. Lowering of the blood pressure
   d. A decrease in the end-tidal carbon dioxide level with a profound increase in oxygen saturation

10. The surgical team understands that time is crucial in recognizing and treating an MH crisis. Once recognized, what is the treatment of choice?
    a. Danazol gluconate
    b. Dilantin sodium
    c. Diazepam sulfate
    d. Dantrolene sodium

11. True or false? In an MH crisis, an extremely elevated and uncontrollable body temperature is one of the early signs of a problem.

12. On a separate sheet of paper, identify five of the best practices for a client with malignant hyperthermia.

13. Positioning of the client during surgical procedures is important in preventing postoperative problems. Match the following nursing interventions with the potential complications, which can be prevented with appropriate positioning and monitoring.

Anatomic area/
Complications
___ a. Brachial plexus/Paralysis; loss of sensation
___ b. Radial nerve/Wrist drop
___ c. Medial or ulnar nerves; peroneal nerve/ Hand deformities; foot drop
___ d. Tibial nerve/Loss of sensation on the plantar surface of the foot
___ e. Joints/Stiffness; pain; inflammation

Interventions
1. Support the wrist with padding; do not overtighten wrist straps.
2. Place pillow or foam padding under bony prominences; maintain good body alignment; slightly flex joints and support with pillows, trochanter rolls, and pads.
3. Place a safety strap above the ankle; do not place equipment on lower extremities; place pillow or padding under the knees.
4. Pad the elbow; avoid excessive abduction; secure the arm firmly on an arm board positioned at shoulder level.
5. Place a pillow or padding under the knees; place a safety strap above or below the area.

Case Study: The Intraoperative Client

A 71-year-old man is scheduled to receive orthopedic surgery in 3 hours. The nurse in the holding area receives a report from the preoperative nurse.

Answer the following questions on a separate sheet of paper:

1. What information will be shared and what information will the nurse ask the client during the interview process?

2. This client has his IV catheter inserted and has a surgical shave performed before surgery. The client is expected to be free of injury during surgery. Identify nursing diagnoses that would be appropriate for this client.

3. While this client is in the holding area, members of the surgical team are preparing the surgical suite. Identify factors related to physical safety in the surgical suite and give the rationale for each.

4. Identify three factors related to what the surgical team does to minimize risk of surgical infection for the client; also identify the rationale for each.

5. This client is having regional anesthesia for surgery because of a family history of malignant hyperthermia (MH). Which of the following statements is true about epidural anesthesia?
   a. Regional anesthesia is used when a Certified Registered Nurse Anesthetist (CRNA) will be administering the anesthetic.
   b. The circulating nurse does not have to monitor the client's reactions to the anesthetic.
   c. There is no risk of pulmonary complications with regional anesthetics.
   d. An advantage of regional anesthesia is the ability to retain the epidural catheter for postoperative pain management.

6. What will the nurse's role be for this client during the administration of anesthesia? *Check all that apply.*
   ___ a. Offering information and reassurance.
   ___ b. Positioning the client safely.
   ___ c. Observing for breaks in sterile techniques.

7. The surgeon, nurse, and anesthesiologist have discussed anesthesia options with the client, who agrees that an epidural anesthetic will be a good choice for him. What are potential complications the surgical team should be aware of with this choice? What are the symptoms?

8. If this client had received general anesthesia, what stressors might also trigger an MH crisis?

STUDY GUIDE NUMBER 4.19

Interventions for Postoperative Clients

Study/Review Questions

1. The postoperative period begins with:
   a. Completion of the surgical procedure and arousal of the client from anesthesia.
   b. Discharge planning initiated in the preoperative setting.
   c. Closure of the client's surgical incision.
   d. Completion of the surgical procedure and transfer of the client to the postanesthetic care unit (PACU) or intensive care unit (ICU).

2. What is the primary purpose of a PACU?
   a. Follow-through on the surgeon's postoperative orders
   b. Ongoing critical evaluation and stabilization of the client
   c. Prevention of lengthened hospital stay
   d. Arousal of client following the use of conscious sedation

3. In the list below, which are *not* postoperative complications?
   a. Sedation, sleepiness, incisional pain
   b. Dysrhythmia, congestive heart failure, pulmonary embolism
   c. Hypothermia, hyperthermia, hypovolemic shock
   d. Wound evisceration, wound infection

4. On a separate sheet of paper, identify risk factors in a client that may slow wound healing.

5. If a client experiences a wound dehiscence, which of the following describes what is happening with the wound?
   a. Yellow drainage is present at incision site
   b. Extreme pain at incision site
   c. A partial or complete separation of outer layers at incision site
   d. An immediate separation of outer layers at incision site

6. When a client describes "being able to see internal organs" at the incision site, he is describing:
   a. An infection.
   b. Evisceration.
   c. Poor wound healing.
   d. Split skin sutures.

7. During PACU care, part of the nursing assessment includes the dressing. What characteristics will the nurse be noting?
   a. How much adhesive is in place upon admission into the PACU
   b. The size of the drain used
   c. Amount, color, odor, consistency of drainage on dressing
   d. The reaction of the client when the dressing is assessed

8. On a separate sheet of paper, identify the guidelines for what information is to be included on the report of the client's status upon arrival in the PACU.

Match the following assessment findings that may be noted for clients in the PACU with their corresponding body systems. *Answers may be used more than once. More than one body system may be involved in a finding.*

Assessment Findings	Body Systems
____ 9. Eyes open on command	a. Respiratory
____ 10. Symmetrical chest wall expansion	b. Cardiovascular
____ 11. Foley catheter to facilitate drainage	c. Fluid and electrolyte balance
____ 12. Absent dorsalis pedis pulsations	d. Neurologic
____ 13. Use of accessory muscles	e. Renal/urinary
____ 14. Large amount of sanguineous drainage	f. Gastrointestinal
____ 15. Negative Homan's sign	g. Integumentary
____ 16. IV infusion of dextrose 5% Ringer's lactate	
____ 17. States name when asked	
____ 18. Rounded, firm abdomen	
____ 19. Exhalation felt from nose or mouth	

___ 20. Decreased blood pressure

___ 21. Wound edges approximated

___ 22. Dry mucous membranes

___ 23. Vomiting

___ 24. Pupils constrict equally

___ 25. Sternal retraction

___ 26. Nasogastric tube in place

___ 27. Evisceration

___ 28. Dullness over symphysis pubis

___ 29. Tenting

___ 30. Faint heart sounds

___ 31. Wound dressing dry

___ 32. Absent bowel sounds

___ 33. Vesicular crackles

___ 34. Hand grips equal

___ 35. Simultaneous apical and radial pulsations

___ 36. Dehiscence

___ 37. Snoring

38. Airway assessment is completed immediately upon arrival to the PACU to establish a patent airway and adequate respiratory exchange. On a separate sheet of paper, identify the key points in the respiratory assessment.

39. The client arrives at the PACU and the nurse notes a respiratory rate of 10, with sternal retractions. The report from anesthesia personnel indicated that the client had received Fentanyl during surgery. Number the following nursing interventions to be performed in order of first to last:

___ a. Continue to monitor the client for effects of naloxone for at least 1 hour.

___ b. Have suction available.

___ c. Closely monitor vital signs and pulse oximetry readings until the client responds.

___ d. Do not leave the client unattended until he or she is able to respond fully.

___ e. Observe for significant reversal of anesthesia.

___ f. Administer oxygen as ordered.

___ g. Maintain an open airway.

40. On a separate sheet of paper, identify three common nursing diagnoses and collaborative problems for a client in the PACU.

The health care team determines the client's readiness for discharge from the PACU by noting a postanesthesia recovery score of at least 10. After determining that all criteria have been met, the client is discharged to the hospital unit or home.

41. Review the following client profiles after 1 hour in the PACU. Number the clients in order of anticipated discharge from the PACU area.

___ a. 10-year-old girl, tonsillectomy, general anesthesia. Duration of surgery 30 minutes. Immediate response to voice. Alert to place and person. Able to move all extremities. Respirations even, deep, rate of 20. VS are within normal limits. IV solution is D5RL. Has voided on bedpan. Eating ice chips. Complaining of sore throat.

___ b. 35-year-old woman, cesarean section, epidural anesthesia. Duration of surgery 27 minutes. Awake and alert. Able to bend knees and lift lower extremities. Respirations are 16 breaths/min and unlabored. Foley draining 300 mL urine. IV of RL infusing. VS are within normal limits.

___ c. 55-year-old man, repair of fractured lower left leg. General anesthesia. Duration of surgery 1 hour, 30 minutes. Drowsy, but responds to voice. Nausea and vomiting twice in PACU. No urge to void at this time. IV infusing D5NS. Pedal pulses noted in both lower extremities. VS: T 98.6° F; P 130; R 24; BP 124/76.

___ d. 24-year-old man, reconstruction of facial scar. General anesthesia. Duration of surgery 2 hours. Sleeping, groans to voice command. VS are within normal limits. Respirations are 10 breaths/min. No urge to void. IV of D5RL infusing. Complains of pain in surgical area.

___ e. 42-year-old woman, colonoscopy. IV conscious sedation. Awake and alert. Up to bathroom to void. IV discontinued. Resting quietly in chair. VS are within normal limits.

Anatomy	Physiology	Pathophysiology	History	Physical Exam	Diagnostic Tests	Interventions	Pharmacology

• Lymph system
• Mononuclear—phagocyte system
• Cells
  B-lymphocytes
  T-lymphocytes
• Antigens
	• Phagocytosis
	• Specificity
	• Memory
	• Self-recognition
	• Human leukocyte antigen (HLA)
	• Inflammatory response
	• Immune response
	  Antibody-mediated
	  Cell-mediated
	• Types of immunity
	  Natural
	  Acquired
	  Active
	  Passive
		• Hypersensitivity response
		• Autoimmune response
		• Immunodeficiency
		• Metastasis
		• Neoplasm
		• Inflammation
		• Infection
		• Transplant reaction
		• Tissue degeneration
			• Past history of infections, allergies, malignancies, autoimmune disease
			• Immunization record
			• Family history
			• Social history
			  Occupation
			  Nutrition
				• Liver size and location
				• Spleen
				• Thymus
				• Lymphatic system
				  Nodes
				• Fever
				• Skin rashes
				• Urticaria
				• Itching
				• Fatigue
				• Malaise
				• Infection
				• Respiratory distress
				• Weight loss
				• Joint assessment
				• Cardiovascular system
				• Renal system
					• Complete blood count
					• Carcinoembryonic antigen (CEA)
					• C-reactive protein
					• Immunoglobins IgA, IgG, IgM, IgD, IgE
					• Rheumatoid factor
					• Antinuclear antibody titer
					• Enzyme-linked immunosorbent assay (ELISA)
					• Western blot
					• Skin tests
					• Tumor staging
						• Education
						  Avoidance of infection
						  Avoidance of trigger substances
						• Rest
						• Nutrition
						• Stress management
						• Lifestyle alterations
						• Radiation
						• Bone marrow transplantation
						• Therapeutic exercise
						• Energy conservation
						• Joint protection
						• Skin protection from the sun
						• Joint replacement
						  Total hip
						  Total knee
						• Abduction pillow
						• Continuous passive motion (CPM) machine
						• Postoperative complications
						  Infection
						  Thromboembolitic complications
						  Dislocation
							• Histamine blockers
							• Corticosteroids
							• Hyposensitization
							• Immunosuppressants
							• Chemotherapeutic agents
							• Biologic response modifiers (BRMs)
							• Antibiotics
							• Nonsteroidal anti-inflammatory drugs
							• Opioids

Unit 5 (Chapters 20-26)

Problems of Protection: Management of Clients with Problems of the Immune System

Learning Plan

Chapter 20: *Concepts of Inflammation and the Immune Response*

Learning Outcomes

1. Describe the concept of self-tolerance.
2. Explain the difference between inflammation and infection.
3. Compare and contrast the cells, purposes, and features of inflammation and immunity.
4. Describe the basis for the five cardinal manifestations of inflammation.
5. Interpret a white blood cell count with differential to indicate no immune problems, an acute bacterial infection, a chronic bacterial infection, or an allergic reaction.
6. Explain how complement activation and fixation assists in protection from infection.
7. Compare the cells, function, and protective actions of antibody-mediated immunity and cell-mediated immunity.
8. Compare and contrast the types of antibody-mediated immunity.

Learning Activities

1. Prior to completing the study guide exercises in this chapter, review the following:
   - Anatomy and physiology of the immune system
   - Process of inflammation
   - Process of immunity
   - White blood cells and their activities in the process of inflammation, immunity, and rejection
   - Sequence of the inflammatory response
   - Types of immunity
   - Transplant rejection and management

2. Review the **boldfaced** Key Terms and their definitions in Chapter 20 to enhance your understanding of the content.

3. Go Study Guide Number 5.20 on the following pages and complete the learning exercises for this chapter.

Supplemental Resources

1. Textbook—Chapter 20
2. Other resources:
   - Alam, R. (1998). A brief review of the immune system. *Primary Care: Clinics in Office Practice, 25*(4), 727-738.
   - Any anatomy and physiology textbook
   - Any laboratory resource textbook
   - Any physical assessment textbook
   - Augustine, S. (2000). Heart transplantation: Long-term management related to immunosuppression, complications, and psychosocial adjustments, *Critical Care Clinics of North America, 12*(1), 69-77.
   - Bush, W. (1999). Overview of transplantation and pharmacotherapy of adult solid organ transplant recipients: Focus on immunosuppression. *AACN Clinical Issues, 10*(2), 253-269.
   - Coelman, C. (1998). Overview of biotherapy and nursing considerations. *Journal of Intravenous Nursing, 21*(6), 367-373.
   - Guton, A. & Hall, J. (2001). *Textbook of medical physiology* (10th ed.). Philadelphia: W.B. Saunders.
   - Nieman, D. (1999). Nutrition, exercise, and immune system function. *Clinics in Sports Medicine, 18*(3), 537-548.
   - United States Pharmacopeia (2000). Drug information for the health care professional (Vol. I, 20th ed.). Englewood, CO: Micromedix.
   - Vasquez, E. & Westin, E. (1999). Transplant immunopharmacology: You CAN fool with mother nature! *Nursing Case Management, 4*(1), 37-48.

Chapter 21: *Interventions for Clients with Connective Tissue Disease*

Learning Outcomes	Learning Activities	Supplemental Resources
1. Compare and contrast the pathophysiology and clinical manifestations of degenerative joint disease (DJD) and rheumatoid disease (RA).	1. Prior to completing the study guide exercises in this chapter, review the following:	1. Textbook—Chapter 20 (Concepts of Inflammation and the Immune Response)
2. Discuss the priority collaborative interventions for postoperative clients with DJD and RA.	• Anatomy and physiology of the musculoskeletal system	2. Textbook—Chapter 21
3. Determine common nursing diagnoses for postoperative clients having total joint replacement surgery.	• Process of inflammation	3. Other resources:
4. Interpret laboratory findings for clients with RA.	• Normal lab values related to immune system	• Any anatomy and physiology textbook
5. Discuss the differences between anti-inflammatory and disease-modifying drugs for clients with RA.	• Assessment of the musculoskeletal system	• Any pathophysiology textbook
6. Identify educational needs for clients with arthritis.	• Postoperative care	• Berman, B.M, Singh, B.B., Lao, L., et al. (1999). A randomized trial of acupuncture as adjunctive therapy to osteoarthritis of the knee. *Rheumatology, 38*(4), 345-354.
7. Identify the pathophysiology and etiology of gout.	• Hazards of immobility	• Eaton, L., & Meiner, S.E. (1999). Marfan syndrome: Identification and management. *MEDSURG Nursing, 8*(2), 113-117.
8. Differentiate between discoid lupus erythematosus and systemic lupus erythematosus.	• Principles of teaching/learning	• Evanoff, A., et al. (1999). Therapeutic touch and osteoarthritis of the knee. *Journal of Family Practice, 48*(1), 11-12.
9. Describe the priority of nursing interventions for clients who have progressive systemic sclerosis.	2. Review the **boldfaced** Key Terms and their definitions in Chapter 21 to enhance your understanding of the content.	• Geier, K. (1998). Perioperative blood management. *Orthopedic Nursing, 17* (1Suppl), 6-36.
10. Identify the pathophysiology and etiology of gout.	3. Go to Study Guide Number 5.21 on the following pages and complete the learning exercises for this chapter.	• Gordon, A, Merenstein, J.H., D'Amico, F., & Hugden, D. (1998). The effects of therapeutic touch on patients with osteoarthritis of the knee. *Journal of Family Practice, 47*(4), 271-277.
11. Explain the differences between polymyositis, systemic necrotizing vasculitis, polymyalgia rheumatica, ankylosing spondylitis, Reiter's syndrome, and Sjogren's syndrome.		• Holcomb, S.S. (2000). Reviewing Marfan syndrome. *Nursing 2000, 30*(5), 32cc10-32cc12.
12. Describe interventions that clients can use to prevent Lyme disease.		• Kee, C.C. (1998). Living with osteoarthritis: Insiders' views. *Applied Nursing Research, 11*(1), 19-26.
13. Identify the primary concern in care for clients with Marfan syndrome.		• Kee, C.C. (2000). Manageable scourge of aging. *Nursing Clinics of North America, 35*(1), 199-208.
14. Describe the common clinical manifestations of fibromyalgia.		• Kettelman, K. (2000). Soothing the ache of joint surgery/ *Nursing 2000, 30*(7), 14.

- Kuper, B.C. & Failla, S. (2000). Systemic lupus erythematosus: A multisystem autoimmune disorder. *Nursing Clinics of North America, 35*(1), 253-266.
- Lash, A.A. (1998). Quality of life in systemic lupus erythematosus. *Applied Nursing Resarch, 11*(3), 130-137.
- Maher, A. B., Salmond, S.W., & Pellino, T.A. (1999). *Orthopedic nursing* (2ⁿᵈ ed.). Philadelphia: W.B. Saunders.
- Matula, P.A. & Shollenberger, D. (1999). Total joint project: Acute care to home care. *MEDSURG Nursing, 8*(2), 92-98.
- Meyers, J. (1998). Lyme disease: A challenge and an opportunity for nurse practitioners. *Journal of the American Academy of Nurse Practitioners, 10*(7), 315-319.
- Mikanowicz, C.K. & Leslie, M. (2000). Polymyalgia rheumatica and temporal arteritis: A case presentation. *Nursing Clinics of North America, 35*(1), 245-252.
- Morris B.A., Colwell, C.W., & Hardwick, M.E. (1998). The use of low molecular weight heparins in the prevention of venous thromboembolic disease. *Orthopedic Nursing, 17*(6), 23-26.
- Pepper, G.A. (2000). Nonsteroidal anti-inflammatory drugs: New perspectives on a familiar class. *Nursing Clinics of North America, 35*(1), 223-244.
- Ritter, M.A., Koehler, M., et al. (1999). Intra-articualar morphine and/or bupivacaine after total knee replacement. *Journal of Bone and Joint Surgery, 81*(2), 301-303.
- Sears, J.R. & Ganger, P.M. (2000). Antibiotics to treat RA. *RN, 63*(1), 41-42.

- Shirkey, N.A., Williams, N.I., & Guerin, J.B. (2000). The role of exercise in the prevention and treatment of osteoporosis and osteoarthritis. *Nursing Clinics of North America, 35*(1), 209-222.
- Yen, P.K. (1999). Diet, complementary therapy, and arthritis. *Geriatric Nursing, 20*(6), 337-338.

Chapter 22: Interventions for Clients with HIV and Other Immunodeficiencies	
Learning Outcomes	**Learning Activities**

1. Compare and contrast primary versus secondary immunodeficiencies for causes and onset of problems.
2. Explain the differences in nursing care required for a client with a pathogenic infection versus a client with an opportunistic infection.
3. Distinguish between the conditions of human immunodeficiency virus (HIV) infection and acquired immunodeficiency syndrome (AIDS) for clinical manifestations and risks for complications.
4. Describe the ways in which HIV is transmitted.
5. Identify techniques to reduce the risk for infection in an immunocompromised client.
6. Develop a teaching plan for condom use among sexually active, non–English-speaking adults.
7. Prioritize nursing care for the client with AIDS who has impaired gas exchange.
8. Identify teaching priorities for the HIV-positive client receiving highly active antiretroviral therapy.
9. Plan a week of meals for the client who has protein-calorie malnutrition.
10. Describe the nursing actions and responsibilities for administration of IV immunoglobulin.
	1. Prior to completing the study guide exercises in this chapter, review the following:
	  • Anatomy and physiology of the immune system
	  • Infection
	  • Complete physical assessment
	  • Grief and loss
	  • Death and dying
	  • Self-concept
	  • Therapeutic communication
	2. Review the **boldfaced** Key Terms and their definitions in Chapter 22 to enhance your understanding of the content.
	3. Go to Study Guide Number 5.22 on the following pages and complete the learning exercises for this chapter.

	Supplemental Resources

	1. Textbook—Chapter 20 (Concepts of Inflammation and the Immune Response)
	2. Textbook—Chapter 22
	3. Other resources:
	  • Any anatomy and physiology textbook
	  • Any laboratory resource textbook
	  • Any pathophysiology book
	  • Any physical assessment textbook
	  • Bjorgen, S. (1998). Clinical snapshot: Herpes zoster. *American Journal of Nursing, 98*(2), 46-47.
	  • Centers for Disease Control (1987). Public Health Service guidelines for counseling and antibody testing to prevent HIV infections and AIDS. *MMWR. Morbidity and Mortality weekly Report, 36*(31), 509-515.
	  • Centers for Disease Control and Prevention (1998a). Public Health Service Guidelines for the management of health-care worker exposure to HIV and recommendations for postexposure prophylaxis. *MMWR. Morbidity and Mortality Weekly Report, 47*(RR-7), 1-32.
	  • Centers for Disease Control and Prevention (1999). *HIV/AIDS surveillance report.* 11(1), Atlanta, GA: Author.

- Center for Disease Control and Prevention (1999). 1999 USPHS/IDSA guidelines for the prevention of opportunistic infections in persons infected with human immunodeficiency virus. *MMWR. Morbidity and Mortality weekly report, 48*(RR-10), 1-66.
- Cochran, A. & Wilson, B.A. (1999). Current management of AIDS and related opportunistic infections. *MEDSUR Nursing, 8*(4), 257-266.
- Dube, M. & Sattler, F. (1998). Metabolic complications of antiretroviral therapy. *AIDS Clinical Care, 10*(6), 41-44.
- Emlet, C. (1997). HIV/AIDS in the elderly. *Home Care Provider, 2*(2), 69-70.
- Evans, B. (1999). Complementary Therapies and HIV infection. *American Journal of Nursing, 99*(2), 42-45.
- Jagger, J. & Perry, J. (1999). Power in numbers: Reducing your risk of blood borne exposures. *Nursing 99, 29*(1), 51-52.
- Kiethley, J. & Swanson, B. (1998). Minimizing HIV/AIDS malnutrition. *MEDSURG Nursing, 7*(5), 256-267.
- Konkle-Parker, D. (1998). Early HIV detection and treatment. *ADVANCE for Nurse Practitioners, 6*(9), 63-66.
- Mitsuyasu, R. (1999). Immune reconstitution in HIV disease. *Disease Management Digest, 3*(3), 2-3.
- Porche, D. (1999). State of the art: Antiviral and prophylactic treatments in HIV/AIDS. *Nursing Clinic of North America, 34*(1), 95-112.
- Sande, M.A. & Volberding, P.A. (1999). The medical management of AIDS (6th ed.). Philadelphia: W.B. Saunders.
- Sowell, R., Moneyham, L., & Aradno-Naranjo, A. (1999). The care of women with AIDS: Special needs and considerations. *Nursing Clinics of North America, 34*(1), 179-197.

- United States Pharmacopeia (2000). *Drug information for the healthcare professional* (Vol I, 20th ed.). Englewood, CO: Micromedex.
- Williams, A. (1999a). Adherence to highly active antiretroviral therapy. *Nursing Clinics of North America, 34*(1), 113-129.
- Williams, A. (1999b). Bridging the gap: Bringing new antiretroviral medications into the clinic. *ADVANCE for Nurse Practitioners, 7*(1), 24-32.
- Wolfe, G. (1999). Anemia-related fatigue in patients with HIV/AIDS. *Journal of Care Management, 5*(3), 86, 88, 93-94, 96, 98.

Chapter 23: *Interventions for Clients with Immune Function Excess: Hypersensitivity (Allergy) and Autoimmunity*

Learning Activities	Supplemental Resources
1. Prior to completing the study guide exercises in this chapter, review the following: • Anatomy and physiology of the immune system • Process of allergens • Anaphylactic shock • Assessment of inflammation and infection 2. Review the **boldfaced** Key Terms and their definitions in Chapter 23 to enhance your understanding of the content. 3. Go to Study Guide Number 5.23 on the following pages and complete the learning exercises for this chapter.	1. Textbook—Chapter 20 (Concepts of Inflammation and the Immune Response) 2. Textbook—Chapter 23 3. Other resources: • Any anatomy and physiology textbook • Any laboratory resource textbook • Any physical assessment textbook • Alam, R. (1998). A brief review of the immune system. *Primary Care: Clinics in Office Practice, 25*(4), 727-738. Online: www.wbsaunders.com/SIMON/ • Augustine, S. (2000). Heart transplantation: Long-term management related to immunosuppression, complications, and psychosocial adjustments. *Critical Care Clinics of North America, 12*(1), 69-77. • Guton, A. & Hall, J. (2001). *Textbook of medical physiology* (10th ed.). Philadelphia: W.B. Saunders.

Learning Outcomes

1. Compare and contrast bases for and manifestations of allergy and autoimmunity.
2. Discuss the nursing responsibility for a client experiencing anaphylaxis.
3. Describe allergy testing techniques.
4. List the defining characteristics of type I, type II, type III, type IV, and type V hypersensitivity reactions.
5. Explain the differences in mechanisms of action between antihistamines and mast cell stabilizers.

- United States Pharmacopeia (2000). *Drug information for the health care professional* (Vol. I, 20th ed.). Englewood, CO: Micromedix.
- Vasquez, E. & Westin, E. (1999). Transplant immunopharmacology: You CAN fool with mother nature! *Nursing Case Management, 4*(1), 37-48.

Supplemental Resources

1. Textbook—Chapter 24
2. Other resources:
   - American Cancer Society (2000). Cancer facts and figures 2000 (Report No. 00-300M No. 5008.00). Atlanta, GA: American Cancer Society.
   - Any anatomy and physiology textbook
   - Any laboratory resource textbook
   - Byers, T., MacDonald, D., Serverin, M., & Fishback, A. (1999). Cancer genetics counseling. *Cancer Practice, 7*(2), 93-95.
   - Haylock, P. (1998). Cancer metastasis: An update. *Seminars in Oncology Nursing, 14*(3), 172-177.
   - Khuri, F. (1999). Chemoprevention of cancer. *Highlights in Oncology Practice, 16*(4), 100-109.
   - Miaskowski, C. & Buchel, P. (1999). *Oncology nursing: Assessment and clinical care.* St. Louis: Mosby.
   - Phillips, J., Cohen, M., & Moses, G. (1999). Breast cancer screening and African-American women: Fear, fatalism, and silence. *Oncology Nursing Forum, 26*(3), 487-494.
   - Sarna, L. (1999). Prevention: Tobacco control and cancer nursing. *Cancer Nursing, 21*(11), 21-28.

Chapter 24: *Altered Cell Growth and Cancer Development*

Learning Outcomes

1. Explain why causes of cancer can be hard to establish.
2. Compare and contrast the characteristics of benign and malignant tumors.
3. List three cancer types associated with exposure to tobacco.
4. Identify cancer types for which primary prevention is possible.
5. Compare and contrast the cancer development processes of initiation and promotion.
6. Describe the TNM system for cancer staging.
7. Explain the differences between a "low-grade" cancer and a "high-grade" cancer.
8. Discuss the roles of oncogenes and suppressor genes in cancer development.
9. Identify four common sites of distant metastasis for cancer.
10. Discuss the role of immunity in protection against cancer.
11. Identify which cancer types arise from connective tissues and which arise from glandular tissues.
12. Describe how genetic predisposition can increase a person's risk for cancer development.
13. Identify behaviors that reduce the risk for cancer development and cancer death.

Learning Activities

1. Prior to completing the study guide exercises in this chapter, review the following:
   - Anatomy and physiology of the immune system
   - Types of prevention
   - Normal cell growth and development
2. Review the **boldfaced** Key Terms and their definitions in Chapter 24 to enhance your understanding of the content.
3. Go to Study Guide Number 5.24 on the following pages and complete the learning exercises for this chapter.

Chapter 25: *Interventions for Clients with Cancer*

Learning Outcomes	Learning Activities	Supplemental Resources
1. Identify the goals of cancer therapy. 2. Differentiate between cancer surgery for cure and cancer surgery for palliation. 3. Discuss how the nursing care needs for the client undergoing cancer surgery compare to those for the client undergoing any other type of surgery. 4. Compare and contrast the purposes and side effects of radiation therapy and chemotherapy for cancer. 5. Prioritize nursing care for the client with radiation-induced skin problems. 6. Prioritize educational needs for the client receiving external beam radiation. 7. Compare the personnel safety issues for working with clients receiving teletherapy radiation versus those receiving brachytherapy radiation. 8. Identify nursing interventions to promote safety for the client experiencing chemotherapy-induced anemia or thrombocytopenia. 9. Prioritize nursing care needs for the client with chemotherapy-induced neutropenia. 10. Prioritize nursing care needs for the client with mucositis. 11. Explain the rationale for hormonal manipulation therapy. 12. Discuss the uses of biologic response modifiers as supportive therapy in the treatment of cancer. 13. Identify clients at risk for oncologic emergencies.	1. Prior to completing the study guide exercises in this chapter, review the following: • Altered cell growth • Immunity and inflammation response in the body • Hematologic norms • Anatomy and physiology of the immune system • Principles of infection • Fluid and electrolytes • Normal cell growth and development • Principles of a complete physical assessment 2. Review the **boldfaced** Key Terms and their definitions in Chapter 25 to enhance your understanding of the content. 3. Go to Study Guide Number 5.26 on the following pages and complete the learning exercises for this chapter.	1. Textbook—Chapter 24 (Altered Cell Growth and Cancer Development) 2. Textbook—Chapter 25 3. Other resources: • American Cancer Society (2000). Cancer facts and figures 1998 (Report No. 00-300M-No.5008.00). Atlanta, GA: American Cancer Society. • Any anatomy and physiology textbook • Any physical assessment textbook • Any pharmacology book with chemotherapy agents • Bennet, M. & Lengacher, C. (1999). Use of complementary therapies in a rural cancer population. *Oncology Nursing Forum, 26*(8), 1287-1294. • Brown, P. (1999). Nutrition and cancer. *MEDSUR Nursing, 8*(6), 333-345. • Burke, C. (1999). Surgical treatment. In C. Miaskowski & P. Buchsel (Eds.). *Oncology nursing: Assessment and clinical care* (pp. 29-58). St. Louis: Mosby. • Hassey, D. (1987). Principles of radiation therapy and protection. *Seminars in Oncology Nursing, 3*, 23-29. • Miaskowski, C. & Buchsel, P. (1999). *Oncology nursing: Assessment and clinical care*. St. Louis: Mosby. • United States Pharmacopoeia (2000). *Drug information for the health care professional* (Vol. I, 20th ed.). Englewood, CO: Micromedix.

Chapter 26: *Interventions for Clients with Cancer*

Learning Outcomes	Learning Activities	Supplemental Resources

1. Explain the chain of infection.
2. Describe the principles of infection control in inpatient and community-based settings.
3. Discuss the risk of gloves and other products made with latex.
4. Interpret the four types of transmission-based precautions.
5. Identify the major complications of infection.
6. Describe the common clinical manifestations of infection for which the nurse should assess.
7. Interpret laboratory test findings related to infections and infectious disease.
8. Evaluate nursing interventions for fever management.
	1. Prior to completing the study guide exercises in this chapter, review the following:
	  • Anatomy and physiology of the immune system
	  • Process of inflammation
	  • Process of immunity
	  • Process of inflammation
	
	2. Review the **boldfaced** Key Terms and their definitions in Chapter 26 to enhance your understanding of the content.
	
	3. Go to Study Guide Number 5.26 on the following pages and complete the learning exercises for this chapter.
		1. Textbook—Chapter 26
		2. Other resources:
		  • Any anatomy and physiology textbook
		  • Any laboratory resource manual
		  • Any physical assessment textbook
		  • Centers for Disease Control (1998). Guidelines for Infection Control in Health Care Personnel, 1998, Table 6. Pregnant health care personnel: Pertinent facts to guide management of occupational exposures to infectious agents. *American Journal of Infection Control, 26,* 322.
		  • Chin, J. (Ed.). (2000). *Control of communicable disease manual* (17th ed.; pp. 20-25, 70-75, 381-387, 455-457). Washington, D.C: American Public Health Association.
		  • Friedman, M.M. & Rhinehart, E. (1999). Putting infection control principles into practice in home care. *The Nursing Clinics of North America.* June 1999, 463, 482.
		  • Gehring, L.L. & Ring, P. (1999). Latex allergy: Creating a safe environment. *MEDSURG Nursing, 8*(6), 358-362.
		  • Kahn, A.S., Sage, M.J., et al. (2000). Biological and chemical terrorism: Strategic plan for preparedness and response. Recommendations of the CDC Stategic Planning Workgroup. *MMWR. Morbidity and Mortality Weekly Report, 49*(RR04), 1-14.

STUDY GUIDE NUMBER 5.20

Concepts of Inflammation and the Immune Response

Study/Review Questions

1. Which of the following is not a purpose of the immune system?
   a. Protect from and eliminate/destroy micro-organisms
   b. Distinguish between non self protein and cells
   c. Reduce leukocytes
   d. Are the only self-tolerance cells

2. Identify the properties of human cells.
   a. _____
   b. _____
   c. _____
   d. _____
   e. _____
   f. _____
   g. _____

3. Identify five areas of the body that can be affected by immune function.
   a. _____
   b. _____
   c. _____
   d. _____
   e. _____

True or False? Write T for true or F for false in the blank provided.

___ 4. Immune cells originate in the bone marrow and are released in the blood at maturity.

5. Identify three processes required for immunity and response to inflammation.
   a. _____
   b. _____
   c. _____

6. Identify the important actions of leukocytes that provide protection.
   a. _____
   b. _____
   c. _____
   d. _____
   e. _____
   f. _____
   g. _____

7. Which of the following statements about the inflammatory response is true?
   a. Response is different with each incident.
   b. Response is the same whether the insult to the body is a burn or otitis media.
   c. Response depends on the location in the body.
   d. Response is not specific to the cell.

8. The inflammatory response is present in which of the following conditions? *Choose all that apply.*
   a. Sprain injuries to joints
   b. Surgical wounds
   c. Poison ivy

9. Cells associated with the inflammatory response that participate in phagocytosis are called:
   a. Neutrophils and eosinophils.
   b. Macrophages and neutrophils.
   c. Macrophages and eosinophils.
   d. Eosinophils and neutrophils.

10. The body produces the most of which type of white cell?
    a. Macrophages
    b. Eosinophils
    c. Neutrophils
    d. Band neutrophils

11. Match the cell characteristics with the types of cells. *Answers may be used more than once.*

Characteristics	Cell Types
___ a. 12 to 18 hours	1. Neutrophil
___ b. 1% to 2% of total WBC	2. Macrophage
___ c. Contains chemicals such as histamine	3. Basophils
___ d. Contains lytic acid	4. Eosinophil
___ e. When mature, capable of phagocytosis	
___ f. Clinical sign of left shift indicates no mature cells being produced	
___ g. Liver and spleen have greatest concentration	
___ h. Vascular leak syndrome	

12. Which of the following statements about phagocytosis is *false*?
    a. It is a process that engulfs invaders and destroys them by enzymatic degradation.
    b. It rids the body of debris and destroys foreign invaders.
    c. It is done in a predictable manner.
    d. All leukocytes perform phagocytosis.

13. When an injury or invasion occurs, which of the following functions will the phagocytic cell *not* perform?
    a. Recognize chemotaxins or leukotaxis
    b. Assist damaged tissue or blood vessels
    c. Act as a chemical magnet
    d. Gain direct contact with the antigen, or invader

True or False? Write T for true or F for false in the blank provided.

___ 14. Opsonization is the process that aids the phagocyte in adhering to the invader.

15. When stimulated, complement activation and fixation is a mechanism of opsonization and phagocytic adherence that includes 20 different inactive protein components that will:
    a. Cause individual complement proteins to activate, join together, surround the antigen, and adhere.
    b. Join together, cause individual complement proteins to activate, surround the antigen, and adhere.
    c. Surround the antigen and adhere to it.
    d. Adherence of cells to each other.

16. Phagocytes are capable of:
    a. Recognizing cells.
    b. Ingesting cells.
    c. Enclosing a target cell.
    d. Producing insulin.

17. Identify the five cardinal signs of inflammation for which the nurse should assess.
    a. _____
    b. _____
    c. _____
    d. _____
    e. _____

18. All the signs of inflammation are present in which stage?
    a. Stage I
    b. Stage II
    c. Stage III
    d. Stage IV

19. What occurs in the body at the time of inflammation is a colony-stimulating factor that stimulates the:
    a. Bone marrow to produce leukocytes in less time.
    b. Bone marrow to produce immature leukocytes.
    c. Bone marrow to release immature leukocytes.
    d. Liver to produce leukocytes.

20. The substance commonly called *pus* is produced by exudate in which stage of inflammation?
    a. Stage I
    b. Stage II
    c. Stage III
    d. Stage IV

21. Neutrophils attack and destroy foreign material and remove dead tissue through the process of:
    a. Phagocytosis.
    b. Adherence.
    c. Cytokines.
    d. Macrophages.

22. B-lymphocytes are part of the antibody-mediated immunity (AMI) that become sensitized to an antigen and will try to:
    a. Adhere to it.
    b. Neutralize, eliminate, or destroy it.
    c. Identify it.
    d. Surround and protect it.

23. Identify seven special actions that take place when a person is exposed to an antigen. *Refer to Figure 20-9.*
    a. _____
    b. _____
    c. _____
    d. _____
    e. _____
    f. _____
    g. _____

24. The steps to antigen recognition are:
    a. Opsonization, presented to T-cell, and process of antigen recognition sites.
    b. Adherence and phagocytosis.
    c. Opsonization, presented to T-cell, and phagocytosis.
    d. Adherence, opsonization, presented to T-cell, and process of antigen recognition sites.

25. Which of the following statements about B-lymphocytes and sensitizing to one antigen is *false*?
    a. Once sensitized, always sensitized to that antigen.
    b. Plasma cell immediately replicates to produce the antigen.
    c. The memory cell is short-lived.
    d. The memory cell lies dormant till next exposure.

26. Humoral immunity is:
    a. Antibodies circulating in body fluid.
    b. Plasma cells.
    c. Memory cells.
    d. Leukocytes.

27. Match the following actions with the antibody-binding reactions.

Actions	Antibody-binding Reactions
____ a. Cell membrane destruction	1. Agglutination
____ b. Large, insoluble antibody molecules formed	2. Lysis 3. Precipitation 4. Inactivation-neutralization
____ c. Clumping-like antibody action	5. Complement fixation
____ d. Can remove or destroy non-self antigens	
____ e. Covers site active site	

28. Which of the following statements is true of natural immunity, or innate-active immunity?
    a. Natural immunity is genetically determined, non-specific, and cannot be developed for transfer.
    b. Natural immunity adapts to exposure and invasion.
    c. Humans are not susceptible to mange, distemper, and hog cholera.
    d. *a* and *c*

29. Identify the two types of immunity.
    a. _____
    b. _____

30. Identify an example of each of the following types of immunity:
    a. Natural active immunity: _____
    b. Artificial active immunity: _____
    c. Natural passive immunity: _____
    d. Artificial passive immunity: _____

31. Identify the three T-lymphocyte subsets that are critically important to cell-mediated immunity (CMI).
    a. _____
    b. _____
    c. _____

32. The 4+ cells or CD4+ antibodies are commercially produced as OKT4 and Leu-3 positive. It is their function to:
    a. Secrete lymphokines to stimulate increased production of stem cells and speed up cell maturation.
    b. Secrete lymphokines to speed up cell maturation only.
    c. Regulate helper/inducer T-cells.
    d. Destroy, eliminate, or neutralize antigens.

33. Match each type of cell with its function.

Function	Cell Type
____ a. Prevents overreaction	1. Suppressor cell
____ b. Binds with infected cell's antigen that results in death of affected cell	2. Natural-killer cell 3. Helper/inducer cell
____ c. Secretes lymphokines that stimulate activities of other cells of the immune system	4. Cytotoxic/cytolytic T-cells 5. Cytokine/lymphokines
____ d. Exerts cytotoxic effect without first undergoing period of sensitization	
____ e. Regulates variety of inflammatory and immune responses	

True or False? Write T for true or F for false in the blanks provided.

____ 34. Cancer and metastasis prevention is controlled by cell-mediated immunity through its surveillance system.

____ 35. Transplanted tissue or organs are destroyed by natural-killer cells and cytotoxic/cytolytic T-cells.

36. Identify three types of graft rejection.

    a. _____

    b. _____

    c. _____

37. Match the descriptors with the types of rejection. *Answers may be used more than once.*

Descriptors	Types of Rejection
___ a. Immediate	1. Hyperacute rejection
___ b. Most common with kidney transplants	2. Acute graft rejection
___ c. Rejection cannot be stopped	3. Chronic rejection
___ d. Occurs over 1 to 3 months	
___ e. Leads to organ destruction	
___ f. Does not mean loss of transplant	
___ g. Accelerated graft atherosclerosis	
___ h. Initiates blood clotting cascade	
___ i. Fibrotic and scar-like tissue	
___ j. Major cause of death in heart clients	
___ k. Accelerated graft atherosclerosis	

38. Nursing interventions regarding maintenance drug therapy after solid organ transplantation include:

    a. Many high-priced drug combinations of specific and nonspecific immunosuppressant and corticosteroids.

    b. Interleukin-2 for kidney transplant clients.

    c. Dosage adjustment for each client.

    d. Monitoring for bacterial and fungal infections.

39. Match the medications on the right with their actions on the left.

Actions	Medications
___ a. Converts to an antimetabolite that inhibits DNA synthesis and cell division in T- and B-lymphocytes and myeloid cells	1. Cyclosporine
	2. Azathioprine
	3. Mycophenolate mofetil
	4. Tacrolimus/ FK506
___ b. Directly cytotoxic to circulating lymphocytes and suppresses bone marrow stem cell proliferation	5. Corticosteroids
	6. Antithymocyte globin
	7. Interleukin-2 receptor antagonist
___ c. Reduces T-lymphocyte production of cytokines that are important in stimulating T-lymphocyte proliferation and activation	8. Muromonab-CD3
___ d. Action similar to cyclosporine	
___ e. Selectively inhibits T- and B-lymphocyte proliferation by interfering with purine synthesis and cell division	
___ f. Binds to the OKT3 receptors on lymphocytes, which regulate the receptor action	
___ g. Depletes existing T-lymphocytes through antigen-antibody binding actions	
___ h. Binds to interleukin-2 receptors; found on activate lymphocytes, especially helper/inducer T-cells, preventing proliferation and limiting activation	

40. Identify each drug with its corresponding descriptor. *Answers may be used more than once.*

Descriptors

___ a. Is a monoclonal antibody raised in a mouse model that has limited duration of action

___ b. Induces general immunosuppression, suppresses adrenal cortical activity, and has numerous metabolic and endocrine side effects

Drug Names

1. Cyclosporine
2. Azathioprine
3. Mycophenolate mofetil
4. Tacrolimus/ FK506
5. Corticosteroids
6. Antithymocyte globulin
7. Interleukin-2 receptor antagonist
8. Muromonab- CD3

___ c. Has fewer side effects than azathioprine and has been demonstrated to be more effective as part of triple therapy in clients after kidney transplantation

___ d. Used as initial induction therapy and not as continuing therapy; is approved as prophylaxis for kidney transplant only

___ e. Has nephrotoxic, neurotoxic, and hepatoxic precautions because blood levels are sensitive to the presence of other drugs

___ f. Is a polyclonal antibody raised in horses; side effects increase on re-exposure; has limited duration of action

___ g. Used primarily in liver transplantation; do not administer with cyclosporine; may be used as rescue agent in kidney rejection

___ h. Has high incidence of nausea and vomiting and suppresses hematologic functions

___ i. Induction of capillary leak syndrome is common

STUDY GUIDE NUMBER 5.21

Interventions for Clients with Connective Tissue Disease

Study/Review Questions

1. Identify these abbreviations commonly used in relation to connective tissue disease.

   CTD _____

   DJD _____

   OA _____

   HRT _____

   ERT _____

   ESR _____

   TJR _____

   THR _____

   DVT _____

   TKR _____

   RA _____

   TMJ _____

   PSS _____

   SLE _____

2. A rheumatic disease is any condition or disease of the:
   a. Blood.
   b. Bone.
   c. Muscle.
   d. Musculoskeletal system.

3. CTDs are characterized by:
   a. Chronic pain.
   b. Muscle spasms.
   c. Decreased function.
   d. *a* and *b*

4. A client describing osteoarthritis or DJD may state that he or she has " _____."

5. Identify the two characteristics of DJD:
   a. _____
   b. _____

6. The most common sites for osteoarthritis are:
   a. Hands, back, hips, and knees.
   b. Hands, elbows, and pelvis.
   c. Hands, back, and pelvis.
   d. Knees, hips, and back.

7. During erosion of the cartilage, which of the following also occurs?
   a. Inflammatory enzymes enhance tissue deterioration.
   b. Fissures, pitting, and ulceration develop.
   c. Pain is decreased.
   d. Joint contractures occur.

8. Identify three types of factors that may be attributed to development of DJD.
   a. _____
   b. _____
   c. _____

9. The occurrence of DJD in the hips and knees is common in clients who are _____.

10. DJD is a universal problem that:
    a. Increases with age.
    b. Has a very high incidence in women.
    c. Has a very high incidence in men.
    d. Is common in thin people.

11. A client would describe crepitus as:
    a. Spasms of surrounding muscles.
    b. Pain with motion.
    c. Continuous grating sensation.
    d. Bony lumps.

12. Characteristics of Heberden's nodes may be which of the following?
    a. Painless but swollen
    b. Painful and swollen
    c. Painful, swollen, and inflamed
    d. Swelling, with or without pain or inflammation

13. Presence of fluid in the knees may be diagnosed as:
    a. Subcutaneous swelling.
    b. Nodules.
    c. Joint effusions.
    d. Joint deformities.

14. DJD may affect the spine as:
    a. Pain at L3-L4, bone spurs, stiffness, muscle spasm.
    b. Radiating pain at L3-L4, C4-C6, stiffness and muscle spasms, bone spurs.
    c. Radiating pain, stiffness, muscle spasm, bone spurs.
    d. Radiating pain throughout spine, stiffness, muscle spasms.

15. Clients with DJD may present with:
    a. Behaviors of the grieving process and depression related to role changes.
    b. Anger, depression, and malaise related to role changes.
    c. Depression, dehydration, malaise and grieving.
    d. Weakness, anger, depression, and euphoria.

16. To determine an alteration in a client's body image and self-esteem, what should the nurse assess? *Check all that apply.*
    ___ a. Personal care of self
    ___ b. Demeanor as happy or sad
    ___ c. Expression feeling of reacting to change

17. Identify and prioritize at least five nursing diagnoses for the client with DJD.
    a. _____
    b. _____
    c. _____
    d. _____
    e. _____

18. For your client with DJD, identify types of analgesia medication and explain their actions. *Use a separate sheet of paper for your answers.*

19. Identify treatments other than medication that this client may receive for arthritis.
    a. _____
    b. _____
    c. _____
    d. _____
    e. _____

20. When educating a client regarding THR or other TJR, the nurse would first:
    a. Ask the client if he or she knows what is going to happen.
    b. Review instructions.
    c. Assess the client's knowledge and begin education if needed.
    d. Ask the client if the doctor has explained the procedure.

21. During the surgery for TJR, a client will *not:*
    a. Receive an intravenous antibiotic.
    b. Receive blood.
    c. Have an antibiotic in the cement.
    d. Have a local anesthetic.

True or False? Write T *for true or* F *for false in the blank provided.*

___ 22. Polymethyl methacrylate is a fixer that holds new prostheses in place but will most likely need replacement in 10 years.

23. Which of the following about noncemented joint prostheses is *false*?
    a. Referred to as a *press fit*
    b. Come in one size
    c. Are computer designed
    d. Take 6 to 12 weeks to "graft"

True or False? Write T *for true or* F *for false in the blank provided.*

___ 24. After a THR, subluxation or total dislocation can occur if the legs are in adduction.

25. Post-THR the signs of dislocation are:
    a. Swelling of leg, shortening of leg, and leg rotation.
    b. Swelling of hip, shortening of leg, and leg rotation.
    c. Hip pain, shortening of leg, and leg rotation.
    d. Swelling in hip, hip pain, and leg rotation.

26. Dislocation of a THR is treated by:
    a. Manipulation and bedrest.
    b. Manipulation and immobilization.
    c. Manipulation and continuation of previous care.
    d. Bedrest and pain medication.

27. Which of the following should be reported to the physician as a possible sign of infection following a THR?
    a. Confusion, excessive or foul drainage
    b. Swelling of the foot and foul drainage
    c. Temperature elevation and complaints of being hungry
    d. Pain in surgical area

True or False? Write T *for true or* F *for false in the blanks provided.*

___ 28. A TJR client's ESR is elevated, which may indicate infection at the site.

___ 29. Initial drainage from the surgical site of the TJR is most likely to be about 250 mL.

30. Post-TJR the drains placed in surgery are removed:
    a. By the surgeon.
    b. By allowing them to fall out.
    c. After 12 to 24 hours.
    d. a and c

31. Your THR or TKR client will need to have hemoglobin and hematocrit monitored for how long?
    a. The operative day only
    b. Only after a transfusion
    c. Only if there is drainage on the dressings
    d. 2 to 3 days postoperatively

32. Which of the following can reduce blood transfusion reactions? *Check all that apply.*
    ___ a. Autologous transfusions
    ___ b. Iron supplementation
    ___ c. Epoetin alfa may be given
    ___ d. Blood salvage

True or False? Write T *for true or* F *for false in the blank provided.*

___ 33. During the first 2 days postoperatively, the TJR client may need epidural analgesia or patient-controlled analgesia.

34. A client with TJR may receive which type of pain medication postoperatively while in the hospital?
    a. Oral opioids
    b. NSAIDs
    c. Ibuprofen
    d. Tylenol

35. Older clients who have TJR sometimes have problems of:
    a. Disorientation and delirium.
    b. Being unable to sleep.
    c. Pain threshold being very high.
    d. Pain threshold being very low.

36. Identify the most common nursing diagnoses for a client that is postoperative TJR.

37. Postoperative THR clients can develop numerous complications; these can be prevented by:
    a. Bedrest with pillow between the legs.
    b. Adequate diet and fluid intake.
    c. Getting out of bed first postoperative day.
    d. Dangling at the bedside.

38. When caring for a THR client, the nurse should be sure the hip is not flexed greater than 90 degrees. This can be accomplished by using a:
    a. Raised toilet seat.
    b. Straight-back chair.
    c. Hoyer lift.
    d. Wing-backed chair.

39. Which of following statements is *false* regarding inserted prostheses?
    a. A client with a cemented implant can tolerate partial weight-bearing immediately.
    b. A client with an uncemented implant needs to wait until bony in-growth occurs before mobilizing the limb.
    c. A cemented implant needs to be x-rayed in 12 weeks.
    d. An uncemented implant can tolerate toe-touch or no weight-bearing.

40. In THR and TKR the risk of deep vein thrombosis is high. Which of the following statements are *false?*
    a. Older adults are at high risk for DVT because of age and compromised circulation.
    b. Thin clients are more at risk than obese clients.
    c. Clients with a history of DVT are at high risk for recurrence.
    d. The thrombus usually forms in the thigh, where it is more life-threatening.

41. Identify three measures used in the hospital to prevent a DVT.
    a. _____
    b. _____
    c. _____

42. To prevent a DVT, several types of anticoagulant medications can be ordered. The most commonly used is:
    a. Aspirin.
    b. Warfarin.
    c. Subcutaneous low-molecular-weight (LMW) heparin.
    d. Ibuprofen.

43. It is important for clients on anticoagulant therapy to have their blood monitored for:
    a. International normalized ratio (INR) of 2.0 to 3.0.
    b. Hemoglobin.
    c. Hematocrit.
    d. RBCs.

Answer the following two questions on a separate sheet of paper.

44. Develop a teaching plan for your client with TJR who is being discharged. *Use Chart 21-4 in the text.*

45. Identify the parts of the total knee prosthesis.

True or False? Write T for true or F for false in the blank provided.

____ 46. Noncemented implants may be used for a TKR.

47. Postoperative care for TKR may include: *Check all that apply.*
    ____ a. Hot compresses to the incisional area.
    ____ b. Continuous passive motion (CPM) used immediately or several days postoperatively.
    ____ c. Ice packs or cold packs to the incisional area.
    ____ d. The use of a CPM machine in the daytime and an immobilizer at night.

48. Dislocation is rare after a TKR, but the client should avoid what postoperatively?
    a. _____
    b. _____

49. Identify the three most common problems associated with a total shoulder replacement postoperatively.
    a. _____
    b. _____
    c. _____

50. Identify what the major problem associated with total elbow replacement is and why.

51. Postoperative care following finger and wrist replacements includes which of the following? *Check all that apply.*
    ____ a. Joint wrapped in a bulky dressing
    ____ b. Splint, brace, cast, or CPM machine
    ____ c. Abduction pillow
    ____ d. Elevation of the arm to prevent edema

52. Identify the nursing diagnosis and major interventions that would be used for joint replacements.
    Nursing Diagnosis: _____
    Interventions: _____
    a. _____
    b. _____
    c. _____

53. An important health teaching point in client education for a client with TJR is:
    a. Do as much as you can.
    b. Push yourself above what the physical therapist has asked.
    c. Protect the joint.
    d. "No pain, no gain."

54. Arthritis is frustrating and incurable; the nurse should encourage the client to:
    a. Try the "curative" remedies.
    b. Check with the Arthritis Foundation for appropriate modalities.
    c. Buy special liniments and creams.
    d. Take herbals and vitamins.

55. When evaluating client outcomes for arthritis and total joint replacement, the nurse should assess what three things?
    a. _____
    b. _____
    c. _____

56. Rheumatoid arthritis, the second most common disease of connective tissue: *Check all that apply.*
    ___ a. Is a chronic, progressive, systemic inflammatory process.
    ___ b. Primarily affects the synovial joints.
    ___ c. Is known to have periods of remission.
    ___ d. Occurs most often in older men and women.

57. Because of the inflammatory process in RA, a pannus forms in the joint which is:
    a. Scar tissue.
    b. Vascular granulation tissue.
    c. Necrotic tissue.
    d. Fluid.

58. The articulator cartilage erodes and destroys the bone in clients with RA. Identify the resulting four bone changes:
    a. _____
    b. _____
    c. _____
    d. _____

59. The client with RA that has lost bone density has secondarily developed _____.

60. Clients with RA may over a lifetime have:
    a. Spontaneous remissions.
    b. Pathologic changes in organs and systems.
    c. Exacerbations.
    d. All of the above

61. The etiology of RA is unknown, but it is considered to:
    a. Be an autoimmune disease.
    b. Have no genetic predisposition.
    c. Have no relationship to female reproductive hormones.
    d. Be the result of infection.

62. RA attacks primarily clients that are:
    a. Men in their early 40s.
    b. Women 35 to 45 years old.
    c. Men and women 30 years old.
    d. Men 25 years old.

63. On a separate sheet of paper, identify the early manifestation of RA. Review Chart 21-9.

64. Your client comes to the office with the following complaints and you suspect RA. Which of these complaints would be typical?
    a. "My hands are stiff, swollen, and tender."
    b. "My right hand is weak."
    c. "My left hand is stiff and swollen."
    d. "My knees are swollen and stiff."

65. When a client has RA of the temporomandibular joint, the major complaint is:
    a. Pain on chewing and opening the mouth.
    b. Headache at the temple.
    c. Toothache.
    d. Earache.

66. Spinal column involvement for a client with RA is commonly in the:
    a. Lumbar spine.
    b. Sacral spine.
    c. Cervical spine.
    d. Thoracic spine.

67. Complications of spinal involvement in RA may be seen as: *Check all that apply.*
    ____ a. Compression of the phrenic nerve that controls the diaphragm.
    ____ b. Resulting subluxation of the first and second vertebrae.
    ____ c. Becoming quadriplegic or quadiparetic.
    ____ d. Bilateral sciatic pain in the legs.

68. Clients with RA may have Baker's cysts located in the:
    a. Ankle.
    b. Wrists.
    c. Popliteal bursae.
    d. Achilles tendon.

69. In late RA, the client may have systemic involvement called "flares," described as:
    a. Moderate-to-severe weight loss.
    b. Fever and fatigue.
    c. Joint pain.
    d. Joint contractures.

70. Which of the following is *not* consistent with a client with RA?
    a. Ischemic
    b. Malfunctional
    c. Small brownish spots in the nail beds
    d. Subcutaneous nodules

71. What are the respiratory complications of advanced RA?
    a. _____
    b. _____
    c. _____
    d. _____

72. What are the two cardiac complications of advanced RA?
    a. _____
    b. _____

True or False? Write T *for true or* F *for false in the blank provided.*

____ 73. In advanced RA, the client can have iritis and scleritis as ocular complications.

74. In clients with advanced RA, Sjögren's syndrome may develop, which is manifested as:
    a. Dry eyes, dry mouth, and dry vagina.
    b. Obstruction of secretory glands and ducts.
    c. Nodules in the lungs.
    d. Enlarged spleen and liver.

75. A psychosocial exam of a client with advanced RA may reveal:
    a. Role changes.
    b. Poor self-esteem and body image.
    c. Grieving and depression.
    d. Loss of control and independence.

76. The test of choice for diagnosing RA is:
    a. Latex agglutination.
    b. CBC.
    c. Rheumatoid factor test.
    d. Rose-Waaler test.

77. Which of the following may be present for a client with an elevated "sed rate," or ESR? *Check all that apply.*
    ____ a. Inflammation or infection in the body
    ____ b. Monitoring for response to drug therapy for an infection
    ____ c. Vasculitis and organ damage
    ____ d. An allergic reaction to drug therapy

78. What CBC lab values would a nurse expect for a client with RA? *Circle* high *or* low *for each value.*

a. Hemoglobin:	High	Low
b. Hematocrit:	High	Low
c. RBC:	High	Low
d. WBC:	High	Low
e. Platelets:	High	Low

79. Athrocentesis being done on a client with RA may reveal which of the following in the synovial fluid of the joint?
    a. Glucose
    b. Inflammatory cells and immune complexes
    c. Protein, such as albumin
    d. Platelet aggregation

80. The common side effect of salicylates and NSAIDs is _____.

81. Match each drug with the possible side effect for which the nurse should be aware in clients with RA.

    Side Effects
    ____ a. Headache, dizziness, drowsiness
    ____ b. Diabetes, infection, HTN
    ____ c. Gastrointestinal problems
    ____ d. Mouth sores, bone marrow suppression
    ____ e. Rash, blood dyscrasias, renal involvement
    ____ f. Injection site reaction infections and headaches
    ____ g. Tinnitus
    ____ h. Retinal toxicity
    ____ i. Low adverse effects and resistance

    Drugs
    1. Salicylates
    2. NSAIDs
    3. Steroids
    4. Antimalarial drugs
    5. Cytotoxic drugs
    6. Minocycine
    7. Analgesics
    8. Etanercept
    9. Gold salts

82. The client with acute inflammation from RA can be given which of the listed treatments during a consultation with a physical therapist?
    a. Hot and cold packs
    b. Paraffin wax dips
    c. Hydraulic lifts and tub chairs
    d. All of the above

83. On a separate sheet of paper, identify eight complementary and alternative therapies that can be used to relieve pain in the RA client.

84. The RA client needs to be as independent as possible; the nurse should help by: *Check all that apply.*
    ____ a. Doing tasks for the client.
    ____ b. Allowing the client to compensate and accomplish tasks.
    ____ c. Allowing the client to use adaptive devices.
    ____ d. Asking family members to assist the client.

    Answer the following four questions on a separate sheet of paper.

85. Identify signs and symptoms the nurse would note in the RA client with fatigue.

86. Identify the nurse's care plan for the RA client with fatigue.

87. Develop a teaching plan for the RA client.

88. Identify the two types of lupus and describe their differences.

89. A client with recently diagnosed SLE can expect:
    a. An acute inflammatory disorder.
    b. Spontaneous remission and exacerbations.
    c. Symptoms limited to arthritis.
    d. Symptoms limited to skin lesions.

90. The most common cause of death in clients with SLE is:
    a. Cardiac failure.
    b. Skin involvement.
    c. Central nervous system involvement.
    d. Renal failure.

91. The clinical manifestations of SLE are many and varied. Use your physical assessment text and Chart 21-13 to list the common manifestations. *Use a separate sheet of paper for your answer.*

92. Discoid lupus can be diagnosed only by doing a

    _____.

93. RA and SLE are treated with like medications and client teaching. Identify three important differences that a client with SLE should know and practice.
    a. _____
    b. _____
    c. _____

94. Review Chart 21-13 and compare symptoms of SLE and PSS.

95. PSS, or "scleroderma," affects the _____ system the most, but death from PSS is usually caused by _____ involvement.

96. Identify the CREST syndrome that is seen in PSS clients with the worst prognosis.
    a. _____
    b. _____
    c. _____
    d. _____
    e. _____

97. A client with scleroderma may have which of the following problems? *Check all that apply.*
    ____ a. Dysphagia, esophageal reflux, hiatal hernia
    ____ b. Esophagitis and ulcerations
    ____ c. Malabsorption problems causing malodorous diarrhea stools
    ____ d. Butterfly lesions on the face and nose

98. Raynaud's phenomenon in the client with sclero-derma may present as: *Check all that apply.*
    ___ a. Digit necrosis.
    ___ b. Excruciating pain.
    ___ c. Autoamputations of digits.
    ___ d. Periungual lesions.

99. On a separate sheet of paper, identify six client teaching instructions for the PSS client.

100. Primary gout: *Check all that apply.*
    ___ a. Results from medications such as diuretics.
    ___ b. Is sodium urate deposited in the synovium.
    ___ c. Affects large joints most commonly.
    ___ d. Affects middle-aged and older men.

True or False? Write T for true or F for false in the blank provided.

___ 101. For clients with secondary gout, it is important to treat the underlying disorder.

102. Identify the four stages of primary gout.
    a. _____
    b. _____
    c. _____
    d. _____

103. The part of the body first affected by gout is most often the:
    a. Fingers.
    b. Knees.
    c. Great toe.
    d. Shoulder.

True or False? Write T for true or F for false in the blanks provided.

___ 104. A client with acute gout cannot tolerate having the joint touched or moved.

___ 105. The client with chronic gout may have tophi on the outer ear.

106. Identify the two medications most commonly ordered for acute gout.
    a. _____
    b. _____

107. A client with polymyositis that has a heliotrope rash with periorbital edema is diagnosed with _____.

108. Clients with dermatomyositis have weakness and muscle atrophy demonstrated as difficulty swallowing and talking, but they also have high incidences of _____.

109. Polymyalgia rheumatica and temporal arteritis present with: *Check all that apply.*
    ___ a. Stiffness, weakness, and arthralgias.
    ___ b. Low-grade fever.
    ___ c. Decreased ESR.
    ___ d. Polycythemia.

110. Clients with anakalosing spondylitis have the threat of:
    a. Compromised respiratory function.
    b. Cardiac involvement.
    c. Hip pain.
    d. Herniated disks.

111. Identify the three common findings associated with Reiter's syndrome.
    a. _____
    b. _____
    c. _____

112. When the nurse sees a client with Marfan's syndrome, she should expect:
    a. Normal height.
    b. Shortened hands and feet.
    c. Short swollen fingers.
    d. Excessive height.

113. Lyme disease is identified early by: *Check all that apply.*
    ___ a. Known bite from deer tick.
    ___ b. Bull's eye rash at onset.
    ___ c. Hardened nodule at the site of the bite.
    ___ d. High fever at onset.

True or False? Write T for true or F for false in the blanks provided.

___ 114. Lyme disease is treated with antibiotics over an extended period of time (more than 7 to 10 days).

___ 115. Pseudo gout is a mimic of gout depositing uric crystals in the joints.

116. Identify the five primary manifestations of fibromyalgia.
    a. _____
    b. _____
    c. _____
    d. _____
    e. _____

117. Clients with fibromyalgia may need what two categories of drugs to get adequate rest?
    a. _____
    b. _____

STUDY GUIDE NUMBER 5.22

Interventions for Clients with HIV and Other Immunodeficiencies

Study/Review Questions

1. Immunodeficiency:
   a. Causes a decrease in the client's risk for infection.
   b. Is always acquired.
   c. Occurs when a person's body cannot recognize antigens.
   d. Is the same as immunosuppression.

2. Matching:
   ___ a. Last stage of HIV
   ___ b. Impaired ability to neutralize, destroy, or eliminate antigen
   ___ c. Birth
   ___ d. Body cannot recognize infectious agent
   ___ e. Injury, exposure to toxins, medical therapy
   ___ f. Chronic condition of immunodeficiency virus

   1. Primary
   2. Secondary (acquired)
   3. Immunocompromised
   4. Immunodeficiency
   5. HIV
   6. AIDS

True or False? Write T for true or F for false in the blank provided.

___ 3. To be diagnosed with HIV, one must have a CD4 or T-lymphocyte level under 200.

4. Using Figure 22-2 in the textbook, identify the clinical classification (a, b, or c) for the following symptoms and diagnoses:
   ___ Bacterial endocarditis
   ___ Toxoplasmosis
   ___ Lymphadenopathy
   ___ Kaposi's sarcoma
   ___ Generalized lymphadenopathy
   ___ Herpes zoster
   ___ Idiopathic thrombocytopenia
   ___ Fever and diarrhea
   ___ Cytomegalovirus retinitis

True or False? Write T for true or F for false in the blanks provided.

___ 5. HIV is acquired faster by sexual contact than by a tainted transfusion.

___ 6. An opportunistic infection and cancer are easily prevented by the use of antibiotics.

7. Define retrovirus and describe its actions.

8. All of the following are true about HIV except:
   a. HIV hides in the macrophages.
   b. RT enzyme replaces DNA.
   c. It replicates in the T-cells and destroys CD4 surfaces.
   d. It hides in the cells until ready to infect.

9. Indicate which of the following are HIV causes:
   a. Lymphocytopenia.
   b. T-cell dysfunction.
   c. Abnormal function of macrophages, receptors for HIV.
   d. Increased production of antibodies.

10. As the incidence of AIDS increases, the fastest growing group has become:
    a. Men having sex with other men.
    b. IV drug users.
    c. Women and minorities.
    d. Asian and African persons only.

11. A nonprogressor has all of the following similarities *except*:
    a. Has been infected for 10 years.
    b. Is asymptomatic.
    c. Has no CD4 or T-lymphocytes.
    d. Has a strong immune system.

12. Women with HIV may have all of the following symptoms *except*:
    a. Vaginal candidiasis.
    b. Herpes.
    c. Nausea and vomiting.
    d. Pelvic inflammatory disease (PID).

13. Older adults are less at risk for being infected with HIV because:
    a. They possess effective immune systems.
    b. They are less sexually active then younger adults.
    c. Of changes in the moistness of vaginal tissue.
    d. HIV only effects young people.

14. HIV can be prevented by:
    a. Engineering.
    b. Education.
    c. Isolation.
    d. Counseling.

15. HIV can be transmitted by:
    a. Viral contact, sexual contact, and parenteral contact.
    b. Parenteral contact, airborne contact, and perinatal contact.
    c. Sexual contact, parenteral contact, and perinatal contact.
    d. Perinatal contact, sexual contact, and viral contact.

True or False? Write T for true or F for false in the blanks provided.

___ 16. HIV is easily transmitted from an infected male to a female through sexual contact.

___ 17. The higher the degree of blood concentration of HIV, the greater the risk of sexual transmission.

18. HAART (highly activated antiretroviral therapy) has:
    a. Caused no change in the HIV virus.
    b. Decreased the viral load.
    c. Increased viral load.
    d. Made HIV more detectable.

19. Describe the procedure for teaching IV drug users to care for equipment.
    a. _____
    b. _____
    c. _____

20. Seroconversion is:
    a. The time of exposure to HIV.
    b. The time lag between exposure and antibody production.
    c. The antibody production rate.
    d. A measure of HIV exposure.

21. When a person has tested positive for HIV, he or she should expect:
    a. Education.
    b. Pre- and post-counseling.
    c. Psychologic support.
    d. Free syringes.

True or False? Write T for true or F for false in the blanks provided.

___ 22. Once diagnosed with HIV, the client needs to have regular health check-ups because of the many ways the disease acts upon the body.

___ 23. Infections detected early in a client with HIV may be treated effectively.

24. When getting a history from a client with HIV, the nurse should be sure to:
    a. Address sexual practices and history of STDs.
    b. Address history of infectious disease: hepatitis and tuberculosis.
    c. Address family history.
    d. Assess knowledge level of diagnosis, treatment, and community resources.

25. Identify seven of the most common symptoms of HIV.
    a. _____
    b. _____
    c. _____
    d. _____
    e. _____
    f. _____
    g. _____

True or False? Write T for true or F for false in the blanks provided.

___ 26. Pathogenic infections are virulent microorganisms that can occur among any people.

___ 27. Opportunistic infections are usually prevented by a properly functioning immune system of the HIV client.

___ 28. An immunosuppressed person can get opportunistic infections that can be quite virulent.

29. Opportunistic infections observed in AIDS can be:
    a. Protozoan or fungal.
    b. Viral.
    c. Bacterial.
    d. All of the above

30. A client with *Pneumocystis carinii* pneumonia usually presents with which of the following symptoms?
    a. Dyspnea, tachypnea, persistent dry cough, and fever
    b. Cough with copious thick sputum, fever, and dyspnea
    c. Low-grade fever, cough, and shortness of breath
    d. Fever, cough, and vomiting

31. A client presenting with toxoplasmosis may have all of the following *except*:
    a. Difficulty with speech, headaches, seizures.
    b. Headaches, confusion, lethargy, and ingestion of rare meat.
    c. Headaches, nausea and vomiting, and has a cat.
    d. Has a cat, headaches, and lethargy.

32. Cryptosporidiosis is a form of gastroenteritis in which diarrhea that can amount to a loss of:
    a. 1 to 2 L/day.
    b. 15 to 20 L/day.
    c. 3 to 5 L/day.
    d. 5 to 8 L/day.

33. Candidiasis can be found anywhere in the body *except* the:
    a. Mouth and esophagus.
    b. Vagina and mouth.
    c. Nose and ears.
    d. Throat, causing retrosternal pain.

True or False? Write T for true or F for false in the blanks provided.

___ 34. Cryptococcosis has the same symptoms as meningitis.

___ 35. Histoplasmosis starts as a respiratory infection; the spleen and liver are not enlarged.

___ 36. Mycobacterium avium-intracelluare complex (MAC) is the most common bacterial infection that infects the respiratory system and genitourinary tract.

___ 37. A negative PPD test for tuberculosis in a person with anergy is common.

38. Cytomegalovirus (CMV) can present as symptoms in the: *Check all that apply.*
    ___ a. Eyes, causing visual impairment.
    ___ b. Gastrointestinal tract, causing colitis.
    ___ c. Respiratory tract, causing pneumonitis.
    ___ d. The kidneys as glomerulonephritis.

39. The herpes simplex virus (HSV) manifests itself in clients with HIV and AIDS as:
    a. Malignant vesicles that can metastasize.
    b. A chronic ulceration when vesicles rupture.
    c. Vesicles located in the perirectal, oral, and genital areas.
    d. Very painful before the vesicle forms.

40. Varicella-zoster virus (VZV) leaves the nerve endings and appears as _____, which is very painful.

True or False? Write T for true or F for false in the blanks provided.

___ 41. Kaposi's sarcoma, the most common malignancy associated with AIDS, has a high incidence among hemophiliacs with HIV.

___ 42. Lesions resulting from Kaposi's sarcoma are painful and have purulent drainage.

43. Lymphomas associated with AIDS include all of the following *except*:
    a. Non-Hodgkin's B-cell lymphomas and Burkitt's lymphoma.
    b. Immunoblastic lymphoma, primary brain lymphoma.
    c. Non-Hodgkin's B-cell lymphoma, immunoblastic lymphoma.
    d. Burkitt's lymphoma, small cell lymphoma.

True or False? Write T for true or F for false in the blanks provided.

___ 44. AIDS dementia complex (ADC) affects the central nervous system, which refers to infection of the cells in the central nervous system by HIV.

___ 45. Neuropathies and myopathies are accompanied by pain, paresthesias, and ataxia.

___ 46. The emaciation of clients affected with AIDS is caused by the wasting syndrome, which has many factors.

___ 47. A client is leukopenic if the WBC is less than 3500 cell/mm^3 and lymphopenic if lymphocytes are below 1500 cell/mm^3.

___ 48. Clients with HIV should know that as CD4 and CD8 counts lower, clinical manifestations increase.

___ 49. HIV antibodies are tested for by enzyme-linked immunosorbent assay (ELISA) first and then the Western blot analysis for confirmation.

___ 50. A positive Western blot test confirms the AIDS diagnosis.

___ 51. The viral load test measures the presence of genetic material in the client's blood and helps with monitoring the disease progression.

52. Quantitative RNA assays help with:
   a. Monitoring the spread of disease.
   b. Clinical management of the disease.
   c. Effectiveness of the drug regimen.
   d. Diagnosing HIV infection in clients with no symptoms.

53. Identify the nine most common nursing diagnoses and collaborative problems associated with AIDS.
   a. _____
   b. _____
   c. _____
   d. _____
   e. _____
   f. _____
   g. _____
   h. _____
   i. _____

True or False? Write T *for true or* F *for false in the blanks provided.*

___ 54. Antiretroviral medications kill the virus to prevent replication.

___ 55. Highly active antiretroviral therapy (HAART) is effective against infections in HIV.

___ 56. Protease inhibitors block the HIV protease enzyme, prevent viral replication, and prevent release of antigen particles.

___ 57. Protease inhibitors make the protease work on the drug rather than on large protein.

___ 58. Ribonucleotide reductase inhibitors are cytotoxic drugs that interfere with DNA synthesis and stop viral replication.

59. Ways to reconstitute the immune system are by: *Check all that apply.*
   ___ a. Bone marrow transplant.
   ___ b. Lymphocyte transfusion.
   ___ c. Administration of interleukin-2.
   ___ d. Radiation therapy.

60. Pentamidine isethionate can be administered to a client with *Pneumocystis carinii* pneumonia (PCP) by all of the following routes *except*:
   a. Orally.
   b. Intravenously.
   c. Intramuscularly.
   d. By aerosol.

61. Severe pain in HIV disease and AIDS is caused by: *Check all that apply.*
   ___ a. Enlarged organs.
   ___ b. Peripheral neuropathy.
   ___ c. Tumors.
   ___ d. High fevers.

True or False? Write T *for true or* F *for false in the blanks provided.*

___ 62. Pain for clients with AIDS is managed by NSAIDs and tricyclic antidepressants.

___ 63. Codeine and morphine are not drugs of choice for moderate-to-severe pain in a client with AIDS.

___ 64. Total parental nutrition can help the client achieve adequate protein intake and nutrition.

___ 65. Lomotil should *not* be given on a regular schedule as an antidiarrheal medication.

66. Kaposi's sarcoma can be treated with: *Check all that apply.*
   ___ a. Radiotherapy.
   ___ b. Chemotherapy.
   ___ c. Cryotherapy.
   ___ d. Surgery.

67. Abscesses should be cleaned by:
   a. Sterile saline and dry dressing.
   b. Hydrotherapy.
   c. Betadine and then allowed to air dry.
   d. Sterile water and sterile dressing.

68. Keeping a client oriented can be done by:
   a. Repeating person, place, and time.
   b. Clocks and calendars.
   c. Giving the MMSE screening test.
   d. Having familiar items present.

69. Malnutrition is common in clients with AIDS and also in the chronically ill. On a separate sheet of paper, identify four points the nurse should keep in mind in relation to malnutrition.

70. Protein-calorie malnutrition is usually manifested by what symptoms?

    a. _____

    b. _____

    c. _____

    d. _____

    e. _____

    f. _____

    g. _____

    h. _____

True or False? Write T for true or F for false in the blanks provided.

____ 71. Obese clients have a higher incidence of infections, impaired cell-mediated immunity, and decreased intracellular killing by neutrophils.

____ 72. Obese clients are *not* malnourished.

____ 73. Immunodeficiencies may be induced by drugs or other treatments as desired for transplantation.

____ 74. Cytotoxic drugs cause immunosuppression by interfering with the ability of lymphocytes to synthesize and release products such as lymphokines and antibodies.

____ 75. Corticosteroids have both anti-inflammatory and immunosuppressive effects.

76. Corticosteroids perform which of the following actions? *Check all that apply.*

    ____ a. Inhibit inflammation by stabilizing vascular membranes and decreasing permeability.

    ____ b. Increase cell production in the bone marrow.

    ____ c. Interfere with immunoglobulin G synthesis and immunoglobulin binding to antigen.

    ____ d. Cause cancer cells to multiply.

True or False? Write T for true or F for false in the blanks provided.

____ 77. Radiation can cause immunodeficiency.

____ 78. Immunosuppression is not as severe if the client is receiving radiation and chemotherapy at the same time.

____ 79. Congenital immunodeficiencies are inherited as an X-linked trait.

____ 80. Bruton's agammaglobulinemia is congenital, is usually seen in girls at 6 months of age, and can be treated with regular administration of immune serum globulin every 3 to 4 weeks.

STUDY GUIDE NUMBER 5.23

Interventions for Clients with Immune Function Excess: Hypersensitivity (Allergy) and Autoimmunity

Study/Review Questions

True or False? Write T for true or F for false in the blank provided.

____ 1. Inflammatory and immune responses can be beneficial for protection and can stimulate cell growth.

2. "Over-reactions" to invaders or foreign antigens can be the result of: *Check all that apply.*

    ____ a. Hypersensitivity.

    ____ b. Allergic response.

    ____ c. An autoimmune response.

    ____ d. Phagocytosis.

3. Hypersensitivity, or allergy, is a state of increased or excessive response to the presence of an antigen. Symptoms may include:
    a. Sneezing, anaphylaxis, and watery eyes.
    b. Itching, sneezing, circulatory collapse, and vomiting.
    c. Watery eyes, constipation, and skin rash.
    d. Watery eyes, asthma, bruising, and anaphylaxis.

4. A type I hypersensitivity reaction, or atopic allergy, causes:
   a. Increased production of platelets, basophils, mast cells, and immunoglobulin E.
   b. Increased production of immunoglobulin E, release of histamine, and vasoactive amine from basophils, eosinophils, and mast cells.
   c. Decreased production of immunoglobulin E, release of histamine, and vasoactive amine from basophils, eosinophils, and mast cells.
   d. An acute inflammatory reaction that occurs without the presence of the antigen.

5. Identify four types of type I hypersensitivity reactions.

6. The most acute and deadly response to an antigen is _____.

True or False? Write T *for true or* F *for false in the blanks provided.*

___ 7. Rhinitis may or may not be an allergic response.

___ 8. "Hay fever" and "seasonal" rhinitis may occur at the same time each year.

9. Match the following reactions with their accompanying symptoms.

Reactions	Symptoms
___ a. Autoimmune destruction of lacrimal, salivary, and vaginal mucus-producing glands	1. Autoimmunity
	2. Allergic rhinitis
	3. Anaphylaxis
	4. Latex allergy
	5. Cytotoxic reaction
	6. Stimulating reaction
___ b. Special autoantibodies directed against self cells or tissue with some foreign protein attached	7. Sjögren's syndrome
___ c. Tissue responding to the autoantibody is "out of control" from the body's normal feedback system of checks and balances	
___ d. Life-threatening hypersensitivity reaction that rapidly and systemically affects multiple organs	
___ e. Hay fever, airborne allergens; may be non-allergic	
___ f. Type I sensitivity reaction to a specific allergen	
___ g. Antibodies and/or lymphocytes are directed against healthy normal cells and tissue	

10. Match the body's reactions with their corresponding causes:

Reactions	Causes
___ a. Increases capillary permeability, nasal and conjunctival mucous secretions, and itching	1. Allergens
	2. Degranulation
	3. Histamine
	4. Rhinorrhea
___ b. Promotes allergic sensitization with IgE	
___ c. Runny nose, clear drainage, and pink mucosa	
___ d. Sensitive skin	

11. Allergy management is treated by all of the following therapies *except:*
    a. Avoidance.
    b. Desensitization.
    c. Conization.
    d. Antibiotics.

12. Identify which of the following methods are used for testing for allergies. *Check all that apply.*
    ___ a. In vitro
    ___ b. Scratch
    ___ c. Intravenous
    ___ d. Intradermal

13. Match the following drug types with their corresponding actions:

Actions	Drug Types
___ a. Competes for histamine at histamine receptor sites	1. Decongestant
	2. Antihistamine
	3. Corticosteroids
	4. Mast cell stabilizers
___ b. Causes vasoconstriction, reducing edema; may be combined with anti-cholinergics	5. Leukotriene antagonist
___ c. Decreases inflammation and immune response in a short time	
___ d. Prevents mast cells from opening when allergen binds with IgE	
___ e. Prevents leukotriene synthesis and blocks leukotriene receptors	

True or False? Write T *for true or* F *for false in the blanks provided.*

___ 14. Desensitization therapy can last 5 years.

___ 15. In desensitization therapy, very small amounts of allergen are injected initially and are too low to bind with IgE but do induce IgE stimulation.

___ 16. Allergens that bind to IgG trigger degranulation and are removed by precipitation.

17. Identify the most common complaints of a client experiencing anaphylaxis.

a. _____

b. _____

c. _____

d. _____

e. _____

f. _____

18. A client in anaphylaxis who is going into respiratory failure will demonstrate which of the following symptoms? *Check all that apply.*

___ a. Laryngeal edema

___ b. Hypoxemia

___ c. Hypocapnia

___ d. Dehydration

19. As nurse for the client with anaphylaxis described above, you would expect to find:

a. Hypertension and rapid pulse.

b. Hypotension and rapid pulse.

c. Hypertension and bounding pulse.

d. Hypotension and bounding pulse.

True or False? Write T *for true or* F *for false in the blanks provided.*

___ 20. Anaphylaxis requires the nurse to inject epinephrine (1:1000) 0.3 to 0.5 mL subcutaneous stat and repeat in 15 minutes, as ordered.

___ 21. The body's response to epinephrine is constriction of the blood vessels, increased myocardial contractions, and dilation of bronchioles.

___ 22. During anaphylaxis, an antihistamine may be given to block histamine and an endotracheal tube may be inserted or a tracheostomy may be performed.

___ 23. The anaphylactic client should be observed for fluid overload.

___ 24. Latex allergies are confined to the skin, so latex-free gloves are the only necessary precaution for those with a latex allergy.

___ 25. A person who is allergic to bananas must be aware of the possibility that he or she could develop a latex allergy.

26. Type II cytotoxic reactions include which of the following? *Check all that apply.*

___ a. Coomb's-positive hemolytic anemias, Goodpasture's syndrome

___ b. Hemolytic transfusion reactions, drug-induced hemolytic anemia

___ c. Systemic lupus erythematosus, rheumatoid arthritis

___ d. Thrombocytopenia purpura, hemolytic disease of the newborn

27. On a separate sheet of paper, define hemolytic transfusion reaction.

28. Your client is experiencing a cytotoxic reaction. As the nurse, what is your first intervention?

True or False? Write T *for true or* F *for false in the blanks provided.*

___ 29. In a type III immune complex reaction, the deposited immune complex activates complement, and tissue and vessel damage results.

___ 30. Rheumatoid arthritis is caused by lodged complexes in the joints that destroy tissue and cause scarring and fibrous changes.

31. Identify clinical manifestations of systemic lupus erythematosus that are caused by immune complex reaction.

a. Vasculitis, nephritis, arthritis

b. Hypertension, anemia

c. Constipation, diarrhea

d. Increased urinary output, cystitis

32. Serum sickness happens because:

a. Vaccines are no longer made from horse and rabbit serum.

b. Clients are less allergic now.

c. Penicillin and related drugs and some animal serum are antitoxins.

d. Of NSAIDs and gold toxicity.

True or False? Write T *for true or* F *for false in the blank provided.*

___ 33. To suppress the immune response after organ transplant, lymphocyte globulin and antithymocyte globulin are used.

34. Identify the type VI delayed hypersensitivity reactions. *Check all that apply.*

___ a. PPD test for tuberculosis, poison ivy

___ b. Insect sting

___ c. Allograft rejections and granulomatous diseases

___ d. Poison ivy

35. _____ is the oral drug of choice for type VI delayed hypersensitivity reactions.

36. On a separate sheet of paper, define type V stimulating response and identify the common form of hyperthyroidism.

37. The most important aspect of treating type V stimulating reactions is:
    a. Medication management.
    b. Removing enough of responding tissue for the organ to return to normal functioning.
    c. Monitoring for other organ involvement.
    d. Surgical removal of responding tissue.

38. On a separate sheet of paper, define autoimmunity.

39. Identify which of the following are types of autoimmune diseases. *Check all that apply.*
    ____ a. Polyarteritis nodosa
    ____ b. Systemic lupus erythematosus
    ____ c. Autoimmune hemolytic anemia
    ____ d. Rheumatic fever
    ____ e. Hashimoto's thyroiditis

40. Clients with connective tissue disorders would typically show signs of all of the following *except*:
    a. Auto antibodies have been detected.
    b. These are organ-specific autoimmunities.
    c. These are organ nonspecific autoimmunities.
    d. Management is dependent on affected organs.

41. Autoimmune diseases occur mostly in:
    a. African-American women.
    b. Asian-American women.
    c. White women.
    d. All nationalities.

42. Sjögren's syndrome appears mostly in:
    a. Men 35 to 40 years of age.
    b. Women younger than 25 years of age.
    c. Women 35 to 40 years of age.
    d. Men and women 35 to 40 years of age.

43. The most common cause of Sjögren's syndrome is:
    a. Bacteria.
    b. Virus.
    c. Inflammation.
    d. Infection.

44. As the nurse, you suspect Sjögren's syndrome because the client has the following complaints:
    a. Blurred vision, thick mattering in the conjunctiva.
    b. Burning and itching of the eyes.
    c. Difficulty swallowing and changes in taste sensation.
    d. All of the above.

45. Physical examination of your client with Sjögren's syndrome reveals which of the following? *Check all that apply.*
    ____ a. Enlarged lymph glands
    ____ b. May have swollen, painful joints
    ____ c. Hypertension

46. As the nurse, you would expect the lab results on a client with Sjögren's syndrome to include: *Check all that apply.*
    ____ a. Increased presence of general antinuclear antibodies.
    ____ b. Elevated levels of IgM rheumatoid factor.
    ____ c. Decreased presence of anti-SS-A or anti-SS-B antibodies.
    ____ d. Decreased erythrocyte sedimentation rate.

47. Match each symptom with the appropriate intervention/treatment. *Some treatments are used for more than one symptom.*

Treatments	Symptoms
____ a. Water-soluble lubricants	1. Dry eyes
____ b. Artificial tears	2. Dry mouth
____ c. Systemic pilocarpine	3. Vaginal dryness
____ d. Corticosteroids	4. Pain control
____ e. Artificial saliva	
____ f. Blocking tear outflow duct	
____ g. NSAIDs	

48. The autoimmune disorder Goodpasture's syndrome is a disorder of autoantibodies against:
    a. Anti-SS-A antibodies.
    b. Anti-SS-B antibodies.
    c. Glomerular basement membrane and neutrophils.
    d. None of the above.

49. The symptoms of Goodpasture's syndrome include: *Check all that apply.*
    ____ a. Hemoptysis.
    ____ b. Increased urine output.
    ____ c. Bradycardia.
    ____ d. Weight loss.
    ____ e. Generalized edema.

50. The cause of death in Goodpasture's syndrome is usually _____.

51. The main form of drug therapy for Goodpasture's syndrome is usually what?

STUDY GUIDE NUMBER 5.24

Altered Cell Growth and Cancer Development

Study/Review Questions

1. Malignant cell growth, or cancer, is ever increasing; it is the nurse's responsibility to:
   a. Make a diagnosis.
   b. Know it can be prevented.
   c. Educate the public.
   d. Treat the client.

2. Identify the cancers being targeted in Healthy People 2010:
   a. Testicular, colorectal, cervical, throat, skin, and alcohol- and tobacco-related
   b. Alcohol- and tobacco-related, cervical, breast, skin, colorectal, and testicular
   c. Colorectal, cervical, skin, throat, breast, and alcohol- and tobacco-related
   d. Lung, liver, throat, breast, colorectal, testicular, skin, and cervical

True or False? Write T for true or F for false in the blank provided.

___ 3. Cell division (mitosis) happens throughout our lives at a well-controlled rate to maintain the tissues and organs.

4. Which of the following statements is true regarding hypertrophy and hyperplasia?
   a. They are the same, except that one is in an organ and the other is in tissue.
   b. Hypertrophy is the expansion of cells; hyperplasia is an increased number of cells.
   c. Hypertrophy is an increase in the number of cells; hyperplasia is the expansion of cells.
   d. Hypertrophy is a decrease in the number of cells; hyperplagia is the shrinkage of cells.

5. A neoplasia: *Check all that apply.*
   ___ a. Is new or continued cell growth that is not needed.
   ___ b. Is always malignant.
   ___ c. Has a parent cell that was normal.
   ___ d. Typically leads to death.

6. Cell mitosis happens: *Check all that apply.*
   ___ a. To develop malignancies.
   ___ b. To replace lost or damaged tissue.
   ___ c. When body conditions and nutrition are decreased.
   ___ d. To develop normal tissue.

True or False? Write T for true or F for false in the blanks provided.

___ 7. Normal body cells are recognized by their appearance, size, and shape.

___ 8. Each cell in the body performs one special function that contributes to homeostasis.

___ 9. All cells produce fibronectin, which binds them closely together so they do not migrate.

___ 10. All cells capable of mitosis have a specific pattern or cycle they follow.

___ 11. Most cells in the body spend their existence in a resting state or GO cycle.

___ 12. Embryonic cells are termed *anaplasia*.

13. Embryonic cells are not committed to a specific cell type, so they can be called:
   a. Pluripotency.
   b. Multipotency.
   c. Totipotency.
   d. All of the above.

True or False? Write T for true or F for false in the blank provided.

____ 14. Proto-oncogenes are present only in the embryonic stage to stop the early rapid growth.

15. When an embryonic cell is given a specific function or is "turned on," it is being:
    a. Repressed.
    b. Suppressed.
    c. Expressed.
    d. Depressed.

16. Characteristics of benign cells include: *Check all that apply.*
    ____ a. Being tissue unnecessary for normal function; following normal growth patterns.
    ____ b. Resembling the parent tissue; adhering to each other.
    ____ c. Having a small nucleus; being nonmigratory.
    ____ d. Performing their differentiated function.

17. Which of the following statements is *true* of cancer cells? *Check all that apply.*
    ____ a. They are slow-growing.
    ____ b. They serve no useful purpose.
    ____ c. They are harmful to the body.
    ____ d. They are abnormal.

18. Cancer cells spread throughout the body because: *Check all that apply.*
    ____ a. They make little fibronectin.
    ____ b. They are able to metastasize.
    ____ c. They are persistent in their growth.
    ____ d. Cell division occurs under adverse conditions.

True or False? Write T for true or F for false in the blank provided.

____ 19. In carcinogenesis and oncogenesis, a normal cell undergoes malignant transformation.

20. The actions of carcinogens include: *Check all that apply.*
    ____ a. Damaging the DNA.
    ____ b. Changing the activity of a cell.
    ____ c. Turning on proto-oncogenes.
    ____ d. Creating allergic reactions.

True or False? Write T for true or F for false in the blanks provided.

____ 21. Initiators start nonreversible mutations in a normal cell.

____ 22. Once a cell has been initiated, it has a latency period that does not last long.

23. The initiated cell response to the promoter may result in:
    a. Promoted or enhanced cell growth.
    b. Shortened latency period.
    c. Lengthened latency period.
    d. *a* and *b*

24. Promoters may include of the following? *Check all that apply.*
    ____ a. Chemicals
    ____ b. Hormones
    ____ c. Drugs
    ____ d. Antibodies

True or False? Write T for true or F for false in the blanks provided.

____ 25. As the tumor cells grow, there are changes within the tumor cells themselves allowing for "selection advantages."

____ 26. The primary tumor is not from the original transformed normal cells.

27. Primary tumors located in vital organs can do which of the following? *Check all that apply.*
    ____ a. "Crowd out" the organ
    ____ b. Lethally damage the organ
    ____ c. Interfere with the organ's functioning
    ____ d. Increase function of the organ initially

True or False? Write T for true or F for false in the blank provided.

____ 28. Primary tumors in the soft tissue usually do not cause death.

29. Metastatic or secondary tumors: *Check all that apply.*
    ____ a. Are caused by cells breaking off the primary tumor and forming remote colonies.
    ____ b. Contain the same original altered tissue.
    ____ c. Rarely occur in humans.
    ____ d. Grow as tissue to the organ they spread to.

30. During metastasis, which of the following actions take place? *Check all that apply.*
    ____ a. The tumor secretes enzymes to open areas and cells use mechanical pressure.
    ____ b. Enzymes open up pores in client's blood vessels.
    ____ c. Clumps of the cells break off for transport.
    ____ d. Cells stop circulating (arrest) and then invade.

True or False? Write T for true or F for false in the blank provided.

____ 31. During metastasis, local seeding takes place near the primary site.

True or False? Write T for true or F for false in the blank provided.

___ 32. Lymphatic spread is usually to primary sites with few lymph nodes.

33. A "high-grade" tumor: *Check all that apply.*
    ___ a. Barely resembles the parent cell.
    ___ b. Is slow growing.
    ___ c. Rapidly metastasizes.
    ___ d. Is the easiest to treat.

34. Grading cells from a tumor is the first most important step because it:
    a. Confirms a diagnosis of cancer.
    b. Helps decide appropriate therapy.
    c. Helps determine a prognosis.
    d. Determines nursing diagnoses.

35. Tumor staging is determined by: *Check all that apply.*
    ___ a. Type of cancer cell.
    ___ b. Exact location.
    ___ c. Degree of metastasis.
    ___ d. Size of the tumor.

36. Clinical staging includes all of the following except:
    a. Clinical signs and tests.
    b. Biopsy.
    c. Major surgery.
    d. Evaluation.

True or False? Write T for true or F for false in the blank provided.

___ 37. Pathologic staging is definitive and done with tissue taken during surgery.

38. The primary factors influencing the development of cancer are: *Check all that apply.*
    ___ a. Environmental exposure to carcinogens.
    ___ b. Gender of the client.
    ___ c. Genetic predisposition.
    ___ d. Immune function.

True or False? Write T for true or F for false in the blanks provided.

___ 39. Primary prevention means cancer can be prevented by avoidance.

___ 40. When exposure to a carcinogen cannot be avoided, it is important to have secondary prevention.

___ 41. Oncogenes are a normal part of every cell.

42. Extrinsic factors for causing cancer can be all of the following *except*:
    a. Chemical.
    b. Physical.
    c. Emotional.
    d. Viral agents.

43. Which cells that undergo mitotic cell division are found in the most common areas for development of cancer? *Check all that apply.*
    ___ a. Brain
    ___ b. Skin
    ___ c. Lining of the gastrointestinal tract
    ___ d. Bone marrow

True or False? Write T for true or F for false in the blank provided.

___ 44. It is rare to see a cancer in the nerve tissue, heart muscle, and skeletal muscles.

45. Tobacco use accounts for 30% of all cancers in North America. The highest exposure to tobacco is from:
    a. Ingesting it.
    b. Inhaling tobacco smoke.
    c. Secondhand smoke.
    d. Chewing it.

True or False? Write T for true or F for false in the blank provided.

___ 46. Two types of physical agents are radiation and chronic irritation.

47. Radiation, even in small doses, can affect cells. Radiation occurs naturally in all of the following except:
    a. Radon.
    b. Uranium.
    c. Radium.
    d. Soil.

48. The most common form of radiation is _____ _____ radiation.

True or False? Write T for true or F for false in the blank provided.

___ 49. Sources of ultraviolet (UV) rays that most commonly cause skin cancer include sun tanning and tanning beds.

50. A few viruses are known carcinogens or oncoviruses because they: *Check all that apply.*
    ___ a. Infect the cell.
    ___ b. Break the DNA chain.
    ___ c. Insert their own genetic material.
    ___ d. Grow slowly.

True or False? Write T for true or F for false in the blank provided.

___ 51. The relationship of cancer and dietary practices is being investigated, and some recommendations have been made to promote better health.

52. The immune system protects the body from cancer by using:
    a. Cell-mediated immunity.
    b. Natural killer cells.
    c. Antibody-mediated immunity.
    d. Helper T-cells.

True or False? Write T for true or F for false in the blanks provided.

___ 53. Children under 2 years of age and adults over 60 years of age have adequate immune systems.

___ 54. Clients taking immunosuppressants do not have a higher rate of cancer.

___ 55. Clients with AIDS have a very high incidence of cancer.

56. The single most important risk factor for developing cancer is _____.

57. The nurse educating the client on cancer detection should:
    a. Teach what the client wants to hear.
    b. Take into consideration whether the client is male or female.
    c. Teach the seven warning signs of cancer.
    d. Ask the client what he or she wants.

58. Using Table 24-14 in the textbook, identify four cancers that have genetic predisposition.

59. The culture with the highest rate of incidence, death rate, and increase in incidence of cancer is:
    a. Whites.
    b. Hispanics.
    c. African Americans.
    d. Asian Americans.

60. The American Cancer Society reports that the cancer incidence and survival rate are related to: *Check all that apply.*
    ___ a. Gender.
    ___ b. Availability of health care services.
    ___ c. Early health care.
    ___ d. Age.

61. Avoidance of potential carcinogens can be practiced by:
    a. Daily exercise.
    b. Protecting skin from UV rays.
    c. Moisturizing the skin.
    d. Avoiding tobacco.

True or False? Write T for true or F for false in the blanks provided.

___ 62. Some cancers can be avoided by modifying diets and changing lifestyles.

___ 63. Chemoprevention, a new form of prevention, uses an exogenous chemical to disrupt cancer development.

___ 64. Chemoprevention agents block the steps in the process of cancer development.

___ 65. Gene therapy is being used to alter cancer cells.

STUDY GUIDE NUMBER 5.25

Interventions for Clients with Cancer

Study/Review Questions

1. Statistics show the following facts about cancer: *Check all that apply.*
    ___ a. Over 50% of people in North America will be diagnosed with cancer.
    ___ b. People rarely die from cancer.
    ___ c. 50% of those diagnosed will be cured.
    ___ d. Surgery is the most effective cure.

2. Untreated cancers can cause: *Check all that apply.*
    ___ a. Impaired immune and hematopoietic function.
    ___ b. Decreased respiratory function.
    ___ c. Altered gastrointestinal tract structure and function.
    ___ d. Motor and sensory deficits.
    ___ e. Death.

3. Which type of cancer puts clients at increased risk for infection? *Check all that apply.*
   ____ a. Breast cancer
   ____ b. Leukemia
   ____ c. Multiple myeloma
   ____ d. Lymphoma

4. Cancer invading the bone marrow can cause: *Check all that apply.*
   ____ a. Decreased potassium and sodium.
   ____ b. Suppressed production of RBCs, WBCs, and platelets.
   ____ c. Suppressed production of RBCs.
   ____ d. Severe anemia and bleeding tendency.

5. Cachexia describes:
   a. Electrolyte imbalance in the cancer client.
   b. Weight loss in the cancer client.
   c. Extreme body wasting and malnutrition in the cancer client.
   d. Poor food intake of cancer client.

6. Nutrition therapy for cancer clients is a controversial topic. Which of the diet regimens below have been proposed as being effective treatment? *Check all that apply.*
   ____ a. The client needs a high-protein, high-carbohydrate diet.
   ____ b. A diet high in protein, carbohydrates, and vitamins contributes to cancer progression.
   ____ c. Clients should be tube-fed in the terminal stages.
   ____ d. Clients believe eating more food, but only foods that are low-fat and high-fiber, is the best diet.

7. Invasion of the bone usually is caused by metastasizes from: *Check all that apply.*
   ____ a. Prostate cancer.
   ____ b. Brain cancer.
   ____ c. Breast cancer.
   ____ d. Leukemia.

8. Cancer metastases to the brain can cause problems in the: *Check all that apply.*
   ____ a. Sensory areas.
   ____ b. Motor areas.
   ____ c. Cognitive areas.
   ____ d. Limbic system.

True or False? Write T for true or F for false in the blanks provided.

____ 9. Cancers of the lungs are obstructive tumors.

____ 10. Clients with lung cancer can develop pulmonary edema and dyspnea.

____ 11. The goal of cancer treatment is to cure the client.

12. What cancer treatment therapy to use for a specific cancer is determined by the: *Check all that apply.*
   ____ a. Individual or combined treatments available.
   ____ b. Physician's preferred protocol.
   ____ c. Type of cancer and extent of disease.
   ____ c. Overall health of the client.

True or False? Write T for true or F for false in the blanks provided.

____ 13. Surgery for a cancer client may be a part of diagnosis or treatment.

____ 14. Prophylactic surgery is a "cure" for cancer most of the time.

15. Diagnostic surgeries done for the purpose of acquiring biopsies are which of the following? *Check all that apply.*
   ____ a. Needle biopsy
   ____ b. Incisional biopsy
   ____ c. Excisional biopsy
   ____ d. Staging

True or False? Write T for true or F for false in the blank provided.

____ 16. An incisional biopsy removes part of the lesion but *not* the adjacent tissue.

17. Cytoreductive surgery is done to:
   a. Remove all tumor cells.
   b. Decrease the number of cells to be treated.
   c. Locate tumor seeding sites.
   d. Cure the cancer.

18. Palliative surgery is done to improve quality of life by: *Check all that apply.*
   ____ a. Relieving pain.
   ____ b. Relieving an obstruction.
   ____ c. Curing the cancer.
   ____ d. Prolonging life.

True or False? Write T for true or F for false in the blank provided.

____ 19. The purpose of "second-look" therapy is to determine the status of the disease and the course of treatment for the cancer client.

20. Reconstructive surgery is for cancer survivors who may need: *Check all that apply.*
   ____ a. Breast reconstruction.
   ____ b. Revision of scars and release of contractures.
   ____ c. Bowel reconstruction or esophageal repairs.
   ____ d. Coronary artery repair.

True or False? Write T for true or F for false in the blank provided.

____ 21. Clients are so relieved to be rid of a cancer that grieving because of a loss is not common after removal of any body part.

22. A nursing diagnosis for a postsurgical client who has lost a body part is:
    a. Anticipatory Grieving.
    b. Disturbed Body Image.
    c. Anxiety.
    d. Chronic Sorrow.

23. Postsurgical care of a cancer client:
    a. Is no different than caring for any other surgery client.
    b. Involves additional psychosocial factors.
    c. Costs more than care after other types of surgery.
    d. Requires a longer time for recovery of the client.

True or False? Write T for true or F for false in the blank provided.

____ 24. The goal of radiation is to destroy cancer cells within the radiation beam.

25. Exposure of ionizing radiation to a cell causes changes in the:
    a. Electrical charge of the cells.
    b. Fluid volume.
    c. Nucleus.
    d. Extracellular energy.

True or False? Write T for true or F for false in the blanks provided.

____ 26. Cell damage occurs with any exposure to radiation, which may cause the cell to die or lose the ability to divide.

____ 27. Use of radiation is commonly determined by cell cycle.

28. Which type of radiation is used for cancer treatment?
    a. Beta
    b. Gamma
    c. Alpha
    d. Delta

True or False? Write T for true or F for false in the blank provided.

____ 29. According to the inverse square law, the distance from the client receiving the radiation to the source of the radiation does not matter.

30. Which factors are used to determine a cancer client's absorbed radiation dose? *Check all that apply.*
    ____ a. Intensity of radiation exposure
    ____ b. Proximity of radiation source to the cells
    ____ c. Duration of exposure
    ____ d. Age of the client

31. Radiation usually damages the DNA of a cell, but whether this damage has occurred can be determined only when the:
    a. Cell attempts to divide.
    b. Cytoplasm shrinks.
    c. Nucleus does not respond.
    d. Cell becomes misshapen.

True or False? Write T for true or F for false in the blank provided.

____ 32. Each cell has its own response to radiation, such as dying, becoming sterile, or repairing self.

33. Fractionation is used to determine:
    a. Amount of exposure.
    b. Amount of each dose.
    c. Amount of damage.
    d. *a* and *b*

True or False? Write T for true or F for false in the blank provided.

____ 34. Dosages for radiation do not vary much from organ to organ except for the size of the tumor.

35. Teletherapy, or beam therapy, requires that the: *Check all that apply.*
    ____ a. Site at which the beam is directed must be exact.
    ____ b. Client is hazardous after exposure.
    ____ c. Client be given help with positioning if needed.
    ____ d. Client is not allowed to be around other people.

True or False? Write T for true or F for false in the blanks provided.

____ 36. Brachytherapy uses isotopes and is placed on or near the cancer tissue, making the client hazardous to others.

____ 37. Unsealed radiation sources can be given orally, intravenously, or as an instillation in a body cavity, making clients and their excrement radioactive for 48 hours.

____ 38. A common example of an unsealed radiation source is the treatment for thyroid cancer.

___ 39. Needles and seed for sealed radiation sources are placed during surgery and may not need to be removed.

40. Radiation has specific side effects of:
    a. Altered taste sensation and fatigue.
    b. Skin changes and permanent local hair loss.
    c. Skin changes and aversion to red meat.
    d. Fatigue.

41. For the client undergoing external radiation therapy, the nurse's instruction should include: *Check all that apply.*
    ___ a. Do not remove the markings.
    ___ b. Do not use lotions or ointments.
    ___ c. Avoid direct skin exposure to sunlight for up to a year.
    ___ d. Use soap and water on the affected skin.

True or False? Write T for true or F for false in the blank provided.

___ 42. Radiation therapy to the head and neck can cause damage to salivary glands, resulting in xerostomia (dry mouth).

43. Chemotherapy is used in cancer treatment for all of the following reasons *except* to:
    a. Cure.
    b. Increase survival time.
    c. Promote nausea and vomiting.
    d. Decrease the risk for a life-threatening complication.

44. Match each type of chemotherapy with the corresponding action.

Action	Type of Chemotherapy
___ a. Cofactor, vitamins or nucleotides and purines considered "counterfeit;" prevents cell division	1. Antimitotic agent 2. Topoisomerase inhibitor 3. Antimetabolites 4. Antitumor agent 5. Alkylating agent
___ b. Causes major damage to DNA and RNA synthesis	
___ c. Cross-links DNA; prevents RNA synthesis	
___ d. A plant source that interferes with formation of microtubules	
___ e. Causes DNA breakage	

45. The lowest level of bone marrow activity and WBCs is called:
    a. Anemia.
    b. Nadir.
    c. Leukopenia.
    d. Immunosuppression.

46. Each chemotherapeutic agent has a specific nadir. In combination therapy, it is important to:
    a. Give two agents with like nadir.
    b. Avoid giving agents with like nadirs at the same time.
    c. Allow for one agent's nadir to rise before giving another agent.

47. Drug dosage is based on total body surface area (TBSA); therefore it is important for the nurse to:
    a. Ask the client height and weight.
    b. Ask the client height but weigh the client.
    c. Accurately weigh and measure the client.
    d. Record the client's intake and output.

48. A course of chemotherapy normally includes: *Check all that apply.*
    ___ a. Rounds every week for a total of 6 weeks.
    ___ b. Variance with clients' responses to therapy.
    ___ c. Timed dosing the therapy to maximize the cancer cell kill and minimize normal cell damage.
    ___ d. A concurrent dose of radiation.

49. Most chemotherapy is administered intravenously, which has the major potential complication of:
    a. Infiltration.
    b. Bruising.
    c. Extravasation.
    d. Swelling.

50. Vesicants are chemicals that cause damage upon direct contact with tissue and also cause: *Check all that apply.*
    ___ a. Pain.
    ___ b. Infection.
    ___ c. Tissue loss.
    ___ d. At times, a need for surgery.

51. The best treatment for extravasation is:
    a. Surgery.
    b. Prevention.
    c. Hot or cold packs.
    d. Antibiotics.

52. The nurse administering a vesicant must be prepared for complications and know:
    a. The antidote.
    b. The effective treatment.
    c. How to use hot or cold packs.
    d. The type of available dressings.

True or False? Write T for true or F for false in the blank provided.

___ 53. Health care workers should use protective clothing when handling or administering chemotherapy.

54. Side effects associated with chemotherapy include:
    a. Alopecia, nausea and vomiting, and mucositis.
    b. Constipation, nausea, and vomiting.
    c. Pain, alopecia, nausea, and vomiting.
    d. Alopecia, pain, and mucositis.

55. Systemic side effects of chemotherapy include: *Check all that apply.*
    ___ a. Dementia.
    ___ b. Immunosuppression.
    ___ c. Anemia.
    ___ d. Thrombocytopenia.

True or False? Write T for true or F for false in the blank provided.

___ 56. Administration of cytoprotectants can offer some protection to normal cells.

57. Alopecia is the loss of hair on the body or, with some chemotherapy drugs, is only the thinning of hair. When thinning or loss of hair is a known side effect of a drug being administered, the nurse should: *Check all that apply.*
    ___ a. Have the client use gentle hair shampoo.
    ___ b. Help the client select wigs, turbans, or scarves.
    ___ c. Instruct the client that hair loss is permanent.
    ___ d. Remind the client to avoid hairwashing.

58. Chemotherapy-induced nausea and vomiting: *Choose all that apply.*
    ___ a. Is a common side effect of emetogenic agents.
    ___ b. Usually lasts for 1 to 2 days after administration.
    ___ c. Lasts as long as 3 weeks postadministration.
    ___ d. Can happen before client is to receive the next dose as a result of anticipation.
    ___ e. All of the above.

True or False? Write T for true or F for false in the blanks provided.

___ 59. Antiemetics can be given before and after chemotherapy to try to control nausea and vomiting, but each person's response is different.

___ 60. The client with nausea and vomiting needs to be observed for dehydration and electrolyte imbalance.

61. Chemotherapy can cause sores in the mucous membranes; this is referred to as: *Check all that apply.*
    ___ a. Mucositis.
    ___ b. Stomatitis.
    ___ c. Gastritis.
    ___ d. Peritonitis

62. Because of the rapid cell division in the gastrointestinal (GI) tract, chemotherapy:
    a. Kills off the cells.
    b. Prevents the body from replacing cells.
    c. Causes cells to be killed more rapidly than they can be produced.
    d. Helps to increase cell division.

63. Oral care for a client with stomatitis should include: *Check all that apply.*
    ___ a. Observation.
    ___ b. Hard-bristled brush.
    ___ c. Saline mouth wash.
    ___ d. Glycerin swabs.

64. Bone marrow suppression will cause all of the following *except:*
    a. Decreased leukocytes.
    b. Decreased electrolytes.
    c. Decreased erythrocytes.
    d. Decreased platelets.

65. Because of the effects of bone marrow suppression, the complaints of the client being treated with bone marrow suppression would include all of the following *except:*
    a. Hypoxia.
    b. Fatigue.
    c. Nausea.
    d. Increased tendency to bleed.

66. Immunosuppression from chemotherapy: *Check all that apply.*
    ___ a. Is life-threatening.
    ___ b. Increases the body's inflammatory response.
    ___ c. Can cause potential for serious infection.
    ___ d. Is always fatal.

True or False? Write T for true or F for false in the blank provided.

____ 67. Biologic-response drugs stimulate the immune system to produce cells.

68. The nurse is responsible for teaching both the immunosuppressed client and the family about health promoting activities. The most important activity is:
   a. Handwashing.
   b. Hygiene.
   c. Cleaning.
   d. Wearing masks.

True or False? Write T for true or F for false in the blank provided.

____ 69. Biologic-response modifiers are cytokines synthesized by mononuclear phagocytes to make the immune system work better by stimulating the immune system to recognize cancer cells and eliminate or destroy them.

70. Match each biologic-response modifier to its action.

   Action
   ____ a. Binds with cell and prevents cell division
   ____ b. Helps immune system recognize and destroy cancer cells
   ____ c. Helps cancer cells revert to original characteristics

   Modifier
   1. Interleukin
   2. Interferons
   3. Monocolonal antibodies

71. The biologic-response modifiers have which positive effect(s) on the client receiving chemotherapy?
   a. Less risk of life-threatening infections
   b. Increased risk of anemia
   c. Client is able to tolerate lower doses of chemotherapy
   d. Euphoria and increased libido

72. Because side effects of interleukin therapy can be dramatic, the client may need to be treated in a critical care unit because of: *Check all that apply.*
   ____ a. Fluid shifts.
   ____ b. Severe inflammatory reaction.
   ____ c. Capillary leaks.
   ____ d. Nausea and vomiting.

73. An immediate reaction to biologic-response modifier therapy can be:
   ____ a. Fever, chills, nausea and vomiting, malaise.
   ____ b. Fever, chills, rigor, malaise.
   ____ c. Fever, nausea and vomiting, rigors.
   ____ d. Chills, nausea and vomiting, rigors.

True or False? Write T for true or F for false in the blank provided.

____ 74. It is best to treat rigors with phenobarbital and Dilantin, and use acetaminophen for the fever.

____ 75. In the chemotherapy client, there is risk of death from septic shock and disseminated intravascular coagulation (DIC).

____ 76. DIC requires close monitoring because it affects the blood clotting mechanism of the body, making the blood clot and then start hemorrhaging until death occurs.

77. The only way to prevent sepsis and DIC is to use:
   a. Strict aseptic technique.
   b. Handwashing.
   c. Gown and gloving.
   d. Standard precautions.

Interventions for Clients with Infection

Study/Review Questions

1. Match words and definitions related to infection.

Definitions

___ a. Cause agent
___ b. Infection recipient
___ c. Ability to cause disease
___ d. Degree of communicability
___ e. Ability to spread
___ f. Characteristic bacteria
___ g. Pathogenic microbes present but no symptoms
___ h. Live at expense of host
___ i. No response to infection

Terms

1. Subclinical infection
2. Parasite
3. Pathogen
4. Pathogenicity
5. Colonization
6. Invasiveness
7. Susceptible host
8. Virulence
9. Normal flora

2. Using Figure 26-1 in the textbook, review the chain of infection. Describe the two types of animate and inanimate reservoirs.
   a. _____
   b. _____

3. Match each type of pathogen with its description.

Description

___ a. Botulism, tetanus, bacteria in the environment
___ b. Typhoid, produced in cell walls and released by cell lysis
___ c. Protein molecules released by bacteria to cause effect at distant sites

Pathogen

1. Toxin
2. Exotoxin
3. Endotoxin

True or False? Write T for true or F for false in the blank provided.

___ 4. The host has many forms of defense from infection; these can be broken down by immunologic deficiencies.

5. Identify the two types of immunity. Explain the differences and give an example of each.

True or False? Write T for true or F for false in the blank provided.

___ 6. The nurse should talk only to the older adult client who has had pneumonia about getting the pneumonia vaccine.

7. Identify the two factors that relate to infection and give examples of each.

8. Match the portal of entry with the method of transmission. *Answers may be used more than once.*

Method of Transmission

___ a. Droplet
___ b. Ingestion
___ c. Intravascular device
___ d. Mucous membranes
___ e. Insect bite
___ f. Catheterization
___ g. Laceration

Portal of Entry

1. Bloodstream
2. Skin/mucous membrane
3. GU tract
4. GI tract
5. Respiratory tract

9. Match the contact for infection to the mode of transmission. *Answers may be used more than once.*

Contact Site

___ a. Skin-to-skin
___ b. Contaminated article or droplet
___ c. Sneezing
___ d. Contaminated food
___ e. Lyme disease

Mode of Transmission

1. Airborne
2. Vehicle
3. Vector
4. Direct
5. Indirect

True or False? Write T for true or F for false in the blank provided.

___ 10. The portal of exit for an infection may be the same as the portal of entry or may be different.

11. Using Table 26-5 in the textbook, describe the tissue action and defense.

True or False? Write T for true or F for false in the blanks provided.

___ 12. Phagocytosis is the actual engulfing, ingesting, killing, and disposing of an invader, which decreases possible infection.

____ 13. Inflammation does not rely on phagocytes to help reduce swelling and prevent infection and pus formation.

____ 14. The body's defense system has the antibody-mediated immune system, which destroys certain microorganisms, and cell-mediated immunity, which is specific to cells.

Answer the following two questions on a separate sheet of paper.

15. Identify the two types of nosocomial infection and provide examples of each type.

16. Identify the three primary goals of infection control in the community.

True or False? Write T for true or F for false in the blanks provided.

____ 17. Proper handwashing includes friction to remove bacteria.

____ 18. In the health care field, most places of employment allow false fingernails but expect proper handwashing.

____ 19. The use of gloves eliminates the need to wash your hands.

20. Match each precaution with an example of its use.

Use

____ a. All body secretions and excretions, most membranes, and tissue, excluding perspiration, are potentially infectious.

____ b. Uses negative airflow rooms, high-efficiency particulate air (HEPA) filters, or ultraviolet (UV) lights

____ c. Infection transmitted by droplet; an example is meningitis

____ d. Transmission by touch of client or environment; examples are methicillin-resistant *Staphylococcus aureus* (MRSA) and vancomycin-resistant *Enterococcus* (VRE)

Precaution

1. Contact precautions
2. Droplet precaution
3. Standard precaution
4. Airborne precaution

True or False? Write T for true or F for false in the blank provided.

____ 21. Bloodborne pathogen transmission among health care workers is most commonly done by needle stick injury.

22. Complications of infection are usually caused by: *Check all that apply.*
____ a. Incorrect choice of antibiotic.
____ b. Poor client compliance.
____ c. Client unable to afford medication.
____ d. The client's overall health condition.

True or False? Write T for true or F for false in the blank provided.

____ 23. Poor compliance or poor drug choice can result in systemic sepsis or septicemia, which then can lead to death.

24. When getting a history from a client with an infection, it is important to ask about: *Check all that apply.*
____ a. Recent travel.
____ b. Recent insect bites.
____ c. Exposure to contaminated food or water.
____ d. Previous infections.

25. Local symptoms of infection may include: *Check all that apply.*
____ a. Pain and redness.
____ b. Swelling and pus.
____ c. Cool and clammy skin.
____ d. Pustules.

True or False? Write T for true or F for false in the blanks provided.

____ 26. Clients with a fever over 100° F are considered to have a systemic infection.

____ 27. Older adult clients may have a severe infection with no fever.

____ 28. A client with an infectious disease may have coping problems because of malaise and fatigue.

29. Match each diagnostic test with its description.

    Description

    ___ a. Pathogen is isolated for identification
    ___ b. Pathogen is tested for antibiotic reactions
    ___ c. Checks WBC, neutrophils, lymphocytes, monocytes, eosinophils, and basophils
    ___ d. Measures rate of RBC fall through plasma; effectiveness of therapy should show a fall in value
    ___ e. X-ray films used to monitor infection
    ___ f. Noninvasive procedure: used particularly for diagnosing heart valve problems
    ___ g. Use of radioactive agents to determine presence of infection
    ___ h. Tissue culture/specimen

    Test

    1. Biopsy
    2. Scanning
    3. Ultraconography
    4. Radiographic studies
    5. Erythrocyte sedimentation rate
    6. Complete blood count
    7. Culture
    8. Sensitivity

30. Identify two nursing diagnoses for a client with infection.

31. In an infectious client, interventions to reduce fever may include: *Choose all that apply.*
    ___ a. Antipyretic drugs such as aspirin or Tylenol.
    ___ b. External cooling, cooling blankets, cool compresses.
    ___ c. Fluid administration, oral and IV.
    ___ d. Antimicrobial therapy with antibiotic, antiviral, or antifungal agents.

32. Antimicrobials act on pathogens by: *Check all that apply.*
    ___ a. Inhibiting cell wall synthesis (penicillin and cephalosporins).
    ___ b. Injuring cytoplasmic membrane (antifungal agents).
    ___ c. Inhibiting biosynthesis or reproduction (erythromycin).
    ___ d. Inhibiting nucleic acid synthesis (actinomycin).

True or False? Write T for true or F for false in the blanks provided.

___ 33. The client with an infection needs education on the specific infection and the route of transmission to understand the need for isolation.

___ 34. Infectious clients staying in their homes and their families may need instruction on effective dishwashing and care of soiled clothes.

___ 35. The nurse should instruct the client on medication administration, including time, dose, therapeutic effects and side effects, and completion of therapy.

UNIT 6 PROBLEMS OF OXYGENATION: RESPIRATORY TRACT ■ Core Concepts Grid

Anatomy	Physiology	Pathophysiology	History	Physical Exam	Diagnostic Tests	Interventions	Pharmacology

• Upper respiratory tract
• Lower respiratory tract
• Alveolar level
• Thoracic structure
	• Ventilation
	• Thoracic pressure
		• Obstruction
		• Inflammation
		• Trauma
		• Hypoxia
		• Infection
		• Fibrosis
		• Tumor
		• Respiratory failure
			• Risk factors
			  Smoking
			  Age
			  Occupation
			  Previous health
			  Socioeconomic status
			• Cardinal symptoms
			  Fatigue
			  Cough
			  Sputum
			  Chest pain
			• Growth and development
				• Respiratory rate, rhythm, depth
				• Breath sounds
				• Dyspnea
				• Cyanosis/pallor
				• Restlessness
				• Irritability
				• Confusion
				• Hoarseness
				• Dysrhythmias
					• Chest x-ray
					• Arterial blood gas (ABG)
					• Pulse oximetry
					• Lung volumes
					• Sputum cultures
					• Acid-fast bacillus
					• Bronchoscopy
					• Thoracentesis
					• Complete blood count
					• V/Q lung scan
						• Positioning
						• Oxygen
						• Incentive spirometry
						• Chest physiotherapy
						• Postural drainage
						• Breathing techniques
						• Intubation
						  Endotracheal
						  Tracheotomy
						  Tracheostomy
						• Suction
						• Chest tubes
						• Mechanical ventilation
						• Lung transplantation
						• Health teaching
							• Antitussives
							• Anti-infectives
							  Antibiotics
							  Antituberculars
							• Bronchodilators
							• Mucolytics
							• Anti-inflammatory drugs
							• Corticosteroids
							• Chemotherapeutic agents
							• Anticoagulants

Unit 6 (Chapters 27-32)

Problems of Oxygenation: Management of Clients with Problems of the Respiratory Tract

Learning Plan

Chapter 27: *Assessment of the Respiratory System*

Learning Outcomes	Learning Activities	Supplemental Resources
1. Compare and contrast the structures and functions of the upper airways to those of the lower airways. 2. Distinguish between normal and abnormal (adventitious) breath sounds. 3. Describe the respiratory changes associated with aging. 4. Calculate the pack-year smoking history for the client who smokes or who has ever smoked cigarettes. 5. Demonstrate proper technique when using observation and auscultation to assess the respiratory system. 6. Demonstrate proper technique when using palpation and percussion to assess the respiratory system. 7. Interpret arterial blood gas values to assess the client's respiratory status. 8. Prioritize educational needs for the client undergoing pulmonary function tests. 9. Prioritize nursing care for the client after a bronchoscopy or open lung biopsy.	1. Prior to completing the study guide exercises in this chapter, review the following: • Anatomy and physiology of the respiratory tract • Process of respiration • Principles of diffusion, perfusion, and ventilation • Techniques for performing a physical assessment • Principles of blood gas analysis • Normal and adventitious breath sounds 2. Review the **boldfaced** Key Terms and their definitions in Chapter 27 to enhance your understanding of the content. 3. Go to Study Guide Number 6.27 on the following pages and complete the learning exercises for this chapter.	1. Textbook—Chapter 27 2. Other resources: • Grap, M. (1998). Pulse oximetry. *Critical Care Nurse, 18*(1), 94-99. • Guyton, A. & Hall, J. (2000). *Textbook of medical physiology* (10th ed.). Philadelphia: W.B. Saunders. • McConnell, E. (1999). Performing pulse oximetry. *Nursing 99, 29*(11), 17. • Obtain a client's blood gas values and practice interpreting the results. • Obtain audio tapes from the laboratory instructor at the school regarding lung sounds. • Observe a bronchoscopy and postprocedure care. • Observe a pulmonary function test being performed. • Observe the procedure for obtaining a blood gas for analysis. • O'Hanlon-Nichols, T. (1998). The adult respiratory system. *American Journal of Nursing, 98*(2), 39-45. • Practice listening to abnormal lung sounds using proper techniques. Validate findings with another health care professional. • Practice listening to normal lungs utilizing proper techniques. • Review an anatomy and physiology textbook for normal anatomy and physiology of the respiratory system. • Review a pathophysiology textbook for abnormal adventitious breath sounds.

- Salzman, S. (1999). Pulmonary function testing: Tips on how to interpret the results. *Journal of Respiratory Diseases, 20*(12), 809-812.
- St. John, R. & Thomson, P. (1999). Noninvasive respiratory monitoring. *Critical Care Nursing Clinics of North America, 1*(4), 423-435.

Chapter 28: *Interventions for Clients with Oxygen Therapy or Tracheostomy*

Learning Outcomes	Learning Activities	Supplemental Resources
1. Compare and contrast the uses and nursing care issues of oxygen delivery by nasal cannula with oxygen delivery by mask. 2. Explain the problems associated with oxygen therapy for those clients whose respiratory efforts are controlled by the hypoxic drive. 3. Analyze changes in clinical manifestations to determine the effectiveness of therapy for the client receiving oxygen. 4. Use laboratory data and clinical manifestations to determine the presence of hypoxemia or hypercarbia. 5. Prioritize educational needs for the client receiving supportive oxygen therapy at home. 6. Prioritize nursing care for the client with a new tracheostomy. 7. Identify techniques to minimize the risk for aspiration when assisting the client with a tracheostomy to eat.	1. Prior to completing the study guide exercises in this chapter, review the following: 　• Principles of sterile technique 　• Assessment of the respiratory system 　• Acid-base balance 　• Concept of respiratory failure 　• Care of a client receiving enteral feedings 　• Assessment of the respiratory system 2. Review the **boldfaced** Key Terms and their definitions in Chapter 28 to enhance your understanding of the content. 3. Go to Study Guide Number 6.28 on the following pages and complete the learning exercises for this chapter.	1. Textbook—Chapter 27 (Assessment of the Respiratory System) 2. Textbook—Chapter 28 3. Other resources 　• Any anatomy and physiology textbook 　• Any physical assessment textbook 　• Audiovisual materials in the learning lab of the nursing school related to administering oxygen and tracheostomy care 　• Consult with a respiratory therapist regarding devices and equipment for oxygen therapy. 　• Dixon, L. & Wasson, D. (1998). Comparing use and cost effectiveness of tracheostomy tube securing devices. *MEDSURG Nursing, 7*(5), 270-274. 　• Hatfield, B.O. (1997). Cost effective trache teaching. *RN, 60*(3), 48-49. 　• McCloskey, J. & Bulechek, G. (2000). *Nursing interventions classification (NIC)* (3rd ed.). St. Louis: Mosby. 　• Visit a respiratory therapy department.

Chapter 29: Interventions for Clients with Noninfectious Upper Respiratory Problems

Learning Outcomes	Learning Activities	Supplemental Resources

1. Compare the clinical manifestations and care needs of a client with an anterior nosebleed to those of the client with a posterior nosebleed.
2. Prioritize nursing care for a client with facial trauma.
3. Identify the potential complications of sleep apnea.
4. Develop a plan of communication for a client who has a disruption of speech and cannot read.
5. Use clinical manifestations and laboratory data to determine airway adequacy in a client with laryngeal or neck injury.
6. Identify the risk factors that predispose a client to the development of head and neck cancer.
7. Develop a teaching plan for the client who is getting ready to go home after undergoing a complete laryngectomy.
	1. Prior to completing the study guide exercises in this chapter, review the following:
	  • Anatomy and physiology of the respiratory system
	  • Principles of oxygen therapy
	  • Concept of body image
	  • Perioperative nursing management
	  • Assessment of the respiratory system
	  • Concept of respiratory failure
	  • Care of clients with trauma or injuries
	  • Tracheostomy care
	
	2. Review the **boldfaced** Key Terms and their definitions in Chapter 29 to enhance your understanding of the content.
	
	3. Go to Study Guide Number 6.29 on the following pages and complete the learning exercises for this chapter.
		1. Textbook—Chapter 27 (Assessment of the Respiratory System)
		2. Textbook—Chapter 28 and facilities policies and procedures related to oxygen therapy and tracheostomy care.
		3. Textbook—Chapter 29
		4. Other resources:
		  • American Cancer Society: http://www.cancer.org/
		  • Any anatomy and physiology textbook
		  • Any physical assessment textbook
		  • Biddle, C. (1999). Sleep apnea and other disordered-breathing syndromes. *Current Reviews for Nurse Anesthetists, 22*(1), 3-8.
		  • Carr, M., Schmidbauer, J., Majaess, L., & Smith, R. (2000). Communication after laryngectomy: An assessment of quality of life. *Otolaryngology-Head and Neck Surgery, 122*(1), 39-43.
		  • Consult a speech therapist to learn more about devices used by patients with total laryngectomy or radical neck surgery.
		  • Consult a dietitian to learn more about foods that clients can eat to prevent aspiration pneumonia, malnutrition, and dehydration in high-risk clients, postoperative clients with facial trauma/surgery, and laryngectomy patients with tracheotomies.
		  • Consult the American Lung Association and ask for literature and programs on smoking cessation.
		  • Depsey, H., Antonitis, J., Gerald, S., & Barbariot, C. (1998). Cold facts about epistaxis. *American Journal of Nursing, 98*(7), 21.
		  • Haynes, V.L. (1996). Caring for the laryngectomy patient. *American Journal of Nursing, 96*, 16B.

- International Association of Laryngectomies: http://www.larynxlink.com
- National Head Injury Foundation, Southborough, MA.

Chapter 30: *Interventions for Clients with Noninfectious Lower Respiratory Problems*

Learning Outcomes	Learning Activities	Supplemental Resources
1. Explain the differences in pathophysiology between asthma and bronchoconstriction and between asthma and inflammation.	1. Prior to completing the study guide exercises in this chapter, review the following:	1. Textbook—Chapter 27 (Assessment of the Respiratory System)
2. Prioritize education needs for the client at step III of on-step therapy for asthma.	• Anatomy and physiology of the lower respiratory tract	2. Textbook—Chapter 30
3. Interpret peak expiratory flow readings for the need for intervention.	• Assessment of the respiratory system including pulse oximetry	3. Other resources:
4. Discuss the complications of chronic oral steroid therapy for treatment of chronic airflow limitations (CAL).	• Process of respiration	• *American Journal of Respiratory and Critical Care Medicine*
5. Compare and contrast the pathophysiology and clinical manifestations of asthma, bronchitis, and emphysema.	• Principles of diffusion, perfusion, and ventilation	• American Thoracic Society: http://www.thoracic.org
6. Identify risk factors for the development of chronic obstructive pulmonary disease (COPD).	• Perioperative nursing management	• American Thoracic Society (1995). Standards for the diagnosis and care of patients with chronic obstructive pulmonary disease. *American Journal of Respiratory and Critical Care Medicine*, 152(5), S78-S121.
7. Prioritize the educational needs for the client with COPD who is receiving oxygen therapy at home.	• Concept of body image	• Any anatomy and physiology textbook
8. Describe interventions for energy conservation for the client with COPD.	• Pulmonary function studies	• Any physical assessment textbook
9. Prioritize nursing care for the client immediately following lung volume reduction surgery.	• Grief and loss	• Bressler, T. (1999). Small cell lung cancer. In C. Miaskowski & P. Buchsel (Eds.). *Oncology nursing: Assessment and clinical care* (pp. 11301-1329). St. Louis: Mosby.
10. Explain the nutritional requirements for the client with severe COPD.	• Signs and symptoms of respiratory failure	• Jablonski, R. (2000). Discovering asthma in the older adult. *Nurse Practitioner*, 25(3), 14, 24-25, 29-39.
11. Use laboratory data and clinical manifestations to determine the effectiveness of therapy for impaired gas exchange in a client with CAL.	• Acid-base balance	• McCloskey, J.C. & Bulechek, G.M. (2000). *Nursing interventions classification (NIC)* (3rd ed.). St. Louis: Mosby.
12. Identify the risk factors that predispose to the development of lung cancer.	2. Review the **boldfaced** Key Terms and their definitions in Chapter 30 to enhance your understanding of the content.	• National Heart, Lung, and Blood Institute; National Institutes of Health: http://www.nhlbi.nih.gov/nhlbi/nhlbi.htm
13. Compare and contrast the side effects of radiation treatment for lung cancer with those of chemotherapy for lung cancer.	3. Go Study Guide Number 6.30 on the following pages and complete the learning exercises for this chapter.	
14. Explain how to troubleshoot the chest tube drainage system in a client 1 day after a thoracotomy.		
15. Develop a teaching plan for the client getting ready to go home after a pneumonectomy.		

Chapter 31: *Interventions for Clients with Infectious Respiratory Problems*

Learning Outcomes	Learning Activities	Supplemental Resources
1. Explain the consequences of an untreated streptococcal infection of the upper respiratory tract.	1. Prior to completing the study guide exercises in this chapter, review the following: • Assessment of the respiratory system • Anatomy and physiology of the lower respiratory tract • Principles of normal defense mechanisms of the body • Principles of infection control and isolation • Incentive spirometry technique • Collecting sputum specimens • Throat culture technique	1. Textbook—Chapter 27 (Assessment of the Respiratory System) 2. Textbook—Chapter 31 3. Other resources: • AIDS resources: http://www.teleport.com/~celinec/aids.shtml • Any anatomy and physiology textbook • Any physical assessment textbook • Centers for Disease Control and Prevention (2000). Update: Influenza activity—United States and worldwide, 1999-2000 season, and composition of the 2000-2001 influenza vaccine. *MMWR. Morbidity and Mortality Weekly Report, 49* (17), 375-38.
2. Identify adult populations at highest risk for contracting influenza.	2. Review the **boldfaced** Key Terms and their definitions in Chapter 31 to enhance your understanding of the content.	• Consult with an infection control nurse at a local hospital regarding collaborative treatment of the client with TB. Inquire about the responsibilities of the health care providers in an acute care setting to protect themselves and others.
3. Develop a teaching plan to prevent influenza in the older adult.	3. Go to Study Guide Number 6.31 on the following pages and complete the learning exercises for this chapter.	• Dimatteo, L. (1999). Managing streptococcal pharyngitis: A review of clinical decision-managing strategies, diagnostic evaluation, and treatment. *Journal of the American Academy of Nurse Practitioners, 11*(2), 57-62.
4. Identify clients for developing community-acquired or hospital-acquired pneumonia.		• Discuss with a community health nurse the initiative in your state relating to Healthy People 2010 in the prevention of TB.
5. Compare the clinical manifestations of pneumonia in the younger client to those exhibited by the older client with pneumonia.		• Discuss with primary health care provider measures they recommend in preventing influenza.
6. Identify adult populations at risk for tuberculosis.		• Finklestein, L. & Petrec, C.A. (1996). Sputum testing for TB: Getting good specimens. *American Journal of Nursing, 96*(2), 14.
7. Interpret correctly the purified protein derivative test results for a person with normal immune function and a person with human immunodeficiency virus/acquired immunodeficiency syndrome.		• Harris, J. & Miller, T. (2000). Preventing nosocomial pneumonia: Evidenced-based practice. *Critical Care Nurse, 20*(1) 51-67.
8. Prioritize educational needs for the client undergoing treatment at home for active tuberculosis.		

- Hospital policy and procedure book regarding isolation and isolation precautions and obtaining sputum specimens
- King, D.E. & Pippin, H.J. (1997). Community acquired pneumonia in adults: Initial antibiotic therapy. *American Family Physician, 56*(2), 544-550.
- Tuberculosis resources: http://www.cpmc.columbia.edu/tbcpp/
- U.S. Department of Health and Human Services, Healthy People 2010: Understanding and Improving Health: http://www.health.gov/healthypeople or call 800-367-4725.

Chapter 32: *Interventions for Critically Ill Clients with Respiratory Problems*

Learning Outcomes	Learning Activities	Supplemental Resources
1. Identify clients at risk for development of pulmonary embolism. 2. Describe the clinical manifestations of pulmonary embolism. 3. Use laboratory data and clinical manifestations to determine the presence of acidosis. 4. Compare and contrast the ventilation-perfusion ratios for respiratory failure of ventilatory origin and respiratory failure of oxygenation origin. 5. Distinguish between normal and abnormal pulmonary capillary wedge pressure readings. 6. Use laboratory data and clinical manifestations to determine the adequacy of ventilatory interventions. 7. Describe the indications for intubation. 8. Prioritize nursing care for the conscious client being mechanically ventilated. 9. Identify clients at risk for development of pneumothorax.	1. Prior to completing the study guide exercises for this chapter, review the following: • Anatomy and physiology of the lower respiratory tract • Process of respiration • Principles of diffusion, perfusion, and ventilation • Interpretation of blood gas measurements • Acid-base balance, acidosis, and alkalosis • Hemodynamic monitoring • Principles of oxygen therapy • Principles of perioperative nursing management • Concepts of body image • Principles of human sexuality • Tracheostomy care and principles of suctioning	1. Textbook—Chapter 27 (Assessment of the Respiratory System) 2. Textbook—Chapter 28 (Interventions for Clients with Oxygen or Tracheostomy) 3. Textbook—Chapter 32 4. Other resources: • Any anatomy and physiology textbook • Any physical assessment textbook • Arcasoy, S.M. & Kreit, J.W. (1999). Thrombolytic therapy of pulmonary embolism: A comprehensive review of current evidence. *Chest, 115*(6), 1695-1707. • Balas, M. (2000). Prone positioning of patients with acute respiratory distress syndrome: Applying research to practice. *Critical Care Nurse, 20*(1), 24-36.

- Burns, S. (1998). Making weaning easier: Pathways and protocols that work. *Critical Care Nursing Clinics of North America, 11*(4), 465-479.
- Calianno, C. (1996). Pneumonia: Repelling a deadly invader. *Nursing 26,* 33.
- Discuss with a critical care clinical nurse specialist the care of a client on a ventilator.
- Discuss with an emergency room clinical nurse specialist the care of clients in the ER in respiratory distress.
- Glass, C., Grap, M., & Battle, G. (1999). Preparing the patient and family for home mechanical ventilation. *MEDSURG Nursing, 8*(2), 99-107.
- O'Hanlon-Nichols, T. (1996). Commonly asked questions about chest tubes. *AJN 96,* 60.
- Pettinicchi, TA. (1998). Trouble-shooting chest tubes, *Nursing, 28,* 58.

2. Review the **boldfaced** Key Terms and their definitions in Chapter 32 to enhance your understanding of the content.

3. Go to Study Guide Number 6.32 on the following pages and complete the learning exercises for this chapter.

STUDY GUIDE NUMBER 6.27

Assessment of the Respiratory System

Study/Review Questions

1. Match each function/description of the airway with the corresponding location.

   Location of Airway
   1. Upper airway
   2. Lower airway

   Function/Description of Airway Segment
   ___ a. Traps particles not filtered by nares
   ___ b. Traps organisms entering nose and mouth
   ___ c. Trachea
   ___ d. Contains cilia to move mucus to trachea
   ___ e. Composed of alveoli for gas exchange
   ___ f. Pharynx, or throat
   ___ g. Place where the trachea divides into the right and left bronchi
   ___ h. Larynx
   ___ i. Dividing point where solid foods and fluids are separated from air
   ___ j. Epiglottis
   ___ k. Pleura
   ___ l. Alveoli

2. Identify the three main functions of the upper respiratory system:
   a. _____
   b. _____
   c. _____

3. a. What is surfactant and where is it found in the lower airway?

   b. Identify three purposes of surfactant in the respiratory process.

4. What is the difference between the pulmonary and bronchial circulatory systems?

5. Match each of the following processes of respiration with its description.

   Description
   ___ a. Movement of air in and out of the lungs
   ___ b. Exchange of oxygen and carbon dioxide in the capillary-alveolar network
   ___ c. Pumping of oxygenated blood through the body

   Process
   1. Diffusion
   2. Perfusion
   3. Ventilation

6. On a separate sheet of paper, develop a concept map relevant to the respiratory system. Consider physiologic, psychosocial, and developmental factors. Identify both subjective and objective data.

Questions 7 to 10 relate to a 64-year-old female client.

7. In obtaining a smoking history, this client reports that she smoked a pack of cigarettes a day for 9 years, quit for 2 years, then smoked 2 packs a day for the last 30 years. Calculate pack years for this client.
   a. 39 years
   b. 69 years
   c. 19.5 years
   d. 41 years

8. As a result of the client's history of smoking, she is scheduled for pulmonary function tests (PFTs) because of complaints of dyspnea and chronic cough. She calls the office and asks to speak to the nurse to learn more about this procedure. On a separate sheet of paper, develop a Deficient Knowledge related to PFT plan for this client.

9. Which of the following will *not* be reported in the PFT test results?
   a. Flow volume curves
   b. Diffusion capacity
   c. Muscle fatigue factor
   d. Lung volumes

10. Match the following pulmonary function tests (PFTs) with their descriptions.

    Pulmonary
    Function Tests
    ___ a. FEV (forced expiratory volume)
    ___ b. FRC (functional residual capacity)
    ___ c. FVC (forced vital capacity)
    ___ d. RV (residual volume)
    ___ e. TLC (total lung capacity)
    ___ f. VC (Vital capacity)
    ___ g. Diffusion

    Descriptions of Pulmonary Function Tests
    1. Maximal amount of forced air that can be exhaled after maximal inspiration
    2. Amount of air in lungs at the end of maximal inhalation
    3. Amount of air remaining in lungs after normal exhalation
    4. Maximal amount of air that can be exhaled over a specific time
    5. Amount of air remaining in lungs at the end of full, forced exhalation
    6. Measure of carbon monoxide uptake across alveolar-capillary membrane
    7. Maximum amount of gas that can be exhaled after maximal inspiration

11. Which pulmonary function test result for this client, being an older adult, will more than likely show a decline as a result of aging and/or respiratory disorders and why?

12. This client is having difficulty with discolored sputum and was scheduled to have a bronchoscopy. She was NPO for several hours before the test. Now, a few hours after the test, she states that she is hungry and would like a meal. You, as a nurse, would do which of the following?
    a. Order a meal since she is now alert and oriented.
    b. Check a pulse oximetry to be sure oxygen saturation has returned to normal.
    c. Check a gag reflex before allowing her to eat.
    d. Assess for nausea as a result of the medications she received for the test.

13. After the bronchoscopy, the client's sputum from her chronic cough contains blood. What is the most appropriate nursing intervention?
    a. Take vital signs and notify the physician of this change in her sputum.
    b. Monitor client to see if blood in the sputum continues.
    c. Send the sputum for cytology for possible lung cancer.
    d. Do nothing. Tell the client this is a normal response after a bronchoscopy.

14. The nurse would perform a respiratory assessment and monitor for a pneumothorax after which of the following procedures?
    a. Bronchoscopy
    b. Laryngoscopy
    c. CT of lungs
    d. Percutaneous lung biopsy

15. Which of the following pulse oximetry readings calls for immediate intervention?
    a. 98%
    b. 93%
    c. 89%
    d. 85%

16. What would the nursing intervention be in the previous question?
    a. Place client in high Fowler's position.
    b. Start oxygen via nasal cannula at 2 L/min.
    c. Notify physician for a stat ABGs.
    d. Encourage coughing and deep breathing exercises.

17. On a separate sheet of paper, describe the physiologic changes that usually occur in the respiratory function of the following when assessing an older adult.
    a. Chest wall
    b. Alveoli
    c. Lungs
    d. Pharynx and larynx
    e. Pulmonary vasculature
    f. Exercise tolerance
    g. Respiratory muscle strength
    h. Immune system

18. The need for vigorous coughing and deep breathing exercises when an older adult is confined to bed is most likely related to which of the following physiologic changes?
    a. Decreased elasticity of lungs
    b. Alveolar surface area decreases and elastic recoil decreases
    c. Decreased effectiveness of cilia
    d. Vocal cord becoming slack

19. Analyze the physiologic changes in the older adult shown in Chart 27-1 of the textbook. Which of the following blood gases would the nurse anticipate to be normal arterial blood gases in a 76-year-old?
    a. Normal pH, normal Pao_2, normal $Paco_2$
    b. Normal pH, decreased Pao_2, normal $Paco_2$
    c. Decreased pH, decreased Pao_2, normal $Paco_2$
    d. Decreased pH, decreased Pao_2, decreased $Paco_2$

20. Match the following adventitious and normal breath sounds with their descriptions. *Breath sounds may have more than one answer.*

    Breath Sounds
    ___ a. Bronchial
    ___ b. Bronchophony
    ___ c. Bronchovesicular
    ___ d. Egophony
    ___ e. Pleural friction rub
    ___ f. Crackles
    ___ g. Rhonchi
    ___ h. Vesicular
    ___ i. Wheezes
    ___ j. Whispered pectoriloquy

    Descriptions
    1. Popping sound as air moves through through moisture in small airways
    2. Normal sounds heard over lung periphery
    3. Grating, scratching sound with respiration
    4. Musical, squeaky sounds related to narrowing of airway
    5. Normal sounds heard over bronchi but abnormal heard elsewhere in the lung
    6. Normal sound heard over trachea
    7. Vocalized "A" is heard as "E" with stethoscope
    8. Abnormal loud transmission of "99" during auscultation
    9. Snoring, rattling sound; coarse, in large airways
    10. Loud sound when client softly says "1, 2, 3."
    11. Cannot be cleared by coughing; sound caused by bronchospasm

21. Answer the following three questions related to the nursing diagnosis of Ineffective Airway Clearance.
    a. Which of the following is *not* an etiology for the nursing diagnosis of Ineffective Airway Clearance for the older adult?
       (1) Loss of elastic recoil of the lungs
       (2) Vocal cords become weak
       (3) Ciliary action has diminished
       (4) Decreased muscle strength and cough

    b. Identify other indications that would cause the nursing diagnosis of Ineffective Airway Clearance.

    c. Identify potential nursing interventions related to this nursing diagnosis for the older adult.

22. The best position in which to place the client when performing a physical assessment of the respiratory system is:
    a. Side-lying.
    b. Semi-Fowler's.
    c. Supine.
    d. Sitting upright.

23. Upon performing a lung sound assessment of the anterior chest, the nurse hears moderately loud sounds on inspiration that are equal in length with expiration. Where in the airway would this lung sound be considered normal?
    a. Trachea
    b. Primary bronchi
    c. Lung fields
    d. Larynx

24. The name that describes the particular lung sound in the previous question is which of the following?
    a. Bronchial
    b. Bronchovesicular
    c. Vesicular
    d. Basilar

25. The lung sound that should be heard throughout the lung fields in the smaller bronchioles and the alveoli is called:
    a. Bronchial.
    b. Bronchovesicular.
    c. Vesicular.
    d. Basilar.

26. Relating to the previous question, which of the following is characteristic of the normal lung sound heard throughout the lung fields?
    a. Short inspiration, long expiration, loud, harsh
    b. Soft sound, long inspiration, short quiet expiration
    c. Mixed sounds of harsh and soft, long inspiration and long expiration
    d. Loud, long inspiration and short, loud expiration

27. Upon assessing the lungs, the nurse hears short, discrete popping sounds in the lower lobes. This assessment would be documented as which of the following?
    a. Rhonchi in bilateral lower lobes
    b. Wheezes in bilateral lower lobes
    c. Fine crackles in bilateral lower lobes
    d. Course crackles in bilateral lower lobes

28. On a separate sheet of paper, explain why the answer for the previous question is *not* (a) rhonchi, (b) wheezes, or (c) course crackles.

29. When the nurse reports that the client is short of breath upon lying down, it would be documented as which of the following terms? What are assessment findings for the incorrect answers?
    a. Orthopnea
    b. Paroxysmal nocturnal dyspnea
    c. Bradypnea
    d. Tachypnea

30. On the diagram below, indicate the correct sequence for percussion and auscultation for the anterior and posterior assessment of the lungs.

31. Identify the three areas of the body that are assessed during a physical examination of the respiratory system.
    a. _____
    b. _____
    c. _____

32. Which of the following clients has an increased risk of respiratory system problems?
    a. A 45-year-old man who breeds and raises racing pigeons
    b. An 18-year-old youth who enjoys body surfing in the ocean
    c. A 68-year-old woman who does needlework for relaxation
    d. A 56-year-old man who ties flies for trout fishing

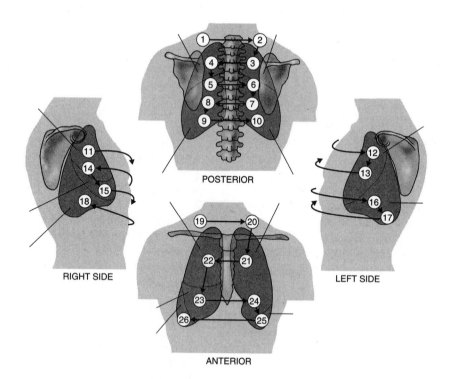

POSTERIOR

RIGHT SIDE

LEFT SIDE

ANTERIOR

33. The following is a partial client history. On a separate sheet of paper, discuss the significance these data have as an assessment of the respiratory system.

    White man, 36 years old; married with two children. History of cigarette smoking for the past 20 years, one pack per day. Works as a machinist in a factory, manufacturing metal tools and molds for tool making. In his current job for 17 years. Completed vocational high school. Hobbies include making model airplanes and model railroading. Denies allergies to any medications. Suffers from seasonal allergies (rhinitis, sneezing). No difficulty with ADLs.

34. Using the data in the previous question, on a separate sheet of paper, document a physical assessment of the respiratory system.

35. When assessing the lungs and thorax, observations would include:
    a. _____
    b. _____
    c. _____

36. Which of the following data is an objective sign of chronic oxygen deprivation?
    a. Complaints of shortness of breath
    b. Baroxysmal nocturnal dyspnea
    c. Chest pain with deep inspiration
    d. Clubbing of fingernails

37. Palpation of the chest is used to assess for:
    a. Retractions or bulging.
    b. Tactile fremitus.
    c. Accessory muscle use.
    d. Friction rub.

38. The laboratory data associated with chronic airflow limitations is decreased levels of:
    a. Hemoglobin.
    b. Neutrophils.
    c. Eosinophils.
    d. Arterial oxygen.

39. The nurse determines there is uneven symmetry on the client's thoracic expansion. What are the steps the nurse would use to palpate this finding?
    a. _____
    b. _____
    c. _____
    d. _____

40. Upon inspection, the nurse would assess an increase in anteroposterior (AP) diameter of the chest when:
    a. There is unequal movement from side to side of the chest.
    b. The client cannot take a deep breath because of changes in aging.
    c. Ratio of the depth of the chest to the width of the chest is equal.
    d. The ribs are horizontal and not sloping downward.

41. Which of the following abnormal findings does percussion determine?
    a. Tracheal deviation
    b. Hyperresonance
    c. Barrel chest
    d. Friction rub

42. The characteristics that best describe the sound heard in the previous question are:
    a. High-pitched, loud and musical.
    b. Thud-like, medium sound.
    c. Normal sound over lung tissue in periphery.
    d. Very loud, long duration, and high pitched.

43. The best position for the client during a thorocentesis is which of the following?
    a. On side, affected side exposed, head slightly raised
    b. Lying flat with arm on affected side across the chest
    c. Sitting up, leaning forward on over-bed table
    d. On stomach with arms above the head

44. After which of the following procedures/tests would the nurse observe for signs and symptoms of a pneumothorax?
    a. Thoracocentesis
    b. PET scan
    c. Lung angiogram
    d. Ventilation-perfusion scan

45. A client was admitted for a deep vein thrombosis (DVT) and later became short of breath. A pulmonary embolus is suspected. What test would be ordered to confirm this diagnosis?
    a. Pulse oximetry
    b. V/Q scan-ventilation and perfusion scanning
    c. Magnetic resonance imaging (MRI)
    d. Chest x-ray

46. Upon inspection, the color of the client's sputum is yellow. This is an indication of:
    a. Infection.
    b. Normal color sputum.
    c. Obstruction.
    d. Unknown problem.

47. The nurse observes the following signs: dusky skin, pale mucous membranes, decreased capillary refill, and poor respiratory rate and chest movement. The nursing diagnosis would be:
    a. Ineffective Airway Clearance.
    b. Ineffective Tissue Perfusion.
    c. Activity Intolerance.
    d. Anxiety related to procedure.

48. When caring for a client, the nurse would assess early signs of decreased oxygenation by using which of the following assessment findings?
    a. Cyanosis
    b. Unexplained restlessness
    c. Cool, clammy skin
    d. Paleness, shortness of breath

49. Demonstrate to your clinical instructor the proper technique for auscultation, palpation, and percussion in a respiratory assessment. Report and document your assessment findings. Validate the findings with your clinical instructor. Complete the remaining steps of the nursing process regarding your assessment findings.

50. A nurse has received a client from the recovery room on hospital unit. The pulse oximetry has dropped from 95% to 90%. The nursing intervention at this time would be to:
    a. Administer oxygen at 2 L by nasal cannula, then reassess.
    b. Have client perform coughing and deep breathing exercises, then reassess.
    c. Administer Narcan to reverse narcotic sedation effect.
    d. Withhold narcotic pain medication to reduce sedation effect.

True or False? Write T for true or F for false in the blank provided. If false, correct the statement.

____ 51. Pulse oximetry, or Pao_2 can determine adequate oxygenation of a client regardless of cardiac status or underlying clinical problems.

52. Which of the following medications warrants further inquiry when collecting subjective data for the respiratory system?
    a. Erythromycin (E-Mycin) for chronic recurrent otitis media
    b. Warfarin sodium (Coumadin) for management of thrombophlebitis of the leg
    c. Lithium carbonate (Lithobid) for management of bipolar disorder
    d. Lovastatin (Mevacor) for hypercholesterolemia

53. In preparing a client for a ventilation-perfusion scan, the nurse explains to the client which of the following? *Correct the wrong answers.*
    a. That NPO before the exam is necessary to prevent aspiration of the dye
    b. That after the test, the client will be in isolation for 8 hours because of the radioactive dye
    c. The need to assess for iodine allergy because of the radioactive dye
    d. That the test is only a screening test for pulmonary embolus; a CT scan will follow if needed

54. A nurse uses a pulse oximeter to measure which of the following?
    a. Oxygen perfusion in the extremities
    b. Mixed venous saturation
    c. Carbon dioxide saturation of the blood
    d. Oxygen saturation in the red blood cells

55. Match the pulmonary function capacities and functions in column B with the correct corresponding information in column A. *Column B answers may be used more than once.*

Column A

____ a. Reduced in clients with obstructive disease and increased with exercise or CHF
____ b. Air left in lung after a forced exhalation
____ c. Largest amount of air the lungs can hold
____ d. After a maximum deep breath, amount of air quickly exhaled
____ e. Not used to measure larger airway obstructions
____ f. After a maximum deep breath, the max amount of air exhaled in the first 1 second

Column B
1. FVC: forced vital capacity
2. FEV1: forced expiratory volume in 1 sec
3. FEF: forced expiratory flow
4. FRC: functional residual capacity
5. TLC: total lung capacity
6. RV: residual volume
7. DLCO: diffusion capacity of carbon monoxide

56. In pulmonary function testing, which of the following would be considered a normal result in the older adult?
    a. Increased forced vital capacity
    b. Decline forced expiratory volume in 1 second
    c. Decrease in diffusion capacity of carbon monoxide
    d. Increased functional residual capacity

57. In the older adult, as a result of loss of elastic recoiling of the lung and decreased chest wall compliance, the nurse may observe which of the following on physical exam?
    a. Thoracic area becomes shorter
    b. Finger clubbing
    c. Increase in anteroposterior ratio
    d. Severe shortness of breath

58. In the older adult, there is a decreased number of functional alveoli; this change in the lungs will result in which of the following?
    a. Decreased Pao_2
    b. Increased Pao_2
    c. False elevation in pulse oximetry
    d. False low value in the pulse oximetry

59. A nurse explains to a client the changes cigarette smoking makes on the lower respiratory tract. Which of the following statements is true?
    a. Clients are more prone to respiratory infection because of the damage to the cilia.
    b. Cigarette smoke affects the ability to effectively cough secretions from the lungs.
    c. Cigarette smoke improves the oxygen saturation of the alveoli.
    d. Clients notice that smoking dilates the large and small airways to increase Pao_2.

60. A client with a pulse oximetry of 80% and a blood gas result of Pao_2 of 62 was started on continuous oxygen therapy. On a separate sheet of paper, describe what assessment findings would indicate that the client is having a positive response to oxygen therapy.

61. A nursing diagnosis for a client is Activity Intolerance, with a pulse oximetry of 99%. Which of the following lab tests contributes to this problem and is related to oxygenation? Would oxygen therapy help this client?
    a. Eosinophils count of 0.6
    b. WBC count of 8.0
    c. Hemoglobin of 9
    d. Glucose 120

62. When performing a respiratory assessment including pulse oximetry, which of the following clients or situations may cause an *artificially* low reading? *Mark Y for yes or N for no, and provide a rationale for your answer.*
    ___ a. Client with peripheral arterial disease
    ___ b. Client with anemia
    ___ c. Client with sickle cell disease
    ___ d. Client with a fever
    ___ e. Client receiving oxygen via nasal cannula
    ___ f. Client in severe shock
    ___ g. Client receiving narcotic pain medication
    ___ h. African-American client
    ___ i. Female clients versus male clients
    ___ j. Client with history of respiratory diseases such as cystic fibrosis or TB
    ___ k. Client with allergies

63. A client who has had neck surgery complains after the operation of being restless, "not being able to breathe very well," with decreased chest movement and elevated pulse. Which of the following tests may be performed by the physician to determine the etiology of this problem? Explain why the other answers are incorrect.
    a. Mediastinoscopy
    b. Direct laryngoscopy
    c. Gastroscopy
    d. Bronchoscopy

64. The nurse prepares the client in the previous question for a bronchoscopy. What client education should the nurse provide?

65. The client returns to the unit after the bronchoscopy. In addition to a respiratory assessment, which of the following would be most important to monitor in order to prevent aspiration?
    a. Sore throat
    b. Position
    c. Chest discomfort
    d. Gag reflex

66. A nurse assesses fine crackles in a lung assessment of a client immediately postoperative. This would more than likely be an indication of which of the following? Explain why the other answers are incorrect. What nursing intervention would help relieve this respiratory problem?
    a. Pneumonia
    b. Atelectasis
    c. Thick secretions
    d. Bronchospasms

67. Which of the following signs of a respiratory assessment is considered the principle, or main, sign of respiratory disease? What questions would the nurse ask in a respiratory assessment regarding this sign?
    a. Sputum production
    b. Cough
    c. Chest movement
    d. Respiratory rate

68. When performing a respiratory assessment, the nurse inquires about the color of the sputum. Which of the following would indicate to the nurse that the client has an infection of the respiratory tract?
    a. Sputum is tan-colored.
    b. Sputum is green.
    c. Sputum is white or clear.
    d. Sputum is gray-colored.

69. A client was admitted for complaints of a sudden onset of sharp pain after sneezing and had a history of a fever and cough. Lung sounds were diminished over the left upper lobe. These clinical assessment findings indicate which of the following?
    a. Bronchitis
    b. Asthma
    c. TB
    d. Pneumothorax

70. Which of the following pathologies is significant to the respiratory system when assessing the family history?
    a. Kyphoscoliosis
    b. Genital herpes simplex
    c. Fibrocystic breast disease
    d. Rheumatoid arthritis

71. During a respiratory assessment for tactile fremitus, the nurse requests the client to:
    a. Breathe deeply three times.
    b. Cough hard.
    c. Whisper.
    d. Say "ninety-nine."

72. On a separate sheet of paper, state the definition of dyspnea.

73. For a healthy adult, the respiratory rate per minute is usually defined as:
    a. 10 to 12.
    b. 12 to 15.
    c. 12 to 20.
    d. 20 or more.

Case Study: Respiratory Tract Assessment

Your adult client reports to the pulmonary clinic with complaints of a productive cough that "won't go away." She is a 62-year-old married housewife whose children are grown. She smoked two packs of cigarettes per day for 20 years, but she has not smoked for the past 10 years. She contracted a "virus" 4 weeks ago, which "settled in her chest." Her usual remedies have not resulted in improvement in her status.

Answer the following questions on a separate sheet of paper:

1. What additional subjective data should the nurse elicit from this client?

2. What physical assessments should the nurse perform on this client?

3. What effect does this client's 10 years of not smoking have on the condition of her lungs?

4. The physician orders a chest x-ray and a sputum specimen. What should the nurse tell this client about these tests?

After 1 week, this client reports no improvement, and the chest x-ray results also indicate that there is no change. A bronchoscopy is scheduled to be done in the outpatient surgical unit the following day. (The physician would prefer to do an MRI, but the client has an inner-ear implant.)

5. Prepare a teaching-learning plan for this client regarding the bronchoscopy. Consider restrictions related to breathing during the procedure.

6. When the client reports to the outpatient surgical units the next morning, what assessments should the nurse make?

7. Both the client and her husband are very anxious. Describe interventions that the nurse should implement to assist the client and her spouse.

Thirty minutes before the procedure, the client is given atropine sulfate 0.6 mg IM. An intravenous infusion is begun with D5 ½ NS, and diazepam (Valium) 10 mg IV is given.

8. Why have these medications been ordered?

9. A topical anesthetic agent is applied to the pharynx immediately before the bronchoscopy is to begin. What is the purpose of this agent?

10. What special actions must the nurse take after the procedure is completed and the client is taken to the PACU? What equipment should be available when she arrives? What are the reasons for this equipment?

STUDY GUIDE NUMBER 6.28

Interventions for Clients with Oxygen or Tracheostomy

Study/Review Questions

1. The following words are used when discussing the care of clients needing oxygen therapy. Briefly describe, in your own words, the meaning of each of the following words.
   a. Hypoxemia
   b. Hypoxia
   c. Hypercarbia
   d. Pulse oximetry
   e. Pao_2
   f. Fio_2

2. Which of the following is not a clinical indication for the use of oxygen therapy?
   a. Decreased arterial Po_2 levels, as in pulmonary edema
   b. Increased cardiac output, as in client with valve replacement
   c. Decreased blood oxygen-carrying capacity, as in anemia
   d. Increased oxygen demand, as in sustained fever

3. True or False? Read the following statements regarding oxygen therapy and decide whether each is true or false. *Write* T *for true or* F *for false in the blanks provided. If the statement is false, correct the statement to make it true.*
   ___ a. Oxygen therapy is needed when the normal 21% oxygen in the air is inadequate and causes hypoxemia and hypoxia.
   ___ b. Examples of conditions that can increase the body's need for more oxygen are infection in the blood, increase in body temperature such as 101° F, Hgb of 9.0, or sickle cell disease.
   ___ c. Hypoxemia and hypoxia can be measured by low Pao_2 and low pulse oximetry.

   ___ d. In order to improve breathing, supplemental oxygen is based on analysis of the client's symptoms.
   ___ e. The primary drive for breathing in most clients is the amount of oxygen in arterial blood.
   ___ f. Oxygen is a fire hazard because it can spontaneously ignite when in use.

4. When a client is requiring oxygen by nasal cannula or mask, which of the following statements should the nurse know regarding oxygen administration?
   a. Adult clients require 2 to 6 L/min by nasal cannula in order for oxygen to be effective.
   b. A minimum of 40% oxygen is used with the venturi mask.
   c. Nurses should be familiar with why the client is receiving oxygen, expected outcomes, and complications.
   d. When administering oxygen, the nurse should know that the highest Fio_2 possible for the particular device being used is the goal.

5. The normal mechanism of the body that stimulates breathing and causes an increase in the respiratory rate is which of the following?
   a. The increase in the CO_2 level as sensed by chemoreceptors in the brain (medulla)
   b. The decreased amount of oxygen saturation in the blood as sensed by the brain (medulla) chemoreceptors
   c. The low levels of carbon dioxide as sensed by the brain (medulla)
   d. The brain recognizes the hypoxemia that occurs with decreased respiration

6. A client with chronic lung disease is admitted to the hospital with oxygen-induced hypoventilation. The nurse needs to be aware that the stimulus to breathe for these clients is which of the following? Provide an explanation for that answer.
   a. Excessively high carbon dioxide (60 to 65 mm Hg) levels in the blood that rose over time
   b. The low level of oxygen concentration in the blood, as sensed by the chemoreceptors in the brain
   c. The low level of oxygen concentration in the blood, as sensed by the peripheral chemoreceptors
   d. CO_2 narcosis in which an elevation of carbon dioxide in the blood turns off the normal mechanism

7. When a nurse administers oxygen to a client who is hypoxic and has chronic high levels of carbon dioxide, the nurse must know that to prevent a decrease in respiratory effort, a:
   a. FIO_2 higher than the usual 2 to 4 L/min nasal cannula is needed.
   b. Venturi mask of 40% is used only to deliver oxygen.
   c. Lower concentration of oxygen (1 to 2 L/min) is provided to minimize worsening of the hypercarbia.
   d. Variable FIO_2 via nasal cannula or mask is used as the client's condition changes.

8. The nurse should perform which of the following interventions for a client who is at high risk or unknown risk for oxygen-induced hypoventilation? Indicate why the other answers are incorrect.
   a. Monitor signs of nonproductive cough, chest pain, crackles, and hypoxemia every 1 to 2 hours.
   b. Monitor change in color from pink, to gray, to cyanotic in the first 30 minutes of administering oxygen.
   c. Monitor for signs and symptoms of hypoventilation rather than hypoxemia.
   d. Monitor for changes in level of consciousness, apnea, improvement in color, and pulse oximetry in the first 30 minutes.

9. When administering a *high concentration* of oxygen to a client, the nurse must be aware of which of the following and why?
   a. Auscultate the lungs every 1 to 2 hours for oxygen toxicity.
   b. Audible wheezes from bronchospasms can occur as a result of absorption atelectasis.
   c. Monitoring the client every 15 to 30 minutes is necessary for observation of side effects.
   d. Crackles and diminished lung sounds can be signs of absorption atelectasis.

10. Oxygen toxicity is related to which of the following?
   ___ a. Oxygen toxicity can result from continuously delivering oxygen greater than 50% concentration.
   ___ b. Delivering a high concentration of oxygen over 24 to 48 hours increases risk.
   ___ c. The degree of lung disease can increase the risk for oxygen toxicity.
   ___ d. The health care provider should order the lowest concentration of oxygen to prevent oxygen toxicity.
   ___ e. The nurse should monitor the client's status for the reduction of oxygen concentration as soon as possible.
   ___ f. Other measures, such as CPAP or PEEP, can be used to reduce the need for a high concentration of oxygen.

11. Which of the following is a classic indication of chronic hypoxemia?
   a. Finger clubbing
   b. Adventitious lung sounds
   c. Anteroposterior ratio increase
   d. Weight gain with even muscle development

12. Humidified oxygen places the client at high risk for which of the following nursing diagnoses?
   a. Risk for Injury related to the moisture in the tube
   b. Risk for Infection related to the condensation in the tubing
   c. Risk for Infection related to the nasal prongs or mask
   d. Risk for Impaired Skin Integrity related to the mask

13. The organism that causes an infection in clients with humidified oxygen is which of the following?
   a. *Escherichia coli*
   b. Streptococcosis
   c. Staphylococcosis
   d. Pseudomonad

True or False? Write T for true or F for false in the blank provided. Give an explanation for your answer.

_____ 14. There are no nursing interventions to prevent infection in clients with humidified oxygen.

15. Which of the following is *not* a hazard of oxygen therapy?
    a. Increased combustion
    b. Oxygen-induced hyperventilation
    c. Oxygen toxicity
    d. Absorption atelectasis

True or False? Write T for true or F for false in the blank provided. Give a rationale for your answer.

_____ 16. In selecting a device for delivery of oxygen, the nurse must be aware of the various devices and not leave it up to the respiratory therapist.

17. A client with an oxygen delivery device would like to ambulate to the bathroom but the tubing is too short. Extension tubing is added. What is the maximum length of the tubing that can be added in order to deliver the amount of oxygen needed for that device?
    a. 25 feet
    b. 35 feet
    c. 45 feet
    d. 50 feet

18. On a separate sheet of paper, briefly describe the difference between a low-flow and high-flow oxygen delivery system.

19. Match the following systems of oxygen delivery with their flow types. *Answers may be used more than once.*

    Oxygen Delivery Systems   **Flow Types**
    _____ a. Aerosol mask   1. Low-flow system
    _____ b. Face tent   2. High-flow system
    _____ c. Nasal cannula
    _____ d. Non-rebreather mask
    _____ e. Partial rebreather mask
    _____ f. Face mask
    _____ g. T-piece
    _____ h. Tracheostomy collar
    _____ i. Venturi mask

20. A client is being discharged from the hospital with home oxygen therapy. As this client's nurse, what nursing interventions would you perform before discharge and what interventions will be ongoing for this client?

21. Indicate the goal for providing discharge planning and teaching for a client receiving home oxygen therapy.

22. Identify and describe the three ways oxygen can be provided to a client on home oxygen therapy.

23. True or False? *Write T for true or F for false in the blanks provided.*
    _____ a. Humidification is absolutely necessary in the home, just as it is in the hospital.
    _____ b. A reservoir-type nasal cannula can be used to reduce oxygen flow by 50%.

24. On a separate sheet of paper, develop and complete a chart on the oxygen delivery systems that is similar to the one on the following page.

25. Which of the following is the correct critical nursing intervention for a client with a non-rebreather mask? Correct the wrong answers.
    a. Maintain liter flow so that the reservoir bag is up to ½ full.
    b. Maintain 60% to 75% FIO_2 at 6 to 11 L/min.
    c. Assure that valves and rubber flaps are patent, functional, and not stuck.
    d. Assess for effectiveness of oxygen and switch to partial rebreather for more precise FIO_2.

26. A client with a face mask at 5 L/min is able to eat. Which of the following nursing interventions would be performed at mealtimes?
    a. Change the mask to a nasal cannula of 6 L/min or more.
    b. Have the client work around the face mask as best as possible.
    c. Obtain a physician order for a nasal cannula at 5 L/min.
    d. Obtain a physician order to remove the mask at meals.

27. A client with respiratory difficulty is using noninvasive positive-pressure ventilation (NPPV). Which of the following statements is correct about this delivery system? Correct the wrong answers.
    a. Only used as an oxygen delivery method.
    b. Used to keep the alveoli open and improve gas exchange.
    c. It is a form of airway intubation.
    d. A system that only uses bi-level positive airway pressure (BiPAP) delivery method.

Oxygen Delivery System	Description and Amount of Oxygen Concentration Delivered to the Client	When Used and Types of Clients Using This System	Key Nursing Interventions
Nasal cannula			
Simple face mask			
Partial rebreather mask			
Non-rebreather mask			
Venturi mask			
Tent and aerosol mask			

28. On a separate sheet of paper, describe the difference between the two NPPV systems of BiPAP and nasal continuous positive airway pressure.

29. A physician orders transtracheal oxygen therapy for a client with respiratory difficulty. This type of oxygen delivery method:
    a. Delivers oxygen directly into the lungs.
    b. Can be inserted into the trachea by any health care provider.
    c. Is used in place of an endotracheal tube.
    d. Does not require any client home care education.

30. A nursing diagnosis for a client receiving oxygen therapy is Risk for Impaired Skin Integrity. Nursing interventions related to prevention include which of the following? *Check all that apply and correct the false statements.*
    ___ a. Assess the client's ears, back of neck, and face at least every 4 to 8 hours for irritation.
    ___ b. Apply padding on tubing to prevent pressure on skin.
    ___ c. Use Vaseline on nostrils, face, and lips to relieve dryness.
    ___ d. Assess nasal and mucous membranes for dryness and cracks.
    ___ e. Obtain an order for humidification when oxygen is being delivered at 6 L/min or more.
    ___ f. Provide mouth care every 8 hours and as needed.
    ___ g. Position tubing so it will not pull on client's ears.

31. A client is receiving oxygen therapy for respiratory problems. According to NIC interventions for administration and monitoring of its effectiveness, a nurse:
    a. Monitors the effectiveness of oxygen therapy at least once every 8 hours.
    b. Monitors for signs of oxygen toxicity and absorption atelectasis.
    c. Instructs the client to replace the oxygen mask when the device is removed.
    d. Delegates monitoring the oxygen liter flow and equipment management to respiratory therapist.

32. The nurse observes a client with "stridor." This indicates which of the following respiratory etiologies?
    a. Pneumonia
    b. Tuberculosis
    c. Atelectasis
    d. Partial obstruction of trachea or larynx

33. Which of the following would be used for a client needing long-term airway maintenance?
    a. Tracheostomy
    b. Nasal trumpet
    c. Endotracheal tube
    d. Continuous positive airway clearance (CPAP)

34. A client is receiving preoperative teaching for a total laryngectomy and will have a tracheostomy post-operative. The nurse explains to the client that a tracheostomy is:
    a. An opening in the trachea that enables breathing.
    b. A surgical incision into the trachea.
    c. A tube that is inserted into an opening in the trachea.
    d. An opening in the neck for placement of an endotracheal tube.

35. Identify the types of clients you would anticipate needing a tracheostomy.

36. Immediately postoperative, the nurse would monitor for which of the following complications of a tracheostomy?
    a. Pneumothorax from the displacement of the tube in the trachea
    b. Septic shock as a result of the secretions and suctioning
    c. Subcutaneous emphysema related to the opening in the trachea
    d. Dislodgment of the tracheostomy tube causing air to enter the tissues

37. Identify possible complications associated with a tracheostomy. On a separate sheet of paper develop a chart with assessment findings and collaborative management with prevention strategies related to the complications.

38. A client with a tracheostomy develops increased coughing, inability to expectorate secretions, and difficulty breathing. These are assessment findings related to:
    a. Airway obstruction.
    b. Tracheoesophageal fistula.
    c. Cuff leak and rupture.
    d. Tracheal stenosis.

39. Which of the following is *false* as relates to post-operative nursing intervention for a client with an artificial airway?
    a. Assuring the tube placement
    b. Auscultating breath sounds bilaterally
    c. Suctioning via a nasotracheal approach
    d. Observing for chest wall movement

40. To prevent accidental extubation of a tracheostomy tube when the client is not on a ventilator, the nurse should implement which of the following interventions?
    a. Continuously restrain the client's arms.
    b. The tube should be secured in place using ties or Velcro holders.
    c. Allow some flexibility in motion of the tube while coughing.
    d. Instruct the client to hold the tube with a tissue while coughing.

41. Equipment that should be kept at the bedside of a client who has a tracheostomy includes:
    a. A pair of wire cutters.
    b. Chest tube with water seal drainage collection device.
    c. Code cart.
    d. A tracheostomy tube with obturator.

42. Match each of the following terms related to a tracheostomy tube with their descriptions.

Terms
___ a. Cuff
___ b. Double-lumen tracheostomy tube
___ c. Faceplate
___ d. Fenestrated tracheostomy tube
___ e. Inner cannula obturator
___ f. Outer cannula obturator
___ g. Single-lumen tracheostomy tube
___ h. Talking tracheostomy tube
___ i. Tracheostomy button

Descriptions
1. Plastic or metal tube with blunted end used during insertion of tracheostomy tube
2. Single-cannula tracheostomy tube
3. Maintains stoma patency while client is in transition from mechanical ventilation to spontaneous breathing
4. Prevents aspiration when inflated
5. Consists of inner and outer tubes and an obturator
6. Provides a means for communication
7. Fits into outer cannula and facilitates cleaning and suctioning
8. Part of outer cannula that anchors tube into the trachea
9. Has precut opening in outer cannula that facilitates speech
10. Fits into the tracheostomy and keeps airway open

43. Tracheostomy cuffs should be deflated to:
a. Allow the client to speak.
b. Permit suctioning more easily.
c. Enable the client to eat or drink.
d. Provide access for tracheostomy care.

44. Which of the following is a nursing intervention to prevent obstruction of a tracheostomy tube? Identify other nursing measures that can be taken.
a. Provide tracheal suctioning
b. Provide oxygen with humidification
c. Inflate the cuff to maximum pressure
d. Suction with a Yankauer's catheter

45. After 72 hours, a client experiences decannulation of the tracheostomy tube. When this occurs, the nurse performs which of the following? What is the nursing intervention if decannulation occurs within the first 72 hours?
a. Notify the physician because this is a medical emergency.
b. Quickly and gently replace the tube.
c. Insert the obturator, administer oxygen, and call the physician.
d. Call the code team and prepare for CPR.

46. On a separate sheet of paper, briefly discuss the following possible complications of a tracheostomy tube.
a. Pneumothorax
b. Subcutaneous emphysema
c. Bleeding
d. Infection

47. Humidification and warming of air are essential for the client with an artificial airway because humidification helps:
a. Prevent tracheal damage.
b. Promote thick secretions.
c. Dry out the airways.
d. Warm the air.

48. Which of the following is *not* a complication related to tracheal suctioning?
a. Hypoxia
b. Tissue trauma
c. Infection
d. Bronchodilation

49. Indicate the sequence the nurse would follow when suctioning a client with an artificial airway by marking the steps 1 through 14.
___ a. Explain procedure to the client.
___ b. Pour sterile saline into sterile container.
___ c. Preoxygenate the client.
___ d. Check suction source for low suction.
___ e. Assemble the necessary equipment.
___ f. Keep catheter sterile; attach to suction.
___ g. Wash hands.
___ h. Insert catheter into trachea without suctioning.
___ i. Assess need for suctioning.
___ j. Lubricate catheter tip in sterile saline solution.
___ k. Open suction kit.
___ l. Withdraw catheter, applying suction and twirling catheter.
___ m. Put on sterile gloves.
___ n. Document procedure after discarding supplies used and washing hands.

50. Briefly describe how to ensure that a tracheostomy tube is never dislodged during tracheostomy care.

51. Indicate the sequence for administering tracheostomy care.
    ____ a. Remove old dressing and excess secretions.
    ____ b. Wash hands.
    ____ c. Suction tracheostomy tube.
    ____ d. Put on sterile gloves.
    ____ e. Reinsert inner cannula into outer cannula.
    ____ f. Open tracheostomy kit and pour peroxide into one side of container and saline into another.
    ____ g. Assemble necessary equipment.
    ____ h. Clean stoma site and plate.
    ____ i. Explain procedure to client.
    ____ j. Rinse inner cannula in sterile saline.
    ____ k. Remove inner cannula.
    ____ l. Change tracheostomy ties if needed.
    ____ m. Place inner cannula in peroxide solution.
    ____ n. Position client.
    ____ o. Place new tracheostomy dressing.
    ____ p. Use brush to clean inner cannula.

52. Nursing interventions for the client with a tracheostomy include which of the following? Indicate why the other answers are incorrect.
    a. Changing the tracheostomy ties daily
    b. Suctioning continuously for 10 to 15 seconds
    c. Providing oral hygiene with glycerin swabs
    d. Cleaning the incision with hydrogen peroxide

53. Discharge instructions for the client with a tracheostomy include teaching about:
    a. Sterile suction technique.
    b. Tap water instillations.
    c. Decreasing humidity in the home.
    d. Wearing a medical alert bracelet.

54. A client with a permanent tracheostomy is interested in developing an exercise regimen. Which of the following activities is *not* appropriate for this client?
    a. Aerobics
    b. Tennis
    c. Golf
    d. Swimming

55. Describe the difference between a tracheostomy collar and a T-piece, both of which are used to deliver oxygen therapy. What are the nursing interventions for clients with these devices?

56. A nurse provides oral hygiene for a client with a tracheostomy by:
    a. Cleansing the mouth with glycerin swabs.
    b. Encouraging the use of mouth washes that alter pH of the oral cavity.
    c. Mixing hydrogen peroxide and sterile water.
    d. Using toothettes or soft bristle brush moistened in water.

57. When the client is able to speak and is not on mechanical ventilation, the nurse would expect the client to have which type of tracheostomy tube and why?
    a. Standard cuffless tube
    b. Standard cuffed tube
    c. Cuffed fenestrated tube
    d. Talking tracheostomy tube

58. Match each type of tracheostomy tube with its description.

Descriptions of Tracheostomy Tubes	Types of Tracheostomy Tubes
____ a. Used with clients who can speak while on a ventilator for a long-term basis	1. Double-lumen tube 2. Single-lumen tube 3. Cuffed tube
____ b. Has a cuff; when inflated seals the airway	4. Cuffless tube 5. Fenestrated tube 6. Cuffed fenestrated tube
____ c. Used for long-term management of clients not on mechanical ventilation or at high risk for aspiration	7. Metal tracheostomy tube 8. Talking tracheostomy tube
____ d. Has three parts—outer cannula, inner cannula, and obturator	
____ e. Used for permanent tracheostomy	
____ f. Used often with clients with spinal cord paralysis or muscular disease who do not require ventilator all the time	
____ g. Has no inner cannula and is used for clients with long or extra thick necks	
____ h. Used when weaning a client from a ventilator; allows the client to speak	

59. How does a nurse determine when the cuff is inflated or deflated on a tracheostomy tube?

60. To prevent tissue damage of the tracheal mucosa of a client with a cuffed tracheostomy tube without a pressure relief valve, the nurse would:
    a. Deflate the cuff every 2 to 4 hours and maintain prn.
    b. Change the tracheostomy tube every 3 days or per hospital policy.
    c. Assess and record cuff pressures each shift using the occlusive technique.
    d. Assess and record cuff pressures each shift using minimal leak technique.

61. Other than high cuff pressure, what other factors should the nurse monitor to prevent tissue damage? What nursing interventions would help minimize the chance of this problem occurring?

62. According to NIC interventions, which of the following interventions is appropriate regarding nursing care of a client with an artificial airway?
    a. Before deflating the cuff, suction the oropharynx and secretions from the top of the tube.
    b. Monitor the cuff pressures every 4 to 8 hours on inspiration.
    c. Provide trachea care once every 24 hours and maintain prn.
    d. Monitor for signs and symptoms of pulmonary edema and fluid overload.

63. To assess whether the client is aspirating food or fluids, the nurse would perform which of the following?
    a. When client is coughing, monitor for increased amount of secretions.
    b. Add food coloring to fluids or enteral feedings and monitor the color of the secretions.
    c. Position the client in high Fowler's position and monitor signs of aspiration.
    d. Obtain an order for a chest x-ray to determine aspiration pneumonia.

64. To prevent aspiration during swallowing, the nurse would perform which of the following interventions? Correct the wrong answers and identify other interventions.
    a. Hyperextend the head to allow food to enter the stomach and not the lungs.
    b. Have the client drink thin liquids because they are the easiest to swallow.
    c. Encourage the client to "dry swallow" after each bite to clear residue from the throat.
    d. Maintain a high Fowler's position during eating and 2 hours afterward.

65. Indicate five nursing interventions to prevent hypoxia in a client with a tracheostomy tube.

66. While being suctioned, a client demonstrated vagal stimulation by a drop in heart rate to 54 and a drop in blood pressure to 90/50. Upon assessment of this client, the nurse would:
    a. Inflate the cuff and "bag" the client with 100% oxygen.
    b. Call a code and be ready to perform CPR.
    c. Stop suctioning, oxygenate with 100% oxygen, and monitor the client.
    d. Stop suctioning and monitor blood pressure and heart rate.

True or False? Write T for true or F for false in the blank provided.

___67. Aspiration cannot occur with a cuffed tracheostomy tube.

68. When the client with a tracheostomy is unable to speak, what nursing interventions can be performed to facilitate communication?

69. Upon discharge from the hospital, the client should be able to perform tracheostomy care, nutritional care, suctioning, and have means for communication. Identify additional information the client with a tracheostomy tube will need to know.

STUDY GUIDE NUMBER 6.29

Interventions for Clients with Noninfectious Upper Respiratory Problems

Study/Review Questions

1. Review the various anatomic structures and their function in the upper respiratory system.

2. The nurse would assess and be prepared for potential interventions in what three primary areas of care for clients with upper respiratory system problems?
   a. _____
   b. _____
   c. _____

3. The nursing priority for the client with any problems of the upper airway is to assess:
   a. Thickness of nasal and oral secretions and encourage ingestion of oral fluids or performing suction.
   b. Anxiety and pain. Provide comfort measures such as sedation and NSAIDs.
   c. Adequacy of oxygenation and ensure an unobstructed air passageway.
   d. For spinal cord injuries and trauma, and obtain order for x-rays.

4. A woman states to the physician that she is concerned that her overweight husband who is a heavy smoker has sleep apnea because of his heavy snoring. Changing sleeping positions and losing weight does not seem to be of help. What other indications would be obtained from the client's history that would lead to a diagnosis of sleep apnea and further testing?

5. The man in the previous question is to have a polysomnograph. The client and his wife are unfamiliar with this study. As the nurse, explain to the client and family the purpose of the test, how it will be performed, and how long it will take to complete.

6. To be diagnosed as having sleep apnea, the client would need to have which of the following criteria?
   a. Apnea for 5 seconds or longer, occurring a minimum of 10 times a night
   b. Apnea for 5 seconds or longer, occurring a minimum of 5 times an hour
   c. Apnea for 10 seconds or longer, occurring a minimum of 10 times a night
   d. Apnea for 10 seconds or longer that occurs a minimum of 5 times an hour

7. The need for diagnosing sleep apnea is related to the complications of:
   a. Side effects of hypoxemia, hypercapnia, and sleep deprivation.
   b. Increase in arterial carbon dioxide levels and sleep deprivation.
   c. Respiratory alkalosis with retention of carbon dioxide.
   d. Irritability, obesity, enlarged tonsils, or adenoids.

8. Various devices are used at home to prevent airway obstruction during sleep. These devices would include which of the following?
   a. CPAP and NPPV breathing assistive device
   b. Oxygen via face mask to prevent hypoxia
   c. Neck brace to support the head in a certain position to facilitate breathing
   d. Nebulizer treatments with bronchodilators

9. When nasal devices are used to treat apnea, what intervention would be of help to the client to prevent dryness of nasal mucosa?
   a. Encourage ingestion of fluids to 3000 mL per day.
   b. Intermittently use the device to decrease irritation.
   c. Use medicated nasal sprays routinely.
   d. Moisturize the nasal mucosa with normal saline sprays.

10. When playing football, a client injured his nose and he suspects there is a simple fracture. The best intervention at this time would be for the client to:
    a. Seek medical attention for a stent placement to keep the airway open.
    b. Monitor the injury for at least 24 hours for swelling and bleeding and apply ice to see whether medical attention is necessary.
    c. Seek medical attention for correction within 24 hours to minimize further complications.
    d. Monitor the symptoms for 24 hours to determine whether medical attention for plastic surgery and nose reconstruction is needed.

11. Briefly explain the term *moustache dressing* and when a client would need this type of dressing. On a separate sheet of paper, describe what observations the nurse and client would make when having this type of dressing.

12. After a client has a rhinoplasty, a family member is instructed by the nurse to monitor the client for postnasal drip by using a flashlight. If bleeding is noticed, the client should be instructed to do which of the following?
    a. Place ice packs on nose and back of neck, and apply pressure on the nose to immediately stop the bleeding.
    b. Hyperextend the neck to facilitate draining the blood, and apply pressure and ice packs as needed.
    c. Notify the physician to seek medical attention for the bleeding problem.
    d. Continue to monitor, and notify the physician if the bleeding continues for more than 24 hours.

13. Clients should be taught that after rhinoplasty, the appearance will be altered by:
    a. A very large dressing on the nose.
    b. Bruising of the eyes, nose, and face.
    c. Swelling that will cause loss of sense of smell.
    d. The nose being three times its normal size for 3 weeks.

14. A client with a history of nosebleeds is admitted to the emergency room. The nurse will attempt to stop the nosebleed by which of the following methods?
    a. Administering sedation/relaxation medication, applying ice packs and pressure to the nose; monitoring respiratory status.
    b. Immediately packing nose, applying ice packs, having client sit with head forward, monitoring amount of bleeding.
    c. Relaxing client, having client sit with head forward, monitoring color and amount of blood, monitoring vital signs, and applying ice pack and pressure to nose.

    d. Applying pressure and ice, having client blow nose hard to remove obstruction of clots, and administering humidified oxygen.

15. A client's nosebleed is not subsiding with the interventions performed in the emergency room. The physician has determined that the bleeding has originated in the posterior region and the client needs further intervention. On a separate sheet of paper, describe how this intervention will be performed by the physician.

16. After being treated in the emergency room for posterior nosebleed, the client is admitted to the hospital. The nursing assessment and interventions for this client would be based on which of the following priority nursing diagnoses?
    a. Risk for Impaired Gas Exchange
    b. Risk for Imbalanced Nutrition
    c. Risk for Anxiety
    d. Acute Pain

17. On a separate sheet of paper, briefly compare and contrast nursing care and discharge instructions for the client with packing from a posterior nosebleed and the client in the emergency room with an anterior nosebleed.

18. True or False? Read the following statements regarding packing for nosebleeds and decide whether each is true or false. Write T *for true or* F *for false in the blanks provided. If the statement is false, correct the statement to make it true.*
    ___ a. Anterior packing involves packing nose, usually with antibiotic gauze.
    ___ b. There is more risk for respiratory failure with posterior packing than anterior packing.
    ___ c. Clients are hospitalized for both posterior and anterior packing.
    ___ d. Packing becomes less uncomfortable over time and NSAIDs are used to control the pain from inflammation.
    ___ e. Packing is usually in for several days.
    ___ f. After removing posterior packing, the nose may be cleaned and lubricated with petroleum jelly.
    ___ g. After posterior packing is removed, the client should not blow the nose very hard, do strenuous lifting, or straining for several weeks to minimize risk of recurrence.
    ___ h. The nursing diagnosis Risk for Infection relates to both types of packing.

19. After a client has a rhinoplasty, postoperative instructions should be given to the client and family. Which of the following should be included in the instructions provided by the nurse?
    a. Avoid constipation the first few days after surgery to prevent pressure on the incision and other complications.
    b. Resume food and fluids as tolerated. Minimize fluids to decrease nasal secretions.
    c. Mild analgesics only, such as Tylenol, Excedrin with Aspirin, and Motrin, should be needed for discomfort.
    d. Swelling and discoloration should be relieved quickly with ice packs placed over the surgical site, eyes, and face.

20. Obstruction of airflow and interference with sinus drainage may result from a deviated septum. The client would require which type of procedure to correct this problem?
    a. Rhinoplasty
    b. Nasoseptoplasty
    c. Submucosusplasty
    d. Open repair of the deviated septum

21. Nursing care of a client after surgery for a deviated septum would include which of the following interventions?
    a. Apply ice to the nasal area and eyes to decrease swelling and pain.
    b. Encourage deep breathing and coughing exercises to prevent atelectasis and clear secretions.
    c. Administer aspirin, NSAIDs, or Tylenol every 4 to 6 hours for pain relief and elevated temperature.
    d. Apply moist heat and humidity to the nasal area to promote comfort and circulation, and drainage.

22. Facial trauma requires emergent care that includes the nurse assessing the following three areas:
    a. _____
    b. _____
    c. _____

23. The nurse monitors a client in the emergency room for signs and symptoms of upper airway obstruction. What signs and symptoms would indicate an upper airway obstruction? Why is early recognition essential?

24. What additional findings, other than upper airway obstruction, would the nurse assess in a client with facial trauma?

25. In addition to clients with facial trauma, identify other types of clients who may experience upper airway obstruction.

26. Management of upper airway obstruction includes:
    a. Repositioning the head and neck so that the head is slightly flexed.
    b. Using Heimlich maneuver on the client with a partial airway obstruction.
    c. Performing a cricothyroidotomy and inserting a hollow tube to maintain patency.
    d. Inserting a nasal airway and administering oxygen by nasal cannula.

27. A client with facial trauma has undergone surgical intervention to wire the jaw shut. Which of the following would be included in discharge teaching and why?
    a. Bleeding, oral care and nutrition, pain control, and activity
    b. Oral care, nutrition, pain, communication, and aspiration prevention
    c. Prevention of airway obstructions, bleeding and oral infection, and pain control
    d. Activity, diet, communication, bleeding, and shock

28. Which of the following symptoms in a client with facial trauma should be reported to the physician immediately?
    a. Asymmetry of the mandible
    b. Bloody drainage from both nares
    c. Nonparallel extraocular movements
    d. Pain upon palpation over the nasal bridge

29. Which of the following foods should be encouraged in the diet of a client who has an inner maxillary fixation?
    a. Milk shakes
    b. Cheeseburgers
    c. Carbonated beverages
    d. Tuna and noodle casserole

30. A client enters the emergency department with dyspnea, inability to produce sounds, hoarseness, and subcutaneous emphysema. These clinical findings indicate:
    a. Vocal cord polyps.
    b. Cancer of the vocal cords.
    c. Laryngeal trauma.
    d. Vocal cord paralysis.

31. A client involved in a motor vehicle accident had a neck injury that resulted in laryngeal trauma. The client is being treated in the emergency department with humidified oxygen and is being monitored every 15 to 30 minutes for respiratory distress. Which of the following assessment findings may indicate the need for further intervention?
    a. Respiratory rate 24, Pao_2 80 to 100, no difficulty with communication
    b. Pulse oximetry 96%, anxious, fatigued, blood in sputum, abdominal breathing
    c. Confused and disoriented because of air hunger, difficulty producing sounds, pulse oximetry 80%
    d. Anxious, respiratory rate 20, explaining the accident, color pink, warm to touch

32. The client in the emergency department with laryngeal trauma has developed shortness of breath with stridor, decreased level of consciousness, restlessness, and decreased oxygen saturation. The nurse should prepare the client and family for which of the following procedures?
    a. Oral or nasal airway
    b. Tracheostomy
    c. Endotracheal tube
    d. Laryngoscopy

33. On a separate sheet of paper, identify those who are at risk for developing vocal cord nodules. Compare these people with those at risk for developing polyps.

34. Clients with vocal cord nodules or polyps should be advised to do which of the following?
    a. Drink plenty of cold liquids.
    b. Talk in a whisper.
    c. Discontinue treatment of allergies because that can exacerbate the problem.
    d. Humidify the air they breathe.

35. Which of the following statements about nasal polyps is correct?
    a. They occur more often in clients with intestinal polyps.
    b. They are removed by application of liquid nitrogen.
    c. They arise more often in clients with viral rhinitis.
    d. They contribute to an increased risk of airway obstruction.

36. Which of the methods of treatment listed below would the nurse expect to perform when treating a client with hypertrophy of the turbinates?
    a. By inhalation
    b. Topically
    c. Orally
    d. Transdermally

37. A postoperative cervical diseconomy client has developed laryngeal edema. The nurse would assess for which of the following?
    a. Eupnea
    b. Crackles
    c. Laryngeal stridor
    d. Cheek-stokes respirations

38. The nurse notifies the physician stat of the assessment of laryngeal edema. Why is this a medical emergency?

39. Which of the following structures in the neck is treated with a tracheostomy if this site is damaged?
    a. Cricoid bone
    b. Thyroid cartilage
    c. Cricoid cartilage
    d. Thyroid gland

40. Initial emergency management for upper airway obstruction as a result of foreign body aspiration includes:
    a. Several sharp blows between the scapulae.
    b. Cardiopulmonary resuscitation.
    c. Nasotracheal suctioning.
    d. Abdominal thrusts (Heimlich maneuver).

41. Identify three causes of neck trauma.
    a. _____
    b. _____
    c. _____

42. As a result of neck trauma, the nurse must monitor for problems related to the: *Check all that apply.*
    ___ a. Esophagus.
    ___ b. Cervical spine.
    ___ c. Carotid artery.
    ___ d. Frontal lobe of the brain.

43. Clients with head and neck trauma or surgery are unable to verbally communicate. Identify at least four methods that such a client can use to communicate.
    a. _____
    b. _____
    c. _____
    d. _____

44. The type of tumor that most commonly affects the head and neck area is which of the following carcinomas?
    a. Adenocarcinoma
    b. Basal cell carcinoma
    c. Squamous cell carcinoma
    d. Melanoma

45. Which of the following statements regarding head and neck cancer is correct?
    a. Metastasizes often to the brain.
    b. Usually develops over a short time.
    c. Often seen as red edematous areas.
    d. Often seen as white patchy mucosal lesions.

46. When performing a nursing history, the nurse would assess for what risk factors that would relate to head and neck cancer? What are the two highest risk factors?

47. Which of the following clients is at risk for developing, specifically, cancer of the larynx?
    a. A 57-year-old male alcoholic
    b. An 18-year-old marijuana smoker
    c. A 28-year-old woman school teacher
    d. A 34-year-old man who snorts cocaine

48. On a separate sheet of paper, identify at least five warning signs of head and neck cancer.

49. To facilitate comfort and breathing for a client with a laryngeal tumor, the nurse would use which type of positioning?
    a. Sims'
    b. Supine
    c. Fowler's
    d. Trendelenburg

50. The one surgical procedure that does *not* put the client at risk postoperatively for aspiration is which of the following and why?
    a. Total laryngectomy
    b. Transoral cordectomy
    c. Supraglottic laryngectomy
    d. Partial laryngectomy

51. The nurse would teach the client to be aware that aspiration can occur as a result of which procedure for treating laryngeal cancer? Indicate other procedures for which the client is at risk for aspiration.
    a. Transoral cordectomy
    b. Laser surgery
    c. Radiation therapy
    d. Supraglottic laryngectomy

52. The client asks the nurse why there is a risk for aspiration as a result of supraglottic laryngectomy. What would be her answer?

53. Explain to a client the steps in performing the supraglottic method of swallowing.

54. Which of the following regarding aspiration precautions is *false*?
    a. Administer pills as whole tablets; they are easier to swallow.
    b. Aspiration with a nasogastric tube is a risk because of an incompetent LES.
    c. Keep head of bed elevated 30 to 45 minutes after feeding.
    d. Follow routine reflux precautions when an NG tube is in place.

55. If frequent aspiration occurs as result of supraglottic laryngectomy, what measures must be taken?

56. The test that is performed to determine a client's ability for swallow rehabilitation and aspiration precautions is a:
    a. Chest x-ray of the neck and chest.
    b. CT scan of head and neck.
    c. Barium swallow under fluoroscopy.
    d. Direct and indirect laryngoscopy.

57. Carotid precautions following radical neck dissection surgery include:
    a. Performing physical therapy exercise.
    b. Monitoring the flap using a Doppler.
    c. Moving the client to an observation bed.
    d. Applying wet to dry dressings to the flap.

58. What measures are available to the client for speech rehabilitation as a result of a total laryngectomy? Indicate what elements need to be in place for these measures.

59. A client is being evaluated by a speech therapist for either esophageal speech or tracheoesophageal fistula. Explain the difference between these two methods.

60. Which of the following is true regarding a radical neck dissection?
    a. Wound drainage tubes are not necessary for this type of surgery because a tracheostomy is in place.
    b. There will not be a permanent tracheostomy tube or stoma opening.
    c. Swallowing will not resume. Client is left with a permanent nasogastric or gastrostomy tube.
    d. Clients will have shoulder muscle weakness and limited range of motion resulting from nerve damage.

61. True or False? Read the following statements regarding head and neck cancers and decide whether each is true or false. *Write T for true or F for false in the blanks provided. If the statement is false, correct the statement to make it true.*
    ____ a. Head and neck cancers can be cured when treated early.
    ____ b. Diagnosis is usually not made until the disease is advanced.
    ____ c. Signs and symptoms of the disease are related to the location of the cancer.
    ____ d. Red velvety patches are called leukoplakia.
    ____ e. Many diagnostic tests are performed. CT scan aides in finding the exact location of a tumor, whereas MRI defines soft tissue invasion.
    ____ f. Radiation treatments are the preferred treatment for all locations and sizes of head and neck cancers.
    ____ g. Physical therapy is for postoperative radical neck surgery clients only.
    ____ h. Discharge teaching for all partial or total laryngectomy clients will include tracheostomy care.
    ____ i. Clients may have tubes removed before they are discharged from the hospital.
    ____ j. Discharge teaching for a total laryngectomy client will include stoma care, which combines wound and airway care.

62. The treatment of small specific tumors and/or early malignancies is which of the following? Develop a client teaching plan for this procedure.
    a. Radical neck dissection
    b. Radiation
    c. Chemotherapy
    d. Partial laryngectomy

63. Which of the following statements regarding client education and radiation therapy is true?
    a. The client's voice will initially be hoarse but should improve over time.
    b. There are no side effects other than a hoarse voice.
    c. Dry mouth after radiation therapy is temporary and short-term.
    d. The throat is unlikely to feel the effects of radiation because it is *not* directly affected by radiation.

64. A client with a partial laryngectomy should be prepared postoperatively for which of the following?
    a. Clients will have permanent swallowing problems after surgery.
    b. Because of postoperative swelling, the client will have a tracheostomy tube and nasogastric tube for feeding.
    c. Communications will not be a problem after the tracheostomy tube is removed because of voice conservation.
    d. The tracheostomy is always permanent and is referred to as a laryngectomy stoma.

65. Complete the table on the following page regarding each of the surgical procedures for laryngeal cancer.

66. Which of the following topics would *not* be included in preoperative teaching for a client scheduled for a total laryngectomy and why?
    a. Airway tube and suctioning
    b. Compensatory method of communication
    c. Drains and tubes
    d. Reconstruction using tissue "flaps"

67. Discharge teaching for clients with tracheotomies includes self-care instructions related to:
    a. Esophageal speech.
    b. Using a table mirror for visibility when suctioning.
    c. Never being able to shower again.
    d. Not being able to eat solid foods.

68. Develop a discharge teaching plan related to a client with total laryngectomy that includes all of the following items. Show your plan to your clinical instructor.
    a. Tracheostomy and stoma care
    b. Method of communication
    c. Activities of daily living
    d. Nutritional support
    e. Psychosocial issues

Surgical Procedures	Description	Resulting Voice Quality
Laser Surgery		
Transoral cordectomy		
Supraglottic partial laryngectomy		
Hemilaryngectomy		
Total laryngectomy		

STUDY GUIDE NUMBER 6.30

Interventions for Clients with Noninfectious Lower Respiratory Problems

Study/Review Questions

1. Match each of the following lower respiratory tract structures with the corresponding function. *Answers may be used more than once.*

   Lower Respiratory Tract Structures
   ___ a. Alveolus
   ___ b. Bronchus
   ___ c. Bronchioles
   ___ d. Carina
   ___ e. Cilia
   ___ f. Hilum
   ___ g. Lung
   ___ h. Parietal pleura
   ___ i. Surfactant
   ___ j. Trachea
   ___ k. Visceral pleura

   Lower Respiratory Tract Functions
   1. Point where trachea bifurcates
   2. Propels mucus for lower airways to trachea
   3. Reduces surface tension in the alveoli
   4. Carries air to each lobe of lungs
   5. Elastic organs that allow for ventilation and air diffusion
   6. Carries air from bronchi to alveolar ducts
   7. Carries air from larynx to bronchi
   8. Covers lung surfaces to decrease friction
   9. Lines inside of thoracic cavity to decrease friction with respiration
   10. Gases are exchanged in this basic unit
   11. Forms the roof of the lungs

2. If problems arise in the lower respiratory tract, they would involve mainly what two principles of respiration?
   a. _____
   b. _____

3. A client has been diagnosed with a chronic airflow limitation (CAL) problem. Which of the following is *not* a disease of CAL?
   a. Bronchiectasis
   b. Bronchial asthma
   c. Chronic bronchitis
   d. Pulmonary emphysema

4. Which of the following statements best character-
izes the long-term effect of asthma and COPD as
chronic diseases of the lower respiratory system?
   a. Asthma and COPD result in acute reversible airway respiratory distress episodes with no permanent alveoli damage.
   b. Asthma and COPD cause acute episodes that
   result in permanent alveoli damage that worsen
   over time causing respiratory failure.
   c. Asthma results in acute reversible airway distress
   with no permanent alveoli damage. COPD
   causes permanent alveoli damage that worsens
   over time.
   d. Asthma causes permanent alveoli damage that
   worsens over time. COPD results in acute
   reversible airway distress with no permanent
   alveoli damage.

5. The narrowing of the airway in either asthma or
COPD is ultimately the result of which of the following?
   a. Constriction from inflammation of the airways
   attributed to different etiologies
   b. Obstruction from thick mucous secretions related
   to infection
   c. Reaction to medications that reverse the effects
   on the airways
   d. Impaired gas exchange in the alveoli affecting
   the bronchial airways

6. Match each of the following pathophysiologic
changes with the corresponding type of disease that
is associated with CAL. *Answers may be used more
than once.*

   Characteristics of
   Diseases of CAL
   ___ a. Affects smaller
   airways
   ___ b. Chronic thickening of bronchial
   walls
   ___ c. Decreased surface area of alveoli
   ___ d. Destruction of alveolar walls
   ___ e. Hypercapnia
   ___ f. Impaired mucociliary clearance
   ___ g. Increased airway resistance
   ___ h. Increased eosinophils
   ___ i. Increased secretions
   ___ j. Affects work of breathing
   ___ k. Intermittent bronchospasm
   ___ l. Intermittent mucosal edema
   ___ m. Intermittent excess mucus production
   ___ n. Loss of elastic recoil
   ___ o. Mast cell destabilization

   Types of Disease
   1. Asthma
   2. Chronic bronchitis
   3. Pulmonary
   emphysema

   ___ p. Proteases break down elastin
   ___ q. Allergies stimulate disease process
   ___ r. Respiratory acidosis can result
   ___ s. Inflammation causes narrowing of the airway lumen
   ___ t. Narrowing of airway from smooth muscle
   constriction occurs in this type
   ___ u. Anti-inflammatory drugs used to treat disease can trigger onset of this disease

7. When exercising, a client with asthma should be
taught to monitor for which of the following problems? What would the nurse recommend to prevent
future episodes of this problem?
   a. Increased peak expiratory flow rates
   b. Wheezing from bronchospasm
   c. Wheezing from atelectasis
   d. Dyspnea from pulmonary hypertension

8. Treatment modalities for emphysema and bronchitis
will be prescribed according to which of the following pathophysiologic changes in the respiratory system?
   a. Hyperinflation and lung elasticity from alveoli
   damage occurs in emphysema. Bronchitis only
   affects the airways.
   b. Emphysema causes a barrel chest resulting from
   bronchospasm, but this does not occur in bronchitis.
   c. Bronchitis affects only the alveoli and not the
   large or small airways. Emphysema affects all
   three areas.
   d. Bronchitis causes the lungs to work hard from
   hyperinflation of the alveoli. Emphysema does
   the same.

9. The classic assessment findings for clients with
CAL are:
   a. Cyanosis, dyspnea, and wheezing.
   b. Cough, dyspnea, and wheezing.
   c. Cough, cyanosis, and dyspnea.
   d. Cough, dyspnea, and tachypnea.

10. For a client who is a nonsmoker, which of the classic assessment findings of CAL is particularly
important in diagnosing asthma?
   a. Cough
   b. Dyspnea
   c. Audible wheezing
   d. Tachypnea

11. A client who is allergic to dogs experiences an
"asthma attack." In addition to audible wheezing,
briefly describe other signs and symptoms that often
occur. *Use a separate sheet of paper for your
answer.*

12. A client newly diagnosed with asthma has a nursing diagnosis of Deficient Knowledge related to treatment interventions. As a nursing intervention, briefly explain to this client the goals for treating asthma and self-care management.

13. The nurse explains to the client that the rationale for what causes a "barrel chest" is the:
    a. Use of accessory muscles increases the front to back ratio of the chest.
    b. Long-term effect of dyspnea as a result of air being trapped in lungs or hyperinflation.
    c. Long-term side effect of chronic hypoxia.
    d. Collapse of the alveoli, increasing the work of breathing.

14. A client with chronic bronchitis often shows signs of hypoxia. The nurse would observe for which of the following clinical manifestations of this problem?
    a. Increased capillary refill
    b. Clubbing of fingers
    c. Pink mucous membranes
    d. Overall pale appearance

15. Match each of the following assessment findings of CAL with the corresponding description.

Assessment Findings	Descriptions
___ a. Abdominal paradox	1. Cachectic emphysemic client
___ b. Asynchronous breathing	2. Increased anteroposterior-to-lateral chest diameter
___ c. Barrel chest	
___ d. Blue bloater	3. Diaphragmatic breathing alternating with abdominal breathing
___ e. Pink puffer	
___ f. Respiratory alternans	4. Use of intercostal and abdominal muscles to breath
	5. Chronic cyanotic bronchitis client
	6. Unorganized chest motion

16. Explain to a client how smoking affects the respiratory tract and why coughing occurs in the morning upon rising.

17. Shortness of breath is often a complaint of clients with chronic pulmonary disease. Which of following best describes the type of breathing that the client experiences? When does this problem usually occur? What relieves the problem?
    a. Paroxysmal nocturnal dyspnea
    b. Orthopnea
    c. Tachypnea
    d. Cheyne-Stokes

18. In chronic bronchitis, impaired gas exchange occurs as a result of which of the following?
    a. Chronic inflammation, thin secretions, and chronic infection
    b. Respiratory alkalosis, decreased $Paco_2$, and increased Pao_2
    c. Chronic inflammation and decreased surfactant in the alveoli and atelectasis
    d. Thickening of the bronchial walls, large amounts of thick secretions, and repeated infections

19. The assessment finding related to the chest x-ray of a client with emphysema would be:
    a. Hypoinflation of the lungs.
    b. A flattened diaphragm.
    c. A mediastinal shift.
    d. No obvious changes.

20. What effect does the work of breathing have on the metabolic demands of the client?
    a. Decreases the need for calories and protein requirements since dyspnea causes activity intolerance.
    b. It has no effect on caloric protein needs, meal tolerance, satiety, appetite, and weight.
    c. Increases metabolism and the need for additional calories and protein supplements.
    d. Creates an anabolic state for building body mass, muscle strength, and easier breathing.

21. In obtaining a history of a client with CAL, which of the following would *not* be related to potentially causing/triggering the disease process?
    a. Cigarette smoking
    b. Occupational and air pollution
    c. Genetic tendencies
    d. Smokeless tobacco

22. The nurse explains that smoking cessation affects the disease process of COPD by:
    a. Completely reversing the damage to the lungs.
    b. Slowing the rate of disease progression.
    c. Stabilizing the effects on the airways and lungs.
    d. Reversing the effects on the airways but not the lungs.

23. Which of the following is *not* a potential complication that can result from COPD?
    a. Respiratory infections
    b. Right-sided heart failure
    c. Left-sided heart failure
    d. Cardiac dysrhythmias

24. When reading a summary of a pulmonary function test, the most significant reading to take note of for obstructive pulmonary disease is the:
    a. FEVI/FVC ratio
    b. Functional residual capacity
    c. Total lung capacity
    d. Residual volume

25. Over time, a decrease in the FEVI/FVC ratio indicates to the nurse that:
    a. The disease process is stable.
    b. CAL is progressing.
    c. CAL is improving.
    d. Further testing is needed to determine effects of disease.

26. Match each pulmonary function test with the corresponding test results that can indicate obstructive or restrictive disease. *There may be more than one answer for each test.*

    Pulmonary Function Test
    ___ a. Forced vital capacity (FVC)
    ___ b. Forced expiratory volume in 1 sec (FEV1)
    ___ c. Functional residual capacity (FRC)
    ___ d. Total lung capacity (TLC)
    ___ e. Residual volume (RV)
    ___ f. Diffusion capacity of carbon monoxide
    ___ g. Peak expiratory flow (PEF)

    Test Results
    1. Often reduced in obstructive disease
    2. Often reduced/decreased in restrictive disease
    3. Increased in obstructive pulmonary disease
    4. Increased in obstructive disease
    5. Reduced/decreased in certain obstructive or restrictive disorders
    6. Normal in restrictive disease
    7. Results improve after use of bronchodilators — classic diagnostic test for asthma

27. The purpose of pulmonary function testing for clients with CAL is to:
    a. Determine the oxygen liter flow rates required by the client.
    b. Measure arterial and venous blood gas levels before bronchodilators are administered.
    c. Evaluate the movement of oxygenated blood from the lung to the heart.
    d. Distinguish airway disease from restrictive lung disease.

28. An adult client with respiratory difficulty has completed the pulmonary function test before starting any treatment. The peak expiratory flow (PEF) is 18% below what is expected for this client's age, gender, and size. This result is:
    a. An indication for further diagnostic tests to confirm asthma.
    b. A confirmed finding in clients with asthma.
    c. High for a client with asthma and COPD.
    d. Confirmation of a respiratory disease of unknown type.

29. Clients with asthma learn to use the PEF/FVC values for determining interventions. Briefly explain how a client uses this information and what options are available.

30. As the nurse, how would you explain to the client how to determine the FEVI/peak flow value?

31. As a result of the analysis of assessment findings, what are the common nursing diagnoses for clients with CAL?

32. Clients with asthma are taught self-care activities and treatment modalities according to the "step method." Which of the following relates to step 3? How does this differ from chronic bronchitis and emphysema?
    a. Symptoms occur frequently; increased use of rescue inhalers.
    b. Symptoms occur daily; daily use of anti-inflammatory inhaler with inhaler bronchodilator; no systemic steroids.
    c. Symptoms occur daily; daily use of CSC and long-acting beta agonist; steroids used for rescue.
    d. Frequent exacerbations with limited physical activity; daily CSC; systemic steroids and methylxanthines.

33. A high-liter flow of oxygen is contraindicated in the client with COPD because:
    a. The client depends often on a hypercapnic drive to breathe.
    b. The client depends on a hypoxic drive to breathe.
    c. Receiving too much oxygen over a short time results in headache.
    d. Response to high doses needed later will be ineffective.

34. In assisting a client with CAL to relieve dyspnea, which of the following positions would *not* be of benefit to the client?
    a. Sitting on edge of chair, leaning forward with arms folded and resting on a small table
    b. Leaning back in a low semi-reclining position with the shoulders back and several pillows under the head
    c. Sitting forward in a chair with feet spread apart and elbows placed on the knees
    d. Leaning back against a support with feet spread apart and shoulders slumped forward

35. Which of the following nursing interventions would *not* be included in the instruction regarding the nursing diagnosis of Deficient Knowledge related to energy conservation measures? Provide a rationale for your answer.
    a. Activities should be at a relaxed paced throughout the day with rest periods.
    b. Avoid working on activities that require using arms at a level higher than the chest.
    c. Eat largest meal when assistance can be provided and eat three large meals a day.
    d. Avoid talking and doing activities at the same time.

36. Identify the main classifications of drugs that are used to treat CAL.
    a. _____
    b. _____
    c. _____
    d. _____
    e. _____

37. Identify and describe the action of the three types of bronchodilators used to treat asthma. Give an example of each type.
    a. _____
    b. _____
    c. _____

38. The lab result for a theophylline level is 18 μ/mL. This would indicate the prescribed dose of theophylline is:
    a. Within therapeutic range.
    b. Too high of a dose.
    c. Too low of a dose.
    d. Questionable; further information is needed.

39. Which of the following information from a client's history would cause a decrease in serum theophylline levels?
    a. Cigarette smoking
    b. Caffeine consumption
    c. Oral contraceptives
    d. Alcohol consumption

40. A client receiving IV theophylline complains of nausea, abdominal pain, headache, and inability to sleep. The nurse would:
    a. Administer Compazine for nausea.
    b. Administer an antacid.
    c. Obtain a physician's order for a theophylline level.
    d. Tell the client that these side effects are normal and not to worry.

41. A client with CAL and pneumonia is admitted to the hospital for exacerbation of COPD. Explain why the nurse has a separate IV line for administering aminophylline to this client.

42. A client with asthma has been prescribed a Flovent inhaler. The nurse explains to the client the purpose of this drug is to:
    a. Relax the smooth muscles of the airway.
    b. Act as a bronchodilator in severe episodes.
    c. Reduce obstruction of the airway by decreasing the inflammation.
    d. Reduce the histamine effect of the triggering agent.

43. In addition to corticosteroid anti-inflammatory inhalers, indicate other types of anti-inflammatory agents used, and give the action of the drugs. Provide an example of the medication for each category.
    a. _____
    b. _____
    c. _____

44. A client is learning to use an inhaler in the treatment of asthma. Briefly describe how the client should use the inhaler correctly.

45. A client asks about the advantages of using the aerosol route for administering corticosteroids. The nurse replies by saying that this route:
    a. Has less of a bronchodilation effect.
    b. Reduces the risk for fungus infections.
    c. Is easier to use and compliance is better.
    d. Is fast acting with fewer systemic side effects.

46. When teaching a client with CAL, which of the following is the correct sequence for administering aerosol treatments?
    a. Steroid should be given immediately after the bronchodilator.
    b. Steroid should be given 5 to 10 minutes after the bronchodilator.
    c. Bronchodilator should be given immediately after the steroid.
    d. Bronchodilator should be given 5 to 10 minutes after the steroid.

47. Which of the following statements about the use of cromolyn sodium for the treatment of asthma is correct?
    a. It acts by strengthening mast cell membranes to increase histamine release and decrease bronchospasm.
    b. It is useful primarily during acute episodes of asthma attacks.
    c. It is not intended for use during acute episodes of asthma attacks.
    d. It acts by weakening mast cell membranes to decrease histamine releases and bronchospasm.

48. Complete the first chart below to compile a comparison of the classes of medications used in the treatment of CAL.

49. Complete the second chart below to compare and contrast the classes of respiratory drugs.

Drug Name	Usual Route/ Dose	Expected Action	Adverse Actions	Nursing Implications
Sympathomimetics				
Methylxanthines				
Anticholinergics				
Corticosteroids				

Drug Name	Usual Route/ Dose	Expected Action	Adverse Actions	Nursing Implications
Antitussives				
Expectorants				
Mucolytics				

50. The nurse instructs the client with COPD in the proper coughing techniques. Which of the following would *not* be a recommended time to perform this technique and why? What is the purpose of coughing at the recommended times?
    a. Upon rising in the morning
    b. Before meals
    c. After meals
    d. Bedtime

Answer the following three questions on a separate sheet of paper.

51. In addition to teaching the client *when* to perform coughing techniques, the nurse teaches the client *how* to cough properly so as to effectively eliminate excessive secretions. Briefly explain the steps for the "controlled coughing" procedure.

52. For a client with CAL, identify at least 10 topics that would be considered for collaborative interventions.

53. Identify appropriate interventions for clients with asthma, including when to seek immediate medical attention.

54. As a result of chronic bronchitis or emphysema, an assessment finding for a client with heart failure, especially cor pulmonale, is:
    a. Left ventricular hypertrophy.
    b. Weak pulse.
    c. Fatigue.
    d. Dehydration.

Answer the following three questions on a separate sheet of paper.

55. Explain how you would instruct a client with a diagnosis of Ineffective Breathing Pattern to perform the diaphragmatic and pursed-lip breathing techniques.

56. Describe the factors that a nurse should assess for when a client with CAL complains of shortness of breath.

57. Develop a teaching plan that includes home care activities for a newly diagnosed adult client with CAL.

58. Assessment findings of respiratory failure for a client with asthma are:
    a. Rales, rhonchi, and productive cough of yellowed sputum.
    b. Tachypnea, dry cough, and chest pain.
    c. Diminished or inaudible breath sounds, wheezing, and use of accessory muscles.
    d. Respiratory alkalosis, slow, shallow respiratory rate.

59. On a separate sheet of paper, develop a concept map relevant to CAL. Consider physiologic, psychosocial, and developmental factors. Identify subjective and objective data.

60. Primary prevention for those employees at high risk for occupational pulmonary disease is which of the following?
    a. Screen all employees by use of chest x-ray films twice a year.
    b. Do not smoke and do use proper masks and ventilation equipment.
    c. Perform pulmonary function tests once a year on all employees.
    d. Perform monthly inspections of areas according to standards.

61. Clients with occupational lung diseases and chronic lung diseases are considered to be at high risk for which of the following?
    a. Tuberculosis
    b. AIDS
    c. Lung cancer
    d. ARDS

62. The most important intervention in the management of dust-related diseases is:
    a. Using masks and having adequate ventilation for prevention.
    b. PFTs to evaluate lung function.
    c. Using supplemental oxygen therapy to alleviate hypoxemia.
    d. Education about using bronchodilators to relieve dyspnea.

63. Match each of the following terms related to occupational lung diseases with the corresponding definition.

    Terms
    ___ a. Pneumoconiosis
    ___ b. Silicosis
    ___ c. Asbestosis
    ___ d. Talcosis
    ___ e. Berylliosis

    Definitions
    1. Interstitial lung fibrosis related to asbestos exposure
    2. Sarcoidosis related to exposure to highly heated or machined metals
    3. Pulmonary fibrosis related to long-term talc dust exposure
    4. A group of chronic respiratory diseases related to occupational inhaling of dust
    5. Chronic fibrosing lung disease related to silica dust inhalation

64. Which of the following statements about lung cancer is correct? *Correct the false statements.*
    a. The death rate for lung cancer is less than prostate, breast, and colon cancers combined.
    b. The overall 5-year survival rate for all clients with lung cancer is 85%.
    c. Survival can be attributed to early diagnosis and treatment of the lung cancer.
    d. The primary prevention for reducing the risk is to stop smoking and avoid secondhand smoke.

65. True or False? Read the following statements regarding lung cancer and decide whether each is true or false. *Write T for true or F for false in the blanks provided. If the statement is false, correct the statement to make it true.*
    ___ a. There are two primary classifications of lung cancer—small cell and non–small cell.
    ___ b. Non–small cell lung cancer is further divided into three types—squamous, adenocarcinoma, and large cell.
    ___ c. Metastasis occurs via three routes—obstruction/direct invasion, blood, and lymph nodes.
    ___ d. Common metastasis sites include bone, liver, brain, and adrenal glands.
    ___ e. Non–small cell lung cancer is often associated with paraneoplastic syndromes.
    ___ f. The risk of lung cancer decreases after 5 years of not smoking.
    ___ g. The number of cigarettes and years of smoking do not contribute to the risk; it is the tar and nicotine that contribute to the risk.
    ___ h. African Americans are at less risk for lung cancer than are whites.
    ___ i. The death rate for lung cancer is the same for African Americans and whites.
    ___ j. Wearing a specialized mask can decrease the risk of developing occupation-related lung cancer.
    ___ k. Women smokers are at a lower risk of developing lung cancer than are men because they have a protective gene.
    ___ l. Onset of symptoms is a positive sign of early disease.
    ___ m. A chest x-ray film is a good screening tool for lung cancer.
    ___ n. Lung cancer is always diagnosed by sputum specimens.
    ___ o. Surgical intervention for non–small cell cancer is the goal for curing the client.
    ___ p. A wedge resection is a form of surgical intervention that removes a small localized section of the diseased lung.

66. A client with sudden onset of a deep vein thrombosis of unknown origin was diagnosed with lung cancer. This type of paraneoplastic syndrome resulting from lung cancer is a sign of:
    a. Good prognosis with surgical intervention of diseased lung.
    b. A lung cancer that can be treated easily with radiation.
    c. The poorest prognosis because of the metastasis.
    d. A good prognosis if the client stops smoking.

67. Match each of the following features of lung cancer with the corresponding type of lung cancer. *More than one answer may apply.*

Features of Lung Cancer	Type of Lung Cancer
___ a. Often located in the large bronchi	1. Small cell
___ b. Slow-growing type of tumor	2. Squamous
___ c. Often associated with lymph metastasis	3. Adenocarcinoma
___ d. Smoking is a high-risk factor	4. Large cell
___ e. Associated with nonsmokers	
___ f. Outcome is a poor prognosis	
___ g. Associated with the classic symptoms of lung cancer	
___ h. Not a good surgical candidate because of metastasis on diagnosis	
___ i. Surgical intervention is effective, especially in early stages	
___ j. Type often found in women	
___ k. Incidence is about one third of all types	
___ l. Chemotherapy is used as a adjunct to other treatment	
___ m. Surgery is treatment of choice for stage I and stage II	

68. The common signs and symptoms that are often associated with lung cancer are which of the following?
    a. Insidious onset of blood-tinged sputum, cough, hoarseness, shortness of breath
    b. Short onset of cough, shortness of breath, and blood-tinged sputum
    c. Wheezing, coughing, shortness of breath, and palpitations
    d. High-grade fever, chills, and shortness of breath

69. Radiation therapy differs from chemotherapy in which of the following ways?
    a. Radiation treatments are given daily in "cycles" over the course of several months.
    b. Radiation treatments cause hair loss, nausea, and vomiting for the duration of treatment.
    c. Radiation treatments cause dry skin at the radiation site, fatigue, changes in appetite with nausea.
    d. Radiation is the best method of treatment for systemic metastatic disease.

70. The term used to define the general surgical procedure for lung cancer is which of the following? Define the incorrect answers.
    a. Lobectomy
    b. Thoracotomy
    c. Pneumonectomy
    d. Segmentectomy

71. Which type of surgical intervention for lung cancer does *not* require a chest tube postoperatively and why?
    a. Segmentectomy
    b. Lobectomy
    c. Wedge resection
    d. Pneumonectomy

72. Immediately after a pneumonectomy, the nurse positions the client on the:
    a. Operative side only to allow expansion of the remaining lung.
    b. Non-operative side only to decrease risk of damage to surgical site and improve breathing.
    c. Side or back, rotating periodically to prevent stagnation of fluid.
    d. Back only, with head elevated to improve breathing.

73. Briefly explain the function of each of the chambers/bottles of a three-bottle/chamber water seal drainage system that is used with chest tubes. On a separate sheet of paper, indicate key nursing interventions related to each chamber.
    a. Bottle/chamber 1
    b. Bottle/chamber 2
    c. Bottle/chamber 3

74. Which of the following is a correct nursing intervention for clients with chest tubes?
    a. Clients should be encouraged to cough and do deep breathing exercises frequently.
    b. Vigorous "stripping" of the chest tubes should be done routinely to prevent obstruction by blood clots.
    c. Water level in the suction chamber need not be monitored, just the collection chamber.
    d. Drainage containers can be positioned upright or on the side with tubing in no particular position.

75. Upon observation of a chest tube set-up, the nurse reports to the physician that there is a leak in the chest tube and system. The nurse assesses this problem by noting which of the following?
    a. Drainage in the collection chamber has decreased.
    b. The bubbling in the suction chamber has suddenly increased.
    c. Fluctuation in the water seal chamber has stopped.
    d. Onset of vigorous bubbling in the water seal chamber.

76. For a client with a chest tube, the physician's orders indicate an increase in the suction to 20 mL. To implement this order the nurse would perform which of the following interventions?
    a. Increase the wall suction to medium suction to maintain the bubbling in the suction chamber.
    b. Add water to the water seal chamber to the level of 20.
    c. Stop the bubbling in the suction chamber, add sterile water to level of 20, and resume bubbling.
    d. Have client cough and deep breath and monitor the level of fluctuation to achieve 20 cm.

77. Discharge teaching considerations for clients with a thoracotomy, especially with a pneumonectomy, is:
    a. Prevention of arm immobility problems by use of range-of-motion exercises and increasing the use of the arm.
    b. Protecting the operative site and preventing complications by limiting the motion of the arm/shoulder with a sling.
    c. Resume preoperative activities as soon as possible to promote well-being, independence, and autonomy.
    d. Change pain medication or decrease pain medication to minimize respiratory depression effects of narcotics.

78. On a separate sheet of paper, briefly summarize nursing interventions for a client with a thoracotomy.

79. Which of the following is *not* a factor in the development of lung cancer?
    a. Air pollution
    b. Radon gas exposure
    c. Chronic respiratory disease
    d. Chewing tobacco

80. Identify the nursing diagnoses common to the client with lung cancer.
    a. _____
    b. _____
    c. _____

81. The major complication from treatment with the chemotherapy agent cisplatin is:
    a. Diarrhea.
    b. Nausea.
    c. Flatulence.
    d. Constipation.

82. The most effective intervention for relieving pain resulting from bone metastases caused by lung cancer that still allows for mobility is:
    a. Radiation therapy.
    b. Patient-controlled analgesia.
    c. Continuous morphine infusion.
    d. Oral meperidine hydrochloride (Demerol).

83. A chest tube system that drains by gravity is functioning correctly when the water seal chamber:
    a. Bubbles vigorously and continuously.
    b. Bubbles gently and continuously.
    c. Fluctuates with the client's respirations.
    d. Fluctuates vigorously when the client coughs.

84. Interventions to promote comfort in the client with lung cancer include:
    a. Medicating with analgesics only when requested.
    b. Positioning prone with a pillow under abdomen and shins.
    c. Ventilating with a high tidal volume and PEEP.
    d. Providing supplemental oxygen via cannula or mask.

85. A client with small-cell lung cancer is being discharged from the hospital. Which of the following community resources would the nurse potentially discuss with this client?
    a. The local hospice program
    b. A home health care agency
    c. A vendor of durable medical supplies
    d. All of the above

86. A client with repeated pleural effusions, as a result of lung cancer, is injected with a sclerosing agent. The nurse's role is to:
    a. Assist in positioning the client so that the affected lung is dependent while the drug is being injected.
    b. Clamp the chest tube securely following the instillation of the drug.
    c. Instruct the client to remain very still for at least 1 hour after the drug has been injected.
    d. Notify the respiratory therapist to administer respiratory therapy treatments.

87. A severe complication of pulmonary hypertension is which of the following problems?
    a. Right side heart enlarges, dilates, and fails
    b. Left side of heart enlarges, dilates, and fails
    c. Decreased cardiac output related to left ventricular failure
    d. Narrowing of the pulse pressure

88. The name of the complication defined in Question 87 is called:
    a. Myocardial infarction.
    b. ARDS.
    c. Cor pulmonale.
    d. Stroke.

89. Which of the following is *not* diagnostic of pulmonary hypertension?
    a. Client complains of fatigue and dyspnea
    b. Normal ventilation–perfusion scans (V/Q scan)
    c. Changes in pulmonary function test
    d. Cardiac catheterization of right side heart indicates elevated pulmonary pressures

90. A client has developed pulmonary hypertension. Which of the following is *not* included in the care of this client?
    a. Coumadin
    b. Beta blockers
    c. Oxygen therapy
    d. Diuretics

91. True or False? Decide whether each of the following statements are *true* or *false* regarding pulmonary hypertension. *Write* T *for true or* F *for false in the blanks provided.*
    ___ a. Conditions such as COPD, pulmonary fibrosis, and pulmonary emboli can result in pulmonary hypertension.
    ___ b. When treating cor pulmonale, collaborative management is designed around the underlying cause of pulmonary hypertension.
    ___ c. When medical management fails, heart-lung or lung transplantation might be necessary.

92. Which of the following statements about sarcoidosis is correct?
    a. Sarcoidosis is a chronic disorder of the alveoli characterized by granuloma development.
    b. Sarcoidosis is a group of diseases also known as *interstitial lung disease.*
    c. Sarcoidosis is an acute disorder of the alveoli characterized by granuloma development.
    d. Sarcoidosis is caused by the sarcoid pneumonia bacterium and is highly contagious.

93. Granuloma development in sarcoidosis results from the activation of:
    a. Lymphocytes.
    b. T-lymphocytes.
    c. Macrophages.
    d. Monocytes.

94. Drug treatment of sarcoidosis includes:
    a. Antibiotics.
    b. Bronchodilators.
    c. Corticosteroids.
    d. Chemotherapeutic agents.

95. The similarity between pulmonary fibrosis and sarcoidosis is that both:
    a. Will result in death if a lung transplant is not performed.
    b. Are treated by steroids.
    c. Are progressive with a slow onset.
    d. Are a result of excessive inflammatory response.

96. A client with a history of CAL enters the emergency room with severe dyspnea with noted accessory muscle involvement and neck vein distension, along with severe inspiratory/expiratory wheezing. This respiratory emergency is diagnosed as which of the following life-threatening conditions?
    a. Pulmonary fibrosis
    b. Pulmonary hypertension
    c. Exacerbation of sarcoidosis
    d. Status asthmaticus

97. Status asthmaticus is a potentially life-threatening problem requiring immediate interventions because:
   a. Usual interventions are ineffective; it tends to intensify and progress, and IV fluids with medications are required.
   b. The asthma attack causes a pneumothorax resulting in audible wheezing and need of a chest tube.
   c. Neck vein distention is a signal of imminent left-sided heart failure and decreased cardiac output.
   d. Respiratory arrest will occur without the required intubation and mechanical ventilation.

98. Identify specific nursing interventions for an older adult client with respiratory disorders.

STUDY GUIDE NUMBER 6.31

Interventions for Clients with Infectious Respiratory Problems

Study/Review Questions

1. Every fall season, your adult client, diagnosed with rhinitis, complains of itchy watery eyes and rhinorrhea. Which of the following best explains rhinitis?
   a. Allergic rhinitis and coryza are initiated by sensitivity reactions to antigens.
   b. Viral rhinitis and hay fever are initiated by sensitivity reactions to antigens.
   c. Allergic rhinitis and hay fever are initiated by sensitivity reactions to allergens.
   d. Rhinitis medicamentous is relieved with the use of nose drops or sprays.

2. A client's history of which of the following disorders is a contraindication for drug therapy in providing symptomatic treatment of rhinitis?
   a. Sleep apnea
   b. Diverticulitis
   c. Meniere's disease
   d. Urinary retention

3. When prescribing drugs for treatment of rhinitis and sinusitis, which of the following classes of drugs would *not* be included?
   a. Antihistamines
   b. Antipyretics
   c. Decongestants
   d. Mucolytics

4. An assessment of which of the following would most likely follow or accompany rhinitis?
   a. Pharyngitis
   b. Tonsillitis
   c. Laryngitis
   d. Sinusitis

5. Which of the following statements regarding rhinitis and the older adult is *true*?
   a. Viral rhinitis is self-limiting and rarely leads to complications in the older adult.
   b. Antihistamines and decongestants should be used with caution.
   c. Antipyretics and antibiotics are not used because of risk of toxicity and allergic reactions.
   d. Complementary and alternative therapies are ineffective in the older adult.

6. A client complains of difficulty breathing, facial pain (especially when head is dependent), sneezing or coughing, green or bloody nasal drainage, productive cough, and low-grade fever. The client will be treated with antibiotics for which of the following diagnoses?
   a. Rhinitis
   b. Tonsillitis
   c. Sinusitis
   d. Pneumonia

7. If the client in Question 6 above had an upper airway infection related to a virus, would this client receive antibiotics? Indicate *yes* or *no* and give a reason for your answer.

8. An older adult diagnosed with bacterial pharyngitis may *not* present with which of the following assessment findings?
   a. Cough and rash
   b. High fever and elevated WBC count
   c. Voice characterized by pain on voicing
   d. Erythema of tonsils with yellow exudate

9. A client is seen in the physician's office for pharyngitis. Which of the following assessment findings is most indicative of a bacteria infection versus a viral infection? Identify other key features of acute viral versus bacterial pharyngitis.
   a. Fever
   b. Erythema of throat
   c. Headache
   d. Positive throat culture

10. A client complains of a "sore throat"/pharyngitis pain, temperature of 101.4° F, scarlatiniform rash, and a positive rapid test throat culture. This client will most likely be treated for which type of bacterial infection?
    a. Staphylococcus
    b. Pneumococcus
    c. Streptococcus
    d. Epstein-Barr virus

11. A client complains of a sore throat that is an indication of "strep throat." To prevent complications such as rheumatic heart disease, this client should receive antibiotic treatment within what time frame?
    a. 24 hours
    b. 48 hours
    c. 1 week
    d. 1 month

12. A priority nursing intervention for the nursing diagnosis of Deficient Knowledge related to the treatment of Group B streptococcus infection would include which of the following?
    a. Administration of penicillin or penicillin-like antibiotics
    b. Gradually resuming activity until there are no physical complaints
    c. Full liquid supplemental diet such as Ensure
    d. Observe for signs and symptoms of glomerulonephritis and rheumatic heart disease

13. A few weeks after having a Group A beta-hemolytic streptococcal pharyngitis, a client complains of joint pain, weakness, and a rash of the inner aspects of the upper arm and thigh. These assessment findings are indicative of which complication of Group A streptococcal infection?
    a. Acute glomerulonephritis
    b. Arthritis
    c. Rheumatic fever
    d. Scarlet fever

14. A 35-year-old male client with no health problems states that he had a flu shot last year and asks if it is necessary to have a flu shot again this year. The best response by the nurse would be:
    a. No, because once you get a flu shot, it lasts for several years and is effective against many different viruses.
    b. Yes, because the immunity against virus wears off, increasing your chances of getting the flu.
    c. Yes, because the vaccine guards against a specific virus and reduces your chances of acquiring flu.
    d. No, flu shots are only for high-risk clients and you are not considered to be at high risk.

15. An active 45-year-old schoolteacher with COPD taking the medication prednisone inquires about getting flu shots. The best response by the nurse would be:
    a. Yes, flu shots are highly recommended for a client with chronic illness and/or receiving immunotherapy.
    b. No, flu shots are only recommended for clients 50 years old and older.
    c. Yes, it will help minimize the risk of triggering an exacerbation of COPD.
    d. No, the client is active, is not living in a nursing home, and is not a health care provider.

16. The body structure primarily affected by pneumonia is which of the following?
    a. Bronchi
    b. Pharynx
    c. Alveoli
    d. Trachea

17. Identify three pathologic results that occur in the lung as a result of pneumonia.
    a. _____
    b. _____
    c. _____

18. Number the following events in sequential order as pertains to the pathophysiologic process of pneumonia.
    ___ a. Atelectasis
    ___ b. Possible septicemia
    ___ c. Decreased surfactant production and compliance
    ___ d. Arterial hypoxemia
    ___ e. Edema formation and inflammation
    ___ f. Tachypnea and tachycardia
    ___ g. Migration of white blood cells (WBCs) to alveoli
    ___ h. Spread of organisms to other alveoli
    ___ i. Shunting of unoxygenated blood
    ___ j. Thickening of alveolar wall and stiffening of lung
    ___ k. Diminished capillary blood flow in alveoli
    ___ l. Invasion of pulmonary tissue by pathogens

19. Decreased lung compliance in pneumonia is the result of which of the following pathologic problems?
    a. Occlusion of the bronchi and alveoli
    b. Inflammatory edema and decreased surfactant production
    c. Inflammatory edema and a ventilation-perfusion defect
    d. Atelectasis and WBC migration to the affected area

20. Which of the following clients are at the highest risk of developing pneumonia?
    a. Any hospitalized client between the ages of 18 and 65 years
    b. A 32-year-old trauma client on a mechanical ventilator
    c. A disabled 54-year-old client living at home with osteoporosis
    d. Any client who has not received the vaccine for pneumonia

21. After being seen at the doctor's office, a client states, "the doctor said I have pneumonia." The nurse explains to the client that pneumonia is:
    a. An infection of just the "windpipe" because the lungs are "clear" of any problems.
    b. Best explained as a serious inflammation of the bronchioles from various causes.
    c. Only an infection of the lungs with mild-to-severe effects on the breathing.
    d. An inflammation resulting from lung damage from long-term smoking.

22. For the client in Question 21, more than likely the first diagnostic test performed would be a:
    a. Lung scan.
    b. Pulmonary function test.
    c. Fluorescein bronchoscopy.
    d. Sputum Gram stain.

23. Which of the following is a common lab value finding as a result of pneumonia? What group of clients are exceptions to this finding?
    a. Increased erythrocyte maturation
    b. Increased number of RBCs
    c. Decreased number of WBCs
    d. Increased number of WBCs

24. A client with impaired gas exchange and pneumonia has a primary problem with which of the following? Identify a nursing intervention to correct this problem.
    a. Hypoxemia
    b. Hyperemia
    c. Hypocapnia
    d. Hypercapnia

25. Match each commonly seen organism to the corresponding type of pneumonia. *Answers may be used more than once.*

Organisms	**Type of Pneumonia**
___ a. *Legionella pneumophila*	1. Community-acquired pneumonia
___ b. *Pseudomonas aeruginosa*	2. Nosocomial pneumonia
___ c. *Staphylococcus aureus*	3. Opportunistic pneumonia
___ d. *Klebsiella pneumoniae*	
___ e. *Mycoplasma pneumoniae*	
___ f. *Streptococcus pneumoniae*	
___ g. *Candida albicans*	
___ h. *Pneumocystis carinii*	

26. A client with acquired immune deficiency syndrome (AIDS) is diagnosed with *Pneumocystis carinii* pneumonia. Identify the clinical manifestations that a nurse would assess.

27. A history, physical exam, and chest x-ray indicate pneumonia. The physician would suspect community-acquired pneumonia based on what assessment finding?
    a. A dry cough
    b. Slow onset of symptoms
    c. Abrupt onset of fever and chills
    d. Sudden change in mental status

28. Which of the following clients is the least likely to be at risk for developing pneumonia? On a separate sheet of paper, explain why you chose your answer.
    a. A client with a 5-year history of smoking
    b. A renal transplant client
    c. A postoperative client walking in the halls
    d. A postoperative client with a hip replacement

29. An essential diagnostic test for pneumonia in the older adult is which of the following tests?
    a. Pulse oximetry because of the older adults' normal decreased lung compliance
    b. Sputum specimen for accuracy of antibiotics to decrease risk of renal failure
    c. Elevated white blood cell count confirming findings of pleuritic chest pain, chills, fever, cough, and dyspnea
    d. Chest x-rays because assessment findings can be vague and resemble other problems

30. A client is admitted to the hospital because of pneumonia. The nurse would expect the chest x-ray results to reveal which of following?
    a. Patchy areas of consolidation
    b. Tension pneumothorax
    c. Thick secretions causing airway obstruction
    d. Stenosed pulmonary arteries

31. For most hospitalized clients, prevention of pneumonia is accomplished by which of the following nursing interventions?
    a. Monitoring chest x-rays for early signs of pneumonia
    b. Monitoring lung sounds every shift and forcing fluids
    c. Teaching the client coughing and deep breathing exercises and incentive spirometry
    d. Assuring respiratory therapy treatments are being performed every 4 hours

32. Education of clients in practices that prevent pneumonia would include which of the following nursing interventions?
    a. Administering vaccines to clients at risk
    b. Implementing strict bedrest for debilitated clients
    c. Restricting food and fluids in immunosuppressed clients
    d. Decontaminating respiratory therapy equipment weekly

33. The rationale for health care providers differentiating between nosocomial versus community-acquired pneumonia is useful because:
    a. Nosocomial infections are more likely to respond to antibiotics.
    b. Nosocomial infections, although common, are caused by organisms that are more resistant to treatment.
    c. The mortality rate is high in individuals with community-acquired pneumonia.
    d. Nosocomial pneumonia often occurs in clients in the fall and winter months after they have had a viral infection.

34. Identify three ways that an individual can develop pneumonia:
    a. _____
    b. _____
    c. _____

35. The key to effective treatment for the nursing diagnosis of Risk for Sepsis is administration of antibiotics. Initial antibiotic therapy is based on which of the following factors?
    a. Gram stains, sputum culture, chest x-ray film
    b. Client's signs and symptoms and type (nosocomial or community-acquired) of pneumonia
    c. Clinical assessment findings with elevated white blood cells
    d. Client's history, physical, and chest x-ray film results

36. A client hospitalized for pneumonia has a nursing diagnosis of Ineffective Airway Clearance related to fatigue, chest pain, excessive secretions, and muscle weakness. The nursing intervention to correct these problems includes which of the following?
    a. Administer oxygen to prevent hypoxemia and atelectasis.
    b. Push fluids to greater than 3000 mL/day to ensure adequate hydration.
    c. Administer respiratory therapy in a timely manner to decrease bronchospasms.
    d. Maintain semi-Fowler's position to facilitate breathing and prevent further fatigue.

37. A client is admitted to the hospital for treatment of pneumonia. Which of the following nursing assessment findings best indicates that the client is responding to the antibiotic?
    a. Wheezing, oxygen at 2 L, respiratory rate 26, no shortness of breath or chills
    b. Temp 99° F, lung sounds clear, pulse oximetry on 2 L at 98%, cough with yellow sputum
    c. Complains of cough, white sputum, temp 99° F, pulse oximetry at 96% on room air
    d. Complains of feeling tired, respiratory rate 28 on 2 L of oxygen, loud clear breath sounds

38. Which of the following lab values may *not* be seen in the older adult diagnosed with pneumonia?
    a. RBC 4.0 to 5.0
    b. Hgb 12 to 16
    c. Hct 36 to 48
    d. WBC 12 to 18

39. A client is admitted to the hospital to rule out pneumonia. Regarding isolation technique, the nurse would maintain which of the following nursing interventions?
    a. Strict respiratory isolation and use of a specially designed face mask only
    b. Respiratory isolation and contact isolation for sputum only
    c. Respiratory isolation with the stock surgical mask
    d. Standard precautions and no respiratory isolation

40. Upon admission, a critical concern of a client is often related to impaired gas exchange caused by inadequate ventilation. Which of the following values would indicate to the nurse that oxygen and incentive spirometry need to be administered?
    a. Pao_2 is 64 and clear lung sounds
    b. Pao_2 is 64 with atelectasis
    c. Pco_2 is 38 with crackles
    d. Pco_2 is 38 with atelectasis

41. The client with pneumonia with ineffective airway clearance has developed bronchospasms. The appropriate nursing intervention would be to:
    a. Increase the number of liters of oxygen and deliver humidified oxygen.
    b. Notify the physician of the need for an order for round-the-clock aerosol nebulizer bronchodilator treatments.
    c. Notify the physician of client status and get an order of hand-held bronchodilator inhaler prn.
    d. Notify the physician of the need for prednisone via inhaler or IV to reduce the inflammation causing the spasms.

42. A client is admitted to the hospital because of pneumonia. Which of the following is *true* regarding administration of antibiotics?
    a. Obtain a sputum culture before starting any antibiotic therapy.
    b. Broad spectrum IV antibiotic therapy should be started without any delays to improve client outcomes.
    c. Wait for sputum culture results with specificity before starting antibiotic therapy.
    d. Obtain at least three sputum specimens before starting IV antibiotics to reduce risk of toxicity.

43. An older adult client asks the nurse how often one should receive the pneumococcal vaccine for preventing pneumonia. The nurse's best response would be which of the following?
    a. Every year, when the client is receiving the "flu shot."
    b. The standard of care for clients is every 3 years.
    c. The recommendation is every 5 years; however, older adults may need it more frequently.
    d. There is no standard; it depends on the client's history and risk factors.

44. A client who was hospitalized for pneumonia is being discharged to home. On a separate sheet of paper, write a plan of care for the nursing diagnosis of Deficient Knowledge related to prevention of upper respiratory infections.

45. A nurse is providing discharge instructions to a client and family. Which of the following is the correct discharge instruction regarding pneumonia?
    a. Complete antibiotics as prescribed; rest; drink fluids; and minimize contact with crowds.
    b. Take all antibiotics as ordered; resume diet and all activities as before hospitalization.
    c. No restrictions regarding activities, diet, and rest because the client is fully recovered when discharged.
    d. Continue antibiotics only until no further signs of pneumonia are seen.

46. Which of the following medications would be given to the client with Ineffective Airway Clearance related to productive, prolonged coughing?
    a. Guaifenesin with 3.5% alcohol (Robitussin)
    b. Benzonatate (Tessalon)
    c. Oxtriphylline with guaifenesin (Brondecon)
    d. Propylhexedrine (Benzedrex)

47. A client has a nursing diagnosis of Ineffective Air-way Clearance. Interventions that help liquefy secretions for expectoration include which of the following measures?
    a. Performing postural drainage twice a day.
    b. Using an incentive spirometer every 4 hours.
    c. Coughing and deep breathing every 2 hours.
    d. Encouraging a minimum fluid intake of 2500 to 3000 mL a day.

48. Drug agents used in the management of pneumonia would include which of the following?
    a. Cough suppressants
    b. Antibiotics
    c. Mucolytic agents
    d. Corticosteroids

49. Which of the following instructions should be given to the client with pneumonia who is being dis-charged to home care?
    a. "You may discontinue the deep breathing exer-cises after 2 weeks when you stop coughing."
    b. "You will continue to feel tired and will fatigue easily for the next several weeks."
    c. "Try to drink 1 quart of water every day until you have finished all the antibiotics."
    d. "You should be able to return to work full-time in 2 weeks when your energy returns."

50. A complication of pneumonia that creates pain by causing friction between the layers of pleura is which of the following? Identify four other compli-cations and define each of them.
    a. Pleuritic chest pain
    b. Pulmonary emboli
    c. Pleural effusion
    d. Meningitis

Answer the following three questions on a separate sheet of paper.

51. Identify clients who are at risk for developing aspi-ration pneumonia and nursing interventions that can be implemented to prevent aspiration pneumonia.

52. Identify agents that may cause a noninfectious type of pneumonia.

53. A client is admitted to the hospital for pneumonia. What common assessment findings would the nurse expect?

54. A 60-year-old client is admitted to the hospital for treatment of pneumonia. Which of the following antibiotics would be recommended for treatment and why?
    a. Vancomycin
    b. Ampicillin
    c. Levofloxacin
    d. Piperacillin

55. Which of the following clients are at risk for com-munity-acquired pneumonia?
    a. A client on tube feedings
    b. A client with history of tobacco use
    c. A client with poor nutritional status
    d. A client with altered mental status

56. A client with HIV is admitted to the hospital with a temperature of 99.6° F, complaints of bloody spu-tum, night sweats, feeling tired, and shortness of breath. These assessment findings indicate which of the following diagnoses?
    a. Pneumocystic pneumonia (PCP)
    b. Tuberculosis
    c. Superinfection as a result of a low CD4 count
    d. Bacterial pneumonia

57. Which of the following statements regarding trans-mission of tuberculosis (TB) is true?
    a. Exposure to a client with TB results in active dis-ease within 2 to 10 weeks.
    b. The causative agent of TB is transmitted via aerosolization (airborne).
    c. It is considered to be an acute disease with no risk for reoccurrence.
    d. The "exposed/infected" client is considered as being the same as having active TB.

58. Number the following steps of Type IV delayed hypersensitivity reaction to the infectious microbe *Mycobacterium tuberculosis* in sequential order.
    ___ a. Cavity forms involving connecting bronchi.
    ___ b. T cells become sensitized to the tubercle.
    ___ c. A Ghon tubercle forms.
    ___ d. Tubercles enter the respiratory tract.
    ___ e. Fibrosis and calcification of the lesion occur.
    ___ f. Granuloma becomes necrotic and cheesy in appearance.
    ___ g. Lymphokines are released and activate macrophages.
    ___ h. A multinucleated giant cell (granuloma) forms.

59. Which of the following clients is at the greatest risk for developing TB?
    a. A 22-year-old college woman living in a double room in a dormitory
    b. A 62-year-old retired schoolteacher living in a house with her widowed sister
    c. A 42-year-old alcoholic homeless man who occasionally stays in a shelter
    d. A 53-year-old housewife who does volunteer work in a shelter for the homeless

60. The most substantial impact in incidence of TB is from which of the following high-risk populations?
    a. Older adults, the homeless, minorities
    b. Lower socioeconomic groups
    c. Those in constant frequent contact with untreated individuals
    d. Those with immune dysfunction, particularly HIV

61. After several weeks of "not feeling well," a client is seen in the physician's office for possible TB. The assessment findings include which of the following if TB is present?
    a. Fatigue, night sweats, and low-grade fever
    b. Weight gain, bloody streaked sputum, and night sweats
    c. Hemoptysis, loss of appetite, and high fever
    d. Nonproductive cough, fatigue, and anorexia

62. Which of the following test results indicate the client has clinically active TB?
    a. Induration of 12 mm and positive sputum
    b. Positive chest x-ray for TB only
    c. Positive chest x-ray and clinical symptoms
    d. Client complaints of signs and symptoms

63. After receiving the subcutaneous Mantoux skin test, a client with no risk factors returns to the clinic in the required 48 to 72 hours for a reading of the test. Assessment findings of which of the following would indicate a positive test result?
    a. The test area is red, warm, and tender to touch.
    b. There is induration or a hard nodule of any size at the sight.
    c. The induration/hardened area measures 5 mm or greater.
    d. The induration/hardened area measures 10 mm or greater.

64. A client has a positive skin test result. What explanation does the nurse give to the client?
    a. There is active disease but client is not yet infectious to others.
    b. There is active disease, and client needs immediate treatment.
    c. The client has been infected but that does not mean active disease is present.
    d. A follow-up chest x-ray is necessary because the test could be a false positive result.

65. A client with TB has been prescribed two or more pharmacologic agents. On a separate sheet of paper, briefly explain why this treatment is prescribed.

66. The nurse explains to the client that the minimum treatment time period for TB is:
    a. 7 to 10 days.
    b. 3 weeks.
    c. 3 months.
    d. 6 months.

67. The client is no longer infectious/communicable when which of the following test results are seen?
    a. Negative chest x-ray
    b. No clinical symptoms
    c. Negative skin tests
    d. Three negative sputum cultures

68. In teaching a client about the medication, the best time for a client to take these chemotherapeutic agents for TB is:
    a. Before breakfast.
    b. After breakfast.
    c. At midday.
    d. At bedtime.

69. To prevent TB, clients with HIV infection with less than 10 mm induration on the TB skin test and no clinical symptoms would receive which of the following medications for a period of 12 months?
    a. Bacille Calmette-Guérin (BCG) vaccine
    b. Isoniazid (INH)
    c. Ethambutol
    d. Streptomycin

70. On a separate sheet of paper, briefly describe the *initial* drug protocol for a client with active TB.

71. On a separate sheet of paper, briefly describe the nursing interventions for the nursing diagnosis of Ineffective Health Maintenance related to the client not taking the medication for TB as prescribed.

72. A client diagnosed with TB has been receiving treatment for 3 weeks and has clinically shown improvement. The family asked the nurse if the client is still infectious. The nurse will reply to this question with which of the following statements?
    a. The client is still infectious until the entire treatment is completed.
    b. The client is not infectious but needs to continue treatment for at least 6 months.
    c. The client is infectious until there is negative chest x-ray.
    d. The client may or may not be infectious. A PPD needs to be done.

73. An older adult client complains of loss of hearing and dizziness after 1 month of taking the medication for TB. The nurse would advise the client to:
    a. Continue taking the medication; the symptom will eventually go away.
    b. Consult a physician because this could be a sign of toxicity.
    c. Not be concerned because this symptom is common with all TB medications.
    d. Wait for 3 months, if the symptom continues, consult a physician.

74. Match the following nursing interventions with the medications to treat TB. *Answers may be used more than once.*

    Nursing Interventions
    ___ a. Assess client's hearing before starting medication.
    ___ b. Teach client that urine will be orange in color.
    ___ c. Consult physician for dose reduction when the client complains of blurry vision after starting treatment.
    ___ d. Teach the client not to take medications such as Maalox with this medication.
    ___ e. Obtain baseline and monitor lab values: CPK, LDH, SGOT, and uric acid.
    ___ f. Monitor creatine and BUN lab values.
    ___ g. Teach client to take in morning, preferably before eating unless it causes an "upset stomach."
    ___ h. Teach to take with food to decrease GI upset.
    ___ i. Closely monitor anticoagulant lab values for clients because it may interfere with this medication.
    ___ j. Teach clients to identify changes in the ability to differentiate colors.

    TB Medications
    1. Isoniazid (INH)
    2. Rifampin
    3. Pyrazinamide
    4. Ethambutol
    5. Streptomycin
    6. Amikacin

75. A client with suspected TB is admitted to the hospital. Which of the following nursing interventions is correct relating to isolation procedure? The nurse would maintain a:
    a. Private room, respiratory isolation, and contact isolation for sputum only.
    b. Private room, strict respiratory isolation, and only use specially designed face masks.
    c. Private room, respiratory isolation with hospital surgical masks until diagnosis is confirmed.
    d. Private room, no respiratory isolation is necessary until diagnosis is confirmed.

76. A client is admitted to the hospital to "rule-out" TB. What type of mask should the nurse wear when caring for this client?
    a. Surgical face mask
    b. Surgical face mask with eye shield
    c. HEPA respirator
    d. Any type of mask that covers the nose and mouth

77. A client seen in the outpatient clinic is diagnosed with TB. Which of the following nursing interventions is correct related to public health policy?
    a. Only contact the infection control nurse at the hospital.
    b. There are no regulations since the client was seen in the clinic and not hospitalized.
    c. Contact the public health nurse so that all individuals who have come in contact with client can be screened.
    d. Have the client sign a waiver regarding the hospital's liability for treatment.

78. What interventions can a nurse perform in meeting the Healthy People 2010 objectives for tuberculosis?

79. Which of the following is *not* a diagnostic test for TB?
    a. Chest radiography
    b. Complete blood count
    c. Mantoux skin test
    d. Sputum culture

80. On a separate sheet of paper, identify the subjective data that are relevant to a client with TB.

81. Which of the following is a physical symptom of TB? Identify other physical findings.
    a. Fatigue
    b. Weight gain
    c. High-grade fever
    d. Nonproductive cough

82. The older adult is more prone to respiratory infection because of which of the following etiologies?
   a. Inability to force a cough
   b. Weak chest wall muscles
   c. Decreased alveoli surfactant
   d. Macrophages in alveoli are decreased

 ## Case Study: The Older Client with Tuberculosis

Your client is a 65-year-old woman who shares a three-room inner-city apartment with two of her daughters and their seven children. She comes into the neighborhood walk-in clinic complaining of extreme fatigue, a 30-pound weight loss, and a cough of 4 months duration. A Mantoux test, sputum culture, and chest x-ray confirm a diagnosis of tuberculosis. She is to begin a 12-month course of medication therapy with isoniazid (INH) 300 mg PO qd and rifampin (Rifadin) 600 mg PO qd.

Answer the following questions on a separate sheet of paper:

1. Discuss why one or more pharmacologic agents are used to treat tuberculosis.

2. When is the best time for this client to take the chemotherapeutic agents to minimize the side effects?

3. Why should rifampin (Rifadin) be taken on an empty stomach?

4. What type of follow-up care should be planned for this client?

5. How long will this client be considered contagious?

6. What measures should be taken with the other family members? Explain your answer.

7. Develop a teaching-learning plan for this client.

Three weeks after diagnosis, the client returns to the clinic stating that she has stopped taking her medications because they make her sick to her stomach. She is unable to eat and has continued to lose weight.

8. Identify the relevant nursing diagnoses for this client based on the above data.

9. Discuss what the nurse should do to assist this client in taking her medications and eating a balanced diet.

Case Study: The Young Client with Tuberculosis

Your client is a 25-year-old inner-city woman with AIDS. She is hospitalized now for active TB. She has four young children who are currently being cared for by her mother, a 42-year-old unemployed woman with diabetes mellitus.

Answer the following questions on a separate sheet of paper:

1. What kind of isolation must this client be placed in, and why?

2. Sputum cultures for AFB are ordered. When is the best time to collect sputum? Can you send sputum that contains saliva to the laboratory?

3. Before the client is discharged, what interventions need to be done at her home in preparation for her return?

Case Study: The Client with Pneumonia

A 75-year-old married woman reports to the outpatient clinic with her husband. She has had a severe cough, says that she has had left-sided chest pain, and holds her left side while coughing. She appears anxious. Her face is flushed. Vital signs are temperature 102.6° F, pulse 118, apical; respirations 32, shallow, and blood pressure 120/80. A diagnosis of pneumonia is suspected. A sputum specimen, chest x-ray, arterial blood gases, and CBC are ordered.

Answer the following questions on a separate sheet of paper:

1. What should the nurse teach this client and her husband about the sputum collection and x-ray?

2. What will the nurse probably hear when she auscultates the client's lungs? Explain your answer.

A diagnosis of pneumonia is confirmed by the chest x-ray and sputum cultures. Because the client's blood gases are within normal limits, she will be managed on an outpatient basis.

3. Identify the relevant nursing diagnoses for this client based on above data.

The physician orders cefaclor (Ceclor) 500 mg PO every 8 hours and wants the client to return to the clinic in 1 week. If her condition does not improve within 48 hours or she becomes short of breath, she should call or return to the clinic.

4. Develop teaching-learning and discharge care plans for the client and her husband.

Interventions for Critically Ill Clients with Respiratory Problems

Study/Review Questions

1. A postoperative client complains of sudden onset of shortness of breath and pleuritic chest pain. Assessment findings include diaphoresis, hypotension, crackles in the left lower lobe, and pulse oximetry of 85%. The nurse interprets these findings as possible:
   a. Bacterial pneumonia.
   b. Pneumothorax.
   c. Pulmonary embolism.
   d. Atelectasis.

2. Indicate which of the following clients the nurse would monitor for a pulmonary embolus and provide preventive measures. *Mark Y for yes or N for no; then briefly explain the rationale for your answer. Use a separate sheet of paper for your rationales.*
   ___ a. Client with total hip or knee replacement, postoperative
   ___ b. Client with low protein S or protein C value
   ___ c. First day postoperative client with cervical diskectomy
   ___ d. Client with previous history of deep vein thrombosis
   ___ e. Hospitalized dehydrated older adult client
   ___ f. Client with sickle cell anemia
   ___ g. Pneumonia client, out of bed in chair
   ___ h. 5'5" Adult weighting 250 pounds
   ___ i. Pregnant woman
   ___ j. Woman in labor about to deliver
   ___ k. Client with aspiration pneumonia
   ___ l. Client with abdominal surgery, postoperative
   ___ m. Client with atrial fibrillation
   ___ n. Client with spinal cord injury and paralysis
   ___ o. All clients with the nursing diagnosis Impaired Mobility

3. The most common site of origin for a pulmonary embolism (PE) is:
   a. Clots in the right side of the heart.
   b. Arterial microemboli such as amniotic fluid.
   c. Fat particles in venous system.
   d. Thrombi in deep veins in the legs or pelvis.

4. The most common risk factor for a PE is which of the following?
   a. Hypercoagulability
   b. Heparin therapy
   c. Superficial phlebitis
   d. Minor trauma

5. Which of the following is true regarding the assessment findings (signs and symptoms) of a client with a PE?
   a. Manifestation of a PE is the same for all clients.
   b. Subtle or severe assessment findings depend on the location and type of clot.
   c. In most cases, signs and symptoms are dyspnea, cough, changes in lung sounds, and skin color.
   d. Signs and symptoms are slow in developing over time and insidious in nature.

6. In clients at high-risk for a PE, a unique assessment finding for a small clot in the lung is which of the following?
   a. Respiratory distress
   b. Sudden dry cough, possible chest pain
   c. ECG changes
   d. Changes in lung sounds

7. What assessment findings would indicate to the nurse that the client has developed a PE? Write your answer on a separate sheet of paper, listing the findings from the most common to the most severe.

8. A nurse suspects a client has a PE and prepares the client for which of the following tests to confirm the diagnosis?
   a. Blood gases, pulse oximetry, CT scan of the chest, echocardiogram
   b. Pulmonary angiography and/or ventilation-perfusion scan
   c. Blood gases, and pulse oximetry, stat 12-lead ECG, and portable chest x-ray
   d. Blood gas, chest x-ray, and cardiopulmonary catheterization

9. Upon diagnosis of a PE in a client, the nurse should expect to perform which of the following therapeutic interventions? Provide a rationale for your answer.
   a. Oral anticoagulant therapy
   b. Bedrest in the supine position and monitor respiratory status prn
   c. Oxygen therapy via mechanical ventilator
   d. Parenteral anticoagulant therapy

10. The client with a PE asked for an explanation of heparin therapy. Which of the following statements is correct?
    a. It keeps the clot from getting larger by preventing platelets from sticking together to improve blood flow.
    b. It will improve your breathing and decrease the chest pain by dissolving the clot in your lung.
    c. It promotes the absorption of the clot in your leg that originally caused the PE.
    d. It increases the time it takes for blood to clot, therefore preventing further clotting and improving blood flow.

11. Which of the following nursing interventions pertains to Risk for Injury (bleeding) related to anticoagulation therapy?
    a. Monitor labs for any elevation of PT or PTT value and notify a physician stat.
    b. Monitor PTT values for greater than 2.5 times the control and/or client for bleeding.
    c. Monitor client for a pulmonary infarction by blood in sputum and notify a physician stat.
    d. Monitor PT values for international normalized ratio (INR) for a therapeutic range of 2 to 3 and/or client for bleeding.

12. When PTT values are above the therapeutic range for heparin therapy, the nurse would obtain a physician's order to:
    a. Temporarily stop heparin infusion or slow the rate of administration.
    b. Change the concentration of heparin in the IV bag.
    c. Administer the antidote protamine sulfate stat.
    d. Administer a dose of vitamin K by IM injection.

13. Nursing care of a client with a pulmonary embolus would include monitoring for: *Check all that apply.*
    ___ a. Nausea and vomiting.
    ___ b. Symptoms of respiratory failure.
    ___ c. Chest pain.
    ___ d. Dehydration.

14. After receiving heparin anticoagulant therapy, clients should not be discharged from the hospital without a prescription and instructions regarding:
    a. Dobutamine (Dobutrex).
    b. Antianxiety agents.
    c. Coumadin.
    d. Vasodilators.

15. Nursing responsibilities for a client on Coumadin who has not yet been discharged from the hospital include:
    a. Having the antidote protamine sulfate available.
    b. Administering NSAIDs or aspirin for pain and fever.
    c. Teaching the client about foods high in vitamin K.
    d. Monitoring platelets for thrombocytopenia.

16. The lab test used to determine the therapeutic range for Coumadin is:
    a. PTT level.
    b. Platelets.
    c. PT and INR.
    d. Coumadin peak and trough.

17. The INR therapeutic range for a client with a new onset PE should be:
    a. 1.0 to 1.5 times the normal.
    b. 2.5 to 3.0 times the normal.
    c. 3.0 to 4.5 times the normal.
    d. 5 times the normal value.

18. Develop a discharge teaching plan for a client after hospitalization for a pulmonary embolus.

19. Arterial blood gas results from the early stage of a PE would probably indicate which of the following? Provide a rationale for your answer.
    a. Respiratory alkalosis
    b. Respiratory acidosis
    c. Metabolic acidosis
    d. Metabolic alkalosis

20. As a nurse, you are employed on an adult medical-surgical unit and frequently encounter clients who are at risk for a DVT and PE. Copy the chart below to a separate sheet of paper, and indicate independent and dependent preventive nursing interventions for these clients.

Independent Nursing Functions to Prevent DVT/PE	Dependent Nursing Functions to Prevent DVT/PE

21. Explain the difference between alteplase (tPA), streptokinase, and urokinase in the treatment of a PE.

22. Which of the following clients are at risk for pulmonary contusion?
    a. Client with gun shot wound to the chest
    b. Client with stab wound to the chest
    c. Client with blunt trauma to the chest
    d. Client with rib fracture

23. A client enters the emergency department with a chest injury that resulted from a motor vehicle accident; client has decreased breath sounds, crackles, wheezing, and blood in the sputum but no open wounds. The nurse would suspect which of the following diagnoses?
    a. Flail chest
    b. Hemothorax
    c. Pneumothorax
    d. Pulmonary contusion

24. Which of the following statements regarding pulmonary contusion is correct? *Correct the wrong answers.*
    a. It is often a result of a flail chest.
    b. Treatment may require mechanical ventilation with PEEP.
    c. It is treated with aggressive fluids to prevent shock.
    d. Clinical manifestations develop rapidly.

25. Pulmonary contusion is a potentially lethal chest injury because of:
    a. Broken ribs and flail chest.
    b. Laryngospasm.
    c. Respiratory failure that can occur over time rather than instantly.
    d. High risk of infection from chest tubes.

26. A client with a rib fracture is primarily treated with:
    a. Mechanical ventilation.
    b. Tight bandage around chest.
    c. Conservative respiratory treatment, e.g., cough and deep breathing.
    d. Potent analgesics and muscle relaxants.

27. A client can develop a tension pneumothorax when:
    a. Blood is lost into the thoracic cavity as a result of blunt trauma.
    b. An air leak in the lung or chest wall causes the lung to collapse.
    c. Air accumulates in the pleural space causing a rise in intrathoracic pressure.
    d. There is an infectious process that leads to the accumulation of pus in the pleural space.

28. A significant assessment finding in a client with a tension pneumothorax is:
   a. Tracheal deviation to the unaffected side.
   b. Inspiratory stridor and respiratory distress.
   c. Diminished breath sounds over the affected hemithorax.
   d. Hyperresonant percussion note over the affected side.

29. During a physical assessment of a client with a hemothorax, percussion of the affected side results in what type of chest sound?
   a. Hypertympanic
   b. Dull
   c. Hyperresonant
   d. Crackles

30. Which of the following is the treatment for a pneumothorax?
   a. Inserting a large bore needle into the intercostal space on the unaffected side
   b. Placement of a chest tube mid sternum to reduce a cardiac tamponade
   c. Attaching the chest to continuous gravity drainage bag
   d. Inserting a large bore needle into the intercostal space on the affected side

31. A 19-year-old male was seen in the emergency room after a motorcycle accident for multiple rib fractures that resulted in free-floating ribs, paradoxical breathing, and impaired gas exchange. This condition is called:
   a. Tension pneumothorax.
   b. Flail chest.
   c. Pulmonary contusion.
   d. Subcutaneous emphysema.

32. Before suctioning a client with an endotracheal or tracheostomy tube, the nurse preoxygenates the client with _____% oxygen.
   a. 21
   b. 40
   c. 70
   d. 100

33. The maximum length of time that suction should be applied to the chest is:
   a. 5 to 10 seconds.
   b. 10 to 15 seconds.
   c. 20 to 30 seconds.
   d. 40 to 60 seconds.

34. The most common cause of ventilatory failure is:
   a. Ventilation-perfusion mismatching.
   b. Impaired respiratory muscle function.
   c. Impaired diffusion at the alveolar level.
   d. Abnormal hemoglobin that does not absorb oxygen.

35. Oxygenation failure occurs when:
   a. Blood shunts from right to left in pulmonary vessels.
   b. The client breaths air that is too concentrated with oxygen.
   c. The respiratory control center in the brain malfunctions.
   d. There is a mechanical abnormality of the chest wall or lungs.

36. Match each of the following disorders or events that can cause clients to be at risk for acute respiratory failure with the corresponding type of respiratory failure. *Answers may be used more than once.*

Disorders and Events That Cause Respiratory Failure

____ a. Lung tumors
____ b. Cerebral edema
____ c. Bronchial asthma
____ d. Near drowning
____ e. Sleep apnea
____ f. Multiple sclerosis
____ g. Pneumonia
____ h. Chronic bronchitis
____ i. Atelectasis
____ j. Gross obesity
____ k. Poliomyelitis
____ l. Smoke inhalation
____ m. Myasthenia gravis
____ n. Meningitis
____ o. Pulmonary emphysema
____ p. Carbon monoxide poisoning
____ q. Opioid overdose
____ r. Guillain-Barré syndrome
____ s. Liquid aspiration

Types of Respiratory Failure

1. Ventilatory failure
2. Oxygenation failure
3. Combination of ventilatory and oxygenation failure

37. Which of the following conditions is a signal to the nurse of impending acute respiratory failure?
   a. Orthopnea
   b. Tachypnea
   c. Dyspnea on exertion
   d. Status asthmaticus

38. For the client with status asthmaticus, indicate the signs and symptoms of respiratory failure. *Use a separate sheet of paper for your answer.*

39. Which of the following is *not* an initial nursing intervention for the client in Question 38 with respiratory failure?
    a. Administer cromolyn sodium by inhaler.
    b. Administer bronchodilator treatments.
    c. Provide energy conservation measures.
    d. Administer oxygen therapy.

40. The major site of injury for ARDS in the respiratory tract is the:
    a. Mainstem bronchi.
    b. Respiratory bronchioles.
    c. Alveolar-capillary membrane.
    d. Tracheobronchial tree.

41. Which of the following clients is at greatest risk of developing ARDS?
    a. A 74-year-old client who aspirates a tube feeding
    b. A 34-year-old client who has nearly drowned
    c. A 26-year-old client with an electrical burn injury
    d. An 18-year-old client with a fractured femur

42. Early assessment findings for a client with ARDS include:
    a. Adventitious lung sounds.
    b. Hyperthermia and hot, dry skin.
    c. Intercostal and suprasternal retractions.
    d. Increased mental acuity and surveillance.

43. Management of ARDS involves:
    a. Oxygen therapy via CPAP.
    b. Mechanical ventilation and endotracheal tube.
    c. Antibiotics.
    d. A tracheostomy tube.

44. Identify four reasons a client would require intubation.
    a. _____
    b. _____
    c. _____
    d. _____

45. Match the following parts of an endotracheal tube with their descriptions.

Description	Parts of Endotracheal Tube
____ a. Device to provide a seal between the trachea and tube	1. Shaft
	2. Cuff
	3. Pilot balloon
____ b. Device to allow attachment of ET tube to ventilation source	4. Universal adapter
____ c. Hollow tube extending from naso-oral cavity to just above the carina	
____ d. Access site for inserting air into the cuff	

46. A client in a critical care unit requires an emergency ET intubation. What supplies are needed to perform this procedure?

47. After the insertion of an ET tube, correct placement is conclusively verified when:
    a. Chest excursion is asymmetrical.
    b. Air emerges from the ET tube on expiration.
    c. Breath sounds are bilaterally equal.
    d. The chest x-ray indicates correct placement.

48. The tape on an endotracheal tube of a client is loose. Describe methods for taping an endotracheal tube and a method to detect tube dislodgment.

49. Which of the following statements relating to nursing care of clients on a ventilator is *false*?
    a. Deflating the cuff on the ET tube to check placement
    b. Applying soft wrist restraints as ordered
    c. Suctioning to prevent complications
    d. Maintaining the correct placement of the ET tube

50. Match the following characteristics of ventilators with their types. *Some characteristics may apply to more than one type of ventilator. Indicate all types to which a characteristic applies.*

Characteristics of Ventilators

____ a. Positive-pressure ventilator

____ b. Administers consistent volume and gas (oxygen concentration) regardless of the client's lung status until preset tidal volume is reached

____ c. Preset inspiration and expiration rate with possible variation of tidal volume and pressure

____ d. Pushes air into the lungs until preset airway pressure is reached

____ e. Needs an artificial airway such as a tracheostomy or endotracheal tube

____ f. Tidal volumes and inspiratory time are variable

Types of Ventilators

1. Pressure-cycled
2. Time-cycled
3. Volume-cycled

51. Match the following ventilator terms and settings with their descriptions.

Descriptions

____ a. Volumes of air that are 1.5 to 2 times tidal volume

____ b. Positive pressure throughout the entire respiratory cycle to prevent alveolar collapse

____ c. Number of ventilations delivered per minute

____ d. Volume of air the client receives with each breath

____ e. Set tidal volume and set rate delivered to the client

____ f. Positive pressure exerted during expiration to keep lungs partially inflated

____ g. Oxygen concentration delivered to the client

____ h. Ventilator takes over the work of breathing for the client and delivers a set tidal volume

____ i. Client breathes at own rate, but machine breathes for client as needed

____ j. Pressure needed to deliver a set tidal volume

____ k. Ventilator delivers mandatory breaths at a preset rate and allows the client to breathe spontaneously between set rate

Terms and Settings

1. Assist-control mode (AC)
2. Breaths per minute (BPM)
3. Continuous positive airway pressure (CPAP)
4. Controlled ventilation
5. Fraction of inspired oxygen (FIO_2)
6. Peak airway inspiratory pressure (PIP)
7. Positive end-expiratory pressure (PEEP)
8. Sighs
9. Synchronized intermittent mandatory ventilation (SIMV)
10. Tidal volume (V1)
11. Intermittent mandatory ventilation (IMV)

52. Identify the acid-base problems and the necessary interventions for each set of ABG data given below.
   a. pH = 7.40, Po_2 = 74 mm Hg, Pco_2 = 40 mEq/L
   b. pH = 7.30, Po_2 = 90 mm Hg, Pco_2 = 40 mEq/L
   c. pH = 7.30, Po_2 = 87 mm Hg, Pco_2 = 50 mEq/L
   d. pH = 7.60, Po_2 = 94 mm Hg, Pco_2 = 21 mEq/L
   e. pH = 7.43, Po_2 = 92 mm Hg, Pco_2 = 40 mEq/L
   f. pH = 7.28, Po_2 = 59 mm Hg, Pco_2 = 40 mEq/L

53. For each of the following body systems, indicate at least one potential complication of mechanical ventilation.
   a. Cardiac: _____
   b. Pulmonary: _____
   c. Gastrointestinal: _____
   d. Immunologic: _____
   e. Muscular: _____

54. A means to determine when a client is ready to be weaned from a ventilator is which of the following assessment findings? Identify other methods that are used.
   a. No respiratory infection
   b. Showing signs of becoming ventilator-dependent
   c. Able to maintain blood gases within normal limits
   d. Able to request that the ventilator is not necessary anymore

55. Which of the following findings might delay weaning a client from a ventilator?
   a. Hematocrit = 42%
   b. Arterial Po_2 = 70 mm Hg on a 40% FIO_2
   c. Apical heart rate = 72
   d. Oral temperature = 99° F

56. Which of the following clients might take the longest time to wean from a ventilator?
    a. A 54-year-old man with metastatic colon cancer who has been intubated for 6 days
    b. A 32-year-old woman recovering from a general anesthetic following a tubal ligation
    c. A 25-year-old man intubated for 28 hours following an anaphylactic reaction
    d. A 49-year-old man with a gunshot wound to the chest who was intubated for 8 hours

57. While weaning a client from a ventilator, the nurse should:
    a. Assess the monitoring devices regularly from a distance but within client's sight.
    b. Assess the family member's willingness to stay with the client to provide emotional support.
    c. Plan enough time to stay at the bedside as much as possible to maintain ventilator settings.
    d. Plan to suction the client more frequently as secretions build up.

58. A nursing intervention to implement during extubation is to:
    a. Ascertain that the cuff is inflated at all times.
    b. Remove the tube during expiration.
    c. Instruct the client not to cough.
    d. Instruct the client to deep breathe and cough.

59. An expected assessment finding in a recently extubated client is which of the following? Why are the other answers incorrect?
    a. Stridor
    b. Dyspnea
    c. Restlessness
    d. Hoarseness

60. Indicate which of the following are nursing interventions related to care of a client on a mechanical ventilator. Why are the other answers incorrect?
    a. Perform mouth care every 2 to 4 hours
    b. Provide a means of communication
    c. Administer mandatory muscle-paralyzing agents to ensure ventilation
    d. Ensure adequate humidity and air temperature
    e. Empty ventilator tubing back into the cascade
    f. Perform a respiratory assessment only once a shift
    g. Include the client and family in care whenever possible
    h. Monitor for complications such as black tarry stools or constipation
    i. When setting is PEEP, observe the peak airway pressure dial

61. A client on a ventilator coughs, gags, and bites on the ET tube. The nursing intervention for this client would be to:
    a. Administer sedation.
    b. Administer a muscle-paralyzing agent.
    c. Insert an oral airway.
    d. Have physician change tube to a tracheostomy.

62. The nurse notices a gradual increase in peak airway pressure over the last several days. The nursing intervention for this client would be to:
    a. Assess for a reason such as ARDS or pneumonia.
    b. Continue to increase peak airway pressure as needed.
    c. Change to another mode such as IMV.
    d. Make arrangements for permanent ventilatory support.

UNIT 7 PROBLEMS OF CARDIAC OUTPUT AND TISSUE PERFUSION: CARDIOVASCULAR SYSTEM

■ Core Concepts Grid

Anatomy	Physiology	Pathophysiology	History	Physical Exam	Diagnostic Tests	Interventions	Pharmacology
• Heart chambers • Heart valves • Major vessels • Blood flow through the heart • Conduction system SA node AV node His Bundle Purkinje fibers • Peripheral vascular system Arteries Arterioles Capillaries Venules Veins	• Heart rate • Stroke volume • Cardiac output • Cardiac cycle • Blood pressure	• Hypertension • Infarction • Atherosclerosis • Pump failure • Inflammation • Hypertrophy • Infection/sepsis • Hypovolemia	• History of cardiac symptoms • Dyspnea • Fatigue • Paroxysmal nocturnal dyspnea • Orthopnea • Chest pain • Palpitations • Syncope • Cough • Past health history • Medications • Risk factors Age Diet Activity Smoking	• Cyanosis • Petechiae • Edema • Pulses • Heart sounds S1-S4 • Murmurs • Bruits • Blood pressure • Neck vein distention • Skin color • Hair distribution on extremities • Lesions • Clubbing • Dysrhythmias	• Chest x-ray • Electrocardiogram • Cardiac catheterization • Arteriography • Thallium scan • Exercise stress test • CK-MB • Lactate dehydrogenase • Cholesterol • Triglycerides • Lipoproteins • Myoglobin • Troponins • C-reactive protein	• Risk factor modification • Oxygen • Positioning • Pain control • Dysrhythmia monitoring • Diet modification • Heart transplantation • Coronary artery bypass graft (CABG) • MIDCAB • Percutaneous cardiac interventions (e.g., PTCA) • Fluid replacement • Hemodynamic monitoring • Mechanical ventilation • Cardiac rehabilitation • Health teaching	• Inotropic agent • Diuretics • Antidysrhythmics • Beta blockers • Vasodilators • Angiotensin-converting enzyme inhibitors • Calcium channel blockers • Nitrates • Anticoagulants • Antiplatelet agents • Morphine • Antibiotics • Antilipidemic agents

Unit 7 (Chapters 33-38)

Problems of Cardiac Output and Tissue Perfusion: Management of Clients with Problems of the Cardiovascular System

Learning Plan

Chapter 33: *Assessment of the Cardiovascular System*

Learning Outcomes

1. Review the anatomy and physiology of the cardiovascular system.
2. Describe cardiovascular changes associated with aging.
3. Identify factors that place clients at risk for cardiovascular problems.
4. Perform appropriate assessments for clients with cardiovascular problems.
5. Interpret diagnostic test findings for clients with suspected or actual cardiovascular disease.
6. Explain the purpose of hemodynamic monitoring.

Learning Activities

1. Prior to completing the study guide exercises for this chapter, review the following:
   - Anatomy and physiology of the cardiovascular system
   - Techniques for performing a physical assessment
2. Review the **boldfaced** Key Terms and their definitions in Chapter 33 to enhance your understanding of the content.
3. Go to Study Guide Number 7.33 on the following pages and complete the learning exercises for this chapter.

Supplemental Resources

1. Textbook—Chapter 33
2. Other resources:
   - Agency for Healthcare Research and Quality: http://www.ahcpr.gov/
   - Any diagnostic laboratory manual
   - Any physical assessment textbook that includes changes in the older adult
   - Braunwald, E. (1998). The clinical examination. In L. Goldman & E. Braunwald (Eds.). *Primary cardiology* (pp. 27-43). Philadelphia: W.B. Saunders.
   - Contact the American Heart Association for information regarding risk factors, statistics, and related information on cardiovascular diseases.
   - Council on Cardiovascular Nursing
   - Coyne, K.S. & Allen, J.K. (1998). Assessment of functional status in patients with cardiac disease. *Heart and Lung, 27*(4), 263-273.
   - Discuss/collaborate with a critical care clinical nurse specialist regarding care of a client with hemodynamic monitoring.
   - Heartweb: http://heartweb.org/
   - Hogsten, P. (1997). Hemodynamic monitoring. In P.S. Kid (Ed.). *High acuity nursing* (pp. 227-256). Stamford, CT: Appleton and Lange.
   - National Heart, Lung, and Blood Institute; Bethesda, MD: http://www.nhlbi.nih.gov/index.htm
   - Review the cardiovascular system in an anatomy and physiology textbook.

- Sox, H.C. (1998). Screening for coronary artery disease and its risk factors. In L. Goldman & E. Braunwald (Eds.). *Primary cardiology* (pp. 57-69). Philadelphia: W.B. Saunders
- Turner, M.A. (2000). Monitoring hemodynamics noninvasively. *Nursing 2000, 30*(5), 32cc8.
- Wenger, N.K. (1998). *Cardiovascular disease in the elderly and in women* (pp. 70-82). Philadelphia: W.B. Saunders.

Chapter 34: *Interventions for Clients with Dysrhythmias*

Supplemental Resources

1. Textbook—Chapter 33 (Assessment of the Cardiovascular System)
2. Textbook—Chapter 34
3. Other resources:
   - An EKG textbook or online source for interpreting EKGs
   - Any anatomy and physiology textbook
   - Any pathophysiology textbook
   - Dubin, D. (1998). *Rapid interpretation of EKGs* (5th ed.). Tampa, FL: Cover Publishing.
   - Hiller, G.A. (1999). Atrial fibrillation: Soothing the savage beat. *Nursing 99, 29*(2), 26-31.
   - Lazzara, D. (1999). Shocking facts about semiautomatic defibrillation. *Nursing 99, 29*(4), 55-57.
   - Miracle, V. & Sims, J.M. (1999). Easy ECG series: Part I. Making sense of the 12-lead ECG. *Nursing 99, 29*(7), 34-40.
   - Observe a telemetry technician or a nurse and practice interpreting EKG strips.

Learning Activities

1. Prior to completing the study guide exercises for this chapter, review the following:
   - Anatomy and physiology of the heart and vascular system
   - Principles of fluid and electrolyte balance
   - Assessment of the cardiovascular system including changes in the older adult
   - Conduction system of the heart
   - Principles of acid-base balance
   - Principles related to cardiac output
   - Anatomy and physiology of respiratory system
   - Assessment of the respiratory system
   - Principles of cardiac output
2. Review the **boldfaced** Key Terms and their definitions in Chapter 34 to enhance your understanding of the content.
3. Go to Study Guide Number 7.34 on the following pages and complete the learning exercises for this chapter.

Learning Outcomes

1. Correlate the components of the electrocardiogram with the cardiac conduction system.
2. Interpret common cardiac dysrhythmias.
3. Identify typical physical assessment findings associated with common dysrhythmias.
4. Identify priority nursing diagnoses for clients experiencing dysrhythmias.
5. Plan care for clients experiencing common dysrhythmias.
6. Develop a teaching plan for clients experiencing common dysrhythmias.
7. Compare and contrast classes of antidysrhythmic drugs.
8. Compare and contrast types of atrioventricular blocks.
9. Explain the purpose and types of pacing used as interventions for clients with dysrhythmias.
10. Outline the procedure and precautions associated with defibrillation.
11. Plan community-based care for a client after pacemaker or implantable cardioverter/defibrillator insertion.

- Practice reading and interpreting EKG strips for multiple sources.
- Resnick, B. (1999). Atrial fibrillation in the older adult: Presentation and management issues. *Geriatric Nursing, 20(4)*, 188-194.
- Shaffer, R.B. (1999). Keeping pace with permanent pacemakers: Part I. *Nursing 99, 18(5)*, 2-8.
- Squires, A. (2000). Critical care: Teaching patients about telemetry. *Nursing 2000, 30(7)*, 32cc4.
- Taler, M.S. (1999). *The only EKG book you'll ever need* (3rd ed.). Philadelphia: Lippincott Williams and Wilkins.

Supplemental Resources

1. Textbook—Chapter 33 (Assessment of the Cardiovascular System)
2. Textbook—Chapter 35
3. Other resources:
- Alderman, L.M. (2000). Congenital heart disease: More than child's play. *Nursing 2000, 30(5)*, 41-47.
- American Heart Association on Cardiovascular Nursing
- Any anatomy and physiology textbook
- Any pathophysiology textbook
- Any physical assessment textbook that includes changes in the older adult
- Baig, M.K., et al. (1999). The pathophysiology of advanced heart failure. *Heart and Lung, 28(2)*, 87-101.
- Branum, K. Using beta blockers in the treatment of heart failure. *The Nurse Practitioner, 24(7)*, 75-83.
- Dugan, K.J. (1998). Caring for patients with pericarditis. *Nursing 98, 28(50)*, 50-51.

Chapter 35: *Interventions for Clients with Cardiac Problems*

Learning Outcomes

1. Explain the pathophysiology of heart failure.
2. Compare and contrast left-sided and right-sided heart failure.
3. Perform a comprehensive assessment of clients experiencing heart failure.
4. Identify common nursing diagnoses and collaborative problems for clients with heart failure.
5. Evaluate the effects of interventions for reducing preload and afterload.
6. Describe special considerations for older adults with heart failure.
7. Discuss prevention of complications for clients with heart failure.
8. Prioritize nursing care for clients experiencing heart failure.
9. Identify essential focused assessments used by the home care nurse for clients with heart failure.
10. Compare and contrast common valvular disorders.
11. Discuss surgical management for clients with valvular disease.
12. Develop a teaching/learning plan for clients with valvular disease.
13. Differentiate between common cardiac inflammations and infections—endocarditis, pericarditis, and rheumatic carditis.
14. Discuss the legal/ethical aspects related to heart transplantation, including cost of care.

Learning Activities

1. Prior to completing the study guide exercises for this chapter, review the following:
- Anatomy and physiology of the cardiovascular system
- Principles of fluid and electrolyte balance
- Principles of acid-base balance including blood gas values
- Regulation of blood pressure
- Cardiovascular assessment
- Respiratory assessment
- Conduction system of the heart
- Principles related to cardiac output
- Principles of infection
2. Review the **boldfaced** Key Terms and their definitions in Chapter 35 to enhance your understanding of the content.
3. Go to Study Guide Number 7.35 on the following pages and complete the learning exercises for this chapter.

- Heartweb: http://heartweb.org
- Kearney, K. (2000). Emergency: Digitalis toxicity. *American Journal of Nursing, 100*(6), 51-52.
- Khai, P.G., et al. (2000). Infective endocarditis. In T. Nguyen, et al. (Eds.). *Management of complex cardiovascular problems* (pp. 235-250). Armonk, NY: Futura Publishing.
- Krau, S.D. (2000). The evolution of heart transplant. *Critical Care Clinics of North America, 12*(1), 1-9.
- Mended Hearts: http://www.mendedhearts.org
- Nagle, B.M. & O'Keffe, L.M. (1999). Closing in on mitral valve disease. *Nursing 99, 29*(4), 32cc1-32cc7.
- Nagle, B.M. & Taylor, J. (1998). Getting to the heart of aortic valve disease. *Nursing 99, 28*(5), 32cc8-32cc12.
- Piano, M.J. (1999). Familial hypertrophic cardiomyopathy. *Journal of Cardiovascular Nursing, 13*(4), 46-58.
- Ross, G.K. & DeJong, M.J. (1999). Emergency! Pericardial tamponade. *American Journal of Nursing, 99*(2), 35.

Chapter 36: *Interventions for Clients with Vascular Problems*

Learning Outcomes	Learning Activities	Supplemental Resources
1. Explain the pathophysiology of arteriosclerosis and atherosclerosis, including the factors that cause arterial injury. 2. Discuss the role of diet therapy in the management of clients with arteriosclerosis. 3. Describe the differences between essential and secondary hypertension. 4. Develop a plan of care for a client with essential hypertension. 5. Compare drug classifications used to treat hypertension. 6. Identify cultural considerations when caring for clients with hypertension. 7. Evaluate the effectiveness of interdisciplinary interventions to improve hypertension.	1. Prior to completing the study guide exercises for this chapter, review the following: • Anatomy and physiology of the cardiovascular system • Cardiovascular assessment • Assessment of cardiovascular system • Coagulation cascade • Cultural diversity • Low-fat diet	1. Textbook—Chapter 33 (Assessment of the Cardiovascular System) 2. Textbook—Chapter 36 3. Other resources: • Any anatomy and physiology book • Any pathophysiology book • Ayello, E.A. (2000). On the lookout for peripheral vascular disease. *Nursing 2000, 30*(6), 64hh1-64hh4. • Church, V. (2000). Stay on guard for DVT and PE. *Nursing 2000, 30*(2), 34-44.

Learning Outcomes

8. Compare and contrast assessment findings typically present in clients with peripheral arterial and peripheral venous disease.
9. Prioritize postoperative care for clients who have undergone peripheral bypass surgery.
10. Develop a continuing care plan for a client who has undergone an abdominal aortic aneurysm repair.
11. Compare and contrast Raynaud's disease and Buerger's disease.
12. Describe the nurse's role in monitoring clients who are receiving anticoagulants, including unfractionated heparin, low–molecular weight heparin, and warfarin.

Learning Activities

2. Review the **boldfaced** Key Terms and their definitions in Chapter 36 to enhance your understanding of the content.
3. Go to Study Guide Number 7.36 on the following pages and complete the learning exercises for this chapter.

Supplemental Resources

• Contact the American Heart Association for patient and professional education pamphlets regarding hypertension and vascular diseases.
• Discuss with a cardiovascular/critical care clinical specialist the postoperative care of clients after an abdominal aortic aneurysm.
• Fahey, V.A. (1999). *Vascular nursing* (3rd ed.). Philadelphia: W.B. Saunders.
• Gibson, J.M. & Kenrick, M. (1998). Pain and powerlessness: The experience of living with peripheral vascular disease. *Journal of Advanced Nursing, 27*(4), 737-745.
• Kunel, N. & Nelson, K.M. (2000). Getting the skinny on lipid-lowering drugs. *Nursing 2000, 30*(7), 52-53.
• Oertel, L.B. (1999). Monitoring warfarin therapy—How the INR keeps your patient safe. *Nursing 99, 29*(11), 41-44.

Chapter 37: *Interventions for Clients in Shock*

Learning Outcomes

1. Describe the clinical manifestations associated with the compensatory mechanisms for shock.
2. Identify clients at risk for hypovolemic shock.
3. Use laboratory data and clinical manifestations to determine the effectiveness of therapy for shock.
4. Explain the basis for crystalloid versus colloid intravenous therapy for shock.
5. Explain the expected client responses to the drugs used in the treatment of shock.
6. Prioritize nursing care needs for the client experiencing the nonprogressive state of hypovolemic shock.
7. Compare and contrast the pathophysiology and clinical manifestations of the hyperdynamic and hypodynamic phases of septic shock.
8. Identify clients at risk for septic shock.
9. Develop an educational plan for the client at risk for septic shock who lives at home.

Learning Activities

1. Prior to completing the study guide exercises for this chapter, review the following:
   • General adaptation syndrome
   • Fluid and electrolytes
   • Acid-base balance
   • Anatomy and physiology of respiratory, cardiovascular, and renal systems
   • Principles of cardiac output
   • Respiratory and cardiac assessment
2. Review the **boldfaced** Key Terms and their definitions in Chapter 37 to enhance your understanding of the content.
3. Go to Study Guide Number 7.37 on the following pages and complete the learning exercises for this chapter.

Supplemental Resources

1. Textbook—Chapter 33 (Assessment of the Cardiovascular System)
2. Textbook—Chapter 37
3. Textbook Unit 3—Fluid, Electrolyte, and Acid-Base Balance
4. Other resources:
   • American Association of Critical-Care Nurses (AACN): http://www.aacn.org
   • Any pathophysiology book with a discussion of shock
   • Carroll, T. (1999). Monitoring the gut to prevent MODS. *RN, 62*(10), 34-37.
   • DeJong, M. (1997). Clinical snapshot: Cardiogenic shock. *American Journal of Nursing, 97*(6), 40-41.

- Gordon, L. (1999). The sepsis continuum from systemic inflammatory response syndrome to multiple organ dysfunction syndrome. *Nursing in Critical Care, 4*(5), 238-244.
- Grap, M. (1998). Pulse oximetry. *Critical Care Nurse, 18*(1), 94-99.
- http://www.wbsaunders.com/simon/Iggy
- Sandrock, J. (1998). Treating traumatic hypovolemia: Which fluid to choose? *Nursing 98, 32,* cc1.

Chapter 38: *Interventions for Critically Ill Clients with Coronary Artery Disease*

Learning Outcomes

1. Explain the pathophysiology of coronary heart disease (CAD).
2. Compare and contrast stable angina, unstable angina, and myocardial infarction (MI).
3. Identify modifiable and nonmodifiable risk factors for CAD.
4. Interpret physical and diagnostic assessment in clients who have CAD.
5. Describe the psychosocial aspects of CAD.
6. Prioritize nursing care needs for clients who have CAD.
7. Explain the advantages of thrombolysis for a client experiencing an MI.
8. Identify the life-threatening complications of CAD.
9. Describe the postprocedure care for the client who has undergone a percutaneous transluminal coronary angioplasty.
10. Describe the postoperative care for the client who has undergone coronary artery bypass graft (CABG) surgery.
11. Discuss the differences between CABG surgery, minimally invasive direct coronary arterial bypass, and transmyocardial laser revascularization.
12. Develop a discharge plan for the client with CAD.

Learning Activities

1. Prior to completing the study guide exercises for this chapter, review the following:
   - Anatomy and physiology of the cardiovascular system
   - Atherosclerosis
   - Arteriosclerosis
   - Diabetes
   - Hypertension
   - Myocardial infarction
   - Cardiovascular assessment
   - Respiratory assessment
   - Postoperative care
   - Principles of cardiac output
   - Shock, cardiogenic shock
2. Review the **boldfaced** Key Terms and their definitions in Chapter 38 to enhance your understanding of the content.
3. Go to Study Guide Number 7.38 on the following pages and complete the learning exercises for this chapter.

Supplemental Resources

1. Textbook—Chapter 33 (Assessment of the Cardiovascular System)
2. Textbook—Chapter 38
3. Other resources:
   - Any anatomy and physiology textbook
   - Any pathophysiology book
   - Contact the local American Heart Association for patient and health care professional information.
   - Discuss, with a critical care clinical nurse specialist specializing in cardiac disorders, the following items:
     a. Factors that affect the decision regarding intervention for treatment for PTCA versus CABG
     b. Preoperative teaching for cardiac surgery
     c. Postoperative collaborative care
     d. Average length of stay
     e. Postoperative cardiac rehab—who attends, what is involved, when started, length of time, where provided, advantages and disadvantages
     f. Role of the nurse versus clinical nurse specialist

- Halm, M.A. & Penque, S. (1999). Heart disease in women. *American Journal of Nursing, 99*(4), 26-32.
- McAvoy, J.A. (2000). Cardiac pain: Discover the unexpected. *Nursing 2000, 30*(3), 34-40.
- Redeker, N.S. & Wykpisz, E. (1999). Effects of age on activity patterns after coronary artery bypass surgery. *Heart and Lung, 28*(1), 5-14.
- Visit a cardiac rehab unit to observe the roles of the health care providers and the activities of the unit.
- Warren, C. (1999). What is homocysteine? *American Journal of Nursing, 99*(10), 39-41.

STUDY GUIDE NUMBER 7.33

Assessment of the Cardiovascular System

Study/Review Questions

1. What are the three pacemaker sites in the heart? Name the pacer rate for each site.
   a. _SA → 60-100 bpm_
   b. _AV → 40-60 bpm_
   c. _Bundle of his → 20-40 bpm_

2. Which of the following statements about the coronary arteries of the heart is correct?
   a. There are three main coronary arteries: left coronary artery (LCA), right coronary artery (RCA), and circumflex.
   b. In most individuals, the left coronary artery supplies both the sinoatrial (SA) and atrioventricular (AV) nodes.
   c. To maintain adequate blood flow through the coronary arteries, diastolic blood pressure must be at least 60 mm Hg.   _60 - 90 mmHg_
   d. Coronary artery blood flow to the myocardium occurs primarily during systole when coronary vascular resistance is minimal.

3. Catalyzing of which of the following ions causes a chemical interaction within the actin and myosin filaments in the myocardial muscle fibers?
   a. Sodium
   b. Calcium
   c. Potassium
   d. Magnesium

4. Which of the following statements about the cardiac cycle is correct?
   a. Diastole is the shorter of the two phases.
   b. Systole is the longer of the two phases.   _SA valves_
   c. S_1 results from tricuspid and mitral valve closure.
   d. S_2 results from the contraction of the ventricles.

5. Identify the two main properties that determine the function of the cardiovascular system.
   —electrical
   — mechanical

6. Match the following variables that affect cardiac output with their descriptions.

   Descriptions

   _4_ a. Number of times ventricles contract per minute
   _6_ b. Degree of myocardial fiber stretch at end of diastole and just before heart contracts
   _1_ c. Amount of pressure or resistance that the ventricles must overcome to eject blood through the semilunar valves and into the peripheral blood vessels
   _5_ d. Pressure that ventricle must overcome to open aortic valve
   _2_ e. Distensibility of ventricles
   _3_ f. Force of contraction independent of preload

   Cardiac Output Variables
   1. Afterload
   2. Compliance
   3. Contractility
   4. Heart rate
   5. Impedance
   6. Preload

   Answer Questions 7 through 11 on a separate sheet of paper.

7. Answer the following questions that relate to the mechanical properties of the heart.
   a. How is blood flow from the heart into the systemic arterial circulation measured clinically? _CO_
   b. Define *cardiac output (CO)*.
   c. CO is the product of what two variables? _HR × SV_
   d. Define the term *stroke volume* and give the variables that impact it and cardiac output.
   e. Define *preload*.
   f. What is Starling's law of the heart?
   g. Briefly discuss afterload.
   h. Briefly discuss how the heart rate affects the cardiac output.

8. Briefly describe the electrophysiologic property of the heart.

9. Describe the relationship of the left ventricle to maintaining the blood pressure and adequate cardiac output (CO).

10. How is the relationship of the left ventricle to maintenance of blood pressure and adequate CO different in the older adult? Indicate other changes in blood pressure that can occur in the older adult.

11. Briefly explain the three systems/mechanisms and external factors that regulate blood pressure.

12. Identify the three types of sensory receptors in the body that affect the autonomic nervous system in regulating the blood pressure.

13. True or False? Which of the following statements about the various components of blood pressure are true? *Write T for true or F for false in the blanks provided.*

    F a. Systolic blood pressure is the lowest pressure during the relaxation phase of the cardiac cycle.

    F b. Diastolic blood pressure is the highest pressure during contraction of the ventricles.

    T c. Diastolic blood pressure is primarily determined by the amount of peripheral vasoconstriction.

    T d. Pulse pressure is the difference between the systolic and diastolic pressures.

    F e. Venus return to the heart is facilitated by positive intrathoracic pressure generated during exhalation.

    T f. Fluid moves from the vascular system into the interstitial spaces when the capillary endothelium is impaired.

14. The chamber of the heart that can generate the greatest amount of blood pressure is the:
    a. Right atrium.
    b. Right ventricle.
    c. Left atrium.
    d. Left ventricle.

15. Which of the following statements about the peripheral vascular system is correct?
    a. Veins are equipped with valves that permit one-way flow of blood toward the heart.
    b. The velocity of blood flow varies directly with the diameter of the vessel lumen.
    c. Blood flow decreases and blood tends to clot as the viscosity decreases.
    d. The parasympathetic nervous system has the greatest effect on blood flow to various organs.

16. In the older adult, a common assessment finding is which of the following?
    a. S_3 or S_4 heart sound
    b. Leg edema
    c. Pericardial friction rubs
    d. Change in point of maximum impulse location

17. For each of the following structures/functions, identify on a separate sheet of paper, the change that occurs in the older adult and explain what implications those changes have in regard to nursing care.
    a. Cardiac valves
    b. Conduction system
    c. Left ventricle
    d. Aorta and other large arteries
    e. Baroreceptors

18. On the illustration below, what are the sites for auscultation of heart sounds and pulse points?

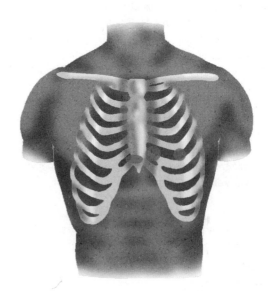

19. The description of S_1 and S_2 refers to:
    a. First and second heart sounds.
    b. Pericardial friction rub.
    c. Murmur.
    d. Gallop.

20. An S_3 or S_4 that is heard on auscultation of the heart refers to a:
    a. Murmur.
    b. Pericardial friction rub.
    c. Gallop.
    d. Normal heart sound.

21. Which of the following clients has an abnormal heart sound?
    a. Split S_1 in an 18-year-old client
    b. S_3 in a 24-year-old client
    c. Split S_2 in a 30-year-old client
    d. S_4 in a 48-year-old client ⟵ *(circled)*

22. Which of the following findings from a cardiovascular assessment is abnormal?
    a. Absence of heaves, lifts, or thrills
    b. Splitting of S_2; decreases with expiration
    c. Jugular venous distention to level of the mandible *(circled)*
    d. Point of maximal impulse (PMI) in fifth intercostal space at midclavicular line

23. On a separate sheet of paper, describe clubbing, how it is assessed, and the indication for a positive result.

24. Which of the following regarding assessment of jugular venous pressure is considered part of best practice?
    a. Elevate the head of the bed to 90 degrees to fully visualize the neck veins.
    b. Shine a light across the client's neck to visualize the internal jugular vein. *(circled)*
    c. CVP is calculated by adding 6 cm to the JVP measurement.
    d. The sternal angle landmark indicates the highest point at which pulsation is visible.

25. Match each source of chest pain with assessment findings. *Each source of chest pain may be used more than once.*

Assessment Findings

- 3 a. Sudden onset
- 6 b. Moderate ache, worse on inspiration
- 4 c. Substernal, may spread to shoulders or abdomen
- 3 d. Intermittent, relieved with sitting upright
- 1 e. Substernal, may spread across chest, back, arms
- 1 f. Usually lasts less than 15 minutes
- 6 g. Continuous until underlying condition is treated
- 2 h. Intense stabbing vice-like pain
- 5 i. Dull ache to sharp stabbing, may have numbness of fingers
- 2 j. Sudden onset, often in early morning
- 5 k. Usually on left side of chest without radiation
- 3 l. Sharp stabbing, moderate to severe
- 4 m. Squeezing, heartburn, variable in severity

Source of Chest Pain

1. Angina
2. Myocardial infarction
3. Pericarditis
4. Esophageal–gastric
5. Anxiety
6. Pleuroplumonary

26. A 50-year-old man with a history of recent cardiac surgery enters the emergency room very anxious and complaining of sudden, sharp, stabbing chest pain that spreads to the left side. He states that he is having a "heart attack." His skin is pink, warm to the touch, and diaphoretic. Capillary refill is within normal limits. No signs of clubbing. HR 110, BP within normal limits. How would you analyze these assessment findings? Is he experiencing a "heart attack"?   MI

27. A client in the emergency department with chest pain has a possible myocardial infarction (MI). Which of the following laboratory tests would be performed to determine this diagnosis?
    a. CK-MB
    b. Lipids
    c. Homocysteine
    d. Lactate dehydrogenase

28. Which of the following laboratory tests is not used to predict a client's risk of coronary artery disease?
    a. Cholesterol level
    b. Triglyceride level
    c. Prothrombin time
    d. Lipoprotein level

29. Which of the following tests would be performed to determine the location and extent of coronary artery disease?
    a. ECG *(circled)*
    b. Echocardiogram
    c. Cardiac catheterization
    d. Chest x-ray

30. Using Gordon's functional health patterns, identify questions a nurse would ask a client in assessing that client's cardiovascular status.

31. On a separate sheet of paper, identify subjective data that would be included in assessment findings related to cardiovascular disease.

32. On a separate sheet of paper, identify objective data that would be included in assessment findings related to cardiovascular disease.

33. One of the most modifiable, controllable risk factors for cardiovascular disease is:
    a. Obesity.
    b. Diabetes mellitus.
    c. Ethnic background.
    d. Family history of cardiovascular disease.

34. On a separate sheet of paper, calculate the number of pack-years for the client who has smoked half a pack of cigarettes per day for 2 years, one pack per day for 4 years, and 2 packs per day for 20 years. Discuss the significance of the number of pack-years and how those data can be used to predict a client's risk for cardiovascular or pulmonary disease.

35. The following is a partial client history. Discuss the significance of these data as they relate to the cardiovascular system.
    White male client, 45 years old. Married with three children. Works as an investment banker. Reports that he feels a lot of pressure to perform his job well. Began to have syncope episodes 3 months ago; feeling lightheaded and sometimes dizzy. Denies loss of consciousness. States that he often skips lunch to continue working through the lunch hour. Entertains clients several times per week by taking them out to lunch or dinner. Commutes to and from work via his own automobile and often gets upset and angry with traffic snarls. Tends to have late dinners with wife at home, consuming several cocktails with meals. Admits to having a "weight problem" off and on. Denies hypertension. His father has had a cerebrovascular accident (CVA).

36. A finding of pallor is indicative of:
    a. Hypoxia.
    b. Anemia.
    c. Dehydration.
    d. Chest pain.

37. The difference between the systolic and diastolic values is referred to as:
    a. Paradoxical blood pressure.
    b. Pulse pressure.
    c. Ankle brachial index.
    d. Normal blood pressure.

38. An ankle brachial index of 0.7 is an indication of:
    a. Normal arterial circulation to the lower extremities.
    b. Moderate arterial disease of the lower extremities.
    c. Severe arterial disease of the lower extremities.
    d. Inconclusive test results.

39. True or False? Decide whether each of the following statements is true or false. *Write* T *for true or* F *for false in the blanks provided.*
    ____ a. Dyspnea can occur with both cardiac disease and pulmonary disease.
    ____ b. Cardinal symptom of heart disease is dyspnea.
    ____ c. Paroxysmal nocturnal dyspnea occurs when the client has been lying down for several hours.
    ____ d. *Orthopnea* is defined as dyspnea on exertion.
    ____ e. *Indigestion, discomfort,* and *heaviness* are terms often used by clients to describe chest pain.

40. True or False? Read the following statements regarding performing a pericardium assessment and decide whether each is true or false. *Write* T *for true or* F *for false in the blanks provided. If the statement is false, correct the statement to make it true.*
    ____ a. The assessment begins with auscultation.
    ____ b. The client is in a supine position with the head of bed elevated for comfort and ease of breathing.
    ____ c. Inspect for point of maximal impulse or pulsations at the apex of the heart.
    ____ d. Heaves and lifts are associated with inspection and also associated with valve disease.
    ____ e. The nurse palpates with fingers and the most sensitive part of the palm of the hand.
    ____ f. When palpating, turn the client to the right side to bring the heart closer to the surface of the chest.
    ____ g. When auscultating, use the diaphragm to listen for low-frequency sounds.
    ____ h. The skill of accurately auscultating sounds requires a good stethoscope and lots of practice.
    ____ i. A Z-pattern is used as a method for listening to heart sounds.

41. Which of the following procedures requires informed consent from the client?
    a. ECG
    b. Use of a Holter monitor
    c. Stress test
    d. Echocardiography

42. Preparation for an ECG includes:
    a. Asking the client to lie on his or her left side.
    b. Applying leads over the client's gown.
    c. Cleaning the client's skin with soap and water.
    d. Placing the leads on as flat an area as possible.

43. Which of the following assessment findings in a client who has had a cardiac catheterization should the nurse report immediately to the physician?
    a. Pain at the catheter insertion site
    b. Catheterized extremity dusky and cool
    c. Small hematoma at the catheter insertion site
    d. Intermittent nonpalpable dorsalis pedis pulse

44. Match each of the following serum lipid values with the serum lipid laboratory test used to determine the value in an adult.

    Name of Lipid Test
    ___ a. Cholesterol
    ___ b. Triglycerides
    ___ c. Plasma high-density lipoproteins (HDLs)
    ___ d. Plasma low-density lipoproteins (LDLs)
    ___ e. HDL:LDL ratio

    Normal Laboratory Value
    1. 57 to 197 mg/dL; over 65 years of age is 92 to 221 mg/dL
    2. Females 39 to 262; males 37 to 286; and older adults is 55 to 260 mg/dL
    3. 122 to 200 mg/dL; older adults is 144 to 280 mg/dL
    4. 3:1
    5. Females 55 to 60; males 45 to 50; older adults is 92 to 221 mg/dL

45. From the list of lipid tests, identify the elevated laboratory values that increase the risk for coronary artery disease.

46. From the list of lipid tests in Question 44, identify the elevated laboratory values that protect against coronary artery disease when the value is elevated.

47. Match each of the following terms related to hemodynamic monitoring with the corresponding description.

    Terms
    ___ a. Central venous pressure (CVP)
    ___ b. Pulmonary artery occlusion pressure (PAOP)
    ___ c. Pulmonary artery wedge pressure (PAWP)

    Descriptions
    1. Reflects the left atrium and left ventricle end-diastolic pressures
    2. Direct measure of right atrial pressure and preload
    3. Measures blood flow to lungs and the state of vascular resistance in lung tissue

48. A CVP reading of less than 3 cm H_2O indicates:
    a. Right-sided heart failure.
    b. Left-sided heart failure.
    c. Cardiac tamponade.
    d. Hypovolemia.

49. Interventions for a client with a pulmonary artery catheter include:
    a. Continuous heparinized flush.
    b. Intermittent heparinized flush.
    c. Continuous normal saline flush.
    d. Heparinized flush prn.

50. A client developed complications from a cardiac catheterization and was admitted to the critical care unit where hemodynamic monitoring (HM) was initiated. On a separate sheet of paper, answer the following questions.
    a. Explain the purpose of HM.
    b. As a critical care nurse, identify the types of HM.
    c. Identify clinical indications, other than a myocardial infarction, for pulmonary artery pressure monitoring.
    d. What are some of the aspects of pulmonary artery catheter monitoring?
    e. How is impedance cardiography different than what was previously discussed regarding conventional HM?

51. A client is scheduled for an angiography. The purpose of this invasive test is to:
    a. Determine the size, silhouette, and position of the heart.
    b. Identify abnormal structures, calcifications, and tumors of the heart by fluoroscopy.
    c. Assess cardiovascular response to an increased workload.
    d. Determine arterial obstruction, narrowing, or aneurysm in specific locations.

52. The most definitive, yet invasive test for studying the right or left side of the heart and the coronary arteries is a _____.

53. It important for the nurse to ask the client who is scheduled for any type of angiography with dye about an allergy to _____ _____.

54. On a separate sheet of paper, explain what you would tell a client about the sensations that may be felt during a cardiac catheterization.

55. On a separate sheet of paper, explain the nursing responsibilities involved in preparing a client for a scheduled cardiac catheterization?

56. The alternative to injecting dye into the coronary arteries is to use a test called _____ _____ that uses a flexible catheter with a miniature transducer at the distal tip to visualize the coronary arteries.

57. Postprocedural care of a client following a cardiac catheterization includes which of the following? *Check all that apply.*
    ____ a. Client is to have bedrest for 12 to 24 hours
    ____ b. Client is to lie flat at all times
    ____ c. Assess dressing for bloody drainage or hematoma
    ____ d. Perform frequent complete neurovascular checks (6 p's) of the legs with vital signs
    ____ e. Asses pain at insertion site; medicate as needed or report to physician
    ____ f. Report to physician any chest pain, nausea, or feelings of lightheadedness
    ____ g. Provide adequate oral and IV fluids for hydration
    ____ h. Monitor intake and output because the dye is an osmotic diuretic

58. To determine valve disease of the mitral valve, left atrium, or aortic arch, the client would be scheduled for:
    a. Transesophageal echocardiogram.
    b. Electrocardiogram (ECG).
    c. Myocardial nuclear perfusion imagining.
    d. Phonocardiography.

59. On a separate sheet of paper, briefly discuss the purpose, client preparation, and procedure for a Holter monitor.

60. True or False? Decide whether each of the following statements is true or false. *Write* T *for true or* F *for false in the blanks provided. If the statement is false, correct it to make it true.*
    ____ a. There is no follow-up care for clients who undergo echocardiograms.
    ____ b. Echocardiograms require an informed consent.
    ____ c. MNPI is a radioactive technique to view cardiovascular abnormalities.
    ____ d. Technetium scanning is effective for diagnosing old infarctions.
    ____ e. After an MNPI, the client is placed in isolation because of radioactive isotopes.
    ____ f. A test that can be done at rest or during an exercise test is thallium imaging.
    ____ g. For clients who cannot perform a treadmill stress test, thallium imaging can be used.
    ____ h. Clients should be aware that thallium can cause flushing, headache, dyspnea, and chest tightness a few moments after the injection.
    ____ i. An echocardiogram is a risk- and pain-free test that uses sound waves to assess cardiac structure and mobility, particularly that of the valves.
    ____ j. There is no pre- or postprocedure care for echocardiograms.
    ____ k. For women, technetium 99m sestamibi rather than thallium is used in exercise stress tests.
    ____ l. MRI is a test using radioisotopes that compares cardiac perfusion and metabolic function.
    ____ m. A PET scan takes 2 to 3 hours and a client may be asked to use a treadmill.

61. Identify reasons a client would be scheduled for a thallium imaging.

Case Study: Assessment of the Cardiovascular System

Your client is a 72-year-old man who had an extensive left ventricular myocardial infarction (MI) at the age of 36 years. At the time of his MI, he was overweight by 50 pounds and smoked two packs of unfiltered cigarettes per day. He had smoked for 20 years. Alcohol consumption was part of his ethnic background; it was customary for him to drink one or two beers per day and several mixed drinks per week. His father had also suffered an MI, at the age of 48, and was a chain smoker. Your client slowly recovered from his MI, gave up smoking, and lost weight. His weight stabilized within 15 pounds of the upper limit of his ideal weight. His wife became an active participant in his recovery by changing her style of cooking and virtually eliminating saturated fats from their diets. He no longer drank beer, but he continued to consume an average of two mixed drinks per day. He began a moderate exercise program that included walking several miles a day at least three times a week. He has had stable angina for many years and has annual physical checkups and ECGs at the cardiologist's office. He took up the hobby of downhill skiing at the age of 66, with his cardiologist's approval. He is a retired accountant with a type A personality. Over the past 6 months, he has experienced infrequent periods of lightheadedness. He has "blacked out" on at least one occasion and was unable to remember any details of what happened. A second episode of loss of consciousness occurred on a clear, cold winter day while he was skiing. He revived spontaneously. The next day, he scheduled an appointment with his physician.

Answer the following questions on a separate sheet of paper:

1. Which lifestyle changes decreased his risk status after his MI? Which habits increased his risk status?

2. Compare and contrast the risk factors of CV disease for a 36-year-old man and a 72-year-old man.

3. The cardiologist performs an ECG and orders blood work drawn for AST, CK and CK-MB, LDH and isoenzymes, and serum potassium. What is the purpose for these tests? What other tests may be ordered?

4. The ECG and blood work are inconclusive, but the physician is concerned about his symptoms. Discuss why there is reason for concern.

5. He is scheduled for an inpatient cardiac catheterization. The physician tells him that, based on the findings at the time of the catheterization, he may go ahead and perform an angioplasty. Develop a teaching-learning plan for this client.

The cardiac catheterization is completed, and a 95% blockage of the left anterior descending (LAD) artery is seen along with an 80% blockage of the circumflex artery. A balloon angioplasty is performed in the catheterization laboratory. After the procedure, the LAD has a 40% blockage, and the circumflex has a 25% blockage.

6. What do these findings mean? What significance does the residual blockage have for this client?

The physician counsels the client to resume activity gradually. A stress test will be scheduled in several weeks for further evaluation of his exercise tolerance and cardiac status.

7. Develop a teaching-learning plan for this client to prepare him for the upcoming tests.

STUDY GUIDE NUMBER 7.34

Interventions for Clients with Dysrhythmias

Study/Review Questions

1. Match the structures of the heart with their descriptions.

   Structures of the Heart
   ___ a. Aortic valve
   ___ b. Atria
   ___ c. Chordae tendineae
   ___ d. Coronary arteries
   ___ e. Mitral valve
   ___ f. Pulmonic valve
   ___ g. Septum
   ___ h. Tricuspid valve
   ___ i. Ventricle

   Descriptions
   1. Muscular wall dividing the heart into halves
   2. Upper heart chamber
   3. Lower heart chamber
   4. Valve between right atrium and ventricle
   5. Valve between right ventricle and pulmonary artery
   6. Valve between left atrium and ventricle, bicuspid value
   7. Filaments that secure the AV valve leaflets
   8. Vessels that supply the heart with oxygenated blood
   9. Valve from the left ventricle to the aorta

2. Match each of the electrophysiologic properties or specialized cells of the cardiac conduction system with its definition.

   Electrophysiologic Properties/Specialized Cells
   ___ a. Contractility
   ___ b. Conductivity
   ___ c. Excitability
   ___ d. Action potential
   ___ e. Automaticity
   ___ f. SA node (sinoatrial node)
   ___ g. Depolarization
   ___ h. Sarcolemma
   ___ i. Atrial kick

   ___ j. Purkinje fibers
   ___ k. AV node (atrioventricular node)

   Definitions
   1. Ability of a cell to respond to an electrical impulse
   2. Extra amount of blood added to ventricles
   3. Heart's primary pacemaker
   4. Ability of the heart to circulate blood; the mechanical response to an impulse
   5. Changing a cell membrane from negatively charged to positively charged
   6. Ability to spontaneously and repeatedly generate a cardiac impulse
   7. Specialized cells in the ventricles
   8. Cell permeability that creates an electrical imbalance
   9. Cardiac cell membrane
   10. Cell-to-cell transmission of impulse
   11. Slows down impulses to the ventricles; secondary pacer

3. The SA node fires at the rate of which of the following times per minute?
   a. Less than 60
   b. 60 to 100
   c. 80 to 100
   d. Greater than 100

4. The electrical impulse of the heart moves through the ventricles from the _____ to _____ _____ to _____.

5. Identify the sequential order of the cardiac tissues that assume the cardiac pacemaker's role if the sinoatrial (SA) node fails to function.
   a. _____
   b. _____
   c. _____

6. Briefly describe the difference between the terms *arrhythmia* and *dysrhythmia*.

7. True or False? Read the following statements regarding characteristics of an ECG complex and decide whether each is true or false. *Write T for true or F for false in the blanks provided. If the statement is false, correct the statement to make it true.*

___ a. The P wave represents atrial depolarization followed by atrial contraction.

___ b. The P-R interval is the period of time from the firing of the SA node to just before ventricular depolarization.

___ c. When depolarization occurs in the ventricles; the T wave is formed on the ECG.

___ d. The period between ventricular depolarization and the beginning of ventricular repolarization is the S-T segment.

___ e. The T wave represents ventricular repolarization.

___ f. Q-T interval is the total time it takes the depolarization and repolarization of atrial and ventricles to occur.

8. ECG signal transmission is enhanced by:

a. Cleaning the skin with povidone-iodine solution before applying the electrodes.

b. Removing excess hair from electrode sites by clipping it closely to the skin.

c. Applying tincture of benzoin to the electrode sites and waiting for it to become "tacky."

d. Abrading the skin by rubbing the electrode sites briskly with a rough surface such as a washcloth.

9. Match the following placements with the limb leads for ECG monitoring.

Placement	Limb Lead
___ a. Right arm (+)	1. Lead I
___ b. Right arm (-), left arm (+)	2. Lead II
___ c. Left arm (-), left leg (+)	3. Lead III
___ d. Left leg (+)	4. aVr
___ e. Left arm (+)	5. aVL
___ f. Right arm (-), left leg (+)	6. aVF

10. On a separate sheet of paper, list in sequence the eight recommended steps for analyzing ECG rhythms.

11. Which of the following statements about ECG waves is correct?

a. The amplitude of the wave reflects the muscular strength of the contraction.

b. Wave duration is measured by a series of vertical lines representing intervals of 0.04 second.

c. Heart rate is estimated by counting the number of wave complexes in a given time if the rhythm is irregular.

d. Assessment of a rapid rhythm is best done by decreasing the recorder speed.

12. Identify the components of a normal electrocardiogram.

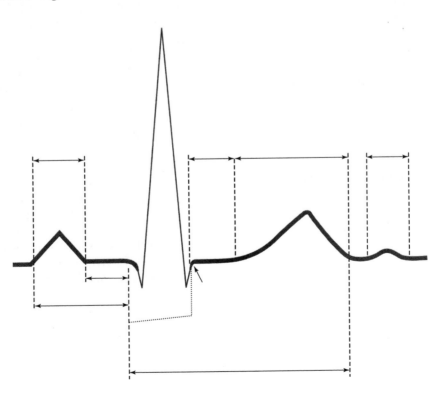

13. With the speed set for 25 mm/second, the segment between the dark lines on a monitor ECG strip represents how many seconds?
    a. 3 seconds
    b. 6 seconds
    c. 10 seconds
    d. 20 seconds

14. ECG waveforms are measured in which of the following?
    a. Pressure and cardiac output
    b. Seconds and minutes
    c. Beats per minute
    d. Amplitude (voltage) and duration (time)

Answer the following two questions on a separate sheet of paper.

15. Calculate the heart rate from an ECG strip when there are 25 small blocks from one R wave to the next R wave.

16. Calculate the heart rate shown on a 6-second ECG strip when the number of R-R intervals is 6. What is this rhythm?

17. How does a nurse interpret the measurement of the P-R interval when it is six small boxes on the ECG strip?
    a. Atrium is taking longer to repolarize.
    b. Longer than normal impulse time from the SA node to the ventricles is shown.
    c. There is a problem with the length of time the ventricles are depolarizing.
    d. This is the normal length of time for the P-R interval, and there is no cause for concern.

18. A wide distorted QRS complex of 0.14 second followed by a p wave is an indication of which of the following?
    a. Wide but normal complex and no cause for concern
    b. A premature ventricular contraction
    c. A problem with the speed set on the ECG machine
    d. A delayed time of the electrical impulse through the ventricles

19. Which of the following statements about sinus dysrhythmias is correct?
    a. A too-rapid heart rate lengthens diastolic filling time and leads to increased cardiac output.
    b. The body attempts to compensate for a decreased stroke volume by decreasing the heart rate.
    c. Sinus bradycardia occurs in trained athletes because the stroke volume is adequate without a higher rate.
    d. Sinus tachycardia is uncommon in the general population and causes symptoms of coronary insufficiency.

20. A client in a cardiac critical care unit has a sustained bradydysrhythmia. Identify key clinical manifestations of this problem.

21. On a separate sheet of paper, identify treatment modalities for the following common dysrhythmias:
    a. Atrial fibrillation
    b. Ventricular tachycardia
    c. Ventricular fibrillation
    d. Premature ventricular contraction (PVC)
    e. Sinus bradycardia
    f. Atrial flutter
    g. Premature atrial contraction
    h. Supraventricular rhythms

22. True or False? Read the following statements regarding heart block and decide whether each is true or false. *Write* T *for true or* F *for false in the blanks provided. If the statement is false, correct the statement to make it true.*
    ____ a. Mobitz type II second degree is a constant block in one of the bundle branches.
    ____ b. First-degree heart block is the complete blockage of impulses from the SA node.
    ____ c. Third-degree AV block results in ventricular rhythm.
    ____ d. Wenckebach is characterized by a progressive prolonged PR interval followed by a dropped beat.
    ____ e. A characteristic feature of third degree block is the P-R interval is not constant.
    ____ f. All heart blocks require interventions.
    ____ g. Clients with first-degree and type I blocks may be asymptomatic, whereas type II blocks may have symptoms.

23. Match each type of dysrhythmia with its description. *Answers may be used more than once.*

Descriptions

_____ a. A straight line on the cardiac monitor

_____ b. Results in the atria and the ventricles contracting independently of one another

_____ c. A ventricular rhythm that in most cases results in loss of consciousness

_____ d. Most common terminal event in sudden cardiac death

_____ e. Results in a QRS complex width that exceeds 0.12 second

_____ f. Results in uncoordination of atrial contraction and decreased cardiac output

_____ g. Can sustain cardiac output indefinitely

_____ h. Atrial rhythm more common than atrial fibrillation

_____ i. Causes the ventricles to quiver, resulting in absence of cardiac output

_____ j. Can be initiated by a single premature ventricular contraction

Types of Dysrhythmias

1. Sinus tachycardia
2. Atrial flutter
3. Atrial fibrillation
4. Atrioventricular dissociation
5. Ventricular tachycardia
6. Ventricular fibrillation
7. Asystole
8. Bundle branch blocks

24. Identify common causes of ectopic foci for cardiac contraction.

25. A client in a critical care unit on telemetry develops the following normal p waves at a regular rate of 88 beats per minute. There is a separate ventricular regular rate of 55 with a normal QRS complex. An AV dissociation exists because the atria and ventricles are independent of each other.
    a. Based on this ECG, what assessment findings might the nurse identify with this dysrhythmia?
    b. What would make a difference in the physical findings?
    c. What type of heart block has been identified?
       (1) 1st degree
       (2) Mobitz type I
       (3) Mobitz type II
       (4) 3rd degree
    d. What intervention is necessary for this client?
    e. Would the client have a temporary or permanent pacemaker? Provide a rationale for your answer.
    f. Indicate nursing interventions including discharge teaching for this client.

26. An adult client with ventricular fibrillation or pulseless ventricular tachycardia will receive which of the following medications? What is the usual dose for this drug? Nursing interventions? Side effects?
    a. Propranolol (Inderal)
    b. Bretylium tosylate (Bretylol)
    c. Diltiazem hydrochloride (Cardizem)
    d. Lidocaine

27. On a separate sheet of paper, differentiate between invasive and noninvasive temporary pacing. Describe the two types of invasive temporary pacing.

28. Identify the three complications that can occur with noninvasive pacemaker therapy.
    a. _____
    b. _____
    c. _____

29. Using a separate sheet of paper, briefly describe what the "demand mode" means in cardiac pacing.

30. Defibrillation for cardioversion is synchronized with which part of the ECG complex?
    a. T wave
    b. Q-T interval
    c. S-T segment
    d. QRS complex

31. All clients who have a dysrhythmia should be instructed to:
    a. Stay at least 4 feet away from a microwave oven that is operating.
    b. Avoid going through any electronic metal detectors, such as those at airports.
    c. Learn the procedure for assessing their apical pulses and have a family member learn the procedure as well.
    d. Wear a medical alert bracelet to inform others of their disability.

32. A nurse observes changes in mental status and orientation and notes client complaints of chest pain while ambulating a client. The nursing diagnosis for this patient would be which of the following?
    a. Activity Intolerance
    b. Decreased Cardiac Output
    c. Acute Confusion
    d. Impaired Gas Exchange

33. When performing external defibrillation, which of the following is a vital step in the procedure?
    a. The gel pads are placed anterior over the apex and posterior for better conduction.
    b. A second shock cannot be administered for 1 minute to allow for recharging.
    c. No one is to be touching the client at the time shock is delivered.
    d. Continue to ventilate the client via endotracheal tube during the procedure.

34. The most life-threatening consequence of cardiac dysrhythmias is:
    a. Severe hypotension.
    b. Sinus bradycardia.
    c. Stroke.
    d. Sudden death.

35. Develop a concept map relevant to dysrhythmias. Consider factors that put clients at risk for atrial and for ventricular dysrhythmias. On a separate sheet of paper, identify subjective and objective data.

36. Based on assessment findings, what is the most common nursing diagnosis for clients with dysrhythmia?

37. Discuss the four factors that are considered when interventions for dysrhythmias are planned.

38. Which of the following statements about antidysrhythmic agents is correct?
    a. Class I agents slow the rate of depolarization and conduction velocity and decrease cardiac rate.
    b. Class II agents control dysrhythmias associated with too much parasympathetic stimulation.
    c. Class III agents decrease the absolute refractory time and help to increase cardiac rate.
    d. Class IV agents impede the flow of sodium into the cell during depolarization and decrease cardiac rate.

39. Which of the following procedures should not be performed on the client who has a dysrhythmia?
    a. Giving an intramuscular injection
    b. Monitoring temperature rectally
    c. Cleaning the mouth using a Water Pik
    d. Assisting transfer to a bedside commode for bowel movement

40. Which of the following statements about sinus dysrhythmias is correct?
    a. A too-rapid rate lengthens diastolic filling time and leads to increased cardiac output.
    b. The body attempts to compensate for a decreased stroke volume by decreasing the heart rate.
    c. Sinus bradycardia occurs in trained athletes because the stroke volume is adequate without a higher rate.
    d. Sinus tachycardia is uncommon in the general population and causes symptoms of coronary insufficiency.

41. Identify the following rhythm pictured in Figure 34-16 in the textbook:
    a. Ventricular tachycardia
    b. Asystole
    c. Multiple premature ventricular contractions (PVCs)
    d. Ventricular fibrillation

42. The priority ACLS intervention for the rhythm in the previous question would be:
    a. Defibrillate immediately.
    b. Administer magnesium IVP.
    c. Administer lidocaine IVP.
    d. Cardioversion.

43. Which of the following drugs would a nurse prepare to administer to a client during a cardiac arrest? *Check all that apply.*
    ____ a. Lidocaine
    ____ b. Epinephrine
    ____ c. Calcium chloride
    ____ d. Sodium bicarbonate
    ____ e. Dopamine
    ____ f. Verapamil (Calan)

44. Which of the following is the correct placement for defibrillator paddles?
    a. The anterior paddle is placed on the client's upper left chest, below the clavicle and to the left of the sternum; the apex paddle is placed on the lower right chest in a mid-axillary line.
    b. The anterior paddle is placed on the client's upper left chest below the clavicle and to the right of the sternum; the apex paddle is placed on the lower right chest in a mid-axillary line.
    c. The anterior paddle is placed on the client's upper right chest below the clavicle and to the right of the sternum; the apex paddle is placed on the client's lower left chest in a mid-axillary line.

45. A client is in ventricular fibrillation. Which of the following actions is correct in regard to defibrillation?
    a. Defibrillate at 360 joules
    b. Defibrillate at 200 joules
    c. Defibrillate at 50 joules
    d. Defibrillate at 100 joules

46. True or False? *Write T for true or F for false in the blanks provided.*
    ___ a. The implantable cardioverter defibrillator (ICD) treats bradyarrhythmia.
    ___ b. Dobutamine is a beta-adrenergic agent used to improve contractility.
    ___ c. Ventricular aneurysms are a complication of myocardial infarction.
    ___ d. A cardioversion shock is synchronized with the T wave.
    ___ e. Class III antidysrhythmics lengthen the absolute refractory period and prolong repolarization.
    ___ f. Confusion, drowsiness, and slurring of speech are signs of lidocaine toxicity.

47. Which of the following is the drug of choice for symptomatic bradycardia?
    a. Epinephrine
    b. Atropine
    c. Calcium
    d. Lidocaine

48. Which of the following class II antiarrhythmic agents controls dysrhythmias associated with excessive beta-adrenergic stimulation by decreasing heart rate and conduction velocity?
    a. Amiodarone
    b. Inderal
    c. Cardizem
    d. Verapamil

49. Identify three important topics to review with clients who have premature beats and ectopic rhythms.
    a. _____
    b. _____
    c. _____

50. On a separate sheet of paper, develop a teaching plan for a client with a pacemaker.

51. On a separate sheet of paper, develop a teaching plan for clients with implantable cardioverters/defibrillators.

52. The older adult is at risk for dysrhythmias because of changes in the cardiac conduction system. Identify at least three nursing interventions that are specific for the older adult.

53. The p wave represents:
    a. Atrial depolarization.
    b. Atrial repolarization.
    c. Ventricular depolarization.
    d. Ventricular repolarization.

54. The normal measurement of the PR interval is:
    a. Less than 0.11 second.
    b. 0.06 to 0.10 second.
    c. 0.12 to 0.20 second.
    d. 0.16 to 0.26 second.

55. The QRS complex normally measures:
    a. Less than 0.12 second.
    b. 0.10 to 0.16 second.
    c. 0.12 to 0.20 second.
    d. 0.16 to 0.24 second.

56. The ST segment is normally:
    a. Isoelectric.
    b. Elevated.
    c. Depressed.
    d. Biphasic.

57. The total time required for ventricular depolarization and repolarization is represented on the ECG by the:
    a. PR interval.
    b. QRS complex.
    c. ST segment.
    d. QT interval.

58. When the myocardium is refractory, it is:
    a. Able to accept another impulse.
    b. Fibrillatory.
    c. Unable to accept another impulse.
    d. Prone to re-entry mechanism.

59. Stimulation of the sympathetic nervous system produces which of the following effects?
    a. Decreased heart rate and decreased force of contraction
    b. Increased heart rate, increased contractility, and dilation of coronary vessels
    c. Has virtually no effect on the ventricles of the heart
    d. Slows the heart rate and slows AV conduction time

60. Which of the following is responsible for the major
    pumping action of the heart?
    a. Endocardium
    b. Myocardium
    c. Epicardium
    d. Pericardium

61. The function of the AV node is to:
    a. Increase the automaticity of the SA node.
    b. Pace the heart at 60 to 100 beats per minute.
    c. Provide structural support for the tricuspid valve.
    d. Delay impulses between the atria and ventricles.

*Interpret the following ECG strips. Write your answers in the
blanks provided.*

62. _____

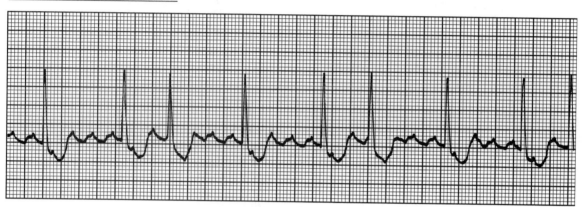

RATE_____   RHYTHM _____   P WAVES _____

PR INTERVAL _____   QRS DURATION _____   INTERPRETATION _____

63. _____

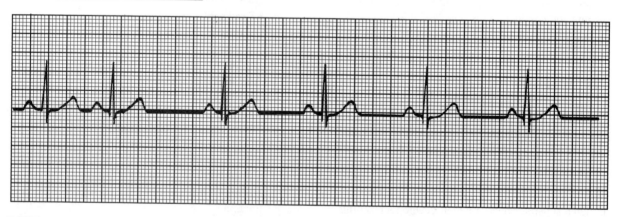

RATE_____   RHYTHM _____   P WAVES _____

PR INTERVAL _____   QRS DURATION _____   INTERPRETATION _____

64. _____

RATE_____   RHYTHM _____   P WAVES _____

PR INTERVAL _____   QRS DURATION _____   INTERPRETATION _____

65. _____

RATE_____   RHYTHM _____   P WAVES _____

PR INTERVAL _____   QRS DURATION _____   INTERPRETATION _____

66. _____

RATE_____   RHYTHM _____   P WAVES _____

PR INTERVAL _____   QRS DURATION _____   INTERPRETATION _____

67. _____

RATE_____ RHYTHM _____ P WAVES _____

PR INTERVAL _____ QRS DURATION _____ INTERPRETATION _____

68. _____

RATE_____ RHYTHM _____ P WAVES _____

PR INTERVAL _____ QRS DURATION _____ INTERPRETATION _____

69. _____

RATE_____ RHYTHM _____ P WAVES _____

PR INTERVAL _____ QRS DURATION _____ INTERPRETATION _____

70. _____

RATE_____   RHYTHM _____   P WAVES _____

PR INTERVAL _____   QRS DURATION _____   INTERPRETATION _____

71. _____

RATE_____   RHYTHM _____   P WAVES _____

PR INTERVAL _____   QRS DURATION _____   INTERPRETATION _____

72. _____

RATE_____   RHYTHM _____   P WAVES _____

PR INTERVAL _____   QRS DURATION _____   INTERPRETATION _____

73. _____

RATE_____ RHYTHM _____ P WAVES _____

PR INTERVAL _____ QRS DURATION _____ INTERPRETATION _____

74. _____

RATE_____ RHYTHM _____ P WAVES _____

PR INTERVAL _____ QRS DURATION _____ INTERPRETATION _____

75. _____

RATE_____ RHYTHM _____ P WAVES _____

PR INTERVAL _____ QRS DURATION _____ INTERPRETATION _____

76. _____

RATE_____   RHYTHM _____   P WAVES _____

PR INTERVAL _____   QRS DURATION _____   INTERPRETATION _____

77. _____

RATE_____   RHYTHM _____   P WAVES _____

PR INTERVAL _____   QRS DURATION _____   INTERPRETATION _____

78. _____

RATE_____   RHYTHM _____   P WAVES _____

PR INTERVAL _____   QRS DURATION _____   INTERPRETATION _____

79. _____

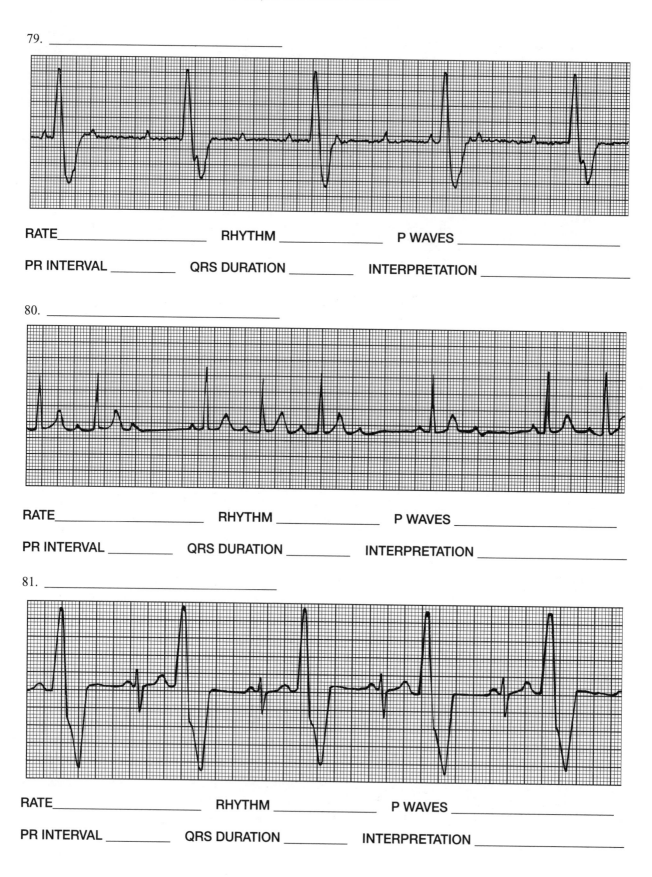

RATE_____ RHYTHM _____ P WAVES _____

PR INTERVAL _____ QRS DURATION _____ INTERPRETATION _____

80. _____

RATE_____ RHYTHM _____ P WAVES _____

PR INTERVAL _____ QRS DURATION _____ INTERPRETATION _____

81. _____

RATE_____ RHYTHM _____ P WAVES _____

PR INTERVAL _____ QRS DURATION _____ INTERPRETATION _____

Case Study: The Client with a Dysrhythmia

A 78-year-old woman is admitted to a telemetry unit directly from her physician's office for evaluation and management of congestive heart failure. She has a history of systemic hypertension and chronic moderate mitral regurgitation. Her medication orders include furosemide (Lasix) 80 mg PO qid, digoxin 0.125 mg PO qd, and diltiazem (Cardizem) 60 mg PO tid. Your initial assessment of the client reveals a pulse rate that is rapid and very irregular. The client is restless and her skin is pale and cool. Her blood pressure is 106/88. She is short of breath and anxious. Her ECG monitor pattern shows uncontrolled atrial fibrillation, with a rate ranging from 150 to 170 beats per minute. Her oxygen saturation level is 90%.

Answer the following questions on a separate sheet of paper:

1. Given the assessment findings, what should you do first?

2. What additional physical assessment techniques would you perform?

3. Because the length of time the client has been in atrial fibrillation is known, what potential problems should be evaluated before attempts to convert the rhythm are implemented?

STUDY GUIDE NUMBER 7.35

Interventions for Clients with Cardiac Problems

Study/Review Questions

1. Indicate which of the following clients are at greatest risk of developing infective endocarditis. *Check all that apply.*
   ____ a. An intravenous drug user
   ____ b. A client with pancreatitis
   ____ c. A client with a myocardial infarction
   ____ d. A client with a prosthetic mitral valve replacement, postoperative
   ____ e. A client with an abscessed tooth and mitral stenosis
   ____ f. An older adult client with urinary tract infection and valve damage
   ____ g. A client with cardiac arrhythmias

2. On a separate sheet of paper, develop a concept map relevant to infective endocarditis. Consider physiologic, psychologic, and developmental factors. Identify subjective and objective data.

3. A client with aortic valve endocarditis complains of fatigue and shortness of breath. Crackles are heard on lung sounds. These assessment findings may indicate:
   a. Emboli to the lung.
   b. Valve incompetence resulting in heart failure.
   c. Pulmonary edema.
   d. Coronary artery disease.

4. A client has an admitting diagnosis of infectious endocarditis. The nurse would anticipate which of the following tests to be performed to confirm a positive diagnosis?
   a. CT scan
   b. MRI
   c. Blood cultures
   d. Echocardiogram

5. Self-care measures for the client who has had infective endocarditis include teaching the client to:
   a. Take an oral temperature reading daily for the remainder of his/her life.
   b. Begin a moderate exercise program to strengthen the myocardium.
   c. Administer prophylactic antibiotics for every invasive procedure including dental care.
   d. Weigh themselves daily to monitor for weight gain, which is then reported to the physician.

6. Which of the following procedures is the client with infective endocarditis most likely to report having had recently?
   a. Teeth cleaning
   b. Urinary bladder catheterization
   c. Chest radiography
   d. Proctoscopy

7. Arterial embolization to the brain resulting from infective endocarditis may cause symptoms such as:
   a. Dysarthria.
   b. Dysphagia.
   c. Atelectasis.
   d. Electrolyte imbalances.

8. Treatment interventions for a client with infective endocarditis would include:
   a. Administration of oral penicillin for 6 weeks or more.
   b. Hospitalization for initial intravenous antibiotics, possibly with a central line.
   c. Complete bedrest for the duration of treatment.
   d. Long-term anticoagulation therapy with heparin.

9. A client has developed endocarditis. On a separate sheet of paper, identify assessment findings related to this disease.

10. Which of the following clients could be at risk for developing viral pericarditis?
   a. 35-year-old woman with tuberculosis
   b. 45-year-old man who has had radiation therapy for lung cancer
   c. 30-year-old man with a respiratory infection
   d. 50-year-old woman with chest trauma

11. True or False? Read the following statements regarding assessment findings of pericarditis and decide whether each is true or false. *Write T for true or F for false in the blanks provided. If the statement is false, correct the statement to make it true.*
   ____ a. A common assessment finding is a grating substernal pain, mainly on inspiration when in supine position.
   ____ b. Initially, pain is best relieved by sitting up and leaning forward and by steroid medications.
   ____ c. Acute pericarditis is usually short-term, lasting approximately 2 to 6 weeks.
   ____ d. Pericardial friction rub is best heard using the diaphragm at the right upper sternal border.
   ____ e. ECG changes are insidious.
   ____ f. Pericardiocentesis is a treatment for pericardial effusion.
   ____ g. Tuberculosis can be a cause of chronic constrictive pericarditis.
   ____ h. Interventions for the client with pericarditis include preparing for a paracentesis if cardiac tamponade develops.
   ____ i. The clinical finding most indicative of rheumatic carditis is precordial pain.

12. A client has been admitted with acute pericarditis. Assessment findings indicate neck vein distention, clear lungs, muffled heart sounds, tachycardia, tachypnea, and a greater than 10 mm Hg difference in systolic pressure on inspiration than on expiration. The nurse's response to these assessment findings would be to:
   a. Continue to monitor client; these are normal signs of pericarditis.
   b. Immediately report findings to the physician, as these are signs of cardiac tamponade.
   c. Administer oxygen and monitor oxygen saturation and seek pain medication order to control symptoms.
   d. Check ECG, administer morphine for pain to slow respiratory rate, and administer diuretic as ordered.

13. Summarize the nursing interventions for a client with pericarditis.

14. A client with rheumatic heart disease needs to understand that signs of rheumatic carditis must be recognized immediately so that the client receives prompt treatment with:
    a. Pericardiocentesis.
    b. Antibiotics for 10 days.
    c. Pain medication for substernal pain control.
    d. Rest with observation for further necessary treatment.

15. The nurse should anticipate the client receiving which medication of choice for treatment of rheumatic carditis?
    a. Antibiotic (penicillin)
    b. NSAIDs
    c. Pain medications (opioids)
    d. Steroids

16. Match each description to the corresponding key feature/finding.

    Key Features/Findings
    ___ a. Janeway's lesions
    ___ b. Osler's nodes
    ___ c. Pleural friction rub
    ___ d. Splinter hemorrhages
    ___ e. Petechiae
    ___ f. Systemic emboli
    ___ g. Pulsus paradoxus
    ___ h. Aschoff's bodies
    ___ i. Cardiac tamponade

    Descriptions
    1. Vegetation fragment in circulation resulting in a CVA or TIA
    2. Red, flat pinpoint spots/lesions in mucous membrane and conjunctive
    3. Nonpainful hemorrhagic lesions on fingers, toes, nose, or earlobes
    4. Painful reddish lesions with a white center
    5. Small red streaks or black longitudinal lines of nail beds
    6. Having a systolic blood pressure higher on expiration than on inspiration
    7. Scratchy, high-pitched sound heard at lower sternal border
    8. Small nodules on myocardium replaced by scar tissue
    9. Fluid around the heart

17. True or False? Which of the following is true regarding cardiac tamponade? *Write T for true or F for false in the blanks provided.*
    ___ a. Cardiac tamponade may occur with as little as 20 to 50 mL fluid.
    ___ b. If fluid accumulates slowly, the pericardium accommodates the fluid by stretching.
    ___ c. This condition is not a medical emergency.
    ___ d. Chest x-ray and echocardiogram can confirm the diagnosis, but hemodynamic monitoring may be necessary.
    ___ e. A pericardiocentesis is performed to remove the fluid.

18. What is the nurse's role before, during, and after a pericardiocentesis?

19. Match each assessment finding with the corresponding inflammatory cardiac disease. *Answers may be used more than once.*

    Assessment Finding
    ___ a. Pulsus paradoxus
    ___ b. Pleural friction rub
    ___ c. Janeway's lesions
    ___ d. Streptococcal infection
    ___ e. Osler's nodes
    ___ f. Cardiac tamponade
    ___ g. Petechiae
    ___ h. Splinter hemorrhage lesions

    Inflammatory Cardiac Disease
    1. Classic late sign of endocarditis
    2. Sign of pericardial effusion; a complication of pericarditis
    3. Classic early sign of endocarditis
    4. An assessment finding for pericarditis
    5. Complication of pericarditis
    6. Common assessment finding for endocarditis
    7. Rheumatic carditis

20. Digitalis, nitrates, and other vasodilators are contraindicated as treatment for which of the following cardiomyopathies?
    a. Nonobstructed
    b. Dilated
    c. Obstructed
    d. Restrictive

21. True or False? Which of the following statements about cardiomyopathies are true? *Write* T *for true or* F *for false in the blanks provided.*
    ___ a. Cardiomyopathy always leads to heart failure with poor prognosis.
    ___ b. Dilated cardiomyopathy is the massive hypertrophy of the ventricles and small ventricular cavities.
    ___ c. Dilated cardiomyopathy results in symptoms of left ventricular failure.
    ___ d. Most clients with hypertrophic cardiomyopathy are asymptomatic until early adulthood.
    ___ e. Sudden death may be the first manifestation of hypertrophic cardiomyopathy.
    ___ f. Restrictive cardiomyopathy results in decreased cardiac output during exercise.
    ___ g. Dilated cardiomyopathy and restricted cardiomyopathy are managed the same as heart failure.
    ___ h. Hypertrophic cardiomyopathy is managed the same as myocardial ischemia.
    ___ i. Heart transplantation is the treatment of choice for severe hypertrophic cardiomyopathy.

22. The client with a heart transplantation will:
    a. Have an increased risk for developing coronary artery disease.
    b. Respond to carotid sinus pressure and vagal stimulation.
    c. Experience numerous episodes of acute organ rejection.
    d. Report episodes of angina with increased activity.

23. A client has decreased cardiac output related to dilated cardiomyopathy and is being considered for heart transplant. Review the section on cardiomyopathy, including criteria for selection for transplantation, along with the legal/ethical issues in health care to formulate your own personal thoughts as a nurse health care provider. *Write your answer on a separate sheet of paper.* Be able to discuss and defend your position on the subject with other health care providers.

24. The most common site of valvular disease is in the:
    a. Aortic valve.
    b. Pulmonary valve.
    c. Tricuspid valve.
    d. Mitral valve.

25. True or False? Read the following statements regarding valvular disease and decide whether each is true or false. *Write* T *for true or* F *for false in the blanks provided. If the statement is false, correct the statement to make it true.*
    ___ a. *Stenosis* is a term referring to the heart valves no longer being able to open fully.
    ___ b. *Regurgitation* is a term referring to the heart valves no longer being able to close completely.
    ___ c. The right side of the heart is more often affected.
    ___ d. The aortic valve is the most common valve affected.
    ___ e. The most common valve disorder is mitral stenosis.
    ___ f. The most common cause of mitral stenosis is rheumatic heart disease.
    ___ g. The tricuspid valve is *not* affected often unless damage occurs after endocarditis resulting from intravenous drug abuse.
    ___ h. Women are diagnosed with mitral regurgitation more often than are men.
    ___ i. Nitrates can cause decreased preload and dizziness with aortic stenosis.
    ___ j. Nonsurgical treatment modality is most concerned with maintaining right side heart function.

26. Which two of the following valve disorders would *not* cause paroxysmal nocturnal dyspnea?
    a. Mitral stenosis
    b. Mitral prolapse
    c. Aortic stenosis
    d. Aortic insufficiency
    e. Mitral insufficiency

27. The most common preventable cause of valvular heart disease is:
    a. Congenital disease or malformation.
    b. Calcium deposits and thrombus formation.
    c. Beta-hemolytic streptococcal infection.
    d. Hypertension or Marfan's syndrome.

28. Pitting edema is a sign for which type of valvular disease?
    a. Mitral valve stenosis and insufficiency
    b. Aortic valve stenosis and insufficiency
    c. Both aortic and mitral valve insufficiency
    d. Mitral valve prolapse

29. The diagnostic test most often performed to assess valvular heart disease is:
    a. Echocardiography.
    b. Electrocardiography.
    c. Exercise testing.
    d. Thallium scanning.

30. Long-term anticoagulant therapy for the client with valvular heart disease includes the drug:
    a. Heparin sodium.
    b. Warfarin sodium (Coumadin).
    c. Tubocurarine chloride.
    d. Protamine sulfate.

31. The most common invasive procedure for a client with valvular heart disease that requires prophylactic antibiotic therapy is:
    a. Intravenous therapy.
    b. Colonoscopy.
    c. Dental cleaning.
    d. Gastroscopy.

32. Match the types of valvular disease with their characteristics. *Answers may be used more than once.*

Characteristics	Types of Valvular Disease
___ a. Fatigue and chronic weakness are first signs, followed by dyspnea	1. Mitral valve stenosis
___ b. Classic signs of dyspnea, angina, and syncope	2. Mitral valve insufficiency
___ c. A first sign is dyspnea and dry cough	3. Mitral valve prolapse
___ d. Blowing type of murmur; "bounding" arterial pulse	4. Aortic stenosis
___ e. Irregular rhythm; atrial fibrillation can cause emboli	5. Aortic insufficiency
___ f. Most clients are asymptomatic	
___ g. Right-side heart failure; later cardiac output fails	
___ h. The client may experience palpitations while lying on left side	
___ i. Symptom-free for decades, later related to left ventricle failure or cardiogenic shock and pulmonary edema	
___ j. Loud apical diastolic murmur	
___ k. Right-sided failure results in neck vein distention	
___ l. Leaflets enlarge and fall back into left atrium during systole	

___ m. Normal heart rate and blood pressure
___ n. Becoming a disorder of aging populations
___ o. Murmur, harsh systolic crescendo-decrescendo

33. On a separate sheet of paper, compare and contrast the pathophysiology and clinical manifestations of each of the following valve disorders.

Valve Disorder	Patho-physiology	Clinical Manifestations
Mitral stenosis		
Mitral insufficiency		
Mitral valve prolapse		
Aortic stenosis		
Aortic insufficiency		

34. The surgical noninvasive intervention of a balloon valvuloplasty is often used for which type of client?
    a. Children with a genetic valve defect
    b. Adults who are nonsurgical candidates
    c. Adults whose open heart surgery failed
    d. Children needing replacement valves

35. Which of the following is a complication of post-valvuloplasty?
    a. Myocardial infarction
    b. Angina
    c. Bleeding and emboli
    d. Infection

36. A client with a prosthetic valve replacement should understand that postoperative care will include life-long:
    a. Antibiotics.
    b. Anticoagulant therapy.
    c. No exercise program.
    d. Aspirin therapy.

37. A client with a xenograft valve must realize that this type of valve does not require anticoagulant therapy but will require which of the following?
    a. Replacement in about 7 to 10 years
    b. An exercise program to develop collateral circulation
    c. Daily temperature check to watch for signs of rejection
    d. Frequent monitoring for pulmonary edema

38. Summarize items that are covered when educating clients and their families about mitral valve disease.

39. The most common nursing diagnosis for a client with valvular heart disease is:
    a. Decreased Cardiac Output.
    b. Ineffective Coping.
    c. Ineffective Breathing Pattern.
    d. Disturbed Body Image.

40. The client undergoing heart valve surgery is instructed to:
    a. Continue taking oral anticoagulants until the time of admission for surgery.
    b. Prepare for a cardiac catheterization, at which time the defective valve will be replaced.
    c. Expect to have open heart surgery and be admitted to an intensive care unit postoperatively.
    d. Refill the prescription for oral anticoagulants because it will be resumed postoperatively.

41. Home care of the client following heart valve surgery includes:
    a. Using an electric toothbrush for regular dental hygiene.
    b. Flossing of teeth daily to prevent plaque formation.
    c. Starting a rehabilitation regimen using weight training.
    d. Using clothing to camouflage the sternal incision.

42. Impaired cardiac function from heart failure results in:
    a. Low ventricular end-diastolic blood pressure.
    b. Reduced systemic diastolic blood pressure.
    c. Decreased pulmonary venous pressure.
    d. Decreased cardiac output.

43. The initial compensatory mechanism of the heart that maintains cardiac output is:
    a. Increased parasympathetic stimulation.
    b. Increased sympathetic stimulation.
    c. The Starling mechanism.
    d. Myocardial hypertrophy.

44. In the table below, describe how each of the following compensatory mechanisms increases cardiac output as a result of heart failure. Indicate the long-term effect of each mechanism.

45. Complete the table below to compare/contrast the classifications of heart failure.

Compensatory Mechanism	Action to Increase CO with Long-Term Damaging Effect
SNS—adrenergic receptors	Action: Long-term effect:
Cardiac dilation	Action: Long-term effect:
Cardiac hypertrophy	Action: Long-term effect:
Hormonal response	Action: Long-term effect:

Heart Failure Classification	Definition	Effect on System
Systolic dysfunction		
Diastolic dysfunction		

46. Which of the following statements about the classification of heart failure is correct?
    a. Forward failure is the result of the heart's inability to maintain cardiac output.
    b. Left ventricular failure is often directly related to right ventricular failure.
    c. High-output failure occurs when the body's metabolic needs are met with an increased cardiac output.
    d. Chronic heart failure develops over time and is caused by a sudden myocardial infarction.

47. The main cause of heart failure is related to which of the following conditions?
    a. Renal failure
    b. Myocardial infarction/coronary artery disease
    c. High-fat diet
    d. Hypertension

48. The client with left ventricular failure is most likely to report:
    a. Nocturia.
    b. Weight gain.
    c. Swollen legs.
    d. Nocturnal coughing.

49. Assessment findings of the client with left-sided heart failure is most likely to include:
    a. S2 splitting.
    b. Jugular venous distention.
    c. Splenomegaly.
    d. Wheezes or crackles.

50. Assessment findings of a client with right-sided heart failure is most likely to include:
    a. Dependent edema.
    b. Weight loss.
    c. Hypotension.
    d. Angina.

51. True or False? Read the following statements regarding older adults and heart failure and decide whether each is true or false. *Write* T *for true or* F *for false in the blanks provided. If the statement is false, correct the statement to make it true.*
    ___ a. A large number of older adults with heart failure are over 60.
    ___ b. Healthy People 2010 includes goals for the older adult such as community support and follow-up care.
    ___ c. Changes with mental status can be an indication of heart failure.
    ___ d. Thyroid studies should be done because hypo- or hyperthyroidism can aggravate heart failure.

___ e. The older client is at high risk for digoxin toxicity, and frequent monitoring is necessary.
___ f. Heart failure of clients older than 80 is often manifested as restlessness and confusion.
___ g. Orthostatic hypotension is a likely side effect of medications in the treatment of heart failure.

52. A client with congestive heart failure is suspected of having pulmonary edema. To diagnose pulmonary edema, the test that is most useful is:
    a. Pulmonary function studies.
    b. Thallium scan.
    c. Chest x-ray.
    d. Lung scan.

53. A client with congestive heart failure develops pulmonary edema. Identify the nursing interventions for this client.

54. Drug therapy for heart failure includes:
    a. Inotropic agents to increase the heart rate.
    b. Sympathomimetics to decrease contractility.
    c. Diuretics to increase the cardiac preload.
    d. Vasodilators to decrease systemic resistance.

55. Clients may receive any of the following medications for the treatment of congestive heart failure. Identify at least two nursing interventions for each of the following drugs:
    a. Captopril (Capoten)
    b. Enalapril (Vasotec)
    c. Loop diuretics—furosemide (Lasix)
    d. Digoxin
    e. Nitroglycerin
    f. Beta blockers

56. A client taking digoxin therapy would be educated to have which of the following laboratory tests to monitor for potential cardiac problems and digoxin toxicity?
    a. Hyper- and hyponatremia
    b. Hyper- and hypokalemia
    c. Hyper- and hypochloremia
    d. Hyper- and hypomagnesemia

57. An outcome for the collaborative problem Potential for Pulmonary Edema would be:
    a. No dysrhythmias.
    b. Clear lung sounds.
    c. Less fatigue.
    d. No disorientation.

58. In addition to oxygen and a diuretic, a drug that is commonly administered to relieve dyspnea resulting from pulmonary edema is:
    a. Beta blockers.
    b. Dopamine.
    c. Morphine sulfate.
    d. Digoxin.

59. Chronic heart failure results in which of the following problems?
    a. Xanthelasma
    b. Leg edema
    c. Hemangioma
    d. Palpitations

60. The best way for a nurse to assess for paroxysmal nocturnal dyspnea is to ask the client about:
    a. Number of times the client voided at night.
    b. Dry hacking coughs.
    c. The use of two or more pillows to sleep.
    d. The inability to breathe well while lying flat in bed.

61. Identify preventive measures for delaying heart failure in clients with pre-existing heart disease.
    a. _____
    b. _____
    c. _____
    d. _____
    e. _____

62. Indicate which of the following medications are used to reduce preload or afterload:
    ___ a. Digoxin
    ___ b. Nitrates
    ___ c. Calcium channel blockers
    ___ d. Ace inhibitors
    ___ e. Diuretics
    ___ f. Beta blockers

63. The client is at risk for developing significant hypotension if which of the following medications is administered by IV?
    a. Nitroglycerin
    b. Loop diuretic (Lasix)
    c. Digoxin
    d. Nitroprusside (Nipride)

64. Discharge planning for the client with heart failure includes:
    a. Teaching the client to take diuretics at bedtime to enhance the effect on increased renal perfusion.
    b. Demonstrating to the client how to monitor an apical pulse and what symptoms to report to the physician.
    c. Determining whether the client has a bathroom scale to monitor weight to facilitate reporting a gain of more than 5 pounds.
    d. Providing the client with dietary exchange lists of food allowed on a low-potassium diet.

65. Correct the *italicized word* in each of the following assessment findings to indicate that heart failure is worsening.
    a. Weight gain of *5 pounds* in a week
    b. Complaints of not being able to perform activities of daily living for *1 week*
    c. Dry cough of *2 days*
    d. Getting up *one time* during the night to urinate
    e. Shortness of breath on *exertion*

66. Which of the following statements is an indication that the client needs more teaching regarding a treatment regimen for heart failure?
    a. "I should only weigh myself once a month and watch for fluid retention."
    b. "I should not take my medications, especially digoxin, if I am nauseated, and I should then call the doctor."
    c. "If my heart feels like it is racing, I should call the doctor."
    d. "I need to consider my activities for the day and take rests as needed."
    e. "I need to have periods of rest and activity and need to avoid activity after meals."

67. Home care for the client with heart failure is a focus for Healthy People 2010. On a separate sheet of paper, summarize areas that the home health nurse assesses in clients with heart failure.

Case Study: The Client with Heart Failure

A 74-year-old woman is admitted to the hospital with heart failure. She had been growing progressively weaker and had ankle edema, dyspnea on exertion, and three-pillow orthopnea. On admission, she is severely dyspneic and can answer questions only with one-word phrases. She is diaphoretic, tachycardiac (pulse 132), and hypotensive (blood pressure 98/70). She is extremely anxious.

Answer the following questions on a separate sheet of paper:

1. Because this client cannot breathe or talk easily, prioritize the immediate nursing assessments upon admission.

2. Considering the process of congestive heart failure, explain the symptoms she is having.

3. Based on assessment, identify nursing diagnoses for this client.

4. The physician orders the following items for this client. Explain the rationale for these medications and treatments.
   - Start an IV stat with DW at KVO
   - Dopamine 3 mg/kg IV
     - Propranolol hydrochloride (Inderal) 80 mg PO q6hr
     - Verapamil hydrochloride (Calan) 10 mg IV stat and then 60 mg PO q6hr
     - Furosemide (Lasix) 40 mg IV stat
     - Digoxin 0.5 mg PO q6hr (4 doses, with ECG before doses 3 and 4)
     - Morphine 2 mg IV stat and then 2 mg q1-2hr IV prn
     - Oxygen 5 L/min per nasal prongs
     - Schedule for an ejection fraction thallium scan

STUDY GUIDE NUMBER 7.36

Interventions for Clients with Vascular Problems

Study/Review Questions

1. Differentiate between the terms *arteriosclerosis* and *atherosclerosis*.

2. Number in sequence the development of atherosclerosis.
   ___ a. Fibrous plaque develops
   ___ b. Intimal layer of artery is injured
   ___ c. Calcification, thrombosis, ulceration of fibrous lesions
   ___ d. Deposit of fatty streak on intimal layer

3. On a separate sheet of paper, describe each of the following as it relates to the development of atherosclerosis.
   a. The characteristics of plaque
   b. Causes of injury to the inner layer of the arterial wall
   c. The rate of progression and factors that influence it
   d. The characteristics of a fatty streak

4. Which of the following has a high incidence and primary risk factor related to atherosclerosis and cardiac and vascular diseases?
   a. Obesity
   b. Stress
   c. Hypertension
   d. Sedentary lifestyle

5. Noted as a result of cholesterol screening, the HDL value for an adult client is greater than 35 with no other cardiac or vascular risk factors. The nurse would advise the client to:
   a. Complete a full-fasting lipoprotein analysis.
   b. Repeat total and HDL cholesterol testing.
   c. Repeat total and HDL cholesterol testing in 6 to 12 weeks.
   d. Repeat total and HDL cholesterol testing in 5 years or with physical examination.

6. Which of the following is a nonmodifiable factor that can be a major factor attributing to injury to the intimal layer?
   a. Smoking
   b. High-fat diet
   c. Hypertension
   d. Aging

7. Generally, the process for developing atherosclerosis in women is:
   a. The same for men and women of all ages.
   b. Less common for premenopausal women than men of the same age.
   c. Greater in postmenopausal women than it is for men of the same age.
   d. Uncertain at this time; more studies need to be done.

8. True or False? Read the following statements regarding atherosclerosis and decide whether each is true or false. *Write* T *for true or* F *for false in the blanks provided. If the statement is false, correct the statement to make it true.*
   ___ a. The exact cause of atherosclerosis is unknown, however, there are theories and risk factors.
   ___ b. Those over 75 years of age have a 5% chance of developing atherosclerosis.
   ___ c. Because of estrogen, atherosclerosis is less common in premenopausal women than it is in men of the same age.
   ___ d. Atherosclerosis progresses for years before clinical manifestations are evident.
   ___ e. An example of a step one diet is 630 calories a day of fat in a 2100 calorie/day diet.
   ___ f. Meats and eggs contain the lowest amount of saturated fats.
   ___ g. Clients with LDL values of 130 to 159 are advised to follow a fat-modified diet.
   ___ h. Cigarette smoking increases the risk by raising the levels of HDLs.
   ___ i. Routine exercises can promote optimal lipid levels, prevent atherosclerosis, and lead to regression of plague.
   ___ j. An NIC intervention for smoking cessation is to encourage the client to "listen to relaxation tapes."
   ___ k. Generally, medications for hyperlipidemia should be taken with meals.

9. On a separate sheet of paper, develop a concept map relevant to atherosclerosis. Consider physiologic, psychosocial, and developmental factors. Identify data that are subjective and data that are objective.

10. Develop a teaching plan to minimize the risk of atherosclerosis for a 62-year-old client with a cholesterol laboratory value of 260 mg/dL, triglyceride laboratory value of 210 mg/dL, and normal blood pressure.

11. Which of the following blood pressure findings for an adult client with no other medical problems should be evaluated further for hypertension?
    a. 124/62
    b. 138/78
    c. 140/96
    d. 142/88

12. On a separate sheet of paper, complete the following table to compare antihypertensive medications.

Category/ Action	Common Drugs	Unique Side Effects	Nursing Implications*
Diuretics:			
Thiazide and thiazide-like			
Loop			
Potassium-sparing			
Carbonic anhydrase inhibitors			
Beta-adrenergic blocking agents			
Calcium channel blockers			
Angiotensin-converting enzyme inhibitors			
Central alpha agonists			
Vasodilators			

*Nursing implications in addition to checking blood pressure before administering the medication.

13. On a separate sheet of paper, identify reasons why a client being treated with antihypertensive medications may *not* be compliant with the prescribed regimen.

14. Which of the following organs are *not* affected by complications of hypertension?
    a. Kidneys
    b. Heart
    c. Brain
    d. Stomach

15. Which of the following items should the client with hypertension have available for home use?
    a. Sphygmomanometer with stethoscope
    b. Exercise bicycle
    c. Weight scale
    d. Food scale

16. Tissue damage as a result of peripheral arterial disease (PAD) is related to which of the following? *Check all that apply.*
    ___ a. Extent of the arterial blockage
    ___ b. Length of time there is decreased blood flow
    ___ c. Location of the arterial blockage
    ___ d. Venous circulation

17. A client who complains of numbness or burning pain that is severe enough to awaken the client at night with dependent rubor is in which of the following stages of PAD? What can the client do to temporarily relieve this pain? What is the implication of these findings?
    a. Stage I
    b. Stage II
    c. Stage III
    d. Stage IV

18. On assessment, a client with PAD is found to have a pulse that is thready, weak, and difficult to detect and easily obliterated by palpation. This assessment would be documented as a grade:
    a. 0.
    b. 1.
    c. 2.
    d. 3.

19. A client diagnosed with peripheral vascular disease is admitted to the hospital. Which of the following assessment findings are indicative of peripheral arterial disease (PAD) and which are indicative of peripheral vascular disease (PVD)? *Write A for arterial and V for venous.*
    ___ a. Decreased peripheral pulses
    ___ b. Reproducible leg pain when walking that is relieved by rest
    ___ c. Neurologic assessment intact in legs
    ___ d. Edema around ankles
    ___ e. Paresthesia
    ___ f. Loss of hair
    ___ g. Skin is cool-to-cold to touch
    ___ h. Skin color is pale, dusky, mottled
    ___ i. Brown pigmentation of the legs
    ___ j. Dependent rubor
    ___ k. Thickened brittle nails
    ___ l. Pain occurs in distal portion of extremity
    ___ m. Aching pain
    ___ n. Pain is relieved in dependent position
    ___ o. Elevation helps relieve discomfort

20. The result of a vascular study related to claudication in the legs indicates a brachial systolic blood pressure of 135 mm Hg with an ankle systolic blood pressure of 105 mm Hg. The ankle-brachial index is _____. Evaluate this finding.

21. A client with a history of vascular disease as a result of diabetes has developed a peripheral neuropathy. This client is at risk for which of the following nursing diagnoses?
    a. Fatigue
    b. Impaired Skin Integrity
    c. Risk for Injury
    d. Disturbed Sensory Perception

22. An assessment finding that indicates arterial ulcers rather than diabetic or venous ulcers is:
    a. Ulcer located over the pressure points of the feet.
    b. Ulcer has deep, pale color with even edges and little granulation tissue.
    c. Severe pain or discomfort at the ulcer site.
    d. Associated ankle discoloration and edema.

23. A complication that can result from severe PAD includes which of the following? *Check all that apply.*
    ___ a. Gangrene
    ___ b. Varicose veins
    ___ c. Septicemia
    ___ d. Amputation

24. A walking program to build collateral arterial circulation in the legs is advised only for clients with:
    a. Severe pain at rest.
    b. Venous ulcers.
    c. Gangrene.
    d. Intermittent claudication.

25. On a separate sheet of paper, develop a teaching plan for a client with PAD.

26. A client has an arterial leg ulcer. What points would you emphasize in your client teaching regarding the dressing change?

27. The client with chronic PAD may be treated with any of the following drugs to promote circulation *except:*
    a. Pentoxifylline (Trental).
    b. Propranolol hydrochloride (Inderal).
    c. Aspirin.
    d. Clopidogrel (Plavix).

28. True or False? A client with PAD is scheduled for a percutaneous transluminal balloon angioplasty. Which of the following statements are true regarding this procedure? *Write* T *for true or* F *for false in the blanks provided.*

___ a. A laser probe is advanced through a cannula into the stenosed/occluded artery to open the vessel lumen by heat from the laser vaporization.

___ b. This procedure is for the purpose of curing the client of any atherosclerosis of the artery.

___ c. Preparation for this procedure is similar to that for a diagnostic angiography.

___ d. The nurse monitors for the primary complication of bleeding at the puncture site.

___ e. Postprocedure, the client is usually on bedrest with the limb straight for 6 to 8 hours.

29. A 77-year-old woman has just had femoral-popliteal bypass surgery to treat severe arterial disease.

a. What are the six P's that are assessed for after femoral-popliteal bypass surgery in relation to arterial flow and lack of oxygenation to the tissues? On a separate sheet of paper, indicate techniques, equipment, and principles that are used by the nurse to assess these findings.

(1) _____

(2) _____

(3) _____

(4) _____

(5) _____

(6) _____

b. Which of the six P's written above is often the first indicator of a graft site occlusion and requires immediate attention from the physician? Give an explanation for your answer.

c. What is the procedure to be followed if a graft occlusion occurs?

30. Which of the following is a postoperative nursing intervention for a client with arterial revascularization?

a. Promote graft patency by maintaining hypotension and hypovolemic state.

b. Having the client bend at the hip or knee is contraindicated.

c. Diet is resumed immediately after surgery for all clients regardless of type of surgery.

d. Cough and deep breathing exercises are contraindicated because of high risk of ruptured grafts.

31. After arterial revascularization, the extremity becomes very edematous with tenseness, pain, decreased sensation, and pulses. The physician is immediately notified regarding a possible

_____.

32. The most common cause of an acute arterial occlusion related to an emboli is:

a. Diabetes.

b. Atherosclerosis.

c. Atrial fibrillation.

d. Hypertension.

33. A client is seen in the physician's office with a recurrence of a superficial ankle ulcer that is pink in color. Pulses are present. There is edema and discoloration of the leg. The client complains of "discomfort" in the leg but no claudication pain.

a. What type of ulcer does this client have? How are these characteristics different from those of an arterial ulcer or a diabetic ulcer? *Write your answers on a separate sheet of paper.*

b. How would the teaching for a client with chronic venous insufficiency differ from teaching for clients with arterial disease?

34. True or False? A client with a venous stasis ulcer has been prescribed an "Unna boot" as a form of treatment. Which of the following statements regarding an Unna boot are true? *Write* T *for true or* F *for false in the blanks provided.*

___ a. It is a type of dressing applied by a health care provider and changed daily.

___ b. It consists of a gauze dressing and is moistened with Betadine or soaked in hydrogen peroxide.

___ c. The Unna boot is covered with elastic wrap that hardens like a cast to promote venous circulation.

___ d. The boot promotes healing by forming a sterile environment for the ulcer.

___ e. The boot is applied from the toes to thigh.

___ f. The ulcer is cleaned with normal saline only before application of dressing.

___ g. Instruct client to assess for signs and symptoms of arterial occlusion if boot is too tight.

35. Indicate whether the following are related to Buerger's disease (B) or Raynaud's phenomenon (R). *Write B or R in the blanks provided.*
    ___ a. Exclusive to smokers and often young males
    ___ b. Episodic, causing white then blue fingers
    ___ c. Both sexes, predominately female
    ___ d. Chronic illness
    ___ e. Triggered by exposure to cold, caffeine, and tobacco
    ___ f. Inflammation of medium and small arteries and veins
    ___ g. Involves the distal upper and lower extremities
    ___ h. Involves small arteries of fingers and toes

36. Match the following physical findings with their related arterial disorders.

Physical Findings	Arterial Disorders
___ a. Blood pressure different in each arm	1. Popliteal entrapment
	2. Subclavian steal
___ b. Unilateral intermittent claudication	3. Thoracic outlet syndrome
___ c. Intermittent neck and shoulder pain	

37. Name two common phenomena that can occur as a result of damage to veins.

38. The greatest risk for a pulmonary embolus is a a result of which venous disorder?
    a. Bilateral varicose veins
    b. Phlebitis of superficial vein
    c. Thrombophlebitis in deep vein of lower extremity
    d. Venous insufficiency throughout the leg

39. Identify the classic signs and symptoms of a deep vein thrombosis (DVT).

40. A client is admitted to the hospital with a deep vein thrombosis. The physician would order which of the following? Give a rationale for your answer.
    a. Heparin 5000 units SQ bid, monitor the partial thromboplastin time international normalized ratio
    b. Loading high dose of Coumadin, monitor the prothrombin time international normalized ratio
    c. Alternate heparin and Coumadin depending on the laboratory values
    d. Heparin IV, then add Coumadin several days later before d/c heparin; monitor partial thromboplastin time and prothrombin time international normalized ratio

41. How would the regimen differ if the client in Question 40 were receiving low-molecular-weight (LMW) heparin and Coumadin?

42. What is the medication regimen and nursing intervention for a client receiving LMW heparin (Enoxaparin)?

43. The antidote for heparin is _____ and for Coumadin is _____.

44. The most definitively preferred noninvasive test to diagnose a DVT is:
    a. Venogram.
    b. Duplex ultrasonography.
    c. X-ray films.
    d. CAT scan.

45. True or False? Read the following statements regarding venous disorders and decide whether each is true or false. *Write T for true or F for false in the blanks provided. If the statement is false, correct the statement to make it true.*
    ___ a. Classic signs and symptoms of a DVT are always present.
    ___ b. Checking for Homan's sign should be done to assess for a DVT.
    ___ c. The focus of treatment for a DVT is to prevent complications and increase in size of the thrombus.
    ___ d. DVTs are often treated medically with rest, anticoagulants, and elevation of leg and compression stockings.
    ___ e. Thrombolytic agents are only effective if administered within the first 24 hours.
    ___ f. To prevent leg edema, elevate legs when in bed or in a chair.
    ___ g. To minimize risk of venous insufficiency after a DVT, clients should wear prescribed compression stockings.

46. Which of the following symptoms in the client with DVT who is receiving heparin therapy should the nurse report to the physician immediately?
    a. Pruritus
    b. Rash
    c. Hematuria
    d. Tinnitus

47. The usual therapeutic range for the prothrombin time in the client receiving warfarin sodium (Coumadin) therapy is:
    a. 1.5 to 2 times normal
    b. 2 to 2.5 times normal
    c. 2.5 to 3 times normal
    d. 3.5 to 4 times normal

48. A client who is prescribed warfarin sodium (Coumadin) should be instructed that the following foods decrease the effect of Coumadin, and therefore, if those foods are eaten, consistency in amount consumed each day is important.
    a. Fresh fruits
    b. Chicken and fish
    c. Green leafy vegetables and cabbage
    d. Milk and cheese

49. In addition to diet and desired laboratory values, indicate additional information a client receiving Coumadin should receive. Write your answer on a separate sheet of paper.

50. Which of the following is *not* included in health teaching for the client with chronic venous stasis?
    a. Frequently elevate the legs when sitting.
    b. Cross legs only at the ankles.
    c. Put on support hose right after rising.
    d. Avoid standing still for any length of time.

51. Which of the following clients are at greatest risk for developing varicose veins?
    a. A 37-year-old mail carrier
    b. A 19-year-old retail store clerk
    c. A 40-year-old operating room scrub technician
    d. A 25-year-old pregnant woman in the first trimester

52. The preferred treatment for phlebitis is:
    a. Dry heat.
    b. Ice packs.
    c. Warm, moist packs.
    d. Compression and elevation.

53. Identify the common types of vascular injury.
    a. _____
    b. _____
    c. _____

54. The type of vascular injury most likely to result from blunt trauma is:
    a. Arteriovenous fistula.
    b. Aneurysm formation.
    c. Dissection.
    d. Incompetent valves.

55. Which of the following clients with vascular trauma is a candidate for immediate surgery?
    a. A 54-year-old with fractured humerus
    b. An 18-year-old with a contusion of the leg
    c. A 36-year-old with a ruptured renal artery
    d. A 67-year-old with a chronic subdural hematoma

56. Identify, in order of priority, the three top principles of management of vascular trauma.
    a. _____
    b. _____
    c. _____

57. An aneurysm is a permanent localized dilation of an artery. Match the following types of aneurysms with their descriptions.

Description	Types of Aneurysms
____ a. Involves the entire circumference of artery	1. Dissecting aneurysm
	2. Saccular
	3. Fusiform
____ b. Involves a distinct portion of the artery	
____ c. Is caused by blood in wall of the artery	

58. The most common location for an aneurysm is:
    a. Abdominal aorta.
    b. Thoracic aorta.
    c. Femoral arteries.
    d. Popliteal arteries.

59. The most common cause of aneurysms is:
    a. Trauma.
    b. Thrombus formation.
    c. Atherosclerosis.
    d. Emboli.

60. A 75-year-old client with atherosclerosis enters the emergency department with a fractured hip. An abdominal aneurysm is suspected. Findings for an abdominal aneurysm would include: *Check all that apply.*
    ____ a. Abdominal, flank, or back pain.
    ____ b. Pulsation of the upper abdomen.
    ____ c. No symptoms; would be found on diagnostic tests.
    ____ d. Increased blood pressure.

61. The client in Question 60 is admitted to the hospital. The physician would order which of the following tests to confirm an accurate diagnosis as well as to determine the size and location of the AAA?
    a. Abdominal x-rays
    b. Ultrasound
    c. Spinal x-ray film
    d. MRI

62. The best nonsurgical intervention to use to decrease the risk of rupture of an aneurysm and to slow the rate of enlargement is:
    a. Maintain adequate blood pressure and control hyperthension.
    b. Bedrest until there is shrinkage of the aneurysm.
    c. Heparin and Coumadin therapy to increase blood flow.
    d. Intra-arterial thrombolytic therapy.

63. The client with a ruptured aneurysm exhibits symptoms of:
    a. Decreased pulse rate.
    b. Increased blood pressure.
    c. Dilated pupils.
    d. Diaphoretic skin.

64. The first action that the nurse should take if a client has a suspected aneurysm rupture is to:
    a. Start an intravenous infusion with a large-bore needle.
    b. Assess baseline measurements of blood pressure and pulse rate.
    c. Insert an indwelling urinary catheter to straight drain.
    d. Assess all peripheral pulses to use as a baseline for comparison.

65. The client with a repair of an abdominal aneurysm is monitored postoperatively for urinary output and renal function studies (creatinine and BUN) because:
    a. The client was probably in shock preoperatively and there may be glomerular damage.
    b. The client is usually in a critical care nursing unit where this is done routinely.
    c. The aorta was clamped during the surgery and the kidneys may have been inadvertently damaged.
    d. Repair of the aneurysm improves renal perfusion and the urinary output should increase.

66. Before surgery to repair an aneurysm, monitoring of which of the following is most important?
    a. Peripheral pulses
    b. Temperature
    c. Blood pressure
    d. Color of extremity

67. Following an aortic aneurysm repair, the nurse would monitor which of the following for several days after surgery? What is the complication that may result?
    a. Cardiac arrhythmias
    b. Blood pressure
    c. Bowel sounds
    d. Respiratory distress

68. Following repair of a thoracic aneurysm, the nurse monitors for and immediately reports:
    a. Shallow respirations and poor coughing.
    b. Increased drainage from the chest tubes.
    c. Sternal pain with coughing and deep breathing.
    d. Increased urinary output from the indwelling catheter.

69. In addition to hemorrhage, clients with repair of thoracic aneurysm are monitored for all of the following *except*:
    a. Cardiac dysrhythmias.
    b. Paraplegia.
    c. Respiratory distress.
    d. Renal failure.

70. Which of the following activities is allowed after discharge of the client who has had an aneurysm repair?
    a. Playing golf
    b. Washing dishes
    c. Raking leaves
    d. Swimming laps

71. On a separate sheet of paper, summarize the discharge teaching for a client with an abdominal aortic aneurysm (AAA) repair.

72. Which statement regarding aortic dissection is true?
    a. It is relatively uncommon in the United States.
    b. It occurs primarily in adults in their 50s and 60s.
    c. There is a high survival rate.
    d. Hypotension and atherosclerosis are the primary causes.

Case Study: The Client with Hypertension

Your client is a 64-year-old African-American man who is diagnosed with hypertension. He is 6 feet tall and weighs 300 pounds. He smokes 2 packs per day.

Answer the following questions on a separate sheet of paper:

1. What type of hypertension does he have? Give a rationale for your answer.

2. What diseases would have made this client at risk for developing secondary hypertension? What initial radiographic test would be performed to evaluate for secondary hypertension?

3. What cultural aspects need to be considered in controlling his hypertension?

4. How does this client's age impact the diagnosis and treatment of hypertension?

5. An interdisciplinary team consult was completed. What assessment findings would indicate successful outcomes have been met?

6. The dietitian working with this client suggests that he eat more of which of the following foods? Why should he not eat the other choices?
   a. Fresh fruits
   b. Canned soups
   c. Luncheon meats
   d. Frozen vegetables

This client was later seen in the emergency department with severe headache, extremely high blood pressure, dizziness, blurred vision, and disorientation.

7. His diagnosis is _____.
   Describe how to administer IV nitroprusside or oral nifedipine to him.

 ## Case Study: The Client with Thrombophlebitis and Pulmonary Embolus

A 58-year-old woman was discharged from the hospital 4 days ago after lower abdominal surgery. She has been readmitted for pain and edema in her right calf. She has a tentative diagnosis of thrombophlebitis.

Answer the following questions on a separate sheet of paper:

1. Discuss the probable etiology of this client's thrombophlebitis.

2. The physician prescribes heparin sodium 1000 units per hour intravenously for this client. Discuss the purpose of this medication, the nursing precautions, and laboratory tests to monitor its effectiveness.

3. How does heparin differ from warfarin in the treatment of thrombophlebitis?

4. This client is placed on strict bedrest with her legs elevated, and a warm, moist pack is to be applied. What are the purposes of these interventions?

5. The following morning, the client complains of leg cramps and asks the nurse to massage her calf because it is "cramping." Should the nurse comply with this request? Why or why not?

6. The client's activated partial thromboplastin prothrombin time is 51 seconds and prothrombin time is 11 seconds. Discuss the significance of these test results.

7. The client's laboratory values are now within therapeutic range, and the client is being discharged from the hospital on Coumadin. Develop a teaching-learning plan for this client.

STUDY GUIDE NUMBER 7.37

Interventions for Clients in Shock

Study/Review Questions

1. As the foundation for understanding the mechanism of shock, complete the following statement related to human physiology. The ability of the organs to deliver oxygen to the tissues is related to the

   _____.

2. Which three factors listed below directly affect mean arterial pressure?
   ____ a. Blood pressure
   ____ b. Total amount of blood in CV system
   ____ c. Heart rate (stroke volume = CO)
   ____ d. Vasodilation and vasoconstriction of arterial and venous systems
   ____ e. Heart rate

3. Which of the three factors identified in Question 2 directly correlates with the MAP when it increases or decreases?

4. Which of the three factors in Question 2 work the opposite of the MAP?

5. Which of the following statements about the control of blood flow is correct?
   a. The most influential factor is the regional control.
   b. The brain can independently control its own blood flow.
   c. The nervous system is the most important factor in blood flow.
   d. Blood flow in all organs is increased at the same rate.

6. During the later phases of shock, anaerobic metabolism causes the following to occur:
   a. _____
   b. _____
   c. _____

7. As a result of pathophysiologic changes, which of the following best describes shock?
   a. A disease state involving the heart, blood vessels, or blood
   b. Abnormal cellular metabolism caused by inadequate delivery of oxygen
   c. Physiologic changes in cardiac output
   d. Lack of oxygenation related to an increase in mean arterial pressure

8. Match the following hormones that are activated during shock with their effects. *More than one answer may apply to each hormone. Answers may be used more than once.*

   Hormones
   ____ a. Renin
   ____ b. Antidiuretic hormone (ADH)
   ____ c. Aldosterone
   ____ d. Epinephrine
   ____ e. Norepinephrine

   Effects of Hormones
   1. Sympathomimetics
   2. Conserves water
   3. Stimulates angiotensin

9. True or False? Read the following statements regarding shock and decide whether each is true or false. *Write* T *for true or* F *for false in the blanks provided. If the statement is false, correct the statement to make it true.*
   ____ a. Regardless of the cause, the pathophysiologic cellular response is the same for all types of shock.
   ____ b. When shock occurs, the body fails and death is the inevitable result.
   ____ c. The older adult and immunosuppressed clients are the only clients who are at risk for shock.
   ____ d. The most reliable indicator that would cause a nurse to suspect shock in a client is changes in the systolic blood pressure.
   ____ e. Anaphylactic shock is a result of an antigen-antibody reaction.
   ____ f. Respiratory failure is the usual cause of death with anaphylactic shock.

___ g. Endotoxins cause vascular changes in phase 1 septic shock that results in increased capillary permeability, decreased systemic resistance with increased cardiac output, clumping platelets, and inflammatory response, all resulting in tissue hypoxia.

___ h. Clinical manifestations of septic shock in phase 1 are difficult to diagnose.

___ i. Phase 2 of septic shock differs from phase 1 in that there is decreased cardiac output with exacerbation of the inflammatory response, decreased count, and decreased PAP.

___ j. Hemodynamic changes associated with cardiogenic shock are decreased cardiac output, decreased pulmonary artery pressure, increased systemic vascular resistance, and increased pulmonary capillary wedge pressure.

___ k. Oxygen administration is appropriate therapy for any type of shock.

___ l. Most clinical manifestations of shock are related to the body's compensatory response to shock and not the cause of shock.

10. The body's ability to initiate the compensatory response for the anaerobic metabolism and decreased MAP is stimulated by which of the following?
   a. Coronary arteries
   b. Carotid and aortic baroreceptors
   c. Respiratory center in the brain
   d. Parasympathetic nervous system

11. On a separate sheet of paper, identify clinical manifestations of shock as they relate to the various body systems.
   a. Cardiovascular manifestations:
   b. Respiratory manifestations:
   c. Neuromuscular manifestations:
   d. Renal manifestations:
   e. Integumentary manifestations:
   f. Gastrointestinal manifestations:

12. True or false? *Write T for true or F for false in the blank provided.*
   ___ Changes in systolic blood pressure are a reliable indicator of initial and nonprogressive stages of shock.

13. In the table below, summarize stages of shock according to the general MAP response, the related compensatory mechanism, and specific clinical manifestations.

14. The major pathophysiologic event in the refractory or irreversible stage is which of the following?
   a. Renal failure
   b. Cardiac failure
   c. Sympathetic nervous system failure
   d. Hormone failure

15. Which of the following is an early sign of shock?
   a. Cool, clammy skin
   b. Decreased urinary output
   c. Restlessness
   d. Hypotension

Stage of Shock	General Body Response, Compensatory Mechanism, and Clinical Manifestations
Initial/early stage	
Nonprogressive/ compensatory stage	
Progressive/ intermediate stage	
Refractory stage of shock/irreversible	

16. Match the overall pathophysiology response that occurs with various types of shock.

Types of Shock	General Pathophysiology Response
___ a. Hypovolemic	1. Indirect pump failure
___ b. Cardiogenic	2. Vascular tone/volume decreased
___ c. Distributive	3. Intravascular volume depleted
___ d. Obstructive	4. Direct pump failure

17. Match each of the following types of clients who may be at risk with the corresponding type of shock. *Answers may be used more than once.*

Types of Clients	Types of Shock
___ a. Client with cardiac tamponade	1. Hypovolemic
	2. Cardiogenic
___ b. Older adult with urinary tract infection	3. Distributive-neurogenic
	4. Obstructive
___ c. Client who recently received a vaccine	5. Distributive-neurogenic
	6. Distributive-septic
___ d. Client who had a myocardial infarction	
___ e. Client who had a ruptured aortic aneurysm	
___ f. Client with a bowel obstruction	
___ g. Client with insect bites	
___ h. Client with ruptured spleen resulting from trauma	
___ i. Client receiving chemotherapy	
___ j. Client with DVT, pulmonary emboli	
___ k. Client receiving heparin therapy	
___ l. Older adult who has a cerebrovascular accident	
___ m. Client with electrolyte imbalance and dehydration	
___ n. Client with diabetes insipidus	
___ o. Older adult with decubitus ulcers	
___ p. Client who has cancer of the head and neck, with a G tube	
___ q. Client with VRE or MRSA	
___ r. Client with congestive heart failure, receiving Lasix therapy	

18. Which of the following assessment findings is most indicative of the early phase of sepsis-induced distributive shock?
    a. Crackles in lung bases
    b. Bounding peripheral pulses
    c. Cool, clammy, and cyanotic skin
    d. Warm, pink, high cardiac output

19. A client has cardiac dysrhythmias and pulmonary problems as a result of receiving an IV antibiotic. What type of shock would this represent?
    a. Hypovolemic
    b. Cardiogenic
    c. Anaphylactic
    d. Septic

20. The most common cause of distributive (septic shock) is:
    a. Gram-negative bacteremia
    b. Gram-positive bacteremia
    c. Viral sepsis
    d. Fungal sepsis

21. The most common cause of hypovolemic shock is:
    a. Traumatic limb amputation.
    b. Ruptured esophageal varices.
    c. Wound dehiscence and evisceration.
    d. Deep lacerations and blunt trauma.

22. The most common cause of anaphylaxis is:
    a. Poisonous snake bites.
    b. Food reaction.
    c. A drug reaction.
    d. Human bites.

23. The most common cause of cardiogenic shock is:
    a. Heart failure.
    b. Myocardial infarction (MI).
    c. Valvular disease.
    d. Cardiac tamponade.

24. An assessment finding that is consistent with hypovolemic shock is:
    a. Pulse pressure of 40 mm Hg.
    b. A rapid, weak, and thready pulse.
    c. Cyanotic, cool extremities.
    d. Increased muscle strength.

25. A life-threatening pulmonary complication of shock is:
    a. Adult respiratory distress syndrome.
    b. Oxygen toxicity from free radicals.
    c. Status asthmaticus with bronchospasm.
    d. Alveolar collapse and altered perfusion.

26. Which of the following clients is at greatest risk for developing cardiogenic shock?
    a. Client with a 25% infarct of the right ventricle
    b. Client who experienced a first heart attack of the left atria
    c. Client with 40% damage to the left ventricle
    d. Client with an infarct of the posterior wall

27. The earliest assessment finding of the client with impending cardiogenic shock is:
    a. Crushing chest pain.
    b. Tachycardia.
    c. Severe hypotension.
    d. Altered mental status.

28. The priority for managing a client with cardiogenic shock is:
    a. Open heart surgery.
    b. Insertion of intra-aortic balloon pump.
    c. Administration of thromboembolic agents.
    d. Determination and treatment of the cause of the shock state.

29. Match either the colloid or crystalloid solution with each of the indications. *Answers will be used more than once.*

Indications	**Solutions**
___ a. Hemorrhagic shock	1. Colloid
___ b. Fluid replacement	2. Crystalloid
___ c. Septic shock	
___ d. Restore osmotic pressure	
___ e. Carries oxygen to peripheral tissues	
___ f. Does not cause allergic reactions	
___ g. Substitute for blood	

30. Ringer's lactate is a common crystalloid solution used in the treatment of shock. In addition to monitoring electrolyte levels, hemoglobin, and hematocrit, what else needs to be monitored with this solution?
    a. Glucose
    b. Liver function
    c. pH
    d. Magnesium

31. When crystalloid solutions are used to maintain adequate fluid and electrolyte balance during shock, the nurse must monitor the clients for:
    a. Allergic reaction.
    b. Peripheral edema.
    c. Renal failure.
    d. Decreased MAP.

32. Which of the following statements about colloids versus crystalloids is correct?
    a. Colloids are less expensive than crystalloids.
    b. Colloids are not as similar to fluids lost as are crystalloids.
    c. Colloids are less readily available than crystalloids.
    d. Colloids need to be administered less often than crystalloids.

33. Which of the following data indicate that a client is responding to treatment for shock?
    a. Blood pH of 7.28
    b. Arterial Po_2 of 65 mm Hg
    c. Distended neck veins
    d. Increased urinary output

34. Which of the following statements about drug therapy for hypovolemic shock is correct?
    a. Vasoconstricting agents stimulate venous return by increasing venous pooling of blood.
    b. Beta$_2$-adrenergic agents increase the contractile response of cardiac muscle cells.
    c. Digoxin (Lanoxin) prolongs ventricular filling time and stimulates the ventricle to contract.
    d. Sodium nitroprusside (Nitropress) dilates coronary blood vessels and causes systemic vasodilation.

35. The nurse's role includes prevention of shock by which of the following interventions?
    a. Frequently assessing vital signs, performing neurologic checks, and monitoring intake and output.
    b. Monitoring all clients at risk for shock.
    c. Instructing clients in lifestyle changes.
    d. Performing blood cultures.

36. Which of the following would not be part of a deficient knowledge teaching plan related to prevention of septic shock in at-risk clients?
    a. Frequent handwashing using antimicrobial soap.
    b. Report temperature over 101° F.
    c. Avoid large crowds or gatherings where people might be ill.
    d. Do not share utensils; wash toothbrush in dishwasher.

37. A 70-year-old man is admitted to the hospital with an infected finger of several days. He is lethargic, confused, and has a temperature of 101.3° F. Other assessment findings were BP of 94/50, HR 105, RR 40, and shallow breathing. Pulmonary arterial wedge pressure (PAWP) was 4 mm Hg. These assessment findings indicate what type of shock?
    a. Hypovolemic
    b. Cardiogenic
    c. Anaphylactic
    d. Septic shock

38. A postsurgical hospitalized client has a falling blood pressure; elevated, thready pulse; shallow respirations of 26; pale skin. The client is in what phase of shock?
    a. Compensatory/nonprogressive
    b. Refractory
    c. Progressive
    d. Multiple organ dysfunction

39. Assessment findings of a client with trauma injuries reveals cool pale skin, complaints of thirst, urine output 100 mm/8 hours, normal BP, HR 100, RR 24 with decreased breath sounds. This client is in what phase of shock?
    a. Compensatory/nonprogressive
    b. Progressive
    c. Refractory
    d. Multiple organ dysfunction

40. Drug therapy specific to distributive (septic) shock management includes:
    a. Inotropics.
    b. Antibiotics.
    c. Vasoconstrictors.
    d. Antidysrhythmics.

41. After discharge from the hospital, a common psychosocial problem faced by the client who has suffered from hypovolemic shock is:
    a. Anxiety about meal preparation.
    b. Fear of recurrence of shock or death.
    c. Inability to perform activities of daily living.
    d. Recognition of resultant limitations.

42. The prioritized treatment modalities for a client with hypovolemic shock include:
    a. _____
    b. _____
    c. _____
    d. _____

43. Identify treatment modalities for a client with septic shock.
    a. _____
    b. _____
    c. _____
    d. _____
    e. _____

44. When dopamine is administered 20 mcg/kg/min IV in the treatment of shock, the nurse will assess for:
    a. Decreased urine output, decreased blood pressure, and headache.
    b. Increased respiratory rate and increased urine output.
    c. Decreased cardiac output, chest pain, and hypertension.
    d. Bradycardia, hypertension, and headache.

45. As a result of administering Levophed, the nurse needs to monitor for:
    a. Decreased tissue perfusion.
    b. Profuse sweating.
    c. High output renal failure.
    d. Chest pain.

46. Which of the following is the best indicator of progressing shock?
    a. Elevated body temperature
    b. Absent peristalsis
    c. Decreasing urine output
    d. Vasodilation

47. A hospitalized client received an antibiotic and developed anaphylactic shock. Which of the following assessment findings indicates this type of shock?
    a. Cool skin, rapid heart rate, abdominal cramping, and changes in mental status
    b. Decreased heart rate, cyanosis, and bronchospasm
    c. Hypertension, distended neck veins, respiratory distress, and bounding pulses
    d. Bronchospasm, abdominal cramping, respiratory distress, and vasodilation

48. In the previous question, the nurse would be ready to administer which type of medication?
    a. Solu-Medrol
    b. Epinephrine
    c. Nebulizer treatment
    d. Atropine

49. A head injury client was treated for a cerebral hematoma. After surgery, this client is at risk for what type of shock?
    a. Anaphylactic
    b. Cardiogenic
    c. Hypovolemic
    d. Neurogenic

50. Identify three common nursing diagnoses associated with hypovolemic shock.
    a. _____
    b. _____
    c. _____

51. A factor that increases the older adult's risk for distributive (septic) shock is:
    a. Reduced skin integrity.
    b. Diuretic therapy.
    c. Cardiomyopathy.
    d. Musculoskeletal weakness.

52. The clinical manifestations in the first phase of sepsis-induced distributive shock results from the body's reaction to:
    a. Leukocytes.
    b. Endotoxins.
    c. Hemorrhage.
    d. Hypovolemia.

53. Identify nursing interventions for a client with hypovolemic shock.

54. Which of the following is typically given intravenously in the treatment of hypovolemic shock due to hemorrhage?
    a. Ringer's lactate
    b. Blood and blood products
    c. Normal saline
    d. D10 ½ NS

55. The nurse would assess which of the following when a client with sepsis is in the compensated stage of shock?
    a. Drop in blood pressure
    b. Dyspnea
    c. Tachycardia with a weak pulse
    d. Anuria

56. Identify the laboratory value that indicates the early stage of compensated shock.

57. True or False? Read the following statements regarding shock and decide whether each is true or false. *Write* T *for true or* F *for false in the blanks provided. If the statement is false, correct the statement to make it true.*
    ___ a. Hypovolemic shock occurs when there is a decrease in blood volume that causes the MAP to decrease, resulting in lack of tissue oxygenation.
    ___ b. Examples of external causes of hypovolemic shock are trauma, wounds, and surgery.
    ___ c. Dehydration, as a result of decreased fluid intake or increased in fluid loss, can cause hypovolemic shock.

    ___ d. Distributive shock is a result of a decrease in the MAP caused by a loss of sympathetic tone, blood vessel dilation, pooling of blood in venous and capillary beds, and increased blood vessel permeability (leak).
    ___ e. Sepsis leading to distributive shock occurs when microorganisms are present in the tissues.
    ___ f. The primary cause of anaphylactic shock is related to drug allergies.
    ___ g. Anaphylactic shock results from large amounts of histamines and other inflammatory substances being rapidly released throughout the circulatory system, causing massive blood vessel dilation and increased capillary permeability.
    ___ h. Age is *not* a concern as a risk factor in the development of sepsis.
    ___ i. During the hyperdynamic phase of septic shock, the endotoxins cause a decrease in cardiac output.
    ___ j. The clinical manifestations of the first phase of septic shock are unique, often opposite to other types of shock, and therefore misinterpreted by the health care provider as a shock state.

58. Death as a result of anaphylactic shock is the result of:
    a. Massive blood vessel permeability and myocardial infarction.
    b. Extreme body hypoxia related to edema, pulmonary obstruction, and inadequate circulation.
    c. Antihistamine and epinephrine release from the adrenal gland.
    d. Renal failure and alternations of blood pressure hormones.

59. Septic shock is the result of: _____
    _____.

60. The goals of interventions for any type of shock are
    (a) _____, (b) _____
    _____, and
    (c) _____
    _____by administering and
    monitoring (d)_____,
    (e) _____, (f) _____,

61. Unlike other types of shock, septic shock has the following two phases: _____
    _____and _____
    _____.

62. The assessment findings of a client suspected of septic shock reveals lethargy, disorientation, tachycardia, changes in white blood cell count, and normal temperature. This client is in which phase of septic shock? Give a rationale for your answer.
    a. Hyperdynamic
    b. Hypodynamic

63. Which of the following is *not* related to the care of a client in septic shock?
    a. Elevate knees with the head flat or elevated 30 degrees
    b. Maintain urine output of at least 20 mL/hr
    c. Administer heparin in phase 2
    d. Provide oxygen therapy and monitor vital signs every 5 minutes until stable

64. Can shock be prevented? Discuss this question with your classmates and instructor.

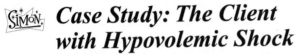

Case Study: The Client with Hypovolemic Shock

A 38-year-old female client returned to the postanesthesia recovery area 2 hours ago after undergoing a tubal ligation by colposcopy (through the back wall of the vagina behind the cervix). Her last documented vital signs, taken 30 minutes ago, were BP = 102/80, pulse = 88, and respirations = 22. You now note that her face is pale, and the skin around her lips has a bluish cast. Her vital signs are now BP = 90/76, pulse = 98, and respirations = 28.

Answer the following questions on a separate sheet of paper:

1. What additional assessment techniques would you perform?

2. Where would you look for the hemorrhage?

3. What other data would you gather?

4. When you reassess her in 15 minutes, you find the following vital signs: BP = 88/70, pulse = 102, and respirations = 30. She awakens when you shake her arm and complains of back pain and thirst. Given these findings, what are your priority actions?

5. What expected outcomes would be specific to this situation?

STUDY GUIDE NUMBER 7.38

Interventions for Critically Ill Clients with Coronary Artery Disease

Study/Review Questions

1. The leading cause of coronary artery disease (CAD) is:
   a. Aging.
   b. Atherosclerosis.
   c. Diabetes.
   d. Hypertension.

2. Which of the following statements best describes the pathophysiology regarding the leading cause of CAD as indicated in the previous question?
   a. There is a blockage of blood that supplies oxygen and nutrients to the cardiac cells.
   b. There is an accumulation of lipids in the intimal layer of the arteries that blocks the flow of blood.
   c. CAD is the result of ischemia and infarction of the myocardium.
   d. CAD occurs when there is an increase in demand of arterial blood flow with activity.

3. When CAD causes chest pain, the coronary artery usually is narrowed to at least:
   a. 60%.
   b. 70%.
   c. 80%.
   d. 90%.

4. Which of the following assessment findings is associated with calcium channel blocker therapy?
   a. Wheezes
   b. Hypotension
   c. Bradycardia
   d. Forgetfulness

Answer the following two questions on a separate sheet of paper.

5. In addition to atherosclerosis, indicate other common causes of a myocardial infarction.

6. Denial is a common reaction of clients with cardiovascular disease. What other reactions should a nurse assess for?

7. Which of the following statements about the heart's physiologic response to an infarction is correct?
   a. The infarcted area shows signs of inflammation after 24 hours.
   b. Neutrophils invade the areas to remove necrotic cells within 6 hours.
   c. Granulation tissue begins to form 8 to 10 days after infarction.
   d. Scar tissue remodeling resembles the original tissue in size and shape.

8. The location of a myocardial infarction (MI) associated with the highest mortality rate is which of the following, and why?
   a. Anterior wall
   b. Lateral wall
   c. Inferior wall
   d. Posterior wall

9. The ECG reading may indicate which of the following as a result of an anterior wall MI?
   a. Bradycardia
   b. PVCs
   c. PAT
   d. Second-degree heart block

10. What complication of an anterior-wall MI may result in an insertion of a pacemaker?
    a. Third-degree heart block
    b. PVCs
    c. Bradycardia
    d. Second-degree AV block

11. Which of the following clients is at greatest risk for having a fatal MI?
    a. A 36-year-old athletic man who smokes
    b. A 72-year-old woman who smokes and is obese
    c. A 24-year-old man with a family history of hypertension
    d. A 32-year-old woman with elevated serum cholesterol levels

12. Which of the following tests is diagnostic for myocardial damage caused by an MI?
    a. Positive chest x-ray
    b. Creatine kinase (CK) elevation
    c. ECG: ST depression, T-wave inversion, wide Q
    d. CK-MB isoenzymes elevation

13. An assessment finding that may indicate heart failure as a result of an MI is which of the following heart sounds?
    a. Murmur
    b. S_3
    c. S_4
    d. S_1, S_2

14. Which of the following regarding thrombolytic therapy is correct?
    a. Streptokinase is the drug of choice for all clients
    b. Monitor for bleeding —laboratory values, stool, urine, CVA, epistaxis
    c. Wait until 12 hours after onset of chest pain to administer medication
    d. Quick, easy to use by all health care providers, no allergic responses expected

15. A client who has been admitted for surgery with a history of angina reports to you, the nurse, symptoms of tightness or pressure in the chest radiating to the left arm. Your assessment also includes cool, clammy skin, BP 150/90, P 100, R 32. *Answer the following questions on a separate sheet of paper.*
    a. What is the priority nursing diagnosis?
    b. Based on the assessment findings, summarize the priority nursing interventions for this client.

16. Using the chart below, compare the following cardiac emergency drugs. *Use a separate sheet of paper for your answers.*

Drug	Action	Indications for Use	Side Effects/ Adverse Reactions	Nursing Implications
Lidocaine				
Epinephrine				
Atropine				
Dopamine				

17. Which of the following diagnostic tests is used to identify the client who may benefit from further invasive management after acute angina or an MI?
    a. Exercise tolerance test
    b. Cardiac catheterization
    c. Thallium scan
    d. Multigated angiogram (MUGA) scan

18. Which of the following statements indicates the client's understanding regarding the effects of angina on sexual activity?
    a. "I will not be able to resume the same level of physical exertion as I did before I had chest pain."
    b. "I will discuss alternative methods with my partner since I will no longer be able to have sexual activity."
    c. "I should stress myself to see if sexual activity is a problem."
    d. "I should take a nitroglycerin tablet just before I engage in sexual activity."

19. On a separate sheet of paper, identify subjective data that would be included in the nursing assessment of a client with CAD.

20. On a separate sheet of paper, identify objective data that would be included in the nursing assessment of a client with CAD.

21. What complication can occur as a result of necrosis of more than 40% of left ventricle failure?
    a. Hypovolemic shock
    b. Cardiogenic shock
    c. Valve regurgitation
    d. PVCs

Answer the following two questions on a separate sheet of paper.

22. Indicate your assessment findings for the complication indicated in Question 21.

23. What treatment modality would you expect for the complication in Question 21, and why?

24. Interventions for the clients with heart failure following an MI include:
    a. Administering digoxin (Lanoxin), 1.0 mg, as a loading dose and then daily.
    b. Infusing intravenous fluids to maintain a urinary output of 60 mL/hr.
    c. Titrating vasoactive drugs to maintain a sufficient cardiac output.
    d. Observing for such complications as hypertension, flushed hot skin, and agitation.

25. A client with angina who is scheduled for PTCA should also sign a consent for:
    a. Intra-aortic balloon pump.
    b. Coronary artery bypass graft (CABG).
    c. Cardiac catheterization.
    d. Carotid endarterectomy.

Answer the following two questions on a separate sheet of paper.

26. Identify the primary indications for CABG and give examples of clients who would be candidates for this surgery.

27. A client is not responding to drug therapy to improve tissue perfusion from cardiogenic shock and requires an intra-aortic balloon pump (IABP). Briefly describe IABP and when it is designed to inflate and deflate during systole and diastole.

28. A client with an inferior MI has a 30% chance of developing:
    a. Valve damage.
    b. Atrial fibrillation.
    c. Right ventricular infarction and failure.
    d. Left ventricular infarction and failure.

29. A client has experienced an MI that has resulted in left ventricular failure. On a separate sheet of paper, discuss the assessment findings and collaborative interventions for this client.

30. A post-MI client in phase I cardiac rehabilitation would perform which of the following activities?
    a. Range-of-motion exercises
    b. Modified weight training
    c. Brisk walking
    d. Jogging

31. An MI client has advanced to phase III cardiac rehabilitation. Which activity is indicated for this phase?
    a. Biking in the mountains
    b. Playing doubles in tennis
    c. Working out with weights at a spa
    d. Walking several miles three times a week

32. Identify at least three reasons for treating dysrhythmias.

    a. _____

    b. _____

    c. _____

33. Which of the following statements regarding nitroglycerin is *false*?

    a. Reduces venous return to the heart
    b. Increases coronary artery blood flow
    c. Reduces coronary artery spasm
    d. Increases heart rate and contractility

34. A client is prescribed nitroglycerin tablets. Which of the following should be included in the client education? *Check all that apply. Give a rationale as to why the other choices are wrong.*

    ___ a. If one tablet does not relieve the angina after 5 minutes, take two pills.
    ___ b. You can tell the pills are active when your tongue feels a tingling sensation.
    ___ c. Keep your nitroglycerin in your pocket with your other pills at all times.
    ___ d. The prescription should last you about 6 months before having it refilled.
    ___ e. If the pain doesn't go away, sit down and wait; the medication takes a while to take effect.
    ___ f. The medication causes the blood vessels to dilate or widen in order to let more blood flow to the heart.
    ___ g. It can cause a temporary headache or a flushed face.

35. Interventions for the hospitalized client who is being treated initially with antianginal agents include:

    a. Elevating the head of the bed to 45 degrees.
    b. Monitoring heart rate and rhythm by continuing ECG.
    c. Assisting with use of the bathroom or commode.
    d. Providing oxygen via intermittent positive pressure.

36. A client complains of chest pain that is unrelieved with nitroglycerin. The nurse should prepare to administer:

    a. A sedative IM.
    b. Morphine sulfate IV every 5 to 15 minutes.
    c. Haldol IV push.
    d. Chewable aspirin.

37. Compare and contrast the pain a client experiences with angina versus an infarction.

38. The most sensitive and reliable test for the diagnosis of an MI is:

    a. ECG.
    b. CK laboratory value.
    c. Client complaints.
    d. Cardiac catheterization.

39. A client is being evaluated for thrombolytic therapy. Contraindications for this procedure include which of the following? *Check all that apply.*

    ___ a. CVA within the last 6 months
    ___ b. Pregnancy
    ___ c. Surgery within the last 10 days
    ___ d. Major trauma in the last 3 months
    ___ e. Endocarditis
    ___ f. Pericarditis
    ___ g. DVT

Answer the following two questions on a separate sheet of paper.

40. Before having a CABG, a client is taking a beta blocker, digitalis, and a diuretic. What advice will the physician give to the client regarding these drugs?

41. Identify the complications for which the nurse should monitor in a postoperative client with CABG.

42. A problem that may result in the collapse of a vein graft is:

    a. Cardiac tamponade.
    b. Hypotension.
    c. Hypertension.
    d. Hypothermia.

43. The electrolyte that is closely monitored in a postoperative client with a CABG is:

    a. Sodium.
    b. Potassium.
    c. Chloride.
    d. Magnesium.

44. On a separate sheet of paper, identify how the fluids are regulated in the postoperative client with a CABG to avoid complications.

45. A postoperative client suddenly has an increase in mediastinal drainage, jugular vein distention, pulsus paradoxus, and equalizing PAWP and right atrial pressure. These are signs of which of the following? Indicate the nursing interventions for this problem.

    a. Severe postoperative pain
    b. Occlusion of the venous graft
    c. Cardiac tamponade
    d. Anxiety reaction

46. True or False? Read the following statements and decide whether each is true or false. *Write T for true or F for false in the blanks provided. If the statement is false, correct the statement to make it true.*
    ___ a. One-third of all clients with CABG develop dysrhythmias.
    ___ b. Sternal wound infections develop within 3 days after surgery.
    ___ c. Signs and symptoms of mediastinitis are fever, bogginess of wound, and increased WBCs.

Answer the following two questions on a separate sheet of paper.

47. Identify special considerations for the older adult with a CABG.

48. A client is being discharged from the hospital after a CABG. Indicate topics that would be covered in the discharge teaching for home care and provide an example of what is included for each topic.

49. The most significant risk factor for coronary artery disease (CAD) and one that should be modified to prevent CAD is:
    a. Smoking.
    b. Eating high-carbohydrate foods.
    c. Inactivity.
    d. Hypotension.

50. Develop a teaching plan for preventing CAD. *Use a separate sheet of paper for your answer.*

51. An over-the-counter medication that is often used by clients on a daily basis as a preventive measure for CAD is:
    a. Motrin.
    b. Aspirin.
    c. Tylenol.
    d. Caffeine.

52. A hospitalized client with a history of angina complains of chest pain. On a separate sheet of paper, summarize the nursing interventions for this client.

53. The client in the previous question is being discharged from the hospital. On a separate sheet of paper, tell what information you, as the nurse, would reinforce for this client with CAD.

54. True or False? A client is scheduled to receive a thrombolytic agent to dissolve thrombi in the coronary arteries. Which of the following statements are true regarding this intervention? *Write T for true or F for false in the blanks provided.*
    ___ a. Examples of agents are t-PA and streptokinase.
    ___ b. These agents are most effective when administered within the first 6 hours of the coronary event.
    ___ c. These agents are commonly used throughout the country.
    ___ d. It is indicated when a client has chest pain of duration greater than 1 hour and that is unrelieved by other medication.
    ___ e. The nurse must monitor for bleeding by assessing IV site, laboratory values, and neurologic status, and by observation.

55. A client has arrived at the open-heart surgical intensive care unit after surgery for a triple bypass graft. On a separate sheet of paper, indicate what your responsibilities as nurse would be for this client at this time.

56. Which of the following diagnostic tests is performed after angina or MI to determine ECG changes that are consistent with ischemia, to evaluate medical interventions, and to determine whether invasive intervention is necessary?
    a. Stress test
    b. ECG
    c. Cardiac catheterization
    d. Chest x-ray

57. Identify the common nursing diagnoses for clients with CAD.
    a. _____
    b. _____
    c. _____
    d. _____

58. What is the purpose of administering morphine sulfate IV to relieve chest pain?

59. What are signs of morphine toxicity?

60. After an MI, the drug that is prescribed within 48 hours to prevent the development of heart failure is:
    a. Calcium channel blockers.
    b. ACE inhibitors.
    c. Beta blockers.
    d. Digoxin.

61. When beta blockers are ineffective and the client continues to have chest pain, the drug of choice to enhance vasodilation is:
    a. Calcium channel blocker.
    b. Digoxin.
    c. ACE inhibitor.
    d. Dopamine.

62. After an inferior MI, the client is at risk for developing which of the following dysrhythmias?
    a. Bradycardia and second-degree heart block
    b. PVCs
    c. Third-degree heart block
    d. Bundle branch block

63. A relatively common complication after an MI is _____, and the most severe form of heart failure is _____.

64. When a client is hemodynamically stable, the client should show evidence of this by:
    a. _____
    b. _____
    c. _____
    d. _____
    e. _____

65. Clients with class I heart failure respond best to which of the following medications?
    a. Digoxin
    b. Beta blockers
    c. Calcium channel blockers
    d. Diuretics

66. A client with discrete, proximal, noncalcified lesions of two vessels is more than likely to benefit from which of the following procedures?
    a. PTCA
    b. Stress test
    c. IABP
    d. CPB

67. On a separate sheet of paper, identify the postprocedure care of a client receiving PTCA.

68. Treatment of hypothermia, a common problem after CABG surgery, with warming blankets is necessary because this condition can cause the client to be at risk for:
    a. Hypotension.
    b. Hypertension.
    c. Heart failure.
    d. Loss of consciousness.

69. True or False? Which of the following statements are true regarding the level of consciousness for a client with CABG? *Write* T *for true or* F *for false in the blanks provided.*
    ____ a. It can be transient or permanent.
    ____ b. Permanent deficits may be associated with CVA.
    ____ c. Return to baseline usually occurs within 4 to 8 hours.
    ____ d. 75% of clients experience some form of transient mental status changes.
    ____ e. Signs and symptoms can include slowness of arousal, memory loss, and confusion.

70. Following a CABG, the nurse must be knowledgeable to monitor what areas in order to provide safe quality client care?
    a. _____
    b. _____
    c. _____
    d. _____
    e. _____
    f. _____
    g. _____

Case Study: The Client with Angina

A 68-year-old woman arrives in the emergency department stating, "I think I had a heart attack." She states that she had an episode of chest pain that lasted a couple of minutes during her daily 3-mile walk; the pain was relieved by rest. ECG rhythm is normal sinus rhythm. No abnormal heart sounds or laboratory values. VS are stable. No O_2 needed. She is diagnosed with angina.

Answer the following questions on a separate sheet of paper:

1. How would this client's clinical manifestations be different if she had had an MI?

2. What laboratory test confirmed a diagnosis of angina?

3. How would you explain to the client the diagnosis of angina?

4. What teaching would you provide for this client regarding her diagnosis of angina?

The client is seen by a cardiologist who prescribed nitroglycerin tablets, procardia, and one baby aspirin per day. In the next few months, the client returns to the cardiologist with additional complaints regarding her chest pain. A cardiac catheterization revealed the following results: 50% blockage of the circumflex artery, 60% blockage of the anterior descending (LAD), and 90% blockage of the right coronary artery.

5. What instructions should this client have received regarding managing her chest pain at home?

6. On this client's return appointment, indicate the assessment findings that would have clued in the cardiologist that her angina is now unstable.

7. This client is a 68-year-old woman. Describe the relationship between older adults, particularly older women, and heart disease.

8. Procardia was prescribed for this client. Identify the drug classification of this medication and the pertinent information that a client needs to know about it.

 ## Case Study: The Client with Coronary Artery Disease

Your client is a 40-year-old African-American man with a history of CAD. He smokes one pack of cigarettes per day. He is 5' 8" tall and weights 250 pounds. He takes Procardia for his hypertension. His last serum cholesterol was 220 mg/dL, with the HDL greater than 40. His father died of an MI at age 54 and his mother has hypertension. He works 50 hours a week as a lawyer and exercises 1 day a week on weekends.

Answer the following questions on a separate sheet of paper:

1. What are this client's modifiable risks for CAD? What are his nonmodifiable risks for CAD?

2. What client education would you provide for this client?

3. Explain to this client his risk factors for developing CAD.

UNIT 8 PROBLEMS OF TISSUE PERFUSION: HEMATOLOGIC SYSTEM ■ Core Concepts Grid

Anatomy	Physiology	Pathophysiology	History	Physical Exam	Diagnostic Tests	Interventions	Pharmacology
• Blood cells • Plasma • Lymph system • Bone marrow	• Oxygen transport • Hematopoesis • Phagocytosis • Blood-clotting mechanism	• Hemolysis • Insufficient production • Hyperproduction • Active loss • Defective cells • Hypoxia • Hypoxemia	• History of bleeding • Fatigue • Bruising • Weakness • Weight loss • Behavioral changes • Anorexia	• Bruising • Pallor • Tachycardia • Tachypnea • Hypotension • Pain • Swelling • Purpura • Infection • Decreased level of consciousness • Skin ulcers • Jaundice • Glossitis • Paresthesias	• Hemoglobin • Hematocrit • Red blood cell count (RBC) • White blood cell count (WBC) • Platelet count • Erythrocyte sedimentation rate (ESR) • WBC differential • Prothrombin time (PT) • Partial thromboplastin time (PTT) • Activated partial thromboplastic time (aPPT) • International Normalized Ratio (INR) • Bone marrow biopsy • Iron	• Blood transfusions • Phlebotomy • Radiation • Chemotherapy • Diet modification • Pain control • Fluids (oral and parenteral) • Bone marrow transplantation • Bleeding precautions • Energy conservation • Health teaching	• Iron supplements • Chemotherapy • Anticoagulants • Opioids • Antivirals • Antifungals • Antibiotics

Unit 8 (Chapters 39-40)

Problems of Tissue Perfusion: Management of Clients with Problems of the Hematologic System

Learning Plan

Chapter 39: *Assessment of the Hematologic System*

Learning Outcomes	Learning Activities	Supplemental Resources
1. Describe hematologic changes associated with aging. 2. Explain the process of erythrocyte maturation. 3. Describe the role of platelet hemostasis. 4. Compare and contrast the structure and function of platelet plugs and fibrin clots. 5. Interpret blood cell counts and clotting tests to assess the client's hematologic status. 6. Compare and contrast the actions and uses of anticoagulants and thrombolytics. 7. Prioritize nursing care for the client after bone marrow aspiration.	1. Prior to completing the study guide exercises in this chapter, review the anatomy and physiology of the blood and blood components. 2. Review the **boldfaced** Key Terms and their definitions in Chapter 39 to enhance your understanding of the content. 3. Go the Study Guide Number 8.39 on the following pages and complete the learning exercises for this chapter.	1. Textbook—Chapter 39 2. Other resources: • Any anatomy and physiology textbook • Any laboratory resource book • Any physical assessment textbook • Bennett, J., DiMichele, D., & Haire, W. (1998). Clotting and bleeding: A new understanding. *Patient Care, 32*(11), 87-88. • Beutler, E., Lichtman, M., Coller, B., & Kipps, T. (1995). *William's hematology* (5th ed.). New York: McGraw-Hill. • Oertel, L. (1999). Monitoring warfarin therapy: How the INR keeps your patient safe. *Nursing 99, 29*(11), 41-45. • United States Pharmacopeial Convention, Inc. (2000). Volume I: *Drug information for the health care professional* (20th ed.). Englewood, CO: Micromedix. • Workman, M. (1998). The lymphoid system and its role in maintaining immunocompetence. *Seminars in Oncology Nursing, 14*(4), 248-255.

Chapter 40: *Interventions for Clients with Hematologic Problems*

Learning Outcomes	Learning Activities	Supplemental Resources
1. Identify three clinical manifestations common to clients who have any type of anemia. 2. Explain the pattern of inheritance for sickle cell disease. 3. Prioritize nursing care needs for the client who has sickle cell disease. 4. Plan a diet for a client who has iron deficiency anemia or vitamin B_{12} deficiency anemia. 5. Explain the mechanism of action and potential side effects of epoetin alpha therapy. 6. Compare and contrast the pathologic mechanisms of hemolytic anemia versus aplastic anemia. 7. Compare and contrast leukemia and lymphoma for etiology, pathophysiology, and clinical manifestations. 8. List four risk factors for the development of leukemia. 9. Analyze laboratory data and clinical manifestations to determine the presence of infection in a client who has neutropenia. 10. Compare the purposes and scheduling of induction therapy, consolidation therapy, and maintenance therapy for leukemia. 11. Prioritize nursing interventions for the client with neutropenia. 12. Prioritize nursing interventions for the client with thrombocytopenia. 13. Develop a teaching plan for a client with thrombocytopenia who is at home. 14. Prioritize nursing responsibilities during transfusion therapy. 15. Identify clients at risk for complications of transfusion therapy.	1. Prior to completing the study guide exercises in this chapter, review the following: • Anatomy and physiology of the blood and blood products • Normal lab values for red and white cells • Principles of inflammation and infection • Function of vitamins • Principles of good nutrition 2. Review the **boldfaced** Key Terms and their definitions in Chapter 40 to enhance your understanding of the content. 3. Go to Study Guide Number 8.40 on the following pages to complete the learning exercises for this chapter.	1. Textbook—Chapter 39 (Assessment of the Hematologic System) 2. Textbook—Chapter 40 3. Other resources: • Alcoser, P.W. & Burchett, S. (1999). Bone marrow transplantation: Immune system suppression and reconstitution, *AJN, 99*(6), 26-32. • American Cancer Society (2000). *Cancer facts and figures 2000. 300M No. 5008.00.* Atlanta, GA: Author. • Any anatomy and physiology textbook • Any physical assessment textbook • Cella, D. & Bron, D. (1999). The effect of epoetin alfa on quality of life in anemic cancer patients. *Cancer Practice, 7*(4), 177-182. • Chielens, D. (1999). Chronic myelogenous leukemia. In C. Miaskowski & P. Buchsel (Eds.). *Oncolgy nursing: Assessment and clinical care* (pp. 1239-1250). St. Louis: Mosby. • Cotran, R., Kumer, V., & Robbins S. (1999). *Robbins pathologic basis of disease* (6th ed.). Philadelphia: W.B. Saunders. • Dietz, K. (1999). Acute leukemia. In C. Miaskowski & P. Buchsel (Eds.). *Oncology nursing: Assessment and clinical care* (pp.1223-1237). St. Louis: Mosby. • Gorman, K. (1999). Sickle cell disease: Do you doubt your patient's pain? *AJN 99*(3), 38-44. • Harrahill, M. & Deloughery, T. (1998). Transfusion and blood component therapy: Key facts. *Journal of Emergency Nursing, 24*(4), 368-370. • Ligda, D.S. (1998). Hemophilia case management. *The Journal of Case Management, 4*(3), 12-24. • McBrien, N.J. (1997). Thrombotic thrombocytopenia purpura. *American Journal of Nursing, 97*(2), 28-29.

STUDY GUIDE NUMBER 8.39

Assessment of the Hematologic System

Study/Review Questions

1. The hematologic system is concerned with blood formation and storage. Identify the parts that compose the system.

Answer Questions 2 through 9 on a separate sheet of paper.

2. Define the following terms and abbreviations:
   Hematopoietic
   RBC
   Erythrocytes
   WBC
   Leukocytes
   Stem cells
   Erythropoietin
   Oxygen dissociation
   Hypoxia
   Aggregation
   Macrocytic
   Microcytic
   Hypochromic

3. Identify the hematopoietic organ that is also involved in the immune response.

4. Identify the types of cells produced in the bone marrow.

5. Describe the formation of blood components from fetus to adulthood.

6. Explain how the bone marrow produces blood cells. *Refer to Figure 39-1 in the textbook.*

7. Plasma is the extracellular fluid of the body and carries three to four times the amount of protein in interstitial fluid. Identify the three types of plasma protein and their functions.

8. Describe the RBC and its special features and give the normal range for RBCs.

9. Describe the formation of RBCs. *Use Figures 39-1 and 39-2 in the textbook.*

10. An RBC life span is 120 days; destruction is done by:
    a. Macrophages and the spleen.
    b. A cooperative effort of macrophages, spleen, and liver.
    c. A cooperative effort of WBCs, spleen, and liver.
    d. A cooperative effort of RBCs, spleen, and liver.

Answer the following four questions on a separate sheet of paper.

11. Identify the parts that must be present in the RBC to transport oxygen.

12. The RBC has other functions besides carrying oxygen; identify these.

13. Identify the body organ that controls RBC production and destruction. Describe how it determines the need for production or destruction of RBCs.

14. Identify the seven substances needed to form RBCs and hemoglobin.

15. If any of the above substances are missing from your client's diet, he or she will develop _____ _____.

16. In the formation of platelets, the megakaryocyte:
    a. Is a part of the formation of any cell type.
    b. Breaks into pieces called platelets.
    c. Is necessary for RBC formation.
    d. Does not release platelets.

17. On a separate sheet of paper, describe the functions of a platelet in the body.

18. Platelet production is stimulated by _____.

Answer Questions 19 through 24 on a separate sheet of paper.

19. Describe the life activities of a platelet.

20. Describe the three tissues of the spleen and their functions.

21. Identify the four functions of the spleen.

22. The liver plays an important part in the hematologic process. Identify its functions and relationship to vitamin K.

23. Describe homeostasis.

24. Identify the three-step process of blood clotting.

25. Platelets normally do not stick together until stimulated to _____ .

26. When stimulated to aggregate, the platelets form a _____ .

27. True or False? *Write* T *for true or* F *for false in the blank provided.*
    ____ A platelet plug can form a clot.

Answer the following three questions on a separate sheet of paper.

28. Once a platelet plug is formed, the cascade reaction starts. Explain cascade reaction.

29. Identify the intrinsic events that stimulate platelet aggregation.

30. Review Table 39-2 in the textbook, and identify the clotting factors and cofactors for forming fibrin.

31. Platelets aggregate in response to extrinsic factors that can be described as:
    a. Trauma.
    b. Bacteria.
    c. WBCs.
    d. Antibody-antigen reactions.

Answer the following three questions on a separate sheet of paper.

32. Identify the two specific clotting factors on which the formation of a platelet plug is dependent.

33. Describe the sequence that clotting factors, inactive proteins, result in activating fibrinogen into fibrin. *Use Table 39-2 in the textbook.*

34. Using Figure 39-5 in the textbook, describe fibrin and its role in clot formation.

35. After the fibrin mesh is formed, then:
    a. More platelets and cells stick to the mesh, clotting factor XIII stabilizes it, and the mesh is sealed with serum.
    b. Clotting factor XIII stabilizes it; more platelets, blood cells, and protein form a clot; and it is sealed with serum.
    c. Serum seals it with clotting factor XIII to stabilize it and more platelets and blood cells and protein form a clot.
    d. Heparin is mobilized, clotting factor XIII encircles it, and protein binds to the mesh.

36. On a separate sheet of paper, compare and contrast the structure and function of the platelet plug and fibrin clots.

37. To maintain control of blood flow in the body during formation of the clotting cascade, the body relies on _____ .

Answer the following five questions on a separate sheet of paper.

38. Describe the breakdown of plasminogen into plasmin, and identify what the enzyme digests to break down a fibrin clot. *See Figure 39-6 in the textbook.*

39. Identify the eight changes in the hematologic system in older adults. Review Chart 39-1 in the textbook to learn how to identify some of these changes upon physical assessment of an older adult.

40. Describe how anticoagulants exert their effect on the blood-clotting cascade and identify the categories.

41. Describe the action of thrombolytic agents and identify the four agents used most commonly.

42. Identify the four conditions for which thrombolytic therapy is used.

43. Clots older than 6 hours are *not* recommended for thrombolytic therapy because of:
    a. Cost.
    b. Anoxic tissue.
    c. Large size of clot.
    d. Too many clots.

44. Thrombolytic therapy is *not* used for deep vein thrombosis or massive pulmonary emboli because:
    a. These conditions involve very large clots.
    b. Massive dosing is risky.
    c. It is possible that large-size particles will break off and cause other occlusions.
    d. The cost and length of treatment.

45. When the nurse is taking a history from a client with a clot, it is important that he or she question the client about:
    a. Any chemical exposures or liver function problems.
    b. Bleeding disorders of self and family (hemophilia, sickle cell trait).
    c. Medications, including over-the-counter drugs, antibiotics, and anticoagulants.
    d. Any radiation therapy received.

46. Having the client give the nurse a detailed record of food eaten in 1 week will allow her to assess the client's dietary pattern for _____.

Answer the following three questions on a separate sheet of paper.

47. Identify the major way that alcohol consumption can affect the hematologic system.

48. A person subsisting on a low income may have a diet deficient in what dietary nutrients?

49. When performing a physical assessment, the nurse should question women about their menorrhagia. What questions would the nurse ask to get an estimate and pattern of menorrhagia?

50. The main symptom of anemia is _____.

Answer the following four questions on a separate sheet of paper.

51. Identify five additional symptoms of anemia.

52. Identify sites the nurse would check to assess for pallor and jaundice.

53. Describe the differences between petechiae and ecchymoses.

54. Describe the different looks of the tongue in pernicious anemia, iron deficiency anemia, and nutritional deficiencies.

55. In performing a client examination, the nurse would assess a urine specimen for _____.

56. When assessing the abdomen, the nurse would note the size of the _____ and _____.

Answer the following three questions on a separate sheet of paper.

57. Identify the types of neurologic impairment that can occur with vitamin B_{12} deficiency.

58. Identify the parts of a complete blood count.

59. Describe the difference in mean corpuscular valve being elevated or decreased and the effect on body.

60. An elevated neutrophil count without an accompanying elevation in leukocyte alkaline phosphate is indicative of _____.

Answer the following five questions on a separate sheet of paper.

61. Demonstrate on a classmate a capillary fragility test. Count the petechiae.

62. Identify the drugs monitored by PT levels and state at what level they should be to be therapeutic.

63. International normalized ratio (INR) also is used to monitor warfarin therapy. State the therapeutic range.

64. Heparin is monitored by PTT; state the desirable range.

65. State the missing factors that are produced in the liver that can extend a PTT.

66. Platelet agglutination/aggregation is impaired in _____ disease.

67. True or False? *Write T for true or F for false in the blank provided.*
    ____ Radioisotope imaging can be used to evaluate iron storage sites in bone marrow.

68. On a separate sheet of paper, identify the difference between a bone marrow biopsy and bone marrow aspiration.

69. During a bone marrow biopsy or aspiration procedure, the client may feel the sensation of _____ and possibly even _____.

STUDY GUIDE NUMBER 8.40

Interventions for Clients with Hematologic Problems

Study/Review Questions

1. Red blood cells (RBCs) are the most abundant component of the blood; problems can arise from which of the following?
   a. Production
   b. Destruction
   c. Function
   d. All of the above

2. Anemia is a reduction in what components of the hematologic system?
   a. _____
   b. _____

3. Identify the types of anemia caused by deficiencies.
   a. _____
   b. _____
   c. _____
   d. _____

4. Identify which of the following descriptors relate to RBCs and which relate to sickle cells. *Write R for RBCs or S for sickle cells in the blanks provided.*
   ___ a. 20-day lifespan
   ___ b. 120-day lifespan
   ___ c. Destroyed in spleen
   ___ d. Chronically stimulated bone marrow
   ___ e. HbS
   ___ f. Clumps with hypoxia
   ___ g. May not be able to return to proper shape
   ___ h. Biconcave disk
   ___ i. HbA
   ___ j. Sickle-shaped and twisted

5. On a separate sheet of paper, describe the difference between sickle cell disease and sickle cell trait.

6. When counseling a client with sickle cell disease, the nurse would tell him or her that an offspring would:
   a. *Not* have sickle cell disease.
   b. Have sickle cell trait.
   c. *Not* have sickle cell trait.
   d. Have sickle cell disease.

7. The client with the sickle cell trait may: *Check all that apply.*
   ___ a. Have no problems.
   ___ b. Develop symptoms under stress.
   ___ c. Have problems but not recognize them as sickle cell disease.
   ___ d. Should not have children.

8. Identify six causes of a sickle cell crisis.
   a. _____
   b. _____
   c. _____
   d. _____
   e. _____
   f. _____

Answer the following three questions on a separate sheet of paper.

9. State the major problem of sickle cell disease crisis and describe how it is treated.

10. Identify an assessment finding in a client with sickle cell disease for each body system listed below:
    a. Cardiovascular
    b. Integumentary
    c. Abdominal
    d. Musculoskeletal
    e. Psychosocial

11. Identify four therapies that can be used for sickle cell disease in conjunction with opioids.

12. Clients with sickle cell disease are more susceptible to infections, specifically *Streptococcus pneumonia* and *Haemophilus influenzae,* which can be prevented with: *Check all that apply.*
    ___ a. Consistent good handwashing technique.
    ___ b. Yearly vaccination.
    ___ c. Twice daily oral penicillin.
    ___ d. NSAIDs

13. For a client with multiple organ dysfunction, the nurse will be giving:
    a. IV fluid up to 500 mL/hr.
    b. Oxygen with nebulization.
    c. Transfusions.
    d. Albumin.

14. Transfusions of RBCs are therapeutic except that:
    a. HbA levels are sustained as HbS levels are diluted.
    b. It suppresses erythropoiesis.
    c. It decreases menstrual flow in women.
    d. It decreases incidence of organ dysfunction and stroke.

15. How would the nurse explain the pattern of inheritance of sickle trait and disease to a female teenager affected with sickle cell disease?

Answer the following two questions on a separate sheet of paper.

16. Identify three clinical manifestations common to clients who have any type of anemia.

17. Plan a diet for a client with an iron deficiency anemia or vitamin B_{12} deficiency anemia.

18. Which of the following does *not* relate to polycythemia vera, an RBC cancer?
    a. Has the symptom of hypercellularity
    b. Plethoric appearance of the face
    c. Causes HTN and thrombosis
    d. Can be cured with anticoagulants

19. True or False? *Write T for true or F for false in the blank provided.*
    ____ To prolong the life of a client with polycythemia vera, periodic phlebotomy (two to five times per week) can help.

20. Polycythemia vera has many negative effects on the body. Besides HTN, there can be:
    a. Thrombosis of heart, spleen, or liver.
    b. Hyperkalemia and gout.
    c. Platelet dysfunction.
    d. Gout.

Answer the following four questions on a separate sheet of paper.

21. Identify the more intensive therapies for polycythemia vera.

22. Leukemia can be acute or chronic and affect the WBC. Identify and define the two categories.

23. Describe the pathophysiology of leukemia.

24. According to your text there are several categories of leukemia. Review these and identify a condition or substance that may be a risk factor for each category.

25. True or False? *Write T for true or F for false in the blank provided.*
    ____ Of the four types of leukemias, acute lymphocytic leukemia is most common in children.

26. Which of the following types of leukemia is most common?
    a. Chronic myelogenous leukemia
    b. Acute myelogenous leukemia
    c. Acute lymphocytic leukemia
    d. Chronic lymphocytic leukemia

27. When doing a physical assessment and interviewing a client, it is important to ask about: *Check all that apply.*
    ____ a. Any bleeding problems or prolonged bleeding from cuts.
    ____ b. Fatigue, lethargy, decreased attention span.
    ____ c. Any petechiae, pallor of the face, enlarged lymph nodes.

Answer the following three questions on a separate sheet of paper.

28. Explain what it means when bone marrow is full of blast phase cells.

29. Identify the common nursing diagnoses for an adult client with leukemia.

30. Define autocontamination and cross-contamination.

31. Match the types of therapy with their descriptions. *Answers may be used more than once.*

Descriptions	Types of Therapy
____ a. Aimed at achieving a rapid complete remission	1. Maintenance therapy
	2. Induction therapy
	3. Consolidation therapy
____ b. Prescribed orally, 3 to 5 years	
____ c. Intent to cure repeat of previous treatment therapy	
____ d. Has many side effects, including immunosuppression	

32. The dilemmas associated with leukemia and pregnancy include all of the following *except:*
    a. Chemotherapeutic drugs used in the first trimester can harm the fetus.
    b. Normal live births of babies occur to mothers treated after the first trimester.
    c. Side effects of the drugs are the same regardless of when during the pregnancy they are taken.
    d. Nursing care includes prevention of premature birth and psychosocial support.

33. Drugs used for prophylaxis in the client with leukopenia include: *Check all that apply.*
    ___ a. Antibiotics.
    ___ b. Antifungal-vaginal creams.
    ___ c. Antiviral agents.
    ___ d. Analgesics.

34. On a separate sheet of paper, describe each of the following types of protection that can be provided to a client with leukopenia.
    a. Protective (reverse) isolation
    b. Cross-contamination prevention
    c. Minimal bacteria diet
    d. (HEPA) filtration system

35. Bone marrow transplants are now done during which stage of therapy? *Check all that apply.*
    ___ a. Induction therapy
    ___ b. Consolidation therapy
    ___ c. Maintenance therapy
    ___ d. Therapeutic therapy

36. True or False? *Write T for true or F for false in the blank provided.*
    ___ The aim of bone marrow or stem cell transplantation is to rid the client of all leukemic cells.

37. Along with chemotherapy, the client with leukemia is given:
    a. Antibiotics.
    b. Radiation.
    c. Antivirals.
    d. Analgesics.

38. Match each type of transplant to the source of transplant tissue.

Source	**Type of Transplant**
___ a. From a sibling or HLA match	1. Allogeneic
___ b. From a twin	2. Autologous
___ c. From own stem cells	3. Syngeneic

39. Identify the five phases of transplant procedures.

40. True or False? *Write T for true or F for false in the blank provided.*
    ___ Donor marrow in the amount of 100 to 500 mL is aspirated in the operating suite and processed and immediately given to the client.

41. Donors need to have the aspiration sites monitored and also need:
    a. Fluid for hydration.
    b. Pain management.
    c. Possible RBC infusion.
    d. Psychological counseling.

42. Peripheral blood stems are obtained by pheresis during which stage?
    a. Collection
    b. Reinfusion
    c. Mobilization
    d. Plasmolysis

Answer the following two questions on a separate sheet of paper.

43. Define mobilization.

44. Identify the common complications of pheresis.

True or False? *Write T for true or F for false in the blanks provided.*

___ 45. Conditioning in a bone marrow transplant client makes him or her more violently ill with side effects; late effects can still occur 3 to 10 years post-transplant.

___ 46. The bone marrow transplant is administered as with usual IV fluids over 30 minutes.

47. The nurse should expect and treat all of the following symptoms in a transplant patient *except:*
    a. Fever.
    b. Hypertension.
    c. Premedication.
    d. Red urine.

48. Engraftment is the settling in of stem cells and the beginning of producing new cells. The success of this procedure is not known until:
    a. 8 to 12 hours after infusion.
    b. 8 to 12 days after infusion.
    c. 12 to 28 days after infusion.
    d. *b* or *c*

Answer the following two questions on a separate sheet of paper.

49. Identify the reasons for possible failure of an engraft.

50. Describe graft-versus-host disease (GVHD) and common areas of damage.

51. True or False? *Write* T *for true or* F *for false in the blank provided.*
    ___ The presence of GVHD is a positive sign for the bone marrow transplant client.

52. The client with veno-occlusive disease (VOD) can expect:
    a. Aggressive treatment.
    b. Surgical intervention.
    c. Supportive treatment.
    d. End-of-life care.

53. Early detection enhances the chance of survival for a patient with veno-occlusive disease (VOD). The nurse would monitor this client:
    a. The same as any other client.
    b. The same as a client with hepatic problems.
    c. While he or she is in isolation.
    d. While he or she is on bedrest.

Answer the following three questions on a separate sheet of paper.

54. Explain *nadir.*

55. Referring to Charts 40-10 and 40-11 in the textbook, describe the interventions for bleeding precautions.

56. When would the nurse start to administer a thrombopoietic?

57. True or False? *Write* T *for true or* F *for false in the blank provided.*
    ___ Leukemic cells tend to have a higher metabolism rate and a greater utilization of oxygen.

Answer the following three questions on a separate sheet of paper.

58. Explain the mechanism of action and the potential side effects of epoetin alpha therapy.

59. Identify the needs of a post–marrow transplant client being discharged home.

60. Compare and contrast leukemia and lymphoma in regard to etiology, pathophysiology, and clinical manifestations.

61. Match each descriptor, symptom, or treatment with the corresponding disease.

Descriptor, Symptom, or Treatment	Disease
___ a. White males over 50	1. Non-Hodgkin's lymphoma
___ b. Sixth most common cause of cancer death	2. Hodgkin's lymphoma
___ c. Mid-to-late twenties; men over 50 years	
___ d. Viral infections and exposure to alkylating chemical agents	
___ e. Twelve subtypes	
___ f. Reed-Sternberg cell	
___ g. Enlarged painless lymph node or nodes	
___ h. Prognosis best in women	
___ i. Stages I and II: treat with radiation; add chemotherapy for more extensive disease	
___ j. Permanent sterility of males	
___ k. Originate from any organ or tissue	
___ l. Follow-up for reoccurrence	

Answer the following two questions on a separate sheet of paper.

62. Prioritize nursing care for the client with thrombocytopenia.

63. Develop a teaching plan for a client who is at home and has thrombocytopenia.

64. Identify which of the following applies to autoimmune thrombolytic purpura (ATP) and which applies to thrombotic thrombocytopenic purpura (TTP). *Write* ATP *for autoimmune thrombolytic purpura or* TTP *for thrombotic thrombocytopenic purpura in the blanks provided.*
    ___ a. Was idiopathic
    ___ b. Platelets clump
    ___ c. Antibodies directed against own platelets
    ___ d. Inappropriate aggregation of platelets
    ___ e. Women aged 20 to 40 years
    ___ f. Preexisting autoimmune condition
    ___ g. Plasma pheresis
    ___ h. Immunosuppressive therapy to reduce intensity
    ___ i. Corticosteroids and azathioprine

65. Coagulation disorders or bleeding disorders can result from all of the following *except*:
    a. Inability to produce a specific clotting factor.
    b. Excess cells in the peripheral blood supply.
    c. Production of insufficient quantities of clotting factor.
    d. Production of a less active form of clotting factor.

66. Common congenital disorders that result in defects of the clotting factor include all but:
    a. Reed-Sternberg disease.
    b. Hemophilia A.
    c. Hemophilia B.
    d. von Willebrand's disease.

67. Disseminated intravascular coagulation (DIC) is an acquired clotting disorder closely related to:
    a. Hemophilia.
    b. Septic shock.
    c. von Willebrand's disease.
    d. Leukemia.

68. Hemophilia A is considered classic hemophilia; hemophilia B is called:
    a. Easter disease.
    b. Christmas disease.
    c. Advent disease.
    d. Hallow disease.

69. The genetic transmission of the X-linked recessive genes of hemophilia is transferred:
    a. From the mother to all of her daughters and sons.
    b. From the mother to all of her sons.
    c. Such that the mother transmits gene trait to half of her daughters and disease trait to half of the sons.
    d. Such that all sons will inherit disease from mother.

70. The clinical characteristics of hemophilia A and hemophilia B are alike *except* that:
    a. Hemophilia A is deficient in factor VIII.
    b. Hemophilia B is deficient in factor IX.
    c. Hemophilia B is deficient in factor X.
    d. *a and b*

True or False? *Write* T *for true or* F *for false in the blanks provided.*

71. ___ Clients who have hemophilia are able to form platelet plugs at the bleeding site when injured.

72. ___ In clients with hemophilia, the missing clotting factor impairs the ability to form a fibrin clot.

73. Common history of the client with hemophilia is: *Check all that apply.*
    ___ a. Excessive hemorrhage from minor cuts.
    ___ b. Joint and muscle hemorrhages.
    ___ c. Easily bruised.
    ___ d. Potential for postoperative hemorrhage.

74. The laboratory tests for a client with hemophilia will include all of the following *except:*
    a. Normal range.
    b. Prolonged partial thromboplastin.
    c. Normal prothrombin time.
    d. Normal bleeding time.

Answer the following two questions on a separate sheet of paper.

75. What two therapies are used for the client with hemophilia A to control bleeding?

76. What is the most common health problem of the client with hemophilia?

77. Nursing actions performed during transfusion of a client are aimed at: *Check all that apply.*
    ___ a. Documentation.
    ___ b. Prevention of adverse transfusion reaction.
    ___ c. Early recognition of adverse transfusion reaction.

78. What are the necessary components of a physician's order for transfusion therapy? *Use a separate sheet of paper for your answer.*

79. True or False? *Write* T *for true or* F *for false in the blank provided.*
    ___ A separate consent form is signed for the administration of a blood transfusion.

80. On a separate sheet of paper, explain the reason for typing and crossmatching blood.

81. When administering a blood transfusion, be sure to use a:
    a. 22-gauge needle.
    b. 20-gauge needle.
    c. 19-gauge needle or larger.
    d. Butterfly needle.

82. True or False? *Write* T *for true or* F *for false in the blank provided.*
    ___ A blood filter is required for a transfusion and a new filter is used with each new bag.

83. The protocol for giving blood calls for the use of what solution with the blood?
    a. Ringers lactate
    b. Saline
    c. Dextrose in water
    d. Dextrose in saline

84. Solutions that are contraindicated when giving blood:
   a. Cause hemolysis of blood cells.
   b. Dilute the cells.
   c. Shrink the blood cells.
   d. Cause blood cells to swell.

True or False? Write T for true or F for false in the blanks provided.

___ 85. It is acceptable to add medications to blood products.

___ 86. When a blood transfusion is given, usual protocol includes two nurses verifying the physician's order.

87. Any severe reactions from a blood transfusion usually occur within the first:
   a. 15 minutes.
   b. 50 mL of blood.
   c. Hour.
   d. 100 mL of blood.

88. Vital signs for the client receiving a transfusion should be checked:
   a. Every 15 minutes throughout the transfusion.
   b. Every 15 minutes times 2, and then every hour throughout the infusion.
   c. Every 15 minutes times 4, and then every hour throughout the infusion.
   d. Every 15 minutes times 2, and then every 2 hours throughout the infusion.

True or False? Write T for true or F for false in the blanks provided.

___ 89. Other blood components without RBCs require the same protocol as blood.

___ 90. A blood transfusion is a transplantation of tissue from one person to another.

Answer the following two questions on a separate sheet of paper.

91. Identify the blood types and their antigen.

92. Explain the mechanism of the Rh antigen system and state who can receive Rh+ blood.

93. The treatment for possible sensitization to Rh+ during a pregnancy and giving birth is given by administering _____.

94. Platelets are given quickly with a special filter and short tubing. On a separate sheet of paper, explain why.

95. The client may be premedicated to prevent reaction with:
   a. Demerol.
   b. Hydrocortisone.
   c. Benadryl.
   d. *a and b*

True or False? Write T for true or F for false in the blanks provided.

___ 96. If a client is receiving amphotericin B, the infusion should be stopped because it is not compatible with blood components.

___ 97. Fresh frozen plasma is infused immediately after thawing to be sure it has viable clotting factor.

98. On a separate sheet of paper, identify different reactions a client can have to a blood transfusion; identify the clinical signs of hemolytic transfusion reaction.

99. True or False? *Write T for true or F for false in the blank provided.*
   ___ An allergic reaction can happen up to 24 hours after the infusion, and the nurse must be aware of complaints of urticaria, itching, bronchospasm, and occasionally anaphylaxis.

100. On a separate sheet of paper, identify the symptoms of and care to be provided for a client who has a reaction to a febrile transfusion.

101. A client experiencing bacterial transfusion reaction needs to be treated for:
   a. Allergic reaction.
   b. Anaphylaxis.
   c. Septic shock.
   d. Infection only.

Answer the following two questions on a separate sheet of paper.

102. Identify the symptoms of circulatory overload and who is most at risk for this.

103. Describe transfusion-associated graft-versus-host disease.

104. Characteristics of TA-GVHD can:
   a. Indicate host and donor share similar human leukocyte antigens.
   b. Be evident within 1 to 2 weeks.
   c. Have a 90% mortality rate.
   d. All of the above

105. True or False? *Write* T *for true or* F *for false in the blank provided.*
     ___ TA-GVHD can be prevented by administering irradiated blood products.

Answer the following question on a separate sheet of paper.

106. a. Identify the advantages of autologous blood transfusion.
     b. Identify the types of autologous blood transfusion.
     c. Explain intraoperative and postoperative autologous infusions and when they are used.

UNIT 9 PROBLEMS OF MOBILITY, SENSATION, AND COGNITION: NERVOUS SYSTEM ■ Core Concepts Grid

Anatomy	Physiology	Pathophysiology	History	Physical Exam	Diagnostic Tests	Interventions	Pharmacology

• **Central system**
 Brain
   Cerebrum
   Cerebellum
   Limbic
    system
   Brainstem
   Reticular
    activating
    system
    (RAS)
 Spinal cord
 Meninges
 Ventricles
 Sensory
   pathways
 Motor
   pathways
 Reflex arcs
 • **Peripheral system**
 Cranial nerves
 Autonomic
   nervous
   system
	• **Coordination**
	 Movement
	 Equilibrium
	 • **Regulation**
	 • **Mental activity**
	 Consciousness
	 Memory
	 Thinking
	 • **Nerve impulse**
	 Transmission
	 • **Sensation**
		• **Infection**
		 • **Inflammation**
		 • **Obstruction**
		 • **Seizure activity**
		 • **Paralysis**
		 • **Paresis**
		 • **Fasciculations**
		 • **Increased intracranial pressure (ICP)**
		 • **Bradykinesia**
		 • **Tremors**
		 • **Hemorrhage**
		 • **Ischemia**
		 • **Plaques and tangles**
		 • **Tumors**
			• **Past history of neurologic symptoms**
			 • **Past history of neurologic trauma, infections**
			 • **Family history**
			 Familial
			   neurologic
			   diseases
			 • **Social history**
			 Drugs
			 Occupation
			 Age
				• **Mental status**
				 General
				   appearance
				 Orientation
				 Mood/affect
				 Thought content
				 Intelligence
				 Recent/remote
				   memory
				 • **Cranial nerves**
				 • **Motor system**
				 Muscles
				 Balance
				 Coordinated
				   movement
				 • **Sensory system**
				 Light touch
				 Pain
				 Temperature
				 Vibration
				 Position
				 Recognition
				 • **Reflexes**
				 • **Other**
				 Romberg's test
				 Brudzinski's
				   sign
				 Kernig's sign
				 • **Functional assessment**
				 • **Speech and language ability**
					• **Radiologic**
					 Skull, spine
					 Computed
					   tomography
					   (CT)
					 • **Magnetic resonance imaging (MRI)**
					 • **Electroencephalogram (EEG)**
					 • **Lumbar puncture (LP)**
					 • **Cerebrospinal fluid**
					 • **Toxic drug levels**
						• **Environmental modification**
						 Quiet
						 Dim light
						 Padded rails
						 • **Bladder training**
						 • **Bowel training**
						 • **Positioning**
						 • **Nutrition**
						 • **Airway management**
						 • **Lifestyle modification**
						 • **Imunosuppressive therapy**
						 • **Intracranial pressure (ICP) monitoring**
						 • **Rehabilitation (physical and vocational)**
							• **Anticonvulsants**
							 • **Antispasmotics**
							 • **Dopaminergics**
							 • **Anticholinergics**
							 • **Dopamine agonists**
							 • **Anticholinesterases**
							 • **Antibiotics**
							 • **Cholinergics**

Unit 9 (Chapters 41–45)

Problems of Mobility, Sensation, and Cognition: Management of Clients with Problems of the Nervous System

Learning Plan

Chapter 41: *Assessment of the Nervous System*

Learning Outcomes

1. Explain the function of the major divisions of the nervous system.
2. Identify common physiologic changes associated with aging that affect the nervous system.
3. Perform a neurologic history based on Gordon's Functional Health Patterns.
4. Perform a basic neurologic physical assessment.
5. Perform a rapid neurologic assessment.
6. Plan pretest and follow-up care for clients undergoing common neurologic diagnostic tests.

Learning Activities

1. Prior to completing the study guide exercises for this chapter, review the following:
   - The anatomy and physiology of the neurologic system (central and peripheral)
   - The process of nerve conduction
   - The principles of acid-base balance
2. Review the **boldfaced** Key Terms and their definitions in Chapter 41 to enhance your understanding of the content.
3. Go to Study Guide Number 9.41 on the following pages and complete the learning exercises for this chapter.

Supplemental Resources

1. Textbook—Chapter 41
2. Other resources:
   - Neatherlin, J.S. (2000). Foundation for practice: Neuroassessment for neuroscience nurses. *Nursing Clinics of North America 34(3)*, 573-592.
   - O'Hanlon-Nichols, T. (1999). Neurologic assessment. *American Journal of Nursing, 99(6)* 44-50.
   - Shpritz, D. (1999). Neurodiagnostic studies. *Nursing Clinics of North America, 34(3)3*, 593-606.

Chapter 42: *Interventions for Clients with Problems of the Central Nervous System: The Brain*

Learning Outcomes

1. Compare migraine and cluster headaches in terms of assessment findings.
2. Develop a teaching plan for a client diagnosed with migraine headaches.
3. Differentiate the common types of seizures, including presenting clinical manifestations and management.
4. Explain the nurse's role in implementing seizure precautions.
5. Plan and document care for a client experiencing a seizure.
6. Identify collaborative management options for treating clients diagnosed with epilepsy.
7. Outline the priorities for care of clients with meningitis and encephalitis.

Learning Activities

1. Prior to completing the study guide exercises for this chapter, review the following:
   - Anatomy and physiology of the neurologic system (central and peripheral)
   - Process of nerve conduction
   - Principles of acid-base balance
   - Principles of fluid and electrolytes
   - Normal function of the musculoskeletal system, including joint range of motion
   - Process of rehabilitation and related interventions

Supplemental Resources

1. Textbook—Chapter 41 (Assessment of the Nervous System)
2. Textbook—Chapter 42
3. Other resources:
   - Contact the local chapter of the Alzheimer's Association. Learn about resources they offer, programs for day care, and seminars for caregivers.
   - Tappen, R.M., et al. (1999). Persistence of self in advanced Alzheimer's disease. *Image: The Journal of Nursing Scholarship 31(2)*, 121-131.

Learning Outcomes	Learning Activities	Supplemental Resources
8. Describe the pathophysiology of Parkinson's disease. 9. Develop a community-based plan of care for a client with Parkinson's disease. 10. Outline realistic expected outcomes for clients with Alzheimer's disease. 11. Explain the use of drug therapy for clients with Alzheimer's disease. 12. Develop a teaching plan for caregivers of clients with Alzheimer's disease in community-based settings. 13. Analyze legal/ethical concerns related to genetic counseling of children with Huntington's disease.	• Concepts of body image and self-esteem • Concepts of loss, death, and grieving • Pain and pain management, coping, and stress management • Principles of perioperative nursing management 2. Review the **boldfaced** Key Terms and their definitions in Chapter 42 to enhance your understanding of the content. 3. Go to Study Guide Number 9.42 on the following pages and complete the learning exercises for this chapter.	• Wright, L.K., et al. (1999). Emotional and physical health of spouse caregivers of persons with Alzheimer's disease and stroke. *Journal of Advanced Nursing, 30*(3), 552-563.

Chapter 43: *Interventions for Clients with Problems of the Central Nervous System: The Spinal Cord*

Learning Outcomes	Learning Activities	Supplemental Resources
1. Identify risk factors that contribute to back pain. 2. Explain ways to prevent back pain. 3. Plan care for the client who has a diskectomy, laminectomy, and/or spinal fusion. 4. Analyze the common nursing diagnoses and collaborative problems for the client with an acute spinal cord injury (SCI). 5. Describe typical medical complications that are experienced by clients with an SCI. 6. Prioritize the nursing care of the client with an SCI. 7. State the expected outcomes for the client with an SCI. 8. Develop a community-based teaching plan for clients who have an SCI. 9. Identify the clinical manifestations associated with spinal cord tumors. 10. Explain the pathophysiology of multiple sclerosis (MS), including the six basic types. 11. Discuss the role of medications in treating clients with MS. 12. Develop a community-based teaching plan for the client with MS. 13. Compare and contrast the clinical manifestations of MS and amyotrophic lateral sclerosis.	1. Prior to completing the study guide exercises for this chapter, review the following: • Anatomy and physiology of the neurologic system (central and peripheral) • Process of nerve conduction • Principles of acid-base balance • Principles of fluid and electrolytes • Normal function of the musculoskeletal system, including joint range of motion • Process of rehabilitation and related interventions • Concepts of body image and self-esteem • Concepts of loss, death, and grieving • Pain and pain management, coping, and stress management • Principles of perioperative nursing management 2. Review the **boldfaced** Key Terms and their definitions in Chapter 43 to enhance your understanding of the content. 3. Go to Study Guide Number 9.43 on the following pages and complete the learning exercises for this chapter.	1. Textbook—Chapter 41 (Assessment of the Nervous System) 2. Textbook—Chapter 43 3. Other resources: • Contact a rehabilitation hospital in your area and discuss home management of clients with an occupational and physical therapist. Discuss plan of care developed for families and support groups such as for multiple sclerosis. • Halper, J. (1998). The nurse case manager in multiple sclerosis. *The Journal of Care Mangement, 4*(1), 12-24. • Ross, A.P. (1999). Neurologic degenerative disorders. *Nursing Clinics of North America, 34*(3), 725-742.

Chapter 44: *Interventions for Clients with Problems of the Peripheral Nervous System*

Learning Outcomes	Learning Activities	Supplemental Resources
1. Compare and contrast the pathophysiology and etiology of Guillain-Barré syndrome (GBS) and myasthenia gravis.	1. Prior to completing the study guide exercises for this chapter, review the following:	1. Textbook—Chapter 41 (Assessment of the Nervous System)
2. Analyze assessment data for a client with GBS to determine common nursing diagnoses.	• Anatomy and physiology of the neurologic system (central and peripheral)	2. Textbook—Chapter 44
3. Prioritize care for the client with GBS.	• Process of nerve conduction	3. Other resources:
4. Evaluate nursing care for the client with GBS based on expected outcomes.	• Principles of acid-base balance	• Contact a dietitian, speech therapist, occupational therapist, and language pathologist to discuss their roles in planning and implementing meals for the client with myasthenia gravis.
5. Identify common clinical manifestations associated with myasthenia gravis (MG).	• Principles of fluid and electrolytes	• Pascuzzi, R.M. & Fleck, J.D. (1999). Acute peripheral neuropathy in adults: Guillain-Barré syndrome and related disorders. *Neurology Clinics, 15*(3), 529-547.
6. Differentiate between a myasthenic crisis and a cholinergic crisis.	• Normal function of the musculoskeletal system, including joint range of motion	• Sorrell, J. (1999). Taking steps to calm restless legs syndrome. *Nursing 99, 29*(9), 60-61.
7. Develop a community-based plan of care for the client with MG.	• Process of rehabilitation and related interventions	
8. Develop a teaching plan for the client with peripheral neuropathy.	• Concepts of body image and self-esteem	
9. Prioritize postoperative care for the client undergoing peripheral nerve repair.	• Concepts of loss, death, and grieving	
10. Compare and contrast trigeminal neuralgia and facial paralysis.	• Pain and pain management, coping, and stress management	
11. Discuss the role of drug therapy in managing the client with trigeminal neuralgia and facial paralysis.	• Principles of perioperative nursing management	
12. Explain the purpose of surgery for clients with trigeminal neuralgia.	2. Review the **boldfaced** Key Terms and their definitions in Chapter 44 to enhance your understanding of the content.	
	3. Go to Study Guide Number 9.44 on the following pages and complete the learning exercises for this chapter.	

Chapter 45: *Interventions for Critically Ill Clients with Neurologic Problems*

Learning Outcomes	Learning Activities	Supplemental Resources
1. Identify the common types of strokes. 2. Discuss risk factors that increase the likelihood of strokes. 3. Describe typical clinical manifestations associated with stroke. 4. Analyze assessment data to determine common nursing diagnoses that are pertinent to clients with strokes. 5. Identify the purpose of intracranial pressure (ICP) monitoring and signs of increasing ICP. 6. Explain the role of drug therapy in managing clients with strokes. 7. Prioritize nursing care for a client who has experienced a stroke. 8. Discuss the purpose of rehabilitation for the client with a stroke. 9. Develop a teaching plan for the client who has experienced a stroke. 10. Differentiate the common types of traumatic brain injury (TBI). 11. Explain the pathophysiologic changes that can result from a moderate or severe TBI. 12. Describe the psychosocial and behavioral manifestations associated with TBI. 13. Prioritize nursing care for the client with TBI. 14. Describe common complications of brain tumors. 15. Develop a postoperative plan of care for a client having a craniotomy.	1. Prior to completing the study guide exercises for this chapter, review the following: • Anatomy and physiology of the neurologic system (central and peripheral) • Process of nerve conduction • Principles of acid-base balance • Principles of fluids and electrolytes • Normal function of the musculoskeletal system, including joint range of motion • Process of rehabilitation and related interventions • Concepts of body image and self-esteem • Concepts of loss, death, and grieving • Pain and pain management, coping, and stress management • Principles of perioperative nursing management 2. Review the **boldfaced** Key Terms and their definitions in Chapter 45 to enhance your understanding of the content. 3. Go to Study Guide Number 9.45 on the following pages and complete the learning exercises for this chapter.	1. Textbook—Chapter 41 (Assessment of the Nervous System) 2. Textbook—Chapter 45 3. Other resources: • Contact a speech therapist and discuss aphasia and implementing a family centered plan for management of speech and communication. • McNair, N. (1999). Traumatic brain injury. *Nursing Clinics of North America, 34*(3), 637-659. • Murphy, M.P., et al. (1998). Discharge planning for individuals with neurocognitive barrier. *The Journal of Care Management, 4*(4), 28-35.

STUDY GUIDE NUMBER 9.41

Assessment of the Nervous System

Study/Review Questions

1. The basic unit of the nervous system is the neuron or nerve cell. Which of the following statements about the neuron are true? *Check all that apply.*
   ____ a. Axons, the efferent pathway, may travel great distances from the cell body.
   ____ b. All axons are covered with a myelin sheath that enhances nerve conduction.
   ✓ c. Dendrite processes bring information into the cell body.
   ✓ d. Synaptic knobs are responsible for storing and releasing transmitter substances.

2. A synapse consists of the _knob_, _left_, and receptor on the cell that receives the impulse.

3. On a separate sheet of paper, identify factors that influence transmission of impulses between neurons.

4. The speed of neural transmission depends on the:
   a. Number and intensity of stimuli.
   (b.) Myelination of the axon.
   c. Diameter of the nerve fibers.
   d. Width of the synaptic cleft.

5. Which factors inhibit and which enhance transmission? *Answers may be used more than once.*

   Factors
   3 a. Acetylcholine (Ach)
   1 b. Anoxia
   1 c. Distance from the cell body
   2 d. Aspartic acid
   1 e. GABA
   2 f. CSF alkalosis
   2 g. Tea or coffee

   Action
   1. Inhibit
   2. Enhance
   3. May do either

6. Match each cell type with the role it plays.

   Cell Type
   3 a. Microglia cells
   1 b. Astroglia cells
   2 c. Ependymal cells
   4 d. Oligodendrocytes

   Role
   1. Physical support
   2. Part of blood-brain barrier
   3. Scavengers
   4. Form myelin sheath

7. Identify the two components of the central nervous system.
   a. _brain_
   b. _spinal cord_

8. Which of the following statements about the meninges is *not* correct?
   a. The pia mater is thin and delicate and adheres to the brain.
   b. Cerebrospinal fluid (CSF) fills the arachnoid layer.
   (c.) The dura mater is a single tough membrane that protects the pia mater.

9. The dura mater dips down between the cerebral hemispheres and the cerebrum and the cerebellum. Which of the following statements are true? *Check all that apply.*
   ✓ a. The dura between the hemispheres is called the falx.
   ✓ b. The dura between the cerebellum and the cerebrum is called the tentorium.
   ____ c. The falx enhances transmission of forces between the cerebral hemispheres.

10. Match the following cerebral areas with their functions.

    Cerebral Areas
    3 a. Motor cortex of the frontal lobe
    1 b. Broca's area
    2 c. Occipital lobe
    5 d. Parietal lobe
    7 e. Limbic lobe
    4 f. Wernicke's area
    6 g. Temporal lobe

    Functions
    1. Speech center
    2. Visual center
    3. Initiate voluntary movement
    4. Process language
    5. Spatial perception
    6. Complicated memory patterns
    7. Emotional and visceral patterns

11. Match each area of the diencephalon with its function.

Areas of the Diencephalon	Functions
3 a. Thalamus	1. Point of reference in x-rays
4 b. Hypothalamus	2. Connects to basal ganglion
1 c. Epithalamus	3. Crudely perceives all sensations except smell
2 d. Subthalamus	4. Regulates water metabolism

12. Which of the following are true of the hypophysis? *Check all that apply.*
    - ✓ a. Is also called the *pituitary gland*.
    - ___ b. Regulates the hypothalamus.
    - ✓ c. Is called the "master gland."
    - ✓ d. Has two lobes that secrete specific hormones.

13. The corticospinal tracts, also called the *pyramidal tracts,* cross over in the medulla. This means that:
    a. The RAS (reticular activating system) controls only right-sided functions.
    b. Reflexes are ipsilateral.
    (c.) Motor function is contralateral.
    d. Sensation is interpreted in the medulla.

14. Cerebellar function:
    a. Controls alertness.
    (b.) Is ipsilateral.
    c. Is contralateral.
    d. Initiates voluntary movement.

15. An interruption of the blood supply in the area served by the middle cerebral artery will:
    a. Be evidenced by a loss of vision.
    (b.) Affect upper body movement.
    c. Cause increased intracranial pressure.
    d. Interfere with temperature regulation.

16. Which of the following pass through the blood-brain barrier and which are blocked by the barrier?

Substance	Blood-Brain Barrier Access
1 a. Oxygen	1. Passes through
2 b. Albumin	2. Is blocked
2 c. Most bacteria	
1 d. Alcohol	
1 e. Water	
1 f. Anesthetics	
2 g. Many antibiotics	
1 h. Carbon dioxide	

17. Match the spinal tract with the function of the tract.

Spinal Tract	Function
3 a. Spinothalamic	1. Proprioception
1 b. Spinocerebellar	2. Voluntary movement
2 c. Fasciculus gracilis or cuneatus	3. Carry sensation of pain, temperature, and pressure
4 d. Corticospinal	4. Vibratory sense

18. Identify the parts of the peripheral nervous system (PNS).
    a. ___spinal nerves___
    b. ___cranial nerves___
    c. ___ANS___

19. Which of the following statements about spinal nerves are correct? *Check all that apply.*
    - ✓ a. Loss of sensation and motor function in a specific body area can be caused by a problem with one particular spinal nerve.
    - ✓ b. Lumbar nerves must travel farther than other thoracic nerves before they leave the spinal column.
    - ___ c. The posterior branch transmits impulses to the muscles.
    - ___ d. Sensory receptors do not transmit information on special senses.

20. Reflexes:
    a. Are mediated by the cerebellum.
    b. Are under direct control of the motor cortex and are therefore contralateral.
    c. Require sensory input from muscles, tendons, skins organs, and special senses.
    d. Involve only the sensory neuron and the motor neuron.

21. Name the components of the autonomic nervous system.
    a. _____
    b. _____

22. Match each statement below to the corresponding part of the autonomic nervous system.

    Statements
    ___ a. Cell bodies in the gray matter of the spinal cord from S-2 to S-4
    ___ b. Lies beside the spinal cord in a chain
    ___ c. Has some sensory function
    ___ d. Part of cranial nerves III, VII, IX, and X
    ___ e. Causes the heart to pump faster
    ___ f. Constricts pupils

    Component of the Autonomic Nervous System
    1. Parasympathetic nervous system (PNS)
    2. Sympathetic nervous system (SNS)

23. Which of the following changes occur in the older adult?
    a. Sense of smell is heightened.
    b. Intellect declines.
    c. Long-term memory seems better than recall.
    d. Early morning wakefulness.

24. On a separate sheet of paper, identify the components relevant to a neurologic assessment.

25. Which of the following chronic conditions can impact neurologic function?
    a. Hypertension
    b. Obesity
    c. Crohn's disease
    d. Coronary artery disease

26. A baseline physical assessment is used to:
    a. Determine a level of function for later comparison.
    b. Show the family what problems the older adult has.
    c. Gain information on past sensory changes.
    d. Determine rehabilitation potential.

27. Match each question that the nurse would pose to the type of information sought.

Questions	**Information Sought**
___ a. Ask client to repeat three unrelated words.	1. Attention span
	2. Recent memory
	3. Remote memory
___ b. What is your birth date?	4. New memory
	5. Language comprehension
___ c. Ask client to follow simple instructions.	6. Cognitive skills
___ d. What health care providers have you seen during the last year?	
___ e. Ask client to repeat a series of numbers.	
___ f. Tell me about your hobbies.	

28. Assessment of sensory function:
    a. Is limited to light touch and pain.
    b. Is done routinely every 4 hours.
    c. Is reserved for clients with problems affecting the spinal cord.
    d. Includes assessment of the hypoglossal nerve.

29. If temperature sensation is intact, which of the following can be omitted from an assessment of nerve function?
    a. Vibration
    b. Pain
    c. Light touch
    d. Pressure

30. Match the component of motor testing with the corresponding test performed.

Test Performed	**Test Component**
___ a. Walk across room, and return	1. Brainstem integrity
___ b. Client stands, eyes open, feet close together	2. Coordination
	3. Muscle strength
	4. Gait
___ c. Client holds arms perpendicular to body, eyes closed	5. Equilibrium
___ d. Client grasps and squeezes nurse's fingers	
___ e. Arms out to side, touch nose 2 to 3 times	

31. Which of the following is *not* a deep tendon reflex?
    a. Achilles tendon
    b. Plantar
    c. Biceps
    d. Brachioradialis

32. Which of the following statements regarding the Glasgow coma scale is *not* true?
    a. It is a rapid neurologic assessment tool.
    b. It establishes a baseline for eye opening, motor response, and verbal response.
    c. It establishes a baseline cognitive function.
    d. It measures the client's best response.

33. Contrast medium can be used in all of the following tests *except:*
    a. MRI.
    b. Computed tomography.
    c. X-rays of skull or spine.
    d. Cerebral angiography.

True or False? *Write T for true or F for false in the blanks provided.*

34. Which of the following statements about lumbar punctures are true?
    ___ a. They are contraindicated for clients with infections at or near the puncture site.
    ___ b. They reduce mild to moderately increased intracranial pressure.
    ___ c. They are done at the T-1 to T-3 spinal level.
    ___ d. They require the client to lie flat for 4 to 8 hours postprocedure.
    ___ e. They are done with the client in the "fetal" position.

35. Which of the following findings in CSF are normal? *Check all that apply.*
    ___ a. Lactic acid 10 to 20 mg/100 mL
    ___ b. Protein less than 15 mg/100 mL
    ___ c. Pressure 70 to 180 mm H_2O
    ___ d. Color yellow
    ___ e. Glucose 45 to 80 mg/100 mL

36. Preparing a client for an EEG would include:
    a. Giving a sedative before bedtime.
    b. Having the client drink coffee or tea before the test.
    c. Keeping the client NPO after midnight.
    d. Keeping the client awake from 2 am to the scheduled test time.

STUDY GUIDE NUMBER 9.42

Interventions for Clients with Problems of the Central Nervous System: The Brain

Study/Review Questions

1. Match each characteristic with the corresponding type of headache.

    Characteristics
    ___ a. Familial disorder
    ___ b. Occurs more often in men
    ___ c. Associated with runny nose and ptosis
    ___ d. Has no known cause
    ___ e. Postulated to be caused by hyperexcitability of nerves
    ___ f. Client may walk or rock

    Type of Headache
    1. Migraine
    2. Cluster headache

    ___ g. May last for several days
    ___ h. Duration limited to 15 to 45 minutes
    ___ i. Occurs at regular intervals with long remission periods
    ___ j. Occurs more often in women

2. The assessment of migraine headaches includes which of the following? *Check all that apply.*
    ___ a. Age of onset of headaches
    ___ b. Presence of mood changes before headache
    ___ c. Presence of aura
    ___ d. Anorexia before onset of the headache

3. A teaching plan for a client with a migraine would *not* include:
   a. Management of urinary incontinence.
   b. Modification of diet.
   c. Plans to decrease pain, such as lying down in a darkened room.
   d. Information on preventive drug therapy.

4. Which of the following is *not* an intervention for cluster headaches?
   a. Modification of diet: eliminating caffeine and chocolate
   b. Providing pain medication
   c. Administering oxygen
   d. Reviewing the need for a consistent sleep-wake cycle

5. Match the type of generalized seizure with the correct terminology.

Definitions	Types of Generalized Seizures
___ a. Brief jerking of extremities, singly or in groups	1. Tonic-clonic
	2. Absence
___ b. Brief period of staring or loss of consciousness	3. Myoclonic
	4. Atonic
___ c. Rigidity followed by rhythmic jerking	
___ d. Sudden loss of body tone	

True or False? *Write T for true or F for false in the blanks provided.*

6. Which of the following statements about partial seizures are true?
   ___ a. They are also called *focal seizures*.
   ___ b. Automatisms may occur.
   ___ c. They involve both cerebral hemispheres.
   ___ d. Medical treatment is more effective for partial seizures than generalized seizures.
   ___ e. The client may report an aura before the seizure.

7. On a separate sheet of paper, identify the subjective data needed for assessment of seizures.

8. Which of the following statements are true for the older adult? *Check all that apply.*
   ___ a. Seizures are likely to be associated with metabolic changes.
   ___ b. Drug monitoring is very important because of changes in metabolism and elimination.
   ___ c. Seizure medication produces fewer adverse reactions.
   ___ d. Drug interactions are of concern.

9. The nurse would do which of the following to institute seizure precautions? *Check all that apply.*
   ___ a. Instruct the family on the use of a padded tongue blade.
   ___ b. Ascertain that airway management equipment is readily available.
   ___ c. Pad the bed rails.
   ___ d. Raise the bed for easy access to the client.
   ___ e. Ensure IV access.

10. Interventions for the client with a seizure include which of the following? *Check all that apply.*
    ___ a. Turning the client to the side.
    ___ b. Restricting the client's movement to prevent injury.
    ___ c. Observing and documenting the seizure.
    ___ d. Administering oxygen as ordered.

11. Status epilepticus is a medical emergency. Which of the following statements are true about this condition? *Check all that apply.*
    ___ a. Education about the necessity for maintaining proper drug therapy can help avoid this condition.
    ___ b. It is characterized by a rapid succession of seizures.
    ___ c. It is a potential complication of atonic seizures only.
    ___ d. It may be treated with IV diazepam.

12. Education for the client and family regarding status epilepticus includes which of the following? *Check all that apply.*
    ___ a. Correcting misinformation about the condition.
    ___ b. Discussion of the type of work done by the client.
    ___ c. Reviewing the importance of continued drug therapy, even if seizures have stopped.
    ___ d. Proper response to a seizure by family members or caregivers.

13. Organisms enter the nervous system through which routes?
    a. _____
    b. _____
    c. _____

14. Match each factor with its associated type of meningitis.

    Factors

    ___ a. Usually self-limiting; full recovery expected.
    ___ b. Manifestations vary according to the state of the immune system.
    ___ c. Cerebrospinal fluid (CSF) is hazy.
    ___ d. No organisms grow from the CSF.
    ___ e. Outbreaks occur in crowded conditions such as dormitories.

    Types of Meningitis

    1. Bacterial meningitis
    2. Viral meningitis
    3. Fungal meningitis

15. Which of the following clinical signs are associated with meningitis? *Check all that apply.*
    ___ a. Nuchal rigidity
    ___ b. Negative Kernig's sign
    ___ c. Positive Brudzinski's sign
    ___ d. Paralysis

16. The nurse can anticipate that which of the following tests will be performed on the client suspected of having meningitis?
    a. X-rays of the mastoid area
    b. Lumbar puncture
    c. Myelography
    d. Cerebral angiogram

17. Which of the following symptoms in a client with meningitis would need to be communicated to the physician?
    a. Capillary refill of 3 seconds
    b. Urinary incontinence
    c. Inability to follow a moving object from side to side
    d. Temperature of 100.6° F orally

18. When considering drug therapy for meningitis, what information must be factored into the decision?
    a. Viral meningitis responds best to ampicillin.
    b. A broad-spectrum antibiotic is given until test results are back.
    c. Rifampin is used as single agent therapy and never given for prophylaxis.
    d. Anticonvulsants must be avoided because they increase intracranial pressure.

19. Vectors that are associated with the spread of encephalitis are which of the following? *Check all that apply.*
    ___ a. Ticks
    ___ b. Mosquitoes
    ___ c. Black flies
    ___ d. Amebae

20. Assessment of the client suspected of having encephalitis may include which of the following questions? *Check all that apply.*
    ___ a. Have you been on a camping trip or spent time out of doors recently?
    ___ b. Are you allergic to any foods?
    ___ c. Have you been exposed to chickenpox recently?
    ___ d. Do you have cold sores?
    ___ e. Have you been swimming in a lake or pond?

21. Signs and symptoms of encephalitis include all but which of the following?
    a. Nausea and vomiting
    b. Stiff neck
    c. Loss of motor reflexes
    d. Symptoms of increased intracranial pressure

22. Interventions for encephalitis include which of the following?
    a. Maintaining a patent airway
    b. Antiviral medication for arboviruses
    c. Placing the client in Trendelenburg position
    d. Administering acyclovir for herpes encephalitis

23. The three cardinal symptoms of Parkinson's disease are:
    a. Muscle rigidity, slow movement, and tremor.
    b. Muscle flaccidity, slow movement, and tremor.
    c. Muscle rigidity, rapid movement, and tremor.
    d. Muscle flaccidity, rapid movement, and tremor.

24. The symptoms of Parkinson's disease are caused by:
    a. An increase in the secretion of dopamine.
    b. Overactive adrenal function.
    c. A decrease in dopamine secretion.
    d. An increase in acetylcholine production.

25. On a separate sheet of paper, identify the key points of assessment for the client with Parkinson's disease.

26. Which of the following statements regarding drug therapy for Parkinson's disease is true?
    a. Dopamine precursors are effective only late in the disease.
    b. Long-term use of dopaminergics is associated with dyskinesia.
    c. Monoamine oxidase inhibitors are used for the depression that accompanies Parkinson's disease.
    d. Drug tolerance is not a problem in Parkinson's disease, although toxicity is.

27. A major goal for the client with Parkinson's disease is to maintain mobility. Achieving this includes doing all of the following *except*:
    a. Encouraging strenuous aerobic exercise.
    b. Maintaining an environment that is conducive to self care.
    c. Including exercises for the face and tongue.
    d. Using adaptive devices for activities of daily living (ADLs).

28. On a separate sheet of paper, describe what structural changes occur in the brain of the client with Alzheimer's disease. (Some of these changes are normal, but are accelerated in Alzheimer's disease.)

29. Which of the following statements about Alzheimer's disease are true?
    ____ a. There is a genetic predisposition to this disease.
    ____ b. Onset is typically in the age group 40 to 50.
    ____ c. It is the leading cause of death among older adults.
    ____ d. Head trauma increases the risk of early onset.

30. Important considerations for the assessment of clients with Alzheimer's include all of the following *except*:
    a. Many disorders, including drug intoxication can mimic this disease.
    b. The client is fully aware of the changes that have occurred.
    c. The most important information concerns onset, duration, and progression of symptoms.
    d. Family history and history of head trauma are important.

31. Match each of the symptoms with its corresponding stage of Alzheimer's disease. *Answers may be used more than once.*

Symptoms of Alzheimer's Disease	Stage of Alzheimer's Disease
____ a. Motor and verbal skills lost	1. Early, or stage I
____ b. Short attention span	2. Middle, or stage II
____ c. Wandering	3. Late, or stage III
____ d. General and focal neurologic deficits	
____ e. Possible depression, agitation	
____ f. Loss of ability to care for self	
____ g. Problems with judgment	

32. There are changes in behavior and personality with Alzheimer's disease. Which of the following is *not* a symptom of Alzheimer's disease?
    a. Increase in aggressiveness
    b. Fatigue
    c. Confusion at night
    d. Mania

33. Laboratory and other diagnostic tests used to diagnose Alzheimer's disease are:
    a. Mainly used to rule out other treatable conditions.
    b. Specific for Alzheimer's, if done early in the disease.
    c. Genetic in nature and fully predictive of the disease.
    d. Used over time to track improvement.

34. Which of the following nursing interventions is *not* suitable for chronic confusion?
    a. Providing a structured environment.
    b. Providing stimulation to enhance cognition.
    c. Providing consistency.
    d. Providing reality orientation.

35. Which of the following statements about drug therapy are correct? *Check all that apply.*
    ____ a. There are no curative drugs for this condition.
    ____ b. Acetylcholinesterase inhibitors may delay the onset of cognitive decline.
    ____ c. Depression is best treated with amitriptyline.
    ____ d. Antipsychotic drugs are useful for treating agitation.

36. Education for the family of a client with Alzheimer's would *not* include:
    a. Sleep disturbance is common; frequent naps during the day are to be encouraged.
    b. Caregivers need to be aware of the effects of stress on their own physical well-being.
    c. Restlessness can be diminished by frequent walks.
    d. The need to keep the client's room free from clutter.

37. The diagnosis of Huntington's disease is made based on which of the following? *Check all that apply.*
    ____ a. Family history
    ____ b. A brain biopsy
    ____ c. Presenting symptoms
    ____ d. A positive EEG test

STUDY GUIDE NUMBER 9.43

Interventions for Clients with Problems of the Central Nervous System: The Spinal Cord

Study/Review Questions

1. Acute back pain usually results from trauma. On a separate sheet of paper, identify other factors that contribute to the occurrence of back pain.

2. On a separate sheet of paper, identify what additional factors contributing to back pain are found in the older adult.

3. Which of the following statements is true about back pain?
   a. The pain follows the dermatome of the affected nerve.
   b. Opiates are more effective in relieving pain than nonsteroidal anti-inflammatory medications.
   c. Sensation is often heightened in the extremity affected by the pain.
   d. Straight leg raising alleviates pain.

4. On a separate sheet of paper, identify the nonsurgical interventions used for back pain.

5. Which of the following surgical procedures is used when the spine is unstable?
   a. Laparoscopic discectomy
   b. Spinal fusion
   c. Laminectomy
   d. Traditional disectomy

6. Which of the following postoperative findings should be reported to the surgeon immediately?
   a. Minimal drainage in the surgical drain after 8 hours
   b. Pain at the operative site
   c. Swelling or bulging at the operative site
   d. Altered sensation in the affected limb

7. Identify the intervention done postoperatively on a fusion that is not done on a laminectomy.
   a. Log roll the client every 2 hours
   b. Have client dangle legs on the evening of surgery
   c. Have client wear a brace when out of bed
   d. Do a neurologic assessment and check vital signs

8. Which of the following statements indicates that the client does *not* understand the postoperative instructions he or she was given?
   a. "I use ice on my back for pain."
   b. "I put a piece of plywood under my mattress."
   c. "Dieting is difficult but important."
   d. "I have a new ergonomic chair at work."

9. Match each of the following symptoms with its corresponding complication.

Symptoms	Complications
___ a. Hypertension	1. Spinal shock
___ b. Flaccid paralysis	2. Autonomic dysreflexia
___ c. Hypotension	
___ d. Severe headache	
___ e. Loss of reflexes below the injury	
___ f. Blurred vision	

10. On a separate sheet of paper, describe the four major mechanisms of spinal cord injury and their causes.

11. Match each type of partial cervical spinal cord lesion with the corresponding physical findings.

    Physical Findings
    ___ a. Motor function is lost on the same side of the body as the injury.
    ___ b. Motor function is lost below the injury.
    ___ c. Motor function remains intact; sensory function is lost.

    Type of Spinal Cord Lesion
    1. Anterior cord injury
    2. Posterior cord injury
    3. Brown-Séquard's syndrome

12. When completing an assessment of a client with a cervical SCI, all of the following information is important with the exception of:
    a. Previous respiratory problems
    b. History of arthritis
    c. Previous back or neck surgeries
    d. Previous use of nonsteroidal anti-inflammatory medications

13. Autonomic dysreflexia may be avoided by:
    a. Careful attention to urinary output.
    b. Keeping the room warm.
    c. Using an elastic corset to raise blood pressure.
    d. Frequent ambulation.

14. Autonomic dysreflexia can lead to:
    a. Heat stroke resulting from loss of thermoregulation.
    b. Paralytic ileus.
    c. Hypertensive stroke.
    d. Aspiration and pneumonia.

15. Match each of the following medications with the corresponding indication/effect.

    Medications
    ___ a. Methylprednisolone
    ___ b. Dextran
    ___ c. Atropine
    ___ d. Dopamine
    ___ e. Dantrolene

    Indications/Effects
    1. Increases heart rate
    2. Relieves spasticity
    3. Increases capillary blood flow
    4. Anti-inflammatory
    5. Regulates blood pressure

16. Nursing interventions to maintain a patent airway include which of the following? *Check all that apply.*
    ___ a. Encourage the use of an incentive spirometer.
    ___ b. Perform oral or nasal suctioning as needed.
    ___ c. Assist the client to cough.
    ___ d. Give prescribed pain medication.

17. On a separate sheet of paper, identify the major complications of prolonged immobility.

18. When implementing bowel and bladder retraining, the nurse should do all the following *except:*
    a. Ensure that the client gets a sufficient quantity of fluid each day.
    b. Assist the client in developing a schedule.
    c. Teach the client about high-fiber foods.
    d. Teach the client that regaining continence is dependent upon how well the spinal cord heals.

19. On a separate sheet of paper, identify the major area of education for the client with a spinal cord injury.

20. The key to successful rehabilitation of a client with spinal cord injury is psychosocial adaptation. The nurse assists the client with this by: *Check all that apply.*
    ___ a. Role-playing about questions that might be asked.
    ___ b. Allowing the client to verbalize feelings about self image.
    ___ c. Arranging for the family to take the client to the hospital lobby.
    ___ d. Allowing the client to act out his or her frustrations.

21. Which of the following statements about spinal cord tumors are correct? *Check all that apply.*
    ___ a. The majority are malignant.
    ___ b. They occur mostly in the thoracic area.
    ___ c. More men than women develop spinal cord tumors.
    ___ d. The symptoms vary by location of the tumor and its rate of growth.

22. The major pathologic feature of multiple sclerosis (MS) is:
    a. Destruction of the dendrite processes on nerve cells.
    b. Destruction of the myelin sheath.
    c. Destruction of the axon.
    d. Destruction of the cell body.

23. Which of the following statements about MS are true? *Check all that apply.*
    ___ a. It is a chronic progressive disease.
    ___ b. It has a defined genetic cause.
    ___ c. It is more prevalent in the 20- to 40-year age group than in any other.
    ___ d. Life expectancy is prolonged if the client moves to an area of low prevalence.

24. Which of the following tests may aid in diagnosing MS?
    a. EMG
    b. EEG
    c. MRI
    d. CT scan

25. Educational topics for a client with MS include:
    a. Support services for the family.
    b. Planning activities and rest periods.
    c. The use of assistive devices.
    d. The role of immunosuppressive therapy.

26. Which of the following statements about amyotrophic lateral sclerosis is false?
    a. It is a progressive disease involving the motor system.
    b. It has no known cause.
    c. It affects mental ability first.
    d. There is no specific treatment.

27. Early symptoms of amyotrophic lateral sclerosis include:
    a. Bowel and bladder incontinence.
    b. Tongue atrophy.
    c. Blurred vision.
    d. Headaches.

STUDY GUIDE NUMBER 9.44

Interventions for Clients with Problems of the Peripheral Nervous System

Study/Review Questions

1. Which statement about Guillain-Barré syndrome (GBS) is correct?
   a. Clients with GBS usually present with an acute respiratory illness or injury.
   b. Males are affected twice as often as females.
   c. Most evidence points to a cell-medicated immunologic reaction as the cause.
   d. The major problem in GBS is the destruction of the muscle receptor site.

2. On a separate sheet of paper, identify the subjective information sought by the nurse from the client in assessing for GBS.

3. Which of the following symptoms are not associated with GBS?
   a. Diplopia
   b. Labile blood pressure
   c. Spasticity
   d. Absent deep tendon reflexes

4. What tests would you expect to be performed on a client with GBS? *Check all that apply.*
   ___ a. Myelogram
   ___ b. Lumbar puncture
   ___ c. Arterial blood gases
   ___ d. Vital capacity
   ___ e. X-rays of the cervical spine

5. Which of the following symptoms would the nurse report to the physician immediately for a client with GBS?
   a. Increasing loss of motor function
   b. Ineffective cough
   c. Dyspnea and confusion
   d. Relief of pain by opiates

6. Interventions for the client with respiratory compromise include which of the following? *Check all that apply.*
   ___ a. Provision of appropriate pain medication to enhance breathing
   ___ b. Auscultation of breath sounds every 2 hours
   ___ c. Checking the vital capacity every 4 hours
   ___ d. Suction as needed using sterile technique

7. Which of the following statements about treatment for GBS is correct?
   a. Immunoglobulins are curative.
   b. Plasmapheresis can be done only once because second treatments have increased risk of side effects.
   c. Treatment is supportive because this disease is usually self-limiting.
   d. Immunoglobulins have no major side effects.

8. On a separate sheet of paper, discuss the goals and intervention for impaired mobility for the client with GBS.

9. Health care teaching for the GBS client:
   a. Should always include a family member or significant other.
   b. May be given in oral form only.
   c. Always includes information on range-of-motion exercises.
   d. Includes information on the need for continued plasmapheresis.

10. Which of the following statements about myasthenia gravis (MG) is correct?
    a. It is a progressive disease marked by a steep decline in function.
    b. Increasing activity delays onset of symptoms.
    c. It is a genetically inherited disease.
    d. Hyperplasia of the thymus gland has been implicated as a cause.

11. On a separate sheet of paper, outline the subjective information gathered by the nurse as part of the client history when assessing for MG.

12. Which of the following statements about Tensilon testing is *incorrect?*
    a. A false-positive test may occur if the muscle is extremely weak.
    b. The drug has a long duration of action, allowing the physician to gauge improvement.
    c. The test can be used to distinguish between a cholinergic crisis and a myasthenic crisis.
    d. A false-negative test can result from increased effort by the client.

13. Which of the following transmitters is deficient in MG?
    a. Serotonin
    b. Acetylcholine
    c. Dopamine
    d. GABA

14. Which of the following symptoms of an MG client should the nurse report to the physician immediately?
    a. Diarrhea
    b. Blurry vision
    c. Inability to swallow
    d. Tinnitus

15. In planning activities for the client with MG, the nurse should remember that the client:
    a. Is weakest in the morning.
    b. Is weakest in the evening.
    c. Should plan activities in relation to medication times.
    d. Will continue to weaken.

16. MG is associated with which of the following diseases?
    a. Diabetes
    b. Peripheral vascular disease
    c. Hyperthyroidism
    d. Hypothyroidism

17. On a separate sheet of paper, identify the objective data gathered by the nurse from the client with MG.

18. Important information about drug therapy in MG is:
    a. If a dose of cholinesterase is missed, a double dose is taken the next day.
    b. Antibiotics such as neomycin and kanamycin have a synergistic effect with cholinesterase inhibitors.
    c. Medications must be taken on an empty stomach.
    d. Drugs containing morphine or sedatives can increase muscle weakness.

19. Clients with MG may develop respiratory compromise. Which of the following statements is *not* a cause of respiratory compromise?
    a. Cholinergic crisis, which causes hyperventilation
    b. Dysphagia, which can result in aspiration
    c. Respiratory infection resulting from inability to cough secondary to weak muscles
    d. Myasthenic crisis, which causes increased muscle weakness

20. Postoperative care for the client with MG consists of which of the following? *Check all that apply.*
    ___ a. Use of an incentive spirometer every 2 hours.
    ___ b. Assessing for onset of chest pain.
    ___ c. Turn, cough, and deep breathe once every 8 hours.
    ___ d. Monitor for decreasing blood pressure or weak, rapid pulse.

21. On a separate sheet of paper, identify the most common causes of polyneuritis.

22. Which of the following statements regarding polyneuritis is true?
    a. All forms of polyneuritis have an inflammatory component.
    b. Polyneuritis usually begins in the hands (glove neuropathy) before going to the legs.
    c. Vitamins in excess of dietary allowances have been found useful in treating polyneuropathies.
    d. Rapid recovery may follow if the toxin causing the polyneuropathy is removed.

23. Which of the following diseases is associated with polyneuropathy?
    a. Raynaud's syndrome
    b. Diabetes
    c. Leukemia
    d. Hyperthyroidism

24. Which of the following would *not* be suited for the client with polyneuropathy?
    a. Checking feet for cuts and reddened areas
    b. Checking bath water for proper temperature
    c. Using a heating pad to keep feet warm
    d. Proper shoe selection

25. Identify the four major ways peripheral nerves can be injured.
    a. _____
    b. _____
    c. _____
    d. _____

26. Which of the following statements about peripheral nerve damage is true?
    a. Successfully remyelinated nerves conduct impulses at 80% of original velocity.
    b. Nerves regenerate at the rate of 10 to 40 mm/day.
    c. After injury, the proximal nerve degenerates within 24 hours.
    d. Some motor function may return before regeneration is complete.

27. On a separate sheet of paper, discuss the subjective data that may be given by the client with peripheral nerve damage.

28. Postoperative care for the client with peripheral nerve damage includes:
    a. ROM exercises for the affected limb to maintain mobility.
    b. Joint extension to keep the nerve properly aligned.
    c. Joint flexion to keep tension off the suture site.
    d. Making sure the skin around the edge of the splint is blanched.

29. Match each statement to the corresponding condition. *Answers can be used more than once.*

Statements	Conditions
___ a. Pain is provoked by stimulation of the trigger zone	1. Trigeminal neuralgia
___ b. More common in women	2. Facial paralysis
___ c. Incidence may be higher in diabetics	
___ d. Thought to be related to brainstem activity	
___ e. Inflammatory in nature	
___ f. Taste is impaired	
___ g. Requires protection of the cornea	
___ h. Surgical procedure removes arterial compression	
___ i. Prednisone is prescribed	
___ j. A soft diet and frequent small meals are encouraged	

STUDY GUIDE NUMBER 9.45

Interventions for Critically Ill Clients with Neurologic Problems

Study/Review Questions

1. A stroke is defined as:
   a. Pressure on central neurons caused by swelling.
   b. Interruption of blood flow.
   c. Severing of pyramidal tracts.
   d. Hydrocephalus.

2. Which of the following statements about stroke are true? *Check all that apply.*
   ___ a. Incidence of stroke has been increasing.
   ___ b. Strokes are the third leading cause of death in the United States.
   ___ c. Clinical pathways have not been developed for stroke victims because of the variety of causes.
   ___ d. Indirect costs of strokes include loss of wages.

3. Strokes cause damage:
   a. Within minutes of occurring.
   b. When the stored oxygen in the brain is depleted.
   c. When too much glucose is delivered to the brain.
   d. When the glia cells constrict.

4. Fill in the following table with the distinguishing features of each type of stroke. *Copy to a separate sheet of paper if necessary.*

Type of Stroke	Thrombotic	Embolic	Hemorrhagic
Feature			
Onset			
Evolution			
Contributing Factors			
Duration			

5. Which of the following statements about stroke are true? *Check all the apply.*
   ___ a. Thrombotic strokes account for over half of all strokes.
   ___ b. Collateral circulation may develop and decrease the effects of an embolic stroke.
   ___ c. The lack of elasticity of the artery is an important feature of a thrombotic stroke.
   ___ d. Bifurcations are protected from thrombus formation because of increased blood flow.

6. A lacunar stroke:
   a. Is a type of thrombotic stroke.
   b. Is a type of embolic stroke.
   c. Causes cavities to develop in the white matter of the brain only.
   d. Always causes severe damage.

7. In embolic stroke, the middle cerebral artery is involved most often. Which of the following deficits are associated with middle cerebral artery occlusion?
   a. Contralateral hemiparesis: arm > leg
   b. Contralateral hemiparesis: leg > arm
   c. Unilateral neglect
   d. Dysconjugate gaze

8. Which of the following statements about the causes of stroke is correct?
   a. Hypertension is the leading cause of embolic stroke.
   b. Rupture of an arteriovenous malformation is the most common cause of hemorrhagic stroke.
   c. Embolic stroke is associated with myocardial infarction.
   d. Transient ischemic attacks last longer than 24 hours and often precede ischemic strokes.

9. Which of the following clients are at increased risk for stroke? *Check all that apply.*
   ___ a. A 66-year-old man with well controlled diabetes
   ___ b. A 35-year-old female cocaine addict
   ___ c. A 77-year-old woman who exercises regularly
   ___ d. A 45-year-old male smoker

10. Factors that are thought to contribute to the stroke belt in the southern United States include which of the following? *Check all that apply.*
    ___ a. Obesity
    ___ b. Race
    ___ c. Average age of the population
    ___ d. Smoking

11. Match each symptom of stroke with the hemisphere most often affected by that symptom. *Answers can be used more than once.*

    Symptoms
    ___ a. Loss of depth perception
    ___ b. Aphasia
    ___ c. Loss of hearing
    ___ d. Cannot recognize faces
    ___ e. Impaired sense of humor
    ___ f. Depression
    ___ g. Denies illness
    ___ h. Frustration and anger
    ___ i. Disoriented to person, place, and time
    ___ j. Poor judgment

    Affected Hemisphere
    1. Left hemisphere
    2. Right hemisphere

12. When assessing motor changes in a client who has had a stroke, it is important to remember that:
    a. Motor deficit is ipsilateral to the hemisphere affected.
    b. Motor deficit is contralateral to the hemisphere affected.
    c. Bowel and bladder function remain intact.
    d. Flaccid paralysis is not an expected finding and should be reported promptly.

13. Match each deficit with its corresponding definition.

    Definitions
    ___ a. Inability to comprehend language
    ___ b. Sensitivity to light
    ___ c. Difficulty writing
    ___ d. Blindness in half of the visual field
    ___ e. Blindness in one eye
    ___ f. Difficulty reading
    ___ g. Drooping eyelid

    Deficits
    1. Ptosis
    2. Hemianopsia
    3. Amaurosis fugax
    4. Receptive aphasia
    5. Agraphia
    6. Alexia
    7. Photophobia

14. Laboratory tests after a stroke may show the following:
    a. Elevated white count caused by inflammation
    b. Elevated hematocrit
    c. A red-tinged CSF specimen
    d. Elevated liver function tests

15. Which of the following tests may be used to establish a diagnosis of stroke and determine the type? *Check all that apply.*
    ___ a. Computed tomography
    ___ b. MRI
    ___ c. EMG
    ___ d. Angiography

16. Which of the following is *not* an indication of intracranial pressure?
    a. Nonreactive pupils
    b. Nausea and vomiting
    c. Hypotension
    d. Seizures

17. Nursing interventions for the client with a stroke include which of the following? *Check all that apply.*
    ___ a. Placing the client in the Trendelenburg position to increase cerebral blood flow.
    ___ b. Spacing care activities to allow for sufficient rest between activities.
    ___ c. Hyperoxygenate before suctioning.
    ___ d. Monitoring vital signs every 8 hours.

18. Which of the following drugs can a nurse expect to give to a client who has had a hemorrhagic stroke?
    a. Enteric-coated aspirin
    b. Warfarin sodium (Coumadin)
    c. Sodium heparin
    d. Docusate (Colace)

19. Which of the following drugs is used to control cerebral vasospasm?
    a. Nimodipine
    b. Phenytoin
    c. Dipyridamole (Persantine)
    d. Clopidogrel (Plavix)

20. On a separate sheet of paper, identify the nursing interventions for a client with a hemorrhagic stroke.

21. Which of the following surgical procedures may be used to treat an ischemic stroke?
    a. Craniotomy to remove clots
    b. Inserting a detachable silicone balloon into the affected artery
    c. Carotid endarterectomy
    d. Craniotomy to clip the artery

22. The client expected outcomes for Impaired Physical Mobility are to increase the client's exercise intolerance, to prevent the client from experiencing the consequences of immobility, and to teach the client to become independent in ADLs. To accomplish these goals, the nurse would do which of the following? *Check all that apply.*
    ____ a. Position the client with a pillow under the knees to decrease spasticity.
    ____ b. Teach the client how to do active and passive ROM exercises.
    ____ c. Splint the arm to prevent contractures.
    ____ d. Apply sequential compression stockings.

23. Match each of the following interventions for a client who has had a stroke to the hemisphere most commonly affected. *Answers may be used more than once.*

    Interventions
    ____ a. Scan side-to-side
    ____ b. Place pictures and familiar objects around client
    ____ c. Approach client from unaffected side
    ____ d. Reorient client frequently
    ____ e. Place objects within the client's field of vision
    ____ f. Establish a structured routine for the client
    ____ g. Teach client to wash both sides of body
    ____ h. Repeat names of objects commonly used

    Affected Hemisphere
    1. Right hemisphere
    2. Left hemisphere

24. If the client has impaired swallowing, the nurse should:
    a. Limit the diet to clear liquids so if aspiration occurs the client still will be able to breathe.
    b. Make sure the client is in semi-Fowler's position for all meals.
    c. Monitor the client's weight.
    d. Make meals more enjoyable by making sure the family is present.

25. To reestablish urinary continence, the nurse should:
    a. Request a Foley catheter.
    b. Offer the urinal to a male client every 4 hours.
    c. Restrict fluid intake to 1500 mL/day.
    d. Determine barriers to continence and correct them.

26. On a separate sheet of paper, identify the areas of education that need to be addressed with the client who has had a stroke.

27. Which of the following statements does not reflect the home management of the client who has had a stroke?
    a. Home caregivers need to plan for respite care.
    b. The home should be evaluated for potential safety risks such as throw rugs.
    c. Teach the family to give the medications used to treat emotional lability.
    d. Have family members give a return demonstration on transfer techniques.

28. Which of the following statements about traumatic brain injury (TBI) are correct? *Check all that apply.*
    ____ a. They are the leading cause of death of persons between the ages of 18 and 34.
    ____ b. They are most often caused by falls.
    ____ c. Although the incidence of injury is higher in the young male, persons over 60 have higher mortality rates.
    ____ d. Even mild brain injury can lead to permanent disability.

29. Match each type of trauma with the corresponding definition.

    Definitions

    ___ a. The head hits a stationary object
    ___ b. A simple, clean break in the skull
    ___ c. Tearing of the cortical surface
    ___ d. The head is in motion
    ___ e. Bone presses inward into brain tissue
    ___ f. CSF leaks from nose or ears
    ___ g. Direct opening to brain tissue
    ___ h. Fragments of bone in brain tissue
    ___ i. Brief loss of consciousness

    Types of Trauma

    1. Laceration
    2. Acceleration
    3. Concussion
    4. Linear fracture
    5. Basilar skull fracture
    6. Comminuted fracture
    7. Depressed fracture
    8. Deceleration
    9. Open fracture

30. On a separate sheet of paper, explain how each of the following causes cerebral edema.
    a. Vasogenic edema
    b. Cytotoxic edema
    c. Interstitial edema

31. Match each type of hematomas with the corresponding description.

    Descriptions

    ___ a. Caused by tearing of small vessels within brain tissue
    ___ b. Occurs between the skull and the dura
    ___ c. May present as acute, subacute, or chronic

    Types of Hematomas

    1. Epidural hematoma
    2. Subdural hematoma
    3. Intracranial hemorrhage

32. Blood flow to the brain remains fairly constant as a result of the process of:
    a. Autostasis.
    b. Automobilization.
    c. Hemodynamic stasis.
    d. Autoregulation.

33. Hydrocephalus is *not:*
    a. Ingestion of too much water caused by the increase in production of antidiuretic hormone.
    b. Caused by dilation of the ventricles.
    c. A result of obstruction of cerebrospinal fluid circulation.
    d. A result of impaired absorption.

34. Obtaining history from a client with traumatic brain injury can be difficult because of all of the following *except:*
    a. Amnesia of events before or after the injury.
    b. Decreased level of consciousness.
    c. Drug-induced coma.
    d. Combative behavior.

35. When obtaining initial history from the client with traumatic brain injury or from the family of the client, it is most important to ask which of the following questions? *Check all that apply.*
    ___ a. Can the client eat shellfish without a problem?
    ___ b. Does the client smoke?
    ___ c. Does the client use alcohol or drugs?
    ___ d. Does the client have glaucoma?

36. Match each type of breathing to the area of the brain that is affected by such breathing.

    Types of Breathing

    ___ a. Cheyne-Stokes
    ___ b. Central neurogenic hyperventilation
    ___ c. Apneustic breathing
    ___ d. Cluster breathing
    ___ e. Ataxic breathing

    Affected Areas of the Brain

    1. Low midbrain, upper pons
    2. Medulla
    3. Cerebral hemispheres, cerebellar
    4. Low pons, high medulla
    5. Mid pons, low pons

37. The first priority in assessment of the client with traumatic brain injury is to determine:
    a. Whether spinal injury is present.
    b. Whether the client is hypotensive.
    c. Whether a patent airway is present.
    d. The level of consciousness using the Glasgow scale.

38. On a separate sheet of paper, identify the indications of intracranial pressure (ICP).

39. Which of the following statements is correct in regard to a client with a traumatic brain injury?
    a. The appearance of abnormal posturing occurs only when the client is not positioned for comfort.
    b. Cushing reflex, an early sign of ICP, consists of severe hypertension, widening pulse pressure, and bradycardia.
    c. Papilledema, edema, and hyperemia of the optic disk are always signs of ICP.
    d. Areas of tenderness over the scalp indicate the presence of contrecoup injuries.

40. Nursing interventions for the client with traumatic brain injury include:
    a. Assessment of vital signs every 8 hours.
    b. Positioning to avoid extreme flexion.
    c. Encouraging fluid intake over the first 48 hours to compensate for diabetes insipidus.
    d. Administration of glucocorticosteroids to prevent ICP.

41. Which of the following nursing interventions are used with clients who have altered sensory functions? *Check all that apply.*
    ___ a. Play tapes for at least 30 minutes to make sure the comatose client has heard them. Sensory input is essential to facilitating response to the environment.
    ___ b. Teach the family to test the water temperature used for bathing.
    ___ c. Position the client upright in bed or in a chair for meals.
    ___ d. Teach the client to place food on the unaffected side of the mouth.

42. On a separate sheet of paper, identify the types of ICP monitoring devices and their major advantages and disadvantages.

43. Identify the most common sites of primary tumors that metastasize to the brain.
    a. _____
    b. _____
    c. _____
    d. _____

44. Which of the following does *not* result in increased ICP in clients with brain tumors?
    a. Vasogenic edema
    b. Hemorrhage into the brain
    c. Obstruction of CSF flow
    d. Pituitary dysfunction

45. Which of the following statements is correct?
    a. Hands-free cellular phones prevent brain tumors.
    b. The exact cause of brain tumors is not known.
    c. Genetics and heredity are important risk factors for brain tumors.
    d. A high-fat diet has been linked to brain tumor development.

46. Match each key feature of brain tumors with the most likely site of the tumor. *Answers may be used more than once.*

Features of Brain Tumors	Site of Tumor
___ a. Vomiting unrelated to food intake	1. Cerebral tumor
___ b. Hemiparesis	2. Brainstem tumor
___ c. Facial pain or weakness	
___ d. Nystagmus	
___ e. Seizures	
___ f. Headache	
___ g. Hoarseness	
___ h. Aphasia	
___ i. Ataxia	
___ j. Hearing loss	

47. Drug therapy for the client with a brain tumor includes all but which of the following?
    a. Glucocorticosteroids for edema
    b. Codeine for pain
    c. Insulin for diabetes insipidus
    d. Histamine-blockers to prevent stress ulcers

48. Which of the following is true of gamma knife therapy?
    a. It is used for easily reached tumors.
    b. It is noninvasive and has fewer complications.
    c. It requires general anesthesia.
    d. It replaces conventional radiation therapy.

49. Education for the client and family concerning craniotomy would *not* include:
    a. Your head will be shaved at the surgical site.
    b. Periorbital edema and bruising may be present.
    c. Drainage of CSF after surgery is normal; blood drainage is not.
    d. The family should bring tapes and pictures postoperatively to help reorient the client.

50. The preferred position for a client who has had an infratentorial craniotomy is:
    a. High-Fowler's position, turned to the operative side.
    b. Head of bed at 30 degrees, turned to the nonoperative side.
    c. Flat in bed, turned to the operative side.
    d. Flat in bed, may turn to either side.

51. Which statements about ICP in the surgical client is correct? *Check all that apply.*
    ___ a. It is the major postoperative complication.
    ___ b. Osmotic diuretics, such as mannitol, may be given.
    ___ c. Cerebral edema, which is frequently present before surgery, subsides within 72 hours.
    ___ d. If not contraindicated, the head of the bed should be at 30 degrees.

52. In regard to respiratory problems, the nurse should remember which of the following points? *Check all that apply.*
    ___ a. Atelectasis and pneumonia can be prevented by proper pulmonary hygiene.
    ___ b. Suctioning and chest physiotherapy should be avoided because they increase intracranial pressure.
    ___ c. Neurologic pulmonary edema occurs frequently.
    ___ d. Incentive spirometry is a useful technique for preventing atelectasis.

53. Health care teaching for a client with brain tumors includes:
    a. Instructing the client on avoiding physical activity.
    b. Teaching the client and family to avoid over-the-counter medications.
    c. Teaching the client and family that seizures may occur in the immediate postoperative period.
    d. Instructing the client on dietary changes needed to prevent recurrence of the tumor.

54. Organisms that cause brain abscesses most often originate from:
    a. _____
    b. _____
    c. _____

55. Septic emboli often originate from:
    a. _____
    b. _____
    c. _____
    d. _____

56. Which of following could be found in the history of a client with a brain abscess?
    a. A family history of Huntington's disease
    b. Recent chemotherapy treatment for cancer
    c. A history of osteoarthritis
    d. Vaccination against influenza

57. Which of the following organisms is found mostly in AIDS clients?
    a. *Streptococcus* species
    b. *Enterobacter* species
    c. *Haemophilus influenzae*
    d. Toxoplasmosis

58. Which of the following statements about diagnostic testing is correct?
    a. The WBC may be normal, even in the presence of infection.
    b. Blood cultures are the only culture likely to grow the causative organism.
    c. MRI is useful late in the course of the disease to identify permanent lesions.
    d. The first test performed will be a lumbar puncture to determine whether the CSF is cloudy.

59. If a client has an abscess that was caused by anaerobic bacteria, the nurse would expect to give the client which of the following medications?
    a. Nafcillin sodium (Nafcil)
    b. Clindamycin (Cleocin)
    c. Metronidazole (Flagyl)
    d. Penicillin G benzathine (Bicillin)

UNIT 10   PROBLEMS OF SENSATION: EYES AND EARS ■ Core Concepts Grid

Anatomy	Physiology	Pathophysiology	History	Physical Exam	Diagnostic Tests	Interventions	Pharmacology
• **Cranial nerves** Optic (II) Oculomotor (III) Trochlear (IV) Trigeminal (V) Abducens (VI) Facial (VII) Vestibulo- cochlear (VIII) • **Ears** External canal Tympanic membrane Middle ear Ossicles Eustachian tube Inner ear Semicircular canals Cochlea Endolymph Perilymph Organ of Corti • **Eyes** Eyelids/eyeballs Conjunctiva Lacrimal glands Cornea Uvea Iris/lens/retina Canal of Schlemm Aqueous/ vitreous humor	• **Sound transmission** • **Light transmission** • **Color discrimination** • **Refraction** • **Accommoda- tion** • **Coordination**	• **Inflammation** • **Obstruction** • **Tinnitus** • **Vertigo** • **Dizziness** • **Hearing loss** • **Hyperopia** • **Myopia** • **Astigmatism** • **Increased intraocular pressure (IOP)** • **Opacity of lens** • **Retinal detachment** • **Hemorrhage** • **Vision loss**	• **Client past medical history** Systemic medical conditoins Past injuries • **Family history** • **Social history** Medications Occupation Gender Diet history Leisure activities Age	• **Ear** Otoscopic examination Light reflex Voice test Watch test Tuning fork Rinne test Weber test • **Eye** Exophthalmos Ptosis Scleral color Aniscocoria Pupillary reaction Snellen chart Visual fields Jaeger card Six cardinal positions of gaze Corneal light reflex Cover/uncover test	• **Cultures** • **Computed tomography (CT)** • **Audiometry** Bone conduction Pure tone Speech • **Tympanometry** • **Slit-lamp examination** • **Corneal staining** • **Tonometry** • **Ophthal- moscopy** • **Gonioscopy**	• **Ear medication installations** • **Removal of ceru- men** • **Removal of for- eign objects from ear canal** • **Ear medication installation** • **Care for the deaf** • **Communication with the deaf** Signing Speech reading • **Eye care** Eye glasses Artificial eyes Contact lenses • **Care for the blind** • **Communication with the blind** Clock TTY Braille	• **Systemic anti- biotics** • **Ear medications** Antibiotic Antifungal Anti-inflammatory • **Antivertigo agents** • **Antiemetics** • **Artificial tears** • **Eye medications** Antibiotic Antifungal Anti-inflammatory • **Midriatics** • **Miotics** Beta blockers Pilocarpine Carbonic anhydrase inhibitors

Unit 10 (Chapters 46-49)

Problems of Sensation: Management of Clients with Problems of the Sensory System

Learning Plan

Chapter 46: *Assessment of the Eye and Vision*

Learning Outcomes	Learning Activities	Supplemental Resources
1. Explain the concept of refraction in relation to how the cornea, lens, aqueous humor, and vitreous humor contribute to vision. 2. Describe age-related changes in the eye, eyelids, and vision. 3. List five systemic disorders that have an impact on the eye and vision. 4. Discuss which elements of a client's history might predict visual impairment later in life. 5. Discuss the educational needs of a client undergoing fluorescein angiography. 6. Explain the relationship between intraocular pressure and eye health. 7. Use proper technique to instill eyedrops.	1. Prior to completing the study guide exercises for this chapter, review the anatomy and physiology of the eye. 2. Review the **boldfaced** Key Terms and their definitions in Chapter 46 to enhance your understanding of the content. 3. Go to Study Guide Number 10.46 on the following pages and complete the learning exercises for this chapter.	1. Textbook—Chapter 46 2. Other resources: • Contact your local chapter of the Lion's Club and discuss client programs for the community. • Gerber, N. (1999). Iris and pupil: Key considerations. *Journal of Ophthalmic Nursing and Technology, 18*(5), 207-218.

Chapter 47: *Interventions for Clients with Eye and Vision Problems*

Learning Outcomes	Learning Activities	Supplemental Resources
1. Describe how to correctly instill ophthalmic drops and ointment into the eye. 2. Explain the consequences of increased intraocular pressure (IOP). 3. Identify common practices that increase intraocular pressure. 4. Prioritize educational needs for the client after cardiac surgery with and without lens replacement. 5. Compare and contrast myopia and hyperopia and the correction needed for each. 6. Describe the pathologic bases, symptoms, and nursing care priorities for primary open-angle glaucoma and acute angle-closure glaucoma. 7. Identify the nursing care priorities for the donor when corneal donation is planned. 8. Explain how diabetes mellitus and hypertension affect vision. 9. Prioritize educational needs for the client after corneal transplantation. 10. Describe the common visual deficits for the client with dry macular degeneration. 11. Identify nursing interventions to promote home safety for the client with impaired vision.	1. Prior to completing the study guide exercises for this chapter, review the following: • Anatomy and physiology of the eye • Installation of eyedrops and ointments • Concept of body image and self-esteem • Concept of loss and grief • Principles of perioperative management 2. Review the **boldfaced** Key Terms and their definitions in Chapter 47 to enhance your understanding of the content. 3. Go to Study Guide Number 10.47 on the following pages and complete the learning exercises for this chapter.	1. Textbook—Chapter 46 (Assessment of the Eye and Vision) 2. Textbook—Chapter 47 3. Other resources: • Jarvis, C. (2000). *Physical examination and health assessment* (3rd ed.). Philadelphia: W.B. Saunders. • Gilbard, J. (1999). Dry eye, blepharitis, and chronic eye irritation: Divide and conquer. *Journal of Ophthalmic Nursing and Technology, 18*(3), 109-115. • Investigate your community for programs developed for clients with impaired vision, and plan to spend a day in their program.

Chapter 48: *Assessment of the Ear and Hearing*

Learning Outcomes	Learning Activities	Supplemental Resources

1. Describe the key elements to inspect when performing assessment of the external ear.
2. Describe age-related changes in the structure of the ear and hearing.
3. Identify 10 drugs that have an impact on hearing.
4. Demonstrate the correct use of an otoscope.
5. Describe the landmarks of the tympanic membrane.
6. Compare and contrast air conduction and bone conduction of sound.
7. Demonstrate the correct use of a tuning fork in performing the Weber and Rinne tests for hearing.
8. Prioritize educational needs for the client about to undergo pure tone audiometry and electronystagmography.
	1. Prior to completing the study guide exercises for this chapter, review the anatomy and physiology of the ear.
	
	2. Review the **boldfaced** Key Terms and their definitions in Chapter 48 to enhance your understanding of the content.
	
	3. Go to Study Guide Number 10.48 on the following pages and complete the learning exercises for this chapter.
		1. Textbook—Chapter 48
		2. Other resources:
		  • Hsu, R. & Levine, S.C. (1998). Sudden hearing loss: How to identify the cause promptly. *Consultant, 38*(1), 23-26, 31-32.
		  • Locate available hearing screening programs in your community.
		  • Stone, C.M. (1999). Clinical outlook: Preventing cerumen impaction in nursing facility residents. *Journal of Gerontological Nursing, 25*(5), 43-45.

Chapter 49: *Interventions for Clients with Ear and Hearing Problems*

Learning Outcomes	Learning Activities	Supplemental Resources

1. Compare and contrast the clinical manifestations and interventions for external otitis and otitis media.
2. Describe how to correctly instill medications into the ear.
3. Explain the procedures to safely remove impacted cerumen from the ear of an older client.
4. Prioritize educational needs for the client with Meniere's disease.
5. Compare and contrast the causes and interventions for conductive versus sensorineural hearing loss.
6. Prioritize nursing care for the client after tympanoplasty.
7. Prioritize educational needs for the client after stapedectomy.
8. Identify an appropriate method for communication with a client who has recently become hearing impaired.
9. Develop a teaching plan for a client who is learning to use a hearing aid.
	1. Prior to completing the study guide exercises for this chapter, review the following:
	  • Anatomy and physiology of the ear
	  • Maintenance of hearing aids
	  • Concepts of body image and self-esteem
	  • Assessment of the ear and hearing
	
	2. Review the **boldfaced** Key Terms and their definitions in Chapter 49 to enhance your understanding of the content.
	
	3. Go to Study Guide Number 10.49 on the following pages and complete the learning exercises for this chapter.
		1. Textbook—Chapter 48 (Assessment of the Ear and Hearing)
		2. Textbook—Chapter 49
		3. Other resources:
		  • Investigate hearing aid providers in your community for fitting practices, costs, and available types.
		  • National Council on Aging (2000). The consequences of untreated hearing loss in older persons. *ORL–Head and Neck Nursing, 18*(1) 12-16.
		  • Shaw, L. (1997). Protocol for detection and follow-up of hearing loss, *Clinical Nurse Specialist, 11*(6), 240-247.

STUDY GUIDE NUMBER 10.46

Assessment of the Eye and Vision

Study/Review Questions

1. Which of the following statements about the optic disk is true?
   a. Nerve fibers and photoreceptor cells are contained in this depressed area on the retina.
   b. It is the clear layer that forms the external coat on the front of the eye.
   c. It is sometimes called the blind spot.
   d. It forms a circular, convex structure behind the iris.

2. Light waves pass through which structures on the way to the retina? Identify them in sequence.
   a. _____
   b. _____
   c. _____
   d. _____

3. Match each characteristic or function of the eye with its associated structure.

Characteristic/Function of the Eye	Structure of the Eye
___ a. Maintains the form of the eyeball	1. Rods
___ b. Is responsible for light refraction	2. Lens
___ c. Spaces between the anterior chamber and the canal of Schlemm	3. Ciliary processes
	4. Vitreous humor
	5. Uvea
___ d. Pigmented, vascular coating of the eye	6. Pupil
	7. Cornea
___ e. Transparent layer over the anterior eye	8. Fovea centralis
___ f. Responsible for peripheral vision	9. Optic disk
	10. Iridocorneal angle
___ g. Secretes aqueous humor	
___ h. Central circular opening	
___ i. Center of the macula	
___ j. Point where optic nerve enters the eyeball	

4. Which of the following muscles is responsible for pulling the eye upward?
   a. Inferior oblique
   b. Lateral rectus
   c. Superior rectus
   d. Superior oblique

5. Match each of the following cranial nerves with their functions.

Nerves	Functions
___ a. Cranial nerve II (optic)	1. Corneal reflex
	2. Visual acuity
___ b. Cranial nerve III (oculomotor)	3. Eyelid closure
	4. Eyelid muscle movements
___ c. Cranial nerve V (trigeminal)	
___ d. Cranial nerve VII (facial)	

6. Name the term used to identify each of the vision problems described below.
   a. A refractive error caused by an irregular curvature: _____
   b. Refraction power is too strong: _____
   c. Loss of accommodation resulting from aging: _____
   d. Insufficient refracting power: _____
   e. Ideal refraction of the eye: _____

7. Match each description with the corresponding name for the eye change associated with aging.

Descriptions	Eye Changes Associated with Aging
___ a. Accumulation of fatty deposits	1. Sunken eyes
	2. Visual acuity decreases
___ b. Decreased ability of iris to dilate	3. Astigmatism
	4. Sclerae become yellow
___ c. Continued growth of lens epithelial layers and water loss from lens	5. Loss of night vision
	6. Color perception decreases
	7. Cataracts
___ d. Loss of subcutaneous fat, skin elasticity, and muscle tone	8. Presbyopia

____ e. Cornea flattens, resulting in irregular curvature

____ f. Weakening of ciliary muscles produces a loss of accommodation

____ g. Lens loses elasticity, becomes more dense

____ h. Lens yellows and absorbs the light waves

8. Identify five ocular signs and symptoms that may be the result of a reaction to a systemic medication.

   a. _____

   b. _____

   c. _____

   d. _____

   e. _____

9. Write a brief answer for why it is important to address each of the following areas of health history with your client when assessing the eyes.

Health History	Reason for Obtaining Information
Family history	
Current medical systemic diseases	
Types of sports activities in which client participates	
All medications	

10. Which of following statements is true?

    a. A client with myopia has smaller pupils.

    b. Normal pupil size is between 1 and 3 mm.

    c. Pupils are larger in older adults.

    d. Anisocoria is normal in 5% of the population.

11. a. Your client complains of not seeing objects in his peripheral vision. Which test would you perform to evaluate this complaint?

    b. Your findings indicate that he has blindness in one half of his field of vision. What is this condition called?

12. Your client, who works in a machine shop, has presented with a suspected foreign body in his eye. What diagnostic test would *not* be done?

13. Match each of the following physical findings with the corresponding related technique.

    Physical Findings

    ____ a. Alignment of anteroposterior axes

    ____ b. Visual acuity

    ____ c. Peripheral vision

    ____ d. Eye muscle strength

    ____ e. Eye drifting

    Related Techniques

    1. Cardinal gaze positions
    2. Cover/uncover test
    3. Corneal light reflex
    4. A Snellen chart
    5. Confrontation

14. Your client is scheduled for a computed tomography (CT) scan. Which of the following statements are true? *Check all that apply.*

    ____ a. This diagnostic method is used to detect hemorrhages in the choroid layer.

    ____ b. The client will need to be positioned in a confined space.

    ____ c. A cross-section image is formed using beams of high intensity x-rays.

    ____ d. There is no pain with this test.

15. When preparing your client for a fluorescein angiography, which of the following statements would be included in your teaching?

    a. An intravenous access is necessary.

    b. Client must avoid sunlight for 2 days.

    c. Urine voided after the test will be bright orange.

    d. Fluids are held for the first 24 hours postprocedure.

16. When instilling ophthalmic drops in a client's eyes, which of the following procedures would *not* be performed?

    a. Check the name, strength, and expiration date of the solution.

    b. Don gloves before instilling the drops for all clients.

    c. Release drops into the conjunctival pocket.

    d. Avoid contaminating the tip of the bottle.

17. Which of the following statements about Tono-Pen XL tonometry are correct? *Check all that apply.*

    ____ a. Exerts a force against the cornea.

    ____ b. Requires a topical anesthetic.

    ____ c. Plunger may abrade the cornea.

    ____ d. High risk of infection with use.

18. When using the ophthalmoscope, which of the following procedures would be *incorrect*? *Check all that apply.*
    ___ a. The nurse comes toward the client's eye from 6 inches away.
    ___ b. The nurse comes toward the client 15 degrees lateral to the client's line of vision.
    ___ c. When examining the OD, the nurse holds the ophthalmoscope in her left hand.
    ___ d. A thumb can be placed on the client's eyebrow to assist the nurse in determining the distance from ophthalmoscope to the client.

19. Which structures or reflexes should be assessed by direct ophthalmoscopy?
    a. _____
    b. _____
    c. _____
    d. _____
    e. _____

20. Which of the following findings in an ophthalmoscopic examination is abnormal?
    a. Red glare from the pupil
    b. Nasal margin of optic disk blurred
    c. Presence of arteriolar or venular nicking
    d. Bright foveal reflection

STUDY GUIDE NUMBER 10.47

Interventions for Clients with Eye and Vision Problems

Study/Review Questions

1. Match each of the following eyelid disorders with the corresponding description.

   Disorder
   ___ a. Ptosis
   ___ b. Ectropion
   ___ c. Blepharitis
   ___ d. Hordeolum
   ___ e. Chalazion
   ___ f. Entropion

   Description
   1. Eyelid margin inflammation
   2. Gland infection at the lid/lash margin
   3. Drooping upper lid
   4. Granulomatous inflammation
   5. Inverted lid margin
   6. Lid eversion

2. Which of the following statements about an entropion are true? *Check all that apply.*
   ___ a. Pain and tearing may be present.
   ___ b. The orbicular muscle can be surgically tightened for correction.
   ___ c. Can be caused by eyelid spasms.
   ___ d. Lacks sufficient tears to wash adequately over the eye.

3. Identify four important safety points to emphasize with clients who will be instilling an ophthalmic ointment.
   a. _____
   b. _____
   c. _____
   d. _____

4. Your client presents with a red swollen area on one eyelid; it is painful and is on the conjunctival side of the eyelid-eyelash margin.
   a. What is the problem?
   b. What would facilitate healing?

5. Which of the following statements about keratoconjunctivitis sicca and its management is true?
   a. Use of antihistamines can stimulate tear production.
   b. Warm, moist compresses help restore moisture to the eye.
   c. HypoTears can be used as often as necessary
   d. Care must be taken to avoid transferring contamination from one eye to the other.

6. Your client has been diagnosed with trachoma. What is the main focus of your nursing interventions?

7. Acute conjunctivitis is associated with:
   a. Significant ocular discharge.
   b. Formation of scales and granulations on the eyelids.
   c. Blurred vision.
   d. Elevated ocular pressure.

8. Which of the following clients are at an increased risk for corneal disorders? *Check all that apply.*
   ___ a. A 60-year-old male with a history of stroke
   ___ b. A 25-year-old skier with protective eye gear
   ___ c. A 5-year-old swimmer with diabetes
   ___ d. A 15-year-old female with recurrent uveitis

9. Identify three nursing care priorities for the donor when a corneal donation is planned.
   a. _____
   b. _____
   c. _____

10. Your client is scheduled for a keratoplasty. What are four possible complications of this surgery?
    a. _____
    b. _____
    c. _____
    d _____

11. Which of the following statements would be true about the postoperative care for a client who has had a keratoplasty?
    a. She should lie on the operative side to reduce intraocular pressure.
    b. Her eye will be covered for 1 week with the initial dressing and shield.
    c. She will require assistance with meals.
    d. The head of the bed must be elevated 15 degrees.

12. On a separate sheet of paper, develop a concept map relevant to corneal disorders. Consider physiologic, psychosocial, and developmental factors. Identify data that are subjective and objective and include significant diagnostic studies.

13. Which of the following statements about cataracts is *not* true?
    a. The degree of reduced vision is determined by the location of the cataract and the density of the opacification.
    b. Cataracts are classified by nature or by onset.
    c. Age-related cataracts are the most common and are characterized by redness and discomfort.
    d. As the cataract matures, visualization of the retina is increasingly difficult.

14. On a separate sheet of paper, develop a concept map relevant to cataracts. Consider physiologic and developmental factors. Identify data that are subjective and data that are objective. Include significant laboratory test findings and other studies.

15. Your client has had cataract surgery and she is ready to go home. What activities should she avoid?
    a. _____
    b. _____
    c. _____
    d. _____
    e. _____
    f. _____
    g. _____
    h. _____

16. The client who has had cataract surgery should know the signs and symptoms of complications. Which signs and symptoms should the client report to her physician?
    a. _____
    b. _____
    c. _____
    d. _____
    e. _____

17. Which of the following statements about glaucoma is *not* true?
    a. Glaucoma is actually a group of diseases resulting in increased intraocular pressure.
    b. Warning signs of glaucoma include gradual loss of central vision.
    c. The most common form of primary glaucoma involves the structure involved in circulation and reabsorption of the aqueous humor, which undergoes direct pathologic change.
    d. Commonly in glaucoma, the increased pressure reduces blood flow to the optic nerve and retina.

18. On a separate sheet of paper, compare and contrast primary open-angle glaucoma and closed-angle glaucoma.

19. Drug therapy for glaucoma focuses on reducing increased ocular pressure through what two mechanisms?

20. Compare the following medications used for glaucoma by completing the chart below.

Drug	Classification	Desired Effect	Nursing Implications
Timolol	1a	1b	1c
Pilocarpine	2a	2b	2c

21. Identify three causes of blood leakage into the vitreous.
    a. _____
    b. _____
    c. _____

22. Which of the following statements about uveitis is correct?
    a. Anterior uveitis is an inflammation of the retina.
    b. Posterior uveitis is an inflammation of the iris.
    c. Symptoms include seeing a red haze or series of floaters.
    d. Adhesions between the iris and the lens are complications.

23. Which of the following conditions are associated with posterior uveitis? *Check all that apply.*
    ____ a. Tuberculosis
    ____ b. Syphilis
    ____ c. Herpes zoster
    ____ d. Rheumatoid arthritis

24. Nursing interventions for a client with uveitis include:
    a. Patching the affected eye.
    b. Offering aspirin and opioids for increased pain.
    c. Darkening the room.
    d. Encouraging light activity such as reading.

25. On a separate sheet of paper, identify the retinal changes that occur in hypertensive retinopathy.

26. What are the two types of diabetic retinopathy?
    a. _____
    b. _____

27. Which of the following statements about retinal detachment is true?
    a. Onset is usually sudden and painful.
    b. It can be directly prevented by prompt intervention.
    c. Clients may suddenly see bright flashes of light.
    d. Hyperopia is directly associated with its occurrence.

28. A client is told by his ophthalmologist that he has a retinal tear and that it should be closed or sealed. What are the three mechanisms for doing this?
    a. _____
    b. _____
    c. _____

29. Following a sclera buckling procedure involving a gas bubble insertion, the client should be positioned:
    a. In high-Fowler's position.
    b. Supine with head to nonoperative side.
    c. Prone with head turned so that the operative eye is facing up.
    d. In Trendelenburg position.

30. The most common early clinical manifestation of retinitis pigmentosa is:
    a. Cataracts.
    b. Night blindness.
    c. Headache.
    d. Vitamin A deficiency.

31. A client states that he has developed problems seeing the exit signs on the highway when he is driving. What should he be checked for?

32. Match the following refractive errors with their definitions.

    Definitions
    ___ a. Short length of the may contribute to this condition.
    ___ b. Curve of the cornea is not even.
    ___ c. Images are bent and fall in front of the retina.
    ___ d. This condition usually appears in people in their 30s and 40s.

    Refractive Errors
    1. Myopia
    2. Astigmatism
    3. Presbyopia
    4. Hyperopia

Answer the following three questions on a separate sheet of paper.

33. Make a chart comparing the surgical management for the treatment of the following refractive errors: radial keratotomy, photorefractive keratectomy (PRK), and laser-in-situ (LASIK).

34. A 10-year-old client was hit in his left eye with a baseball. He has a "black eye," but his vision is not affected and he is applying ice. He wants to know how long the discoloration will last. What would you tell him about the discoloration?

35. What is the most common intraocular malignant tumor in adults?

36. Clients are classified as blind if their best visual acuity with corrective lenses is:
    a. 20/50
    b. 20/100
    c. 20/150
    d. 20/200

37. Clients who have lost their sight may experience: *Check all that apply.*
    a. Hopelessness.
    b. Grieving.
    c. Anger.
    d. Immobility.

38. A client is vision impaired and has been found to be making errors on her medications. On a separate sheet of paper, name what suggestions would help her manage her medicines yet remain independent.

STUDY GUIDE NUMBER 10.48

Assessment of the Ear and Hearing

Study/Review Questions

1. The spiral organ of hearing is the:
   a. Cochlea.
   b. Semicircular canal.
   c. Pinna.
   d. Stapes.

2. The two critical functions of the ear are _____ and maintaining _____.

3. Match each ear structure with the corresponding locations. *Answers may be used more than once.*

   Structures
   ___ a. Mastoid process
   ___ b. Incus
   ___ c. Stapes
   ___ d. Cochlea
   ___ e. Auricle
   ___ f. Organ of Corti
   ___ g. Malleus

   Locations
   1. External ear
   2. Middle ear
   3. Inner ear

4. Identify the events, in sequential order, that lead to the sense of hearing.
   ___ a. Sound waves are transferred to the malleus.
   ___ b. Sound waves are transferred to incus and the stapes.
   ___ c. Vibrations are transmitted to the cochlea.
   ___ d. Neural impulses are conducted by the auditory nerve.
   ___ e. Sound waves strike the mastoid and the movable tympanic membrane.
   ___ f. Sound is processed and interpreted by the brain.

5. Which of the following is a change in the ear that is related to aging?
   a. Hearing for high frequency sound increases.
   b. The pinna becomes shorter and thickened.
   c. Cerumen producing glands increase in number and function.
   d. Bony ossicles have decreased movement.

6. Match the following terms with their definitions.

   Terms
   ___ a. Decibel
   ___ b. Masking
   ___ c. Vestibular hearing loss
   ___ d. Otosclerosis
   ___ e. Sensorineural

   Definitions
   1. Relating to the functions of the ear needed for the sense of balance and position
   2. A unit of sound for expressing loudness
   3. Formation of spongy bone around structures of the middle and inner ear
   4. The process of hiding a specific sound from one ear while the other ear is tested
   5. Hearing loss resulting from neural defects

7. A sensorineural hearing loss results from impairment of which of the following?
   a. Fused bony ossicles
   b. The eighth cranial nerve
   c. The seventh cranial nerve
   d. The first cranial nerve

8. Your adult client is having problems with his hearing. Below are his medications. Which of his medications are ototoxic? *Check all that apply.*
   ___ a. Motrin
   ___ b. Digoxin
   ___ c. Lasix
   ___ d. Synthroid

9. Which of the following statements about an otoscopic assessment is true?
   a. The client's head should be tilted slightly toward the nurse for support.
   b. The nurse holds the otoscope in his or her dominant hand.
   c. The pinna is pulled down and back.
   d. The internal canal is visualized while the speculum is slowly inserted.

10. Upon otoscopic assessment, which of the following findings indicate a normal tympanic membrane? *Check all that apply.*
    ___ a. The membrane is slightly convex in nature.
    ___ b. The membrane is a pink to deep-red color.
    ___ c. The membrane has a mobile pars tensa.
    ___ d. The membrane is opaque or pearly gray.

Answer the following two questions on a separate sheet of paper.

11. Which structures are seen through the normal tympanic membrane?

12. Compare and contrast the air conduction and bone conduction of sound.

13. Which of the following statements about intensity of sound are *false*? *Check all that apply.*
    a. A level of 110 dB is the lowest a young healthy ear can detect.
    b. A hearing loss of 45 to 50 dB renders a person unable to hear without a hearing aid.
    c. A soft whisper is around 20 dB.
    d. Conversational speech is generally around 90 dB.

14. Match the following hearing test terms with their correct definitions.

    Definitions
    1. Measurement of hearing acuity
    2. Test for high frequency sounds
    3. Used to differentiate between conductive and sensorineural hearing losses
    4. Test for detecting central and peripheral disease of vestibular system
    5. Tests for vertigo
    6. A simple acuity test

    Hearing Tests
    ___ a. Voice test
    ___ b. Electronystagmography
    ___ c. DixHallpike test
    ___ d. Audiometry
    ___ e. Watch test
    ___ f. Weber tuning fork test

15. When conducting a Weber tuning fork test:
    a. The fork can be placed above the client's upper lip.
    b. Lateralization is a normal result.
    c. Proper handling of the fork includes grasping the upper part of the fork for stability.
    d. Bone conduction is greater than air conduction.

16. The Rinne tuning fork test: *Check all that apply.*
    ___ a. Assists in differentiating hearing by air conduction and bone conduction.
    ___ b. Involves time responses.
    ___ c. Requires placing the vibrating fork stem on the client's mastoid process.
    ___ d. Requires lateralization.

17. It is important for the nurse to understand the terminology of pure tone audiometry. Match each of the following terms with the corresponding definition.

    Definitions
    ___ a. Lowest level of intensity heard by client (50% of the time)
    ___ b. Expressed in decibels
    ___ c. Highness or lowness of tones
    ___ d. Results of pure tone audiometry testing

    Terms
    1. Frequency (time)
    2. Threshold
    3. Audiogram
    4. Intensity

Answer the following two questions on a separate sheet of paper.

18. A client is scheduled for an electronystagmography (ENG). What should the nurse tell this client to prepare him for this test?

19. The ability to understand speech is the most important aspect of human auditory function. What does speech discrimination testing determine?

20. Tympanometry is helpful in distinguishing:
    a. Middle ear infections.
    b. Outer ear infections.
    c. Furuncles.
    d. Indurated lesions on the pinna.

STUDY GUIDE NUMBER 10.49

Interventions for Clients with Ear and Hearing Problems

Study/Review Questions

1. Which of the following treatments is not used for external otitis?
   a. Application of heat
   b. Oral analgesics
   c. Topical antibiotics
   d. Myringotomy

2. What is the most common fungal organism associated with external otitis?
   a. *Streptomyces albus*
   b. *Aspergillus*
   c. *Streptococcus*
   d. *Staphylococcus aureus*

3. Identify four conditions affecting the external ear.
   a. _____
   b. _____
   c. _____
   d. _____

4. Which of the following statements about necrotizing or malignant external otitis are true? *Check all that apply.*
   ____ a. It is the most virulent form of external otitis.
   ____ b. There is a low mortality rate related to complicating disorders.
   ____ c. It can destroy cranial nerves, especially the facial nerve.
   ____ d. It is a very common problem among younger adults.

5. Your adult client has external otitis. After the inflammation resolves, he should *not:*
   a. Use earplugs while swimming.
   b. Drop diluted alcohol in the ear to prevent recurrence.
   c. Use cotton-tipped applicators to dry the ears.
   d. Use analgesics for pain relief.

6. On a separate sheet of paper, describe the clinical manifestations of a furuncle.

7. Ear irrigation fluid would be least likely to stimulate the vestibule sense at what temperature?
   a. 98° F
   b. 120° F
   c. 110° F
   d. 78° F

8. A female adult client has otitis media. The nurse would expect her chief compliant to be:
   a. Ear pain.
   b. Sensation of fullness in the ear.
   c. Rhinitis.
   d. Dizziness.

9. Your adult client has a history of otitis media. He states that his left ear pain is better, but he has noticed some pus with some blood in that ear.
   a. What does the nurse suspect has happened?
   b. What would reveal an infecting agent?

10. As part of the procedure for instilling ear drops, a nurse would:
    a. Irrigate the ear if the membrane is not intact.
    b. Place the bottle of eardrops in a bowl of warm water for 5 minutes.
    c. Tilt the client's head in the opposite direction of the affected ear.
    d. Use sterile gloves during the procedure.

11. Your adult client has wax in his left ear. When irrigating his ear, you would use no more than _____ mL of solution.
    a. 50 to 70
    b. 150 to 170
    c. 125 to 140
    d. 90 to 120

12. The nurse would stop irrigating the ear if the client complained of:
    a. Headache.
    b. Nausea.
    c. Tingling sensation.
    d. Fatigue.

13. What would the nurse's instructions to the client include after a myringotomy? *Check all that apply.*
    ____ a. Report an excessive drainage to your physician.
    ____ b. Restrict hair washing for several days.
    ____ c. Use a straw for drinking liquids.
    ____ d. Report a fever to your physician.

14. Mastoiditis is an inflammation of the:
    a. Bones in the middle ear.
    b. Temporal bone behind the ear.
    c. Sixth and seventh cranial nerves.
    d. Labyrinth structure.

15. Which of the following statements about tinnitus are true? *Check all that apply.*
    ____ a. It is one of the most common complaints of clients with hearing disorders.
    ____ b. Diagnostic tests cannot confirm the disorder.
    ____ c. This disorder does not have observable characteristics.
    ____ d. Tinnitus can lead to particularly disturbing emotional consequences.

Answer the following two questions on a separate sheet of paper.

16. Identify four causes of tinnitus.

17. A male client has vertigo. What should the nurse advise him to do?

18. Meniere's disease is associated with: *Check all that apply.*
    ____ a. Viral or bacterial infection.
    ____ b. Allergic reactions.
    ____ c. Biochemical disturbances.
    ____ d. Genetic and familiar traits.

19. On a separate sheet of paper, identify the three distinct characteristics of Meniere's disease and give the pathologic changes associated with each.

20. An adult male client has been diagnosed with Meniere's disease. Which of the following would the nurse include in teaching for this client? *Check all that apply.*
    ___ a. Make slow head movements.
    ___ b. Reduce the intake of salt.
    ___ c. Stop smoking.
    ___ d. Take aspirin every 4 hours.

21. An acoustic neuroma is a:
    a. Tumor that is benign and rarely causes a problem.
    b. Malignant tumor that metastasizes quickly.
    c. Benign tumor that can be neurologically damaging.
    d. Benign tumor of cranial nerve VI.

Answer the following three questions on a separate sheet of paper.

22. Identify the causes of conductive hearing loss.

23. Identify the causes of sensorineural hearing loss. Which cause is easily preventable?

24. Presbycusis is a common cause of sensorineural hearing loss associated with aging. What are some physiologic changes associated with this loss?

25. What percentage of the population of clients aged 65 to 75 years suffers hearing loss?
    a. 15%
    b. 40%
    c. 35%
    d. 18%

26. Which of the following actions could prevent ear trauma?
    a. Holding your nose when sneezing to reduce pressure.
    b. Not using small objects to clean your external ear canal.
    c. Occluding one nostril when blowing your nose.
    d. Avoiding washing your external ear and canal.

27. A client has just started to wear a hearing aid. On a separate sheet of paper, indentify what special tips the nurse should offer to help this client adapt more easily to the hearing aid.

28. Which of the following is proper care of a hearing aid?
    a. Cleaning the hearing aid with mild soap and water.
    b. Storing the device with the battery conveniently left in place.
    c. Adjusting the volume at the highest setting to maximize hearing.
    d. Cleaning the debris from the hole in the middle with a pipe cleaner.

29. A tympanoplasty reconstructs the middle ear. Which of the following statements are true? *Check all that apply.*
    ___ a. The goal of a tympanoplasty is to improve hearing caused by conductive hearing loss.
    ___ b. Hearing loss after surgery is usually normal.
    ___ c. General anesthesia is usually required.
    ___ d. Water activities, such as swimming, are never permitted.

30. A client is recovering from ear surgery. On a separate sheet of paper, identify what instructions the nurse should incorporate in the discharge teaching.

31. The client who has had a stapedectomy should be told which of the following? *Check all that apply.*
    ___ a. Hearing is initially worse after surgery.
    ___ b. Success rate is high.
    ___ c. The surgery is low risk for hearing loss.
    ___ d. Hearing is improved immediately after surgery.

32. On a separate sheet of paper, briefly discuss some strategies for communicating with a hearing-impaired client.

UNIT 11 PROBLEMS OF MOBILITY: MUSCULOSKELETAL SYSTEM ■ Core Concepts Grid

Anatomy	Physiology	Pathophysiology	History	Physical Exam	Diagnostic Tests	Interventions	Pharmacology

• **Skeletal System**
Bones
Cartilage
Tendons
Ligaments
Joints
• **Muscular system**
	• Calcium storage
	• Hematopoesis
	• Protection
	• Form/framework
	• Motion
	• Joint articulation
		• Fracture
		• Sprain
		• Contusion
		• Trauma
		• Osteoporosis
		• Infection
			• **Client medical history**
			Injury
			Illness
			  Musculo skeletal
			  Systemic
			• **Family history**
			Congenital problems
			• **Social history**
			Occupation
			Sports
			Nutrition
			Age
			Race
			Gender
			• **Risk factors**
			Diet
			Exercise
				• Joint appearance
				• Gait
				• Range of motion
				• Flexion
				• Extension
				• Hyperextension
				• Abduction
				• Adduction
				• Pronation
				• Supination
				• Circumduction
				• Rotation
				• Inversion
				• Eversion
				• Alignment
				• Bruising/skin trauma
				• Kyphosis
					• Radiologic studies
					• Arthroscopy
					• Magnetic resonance imaging (MRI)
					• Bone scan
					• Serum calcium
					• Serum phosphorus
						• Cast care
						• Traction
						• Neurovascular checks
						• Braces/splints
						• Pin tract care
						• Skin assessment
						• Positioning
						• Logroll turning
						• Range-of-motion exercises
						• Body alignment
						• Lifestyle modifications
						  Diet
						  Exercise
						• Rest
						• Physical rehabilitiation
						• Preventing immobility complications
							• Analgesics
							• Muscle relaxants
							• Nonsteroidal anti-inflammatory drugs (NSAIDs)
							• Antibiotics
							• Calcium
							• Vitamin D
							• Selective estrogen receptor modulators
							• Anticoagulants

Unit 11 (Chapters 50-52)

Problems of Mobility: Management of Clients with Problems of the Musculoskeletal System

Learning Plan

Chapter 50: *Assessment of the Musculoskeletal System*

Learning Outcomes	Learning Activities	Supplemental Resources
1. Recall the anatomy and physiology of the musculoskeletal system.	1. Prior to completing the study guide exercises for this chapter, review the following:	1. Textbook—Chapter 50
2. Perform a musculoskeletal assessment using Gordon's Functional Health Patterns.	• Anatomy and physiology of the musculoskeletal system (muscles, bones, and joints)	2. Other resources:
3. Evaluate important assessment findings in a client with a musculoskeletal health problem.	• Physiology of muscle contraction	• Any anatomy and physiology textbook
4. Explain the use of laboratory testing for a client with a musculoskeletal health problem.	• Active and passive range-of-motion (ROM) exercises for each joint	• Any laboratory and diagnostic test manual
5. Identify the use radiography in diagnosing musculoskeletal health problems.	• Assessment of the musculoskeletal system	• Any pathophysiology textbook
6. Plan follow-up care for clients undergoing musculoskeletal diagnostic testing.	• Normal ROM for each joint	• Any physical assessment textbook
	• Effect of immobility on the musculoskeletal system	• National Association of Orthopaedic Nurses (NAON): North Woodbury Road, Box 56, Pitman, NJ 08071-0056; telephone: (609) 256-2310.
	2. Review the **boldfaced** Key Terms and their definitions in Chapter 50 to enhance your understanding of the content.	• O'Hanlon-Nichols, T. (1998). Basic assessment series: Musculoskeletal system. *American Journal of Nursing, 98*(6), 48-52.
	3. Go to Study Guide Number 11.50 on the following pages and complete the learning exercises for this chapter.	• Patel, P.R. & Lauerman, W.C. (1997). The use of magnetic resonance imaging in the diagnosis of lumbar disc disease. *Orthopedic Nursing, 16*(1) 59-65.
		• Salmond, S.W., et al. (Eds.) (1996). *Core curriculum for orthopaedic nursing* (3rd ed.). Pitman, NJ: National Association of Orthopaedic Nurses.

Chapter 51: *Interventions for Clients with Musculoskeletal Problems*

Learning Outcomes	Learning Activities	Supplemental Resources

1. Explain the risk factors for primary and secondary osteoporosis.
2. Describe ways to decrease the risk for osteoporosis.
3. Discuss the role of drug therapy in the prevention and management of osteoporosis.
4. Compare and contrast osteoporosis and osteomalacia.
5. Identify common assessment findings in clients with Paget's disease of the bone.
6. Differentiate acute and chronic osteomyelitis.
7. Analyze assessment data to determine common nursing diagnoses and collaborative problems for the client with a malignant bone tumor.
8. Discuss the psychosocial aspects associated with a diagnosis of bone cancer.
9. Develop a community-based plan of care for a client with a malignant bone tumor.
10. Evaluate the nursing care of a client with a bone tumor using expected outcome criteria.
11. Evaluate the pathophysiology and risk factors for carpal tunnel syndrome.
12. Discuss treatment options for the client diagnosed with carpal tunnel syndrome.
13. Describe common disorders of the foot, including hallux valgus and plantar fasciitis.
14. Explain the role of the nurse when caring for a client with muscular dystrophy.
	1. Prior to completing the study guide exercises for this chapter, review the following:
	  • Anatomy and physiology of the musculoskeletal system (muscles, bones, and joints)
	  • Perioperative nursing management
	  • Postoperative nursing management
	  • Wound and skin isolation, contact isolation, and drainage precautions
	  • Metabolism of calcium and vitamin D
	  • Parameters of a complete musculoskeletal and neurologic assessment
	  • Principles of IV therapy
	  • Concepts of growth and development
	  • Concept of body image and self-esteem
	  • Concepts of grief, loss, death, and dying
	2. Review the **boldfaced** Key Terms and their definitions in Chapter 51 to enhance your understanding of the content.
	3. Go to Study Guide Number 11.51 on the following pages and complete the learning exercises for this chapter.
		1. Textbook—Chapter 50 (Assessment of the Musculoskeletal System)
		2. Textbook—Chapter 51
		3. Other resources:
		  • Ailinger, R.L. & Emerson, J. (1998). Women's knowledge of osteoporosis. *Applied Nursing Research, 11*(3), 111-114.
		  • Any anatomy and physiology textbook
		  • Any laboratory and diagnostic test manual
		  • Any pathophysiology textbook
		  • Any physical assessment textbook
		  • Epps, C. (1994). *Complications in orthopaedic surgery* (3rd ed.). Philadelphia: J.B. Lippincott.
		  • Hunt, A.H. (1996). The relationship between height and change and bone mineral density. *Orthopaedic Nursing, 15*(3), 57-71.
		  • Kessenich, C.R. & Rosen, C.J. (1996). Vitamin D and bone status in elderly women. *Orthopaedic Nursing, 15*(3), 67-71.
		  • Maher, A.B., et al. (1998). *Orthopaedic nursing* (2nd ed.). Philadelphia: W.B. Saunders.
		  • National Association of Orthopaedic Nurses (NAON): North Woodbury Road, Box 56, Pitman, NJ 08071-0056; telephone: (609) 256-2310.

Chapter 52: *Interventions for Clients with Musculoskeletal Trauma*

Learning Outcomes	Learning Activities	Supplemental Resources

1. Compare and contrast common types of fractures.
2. Discuss the usual healing process for bone.
3. Identify common complications of fractures.
4. Explain the typical clinical manifestations that are seen in clients with one or more fractures.
5. Analyze common nursing diagnoses for the client with a fracture.
6. Describe the nursing care related to care of the client with a cast, including client education.
7. Describe the nursing care related to care of the client in traction.
8. Discuss pain management for the client with a fracture.
9. Prioritize nursing care for the postoperative client who has undergone open reduction with internal fixation of the hip.
10. Evaluate the nursing care of a client with a fracture.
11. Identify common types of amputations.
12. Explain the psychosocial aspects related to amputations.
13. Develop a community-based teaching plan for a client who has undergone an elective amputation.
14. Describe the collaborative management for the client with complex regional pain syndrome.
15. Identify the common types of sports-related injuries and their management.
	1. Prior to completing the study guide exercises for this chapter, review the following:
	  • Anatomy and physiology of the musculoskeletal system
	  • Principles of body mechanics
	  • Normal ROM for joints
	  • Parameters for a complete musculoskeletal and neurologic assessment
	  • Principles of perioperative and postoperative nursing management
	  • Concept of body image
	  • Principles of hot and cold therapy
	  • Concepts of grief and loss
	  • Gaits for crutch and cane walking: use of a walker
	  • Principles of rehabilitation
	
	2. Review the **boldfaced** Key Terms and their definitions in Chapter 52 to enhance your understanding of the content.
	
	3. Go to Study Guide Number 11.52 on the following pages and complete the learning exercises for this chapter.
		1. Textbook—Chapter 50 (Assessment of the Musculoskeletal System)
		1. Textbook—Chapter 52
		2. Other resources:
		  • Any anatomy and physiology textbook
		  • Any physical assessment textbook
		  • Any pathophysiology textbook
		  • Any laboratory and diagnostic test manual
		  • Epps, C. (1994). *Complications in orthopaedic surgery* (3rd ed.). Philadelphia: J.B. Lippincott.
		  • Hefti, D. (1995). Complications of trauma: The nurse's role in prevention. *Orthopaedic nursing, 14*(6), 9-16.
		  • Maher, A.B., et al. (1998). *Orthopaedic nursing* (2nd ed.). Philadelphia: W.B. Saunders.
		  • National Amputation Foundation: 12-45 150th Street, Whitestone, NY 11357.
		  • National Association of Orthopaedic Nurses (NAON): North Woodbury Road, Box 56, Pitman, NJ 08071-0056; telephone: (609) 256-2310.
		  • Taffet, R. (Ed.). (1997). Trauma to the adult pelvis and hips. *Orthopaedic Clinics of North America, 28*(3), 299-477.

STUDY GUIDE NUMBER 11.50

Assessment of the Musculoskeletal System

Study/Review Questions

1. Identify the four common types of bones and give an example of each.
   a. _____
   b. _____
   c. _____
   d. _____

2. Match each of the following musculoskeletal terms with the corresponding description.

   Terms
   ____ a. Cancellous
   ____ b. Cortex
   ____ c. Diaphysis
   ____ d. Epiphysis
   ____ e. Haversian system
   ____ f. Osteoblast
   ____ g. Osteoclast
   ____ h. Osteocyte
   ____ i. Periosteum
   ____ j. Trabeculae
   ____ k. Volkmann's canal

   Descriptions
   1. Living bone cells
   2. Shaft of a long bone
   3. Outer layer of bone tissue
   4. Longitudinal canal network containing blood vessels
   5. End of a long bone
   6. Spongy inner layer of bone
   7. Network connecting bone marrow vessels to outer bone covering
   8. Bone-forming cells
   9. Bone tissue containing marrow
   10. Highly vascular bone covering
   11. Bone-destroying cells

3. Identify the six major functions of the skeletal system.
   a. _____
   b. _____
   c. _____
   d. _____
   e. _____
   f. _____

Describe each of the following types of joints and give an example of each.

4. Synarthrodial joints
   _____
   _____
   _____
   _____

5. Amphiarthrodial joints
   _____
   _____
   _____
   _____

6. Diarthrodial joints
   _____
   _____
   _____
   _____

Read the following statements and decide whether each is true or false. Write T for true or F for false in the blanks provided. If the statement is false, correct the statement to make it true.

____ 7. The knee is considered to be a "ball-and-socket" joint.

____ 8. The elbow is considered to be a "hinge" joint.

____ 9. Pivotal joints allow for flexion and extension only.

____ 10. Biaxial joints allow for gliding movement such as that done with the wrist.

___ 11. Condylar joints allow for flexion and extension only.

Describe each of the following types of muscle tissue and identify their functions

12. Smooth muscle _____
_____
_____
_____

13. Cardiac muscle _____
_____
_____
_____

14. Skeletal muscle _____
_____
_____
_____

15. Match each of the following musculoskeletal terms with the corresponding definition.

Terms
___ a. Atrophy
___ b. Bursa
___ c. Cartilage
___ d. Fascia
___ e. Fasciculi
___ f. Ligament
___ g. Synovium
___ h. Synovial fluid
___ i. Tendon

Definitions
1. Membrane that secretes a lubricating fluid
2. Decrease in size and number of muscle fibers
3. Sac preventing joint friction
4. Band of tough, fibrous tissue attaching muscle to bone
5. Bundles of muscle fibers
6. Lubricating liquid
7. Band of tough, fibrous tissue attaching bone to bone
8. Fibrous tissue surrounding muscle
9. Collagen fibers at bone ends

Read the following statements and decide whether each is true or false. Write T for true or F for false in the blanks provided. If the statement is false, correct the statement to make it true.

____16. As one ages, bone density often increases.

____17. As one ages, synovial joint cartilage regenerates.

____18. Degenerative joint disease, muscle atrophy, slowed movement, and decreased strength are common changes in the musculoskeletal system of the older adult.

For each of the categories of assessment listed below, identify one finding that would indicate a risk factor for an actual or potential problem of the musculoskeletal system.

19. History _____
_____
_____

20. Demographic data _____
_____
_____

21. Women's health _____
_____
_____

22. Personal and family history _____
_____
_____

23. Diet history _____
_____
_____

24. Older adults _____
_____
_____

25. Socioeconomic status _____
_____
_____

26. Cultural _____
_____
_____

27. Current health problem _____
_____
_____

28. Posture _____
_____
_____

29. Gait _____
_____
_____

30. Mobility _____
_____
_____

31. Head and neck _____
_____
_____

32. Spine _____
_____
_____

33. Upper extremities _____
_____
_____

34. Lower extremities _____
_____
_____

35. Muscular system _____
_____
_____

36. Psychosocial _____
_____
_____

37. While the nurse observes the client performing range-of-motion (ROM) exercises, she notes that he can spread his fingers apart. She would document this movement as:
a. Flexion.
b. Adduction.
c. Extension.
d. Abduction.

38. The instrument used to assess joint ROM is:
a. An odometer.
b. An ergometer.
c. A goniometer.
d. A spectrometer.

39. Which of the following is an abnormal finding in the physical assessment of the musculoskeletal system?
a. Upper extremities symmetric, equal muscle mass
b. Gait balanced, stride smooth and regular
c. Flexion, extension, and rotation of the neck
d. Opposition of three of four fingers to the thumb

40. Which of the following is primarily responsible for regulating serum calcium levels?
a. Calcitonin
b. Vitamin D
c. Glucocorticoids
d. Growth hormone

41. Which of the following is present in bone and serum in direct proportion to calcium?
a. Estrogen
b. Phosphorus
c. Thyroxine
d. Insulin

42. Which of the following laboratory results may indicate bone or liver damage, such as metastatic cancer of the bone?
a. Serum calcium 9.0 mg/dL
b. Serum calcium 8.2 mg/dL
c. Serum phosphorus 3.2 mg/dL
d. Alkaline phosphatase 115 U/L

43. Match each of the following radiographic examinations and diagnostic tests with the corresponding definition.

Radiographic Examinations

___ a. Tomography
___ b. Xeroradiography
___ c. Myelography
___ d. Arthrography
___ e. Computed tomography (CT)
___ f. Bone biopsy
___ g. Muscle biopsy
___ h. Electromyography
___ i. Arthroscopy
___ j. Bone scan
___ k. Gallium/thallium scan
___ l. Magnetic resonance imaging (MRI)
___ m. Ultrasonography

Definitions

1. An isotope is administered 1 to 2 days before testing; procedure takes 30 to 60 minutes; client must lie still; mild sedation may be necessary. Test can be used to evaluate cancers of the bone.

2. A contrast may or may not be given; if contrast is given, then client must be kept NPO for at least 4 hours; client cannot be allergic to iodine. Excellent test to detect vertebral column disorders. Claustrophobia and annoyance from clicking sounds are common complaints.

3. Helpful in detailing the musculoskeletal system because it produces planes, or slices, for focusing and blurs the images of other structures.

4. Invasive test that may confirm the presence of infection or neoplasm. A long needle is inserted into the bone cortex, or a small incision is made to reveal the bone tissue. The nurse must monitor the site for bleeding, swelling, hematoma formation, and pain. If an open procedure is used, the nurse must teach the client how to change the dressing daily while inspecting the site for signs of infection.

5. Margins and edges are clearly seen because this test highlights the contrast between structures. A drawback to this test is that it exposes the client to higher doses of radiation and lacks the ability to determine tissue densities.

6. A contrast medium or dye is injected into the subarachnoid space of the spine. The vertebral column, intervertebral disks, spinal nerve roots, and blood vessels all can be visualized. This test is becoming less popular as other less invasive and less painful tests are replacing it.

7. Used for the diagnosis of atrophy (as in muscular dystrophy) and inflammation (as in polymyositis).

8. A fiberoptic tube is inserted into a joint for direct visualization; the knee and shoulder are most commonly evaluated. Multiple incisions may be required. The nurse evaluates the neurovascular status of the client's affected limb frequently after the procedure. The nurse must instruct the client to contact the physician immediately if after discharge the client exhibits severe joint or limb pain.

9. Radioactive material is injected for visualization of the entire skeletal system. This test is used to detect tumors, arthritis, osteomyelitis, vertebral compression fractures, osteoporosis, and unexplained bone pain. The client must void before the test, and the nurse encourages the client to push fluids after the test.

10. Sound waves produce an image of the tissue. This test may be used to visualize osteomyelitis, soft-tissue disorders (such as masses and fluid accumulation), and traumatic injuries. No special preparation or post-test care is indicated.

11. An image is produced through the interaction of magnetic fields, radio waves, and atomic nuclei showing hydrogen density. This test is particularly useful in identifying problems with muscles, tendons, and ligaments. The nurse must ensure that the client removes all metal objects. The nurse must question the client about prior surgical procedures in which surgical clips were used, or if the client has a pacemaker.

12. This test is usually accompanied by nerve conduction studies to determine the electrical potential generated in an individual muscle. It helps to diagnose neuromuscular, lower motor neuron, and peripheral nerve disorders. The nurse informs the client that there may be temporary discomfort while the client is exposed to episodes of electrical current. If the client is taking muscle relaxants, the physician may temporarily discontinue the medication for several days before testing to prevent the medication from having effects on the test results. The nurse must monitor the needle sites for hematoma formation and provide comfort measures.

STUDY GUIDE NUMBER 11.51

Interventions for Clients with Musculoskeletal Problems

Study/Review Questions

1. Briefly describe each of the following metabolic bone diseases. *Use a separate sheet of paper if needed.*

   a. Osteoporosis _____
   _____
   _____
   _____

   b. Primary osteoporosis _____
   _____
   _____
   _____

   c. Secondary osteoporosis _____
   _____
   _____
   _____

   d. Osteomalacia _____
   _____
   _____
   _____

   e. Paget's disease _____
   _____
   _____
   _____

2. Match each of the following musculoskeletal disorders with the corresponding risk factors.

   Musculoskeletal Disorders
   ___ a. Osteoporosis
   ___ b. Osteomalacia
   ___ c. Paget's disease

   Risk Factors
   1. Older adults; vitamin D deficiency; insufficient exposure to sunlight
   2. Possibly a result of latent viral infection
   3. Female; white; menopause; thin; lean; immobilization

3. Describe three ways a person could reduce his or her risk for osteoporosis.

   a. _____
   _____

   b. _____
   _____

   c. _____
   _____

4. Match the following subjective client data with the musculoskeletal disorders they are primarily associated with. *Answers may be used more than once.*

Subjective Client Data	Musculoskeletal Disorders
___ a. Headache	1. Osteoporosis
___ b. Dress hem longer in front	2. Osteomalacia
___ c. Muscle cramps	3. Paget's disease
___ d. Smokes two packs of cigarettes per day	
___ e. Back pain relieved by rest	
___ f. Fatigue	
___ g. Milk intolerance	
___ h. Sedentary lifestyle	
___ i. Pelvic bone pain, worse at night	
___ j. Drinks eight cups of coffee per day	
___ k. Dizziness	
___ l. Muscle weakness in legs	
___ m. Loss of height	

5. Match the following subjective client data with the musculoskeletal disorders they are primarily associated with. *Answers may be used more than once.*

Subjective Client Data	Musculoskeletal Disorders
____ a. Unsteady gait	1. Osteoporosis
____ b. Hip flexion contractures	2. Osteomalacia
____ c. Flushed warm skin	3. Paget's disease
____ d. Vertebral fracture	
____ e. Bone tenderness over rib cage	
____ f. Kyphosis	
____ g. Long bone bowing	
____ h. Discomfort on vertebral palpation	
____ i. Soft skull	

Explain briefly why each of the following drug therapies would benefit the client in the prevention of and/or management of osteoporosis.

6. Estrogen _____

_____

7. Calcium _____

_____

8. Vitamin D _____

_____

9. Biphosphonates (BPs) _____

_____

10. Selective estrogen receptor modulators (SERMs)

_____

_____

11. Calcitonin _____

_____

12. Match each of the following precautions and/or side effects to the appropriate drug therapy.

Precautions/Side Effects	Drug Therapy
____ a. Esophagitis and esophageal ulcers; drug should not be given to clients with poor renal function; hypocalcemia or GERD	1. Calcitonin
	2. Vitamin D
	3. Estrogen
	4. Calcium
	5. SERMs (Evista)
	6. BPs (Fosamax)
____ b. Hypercalcemia; can cause serious damage to the urinary system.	
____ c. Low doses may be prescribed because of the potentially serious side effects, such as endometrial or breast cancer	

____ d. If used intranasally, may cause nasal mucosal irritation

____ e. Should not be given to women with a history of thrombosis

____ f. Hypercalcemia and hyperphosphatemia

13. Osteomalacia can be a complication of the intake of certain drugs. Identify the three drugs commonly associated with this circumstance.

a. _____

b. _____

c. _____

Briefly describe the two major types of osteomyelitis and differentiate between them.

14. Acute osteomyelitis _____

_____

_____

_____

15. Chronic osteomyelitis _____

_____

_____

_____

16. Briefly describe the pathophysiologic process involved in osteomyelitis._____

_____

_____

_____

17. Your adult client is a carpenter. One day he was building a house and using an automatic nailing gun for his work. As he reached up to nail a piece of wood in place, he missed the wood and the nail fired into his hand. This would be an example of which of the following routes that could lead to osteomyelitis?
   a. Acute hematogenous spread
   b. Contiguous spread
   c. Direct inoculation
   d. Indirect inoculation

18. Which of the following is usually not an assessment finding that the nurse would note for the client with acute osteomyelitis?
   a. Fever, usually above 101° F
   b. Sinus tract formation
   c. Erythema of the affected area
   d. Swelling around the affected area

19. Which of the following statements is correct or relevant to antibiotic therapy for the client with osteomyelitis?
    a. Single-agent therapy is the most effective treatment for acute infections.
    b. The optimal drug regimen for chronic osteomyelitis is well established.
    c. Clients usually remain hospitalized to complete the full course of antibiotic therapy.
    d. The infected wound may be irrigated with one or more types of antibiotic solutions.

20. Match each of the following terms related to bone tumors with its corresponding definition.

    Bone Tumors
    ___ a. Chondrogenic
    ___ b. Fibrogenic
    ___ c. Osteogenic
    ___ d. Primary tumor
    ___ e. Sarcoma
    ___ f. Secondary tumor

    Definitions
    1. Tumor originating in bone
    2. Tumor arising from bone
    3. Malignant tumor metastasizing to bone
    4. Tumor arising from cartilage
    5. Tumor arising from fibrous tissue
    6. Malignant bone tumor arising from underlying tissue

21. Match each type of benign tumor with its most common location.

Types of Benign Tumors	**Most Common Locations**
___ a. Chondroma	1. Vertebra
___ b. Giant cell tumor	2. Femur and tibia
___ c. Osteoblastoma	3. Metastasis to lung
___ d. Osteoid osteoma	4. Hands and feet

22. Match each of the following types of malignant bone tumors with the associated signs and symptoms.

Types of Malignant Bone Tumors	**Signs and Symptoms**
___ a. Chondrosarcoma	1. Local tenderness in lower extremity long bones
___ b. Ewing's sarcoma	
___ c. Fibrosarcoma	2. Short-term pain and swelling in distal femur
___ d. Osteosarcoma	

    3. Long-term dull pain near proximal femur
    4. Pain and swelling in lower pelvis

23. Identify the common sites of formation of primary tumors that metastasize to the bone.
    a. _____
    b. _____
    c. _____
    d. _____
    e. _____

24. Identify the common sites for bone tumor metastases.
    a. _____
    b. _____
    c. _____
    d. _____

Read the following nursing assessment findings regarding malignant bone tumors and decide whether each is true or false. Write T for true or F for false in the blanks provided. If the statement is false, correct the statement to make it true.

___ 25. Osteosarcoma is the most common type of malignant bone tumor; the lesion is large and causes pain and swelling of short duration. The involved area is usually warm. This lesion typically metastasizes to the periphery of the lung within 2 years of treatment.

___ 26. Ewing's sarcoma is not as common as the other tumors and therefore is not as malignant. It also causes pain and swelling, as well as fever, leukocytosis, and anemia.

___ 27. Ewing's sarcoma is often confused with osteomyelitis.

___ 28. Chondrosarcoma typically affects the pelvis and proximal femur near the diaphysis. The client typically verbalizes complaints of swelling and constant, severe, throbbing pain.

___ 29. Fibrosarcoma clinically presents slowly and insidiously, without specific manifestations. Local tenderness, with or without a palpable mass, occurs in the long bones of the lower extremity.

Identify the pertinent data in each of the following categories that the nurse would collect in an assessment of the client with suspected metastatic bone disease.

30. History _____
    _____

31. Clinical manifestations _____
    _____
    _____

32. Psychosocial _____
_____

33. Identify two nursing diagnoses and two collaborative problems based on your assessment findings relevant to the client with suspected metastatic bone disease.
Nursing diagnoses: _____
_____

Collaborative problems: _____
_____

34. Match the following radiographic findings with their associated types of bone tumor growths. *Answers may be used more than once.*

Radiographic Findings	Types of Bone Tumors
___ a. Poor margination	1. Benign
___ b. Intact cortices	2. Malignant
___ c. Bone destruction	
___ d. Cortical breakthrough	
___ e. Smooth uniform periosteal bone	
___ f. Irregular new periosteal bone	
___ g. Sharp margins	

35. Identify six interventions for pain management relevant to the client with bone tumors.
a. _____
b. _____
c. _____
d. _____
e. _____
f. _____

36. Which of the following assessment findings in the client who has undergone a bone graft for a tumor should the nurse report to the physician immediately?
a. Extremity distal to operative site warm and pink
b. Cast over operative site cool
c. Blanch response in distal digits lasting longer than 5 seconds
d. Pain in operative extremity relieved by analgesics

37. Interventions to assist the client with a bone tumor who is grieving and anxious include: *Check all that apply.*
___ a. Allowing the client to verbalize feelings.
___ b. Offering to call the client's clergy person or religious leader.
___ c. Preparing the client for death.
___ d. Listening attentively while the client talks.

38. Identify six expected outcomes for the client with a malignant bone tumor, based on identified nursing diagnoses and collaborative problems.
a. _____
b. _____
c. _____
d. _____
e. _____
f. _____

39. Briefly describe the pathophysiology and related risk factors for carpal tunnel syndrome.
a. Pathophysiology _____
_____
_____

b. Risk factors _____
_____
_____

Answer the following two questions on a separate sheet of paper.

40. Briefly describe Phalen's maneuver.

41. What is Tinnel's sign?

42. Identify the two common conservative measures the health care provider may use before surgical intervention as a treatment option for the client with carpal tunnel syndrome. Give an example of each.
a. _____
b. _____

43. Identify and briefly describe the two common surgical procedures for carpal tunnel syndrome.
a. _____
b. _____

44. Match the following characteristics to the hand disorders they are primarily associated with. *Answers may be used more than once.*

Characteristics	Hand Disorders
___ a. Pain worse at night	1. Carpal tunnel syndrome
___ b. Round, cyst-like lesion	2. Dupuytren's contracture
___ c. First three digits affected	3. Ganglion
___ d. Progressive palmar flexion deformity	
___ e. Joint discomfort after strain	
___ f. Median nerve compression	
___ g. Fourth and fifth digits affected	
___ h. Swollen synovium	
___ i. Familial tendency common	
___ j. Colles' fracture or hand burns	
___ k. Occupational hazard	

45. Match each of the following characteristics to the foot disorder it is primarily associated with. *Answers may be used more than once.*

   Characteristics
   ___ a. Dorsiflexion of any MTP joint with plantar flexion of the adjacent PIP joint
   ___ b. A small tumor in a digital nerve of the foot
   ___ c. Often referred to as a bunion
   ___ d. Pain is acute; burning sensation in the web space
   ___ e. Posterior tibial nerve in ankle becomes compressed
   ___ f. Pain in the arch of the foot, especially when getting out of bed
   ___ g. Can occur as a result of poorly fitted shoes
   ___ h. Corns may develop on the dorsal side of the toe
   ___ i. Surgical procedure involves removal of the bony overgrowth and bursa
   ___ j. Diagnosis and treatment are similar to those for carpal tunnel syndrome
   ___ k. Commonly seen in athletes, especially runners
   ___ l. Inflammation of the plantar fascia
   ___ m. Insertion of Kirschner wires for fixation

   Foot Disorders
   1. Hallux valgus
   2. Hammertoe
   3. Morton's neuroma
   4. Tarsal tunnel syndrome
   5. Plantar fasciitis

Read the following statements regarding scoliosis and decide whether each is true or false. Write T for true or F for false in the blanks provided. If the statement is false, correct the statement to make it true.

___ 46. Scoliosis is a C- or S-shaped lateral curvature of the vertebral spine.

___ 47. The abnormal curvature can cause low back pain.

___ 48. Men are affected more than women.

___ 49. Children are typically screened for scoliosis before starting school.

___ 50. Surgical intervention is the least common treatment for adults.

___ 51. Luque and Cotrel-Dubousset instrumentation allows for the client to be able to get out of bed by the end of the day on the day of surgery or the day after surgery.

52. Match each of the following characteristics and physical findings with the associated musculoskeletal disorder. *Answers may be used more than once.*

   Characteristics/ Physical Findings
   ___ a. Muscle atrophy and weakness
   ___ b. Fragile and deformed bones
   ___ c. Cardiac involvement
   ___ d. Presenile deafness
   ___ e. Poor skeletal development

   Musculoskeletal Disorders
   1. Osteogenesis imperfecta
   2. Muscular dystrophy

53. Briefly discuss the role of the nurse when caring for a client with muscular dystrophy.

Case Study: The Client with Osteoporosis

A 67-year-old postmenopausal woman has come to your clinic complaining of lower backache. She states that this pain is interfering with her sleep. She gets together weekly with her friends to play cards, and lately has had to cancel. She says she is afraid her back will give out on her and she will fall. She states that the pain is interfering with her social life and other daily activities and that the episodes are becoming unbearable so she has decided to seek treatment.

Answer the following questions on a separate sheet of paper:

1. You suspect she may have osteoporosis. Identify six questions that you would ask her while performing her assessment.

2. During your assessment you discover that she does not take estrogen. What main question would you ask the client that would be important in determining any contraindications or precautions if the physician decides to place her on estrogen replacement therapy?

3. This client tells you that she does not like milk and rarely drinks it. How could you get her to increase her calcium intake?

4. The physician suspects osteoporosis as well and has ordered x-ray studies of her spine. When the films come back, they appear normal. The client asks you, "How can this be?" How would you respond to her?

5. The client's laboratory studies have returned as well, and you have informed her that her calcium levels were near normal. She says to you, "This is ridiculous. How can I have osteoporosis if I have the right amount of calcium in my blood?" How will you respond to her now and why?

6. Determine appropriate measures to relieve this client's back pain.

7. The client states that she does not exercise. She tells you that the most exercise she gets is going up and down a few stairs to get to and from her car. What advice could you give her in regard to exercise?

STUDY GUIDE NUMBER 11.52

Interventions for Clients with Musculoskeletal Trauma

Study/Review Questions

1. Compare and contrast the following pairs of fracture types. *Use a separate sheet of paper for your answer.*
   a. Complete versus incomplete
   b. Open versus closed
   c. Pathologic versus fatigue
   d. Greenstick versus spiral

2. Match each of the following descriptions to the corresponding type of fracture.

   Descriptions
   ___ a. An adult client was riding his four-wheeler on a country road late one evening. Off in the distance he saw several cows in the middle of the road. He turned

   Types of Factures
   1. Pathologic (spontaneous) fracture
   2. Incomplete fracture
   3. Open (compound) fracture

   sharply to avoid hitting them and spun out of control. His four-wheeler landed on top of him. His lower leg is obviously broken. It is bleeding and bone fragments are protruding from the skin.

   ___ b. One afternoon in her classroom, a schoolteacher slipped on some chalk that had fallen from the blackboard. She did not fall far and seemed to be all right. With the help of a student she was able to walk to the office. The secretary drove her to the emergency room.

   ___ c. Your adult female client has osteoporosis. She plays cards often with her friends. One morning she was opening her car door while on her way to play cards when all of a sudden she fell. She said it was as though her "leg gave way" and caused her to fall.

3. Match each of the following terms related to the fracture healing process with its definition.

   Definitions
   ___ a. Callus
   ___ b. Granulation
   ___ c. Hematoma
   ___ d. Remodeling

   Fracture Terminology
   1. Mass of clotted blood at fracture site
   2. Process of bone building and resorption
   3. Outgrowth of new capillaries
   4. Non-bony union at fracture site

4. Indicate the numeric sequence of bone healing from the beginning.
   ___ a. Callus formation
   ___ b. Bone remodeling
   ___ c. Hematoma formation
   ___ d. Osteoblastic proliferation
   ___ e. Hematoma to granulation tissue

5. Identify the complications associated with fractures.
   a. _____
   b. _____
   c. _____
   d. _____
   e. _____
   f. _____
   g. _____
   h. _____

6. Briefly explain why acute compartment syndrome is a medical emergency. *Answer on a separate sheet of paper.*

7. Identify eight signs and symptoms associated with acute compartment syndrome.
   a. _____
   b. _____
   c. _____
   d. _____
   e. _____
   f. _____
   g. _____
   h. _____

8. Identify four possible complications resulting from acute compartment syndrome.
   a. _____
   b. _____
   c. _____
   d. _____

Answer the following two questions on a separate sheet of paper.

9. Briefly describe a fasciotomy.

10. Identify the type of shock that is a possible complication of fractures.

11. Identify the types of fractures that are primarily associated with fat embolism syndrome.
    a. _____
    b. _____
    c. _____

Answer the following two questions on a separate sheet of paper.

12. What is the earliest manifestation of fat embolism syndrome?

13. Identify the signs and symptoms the client would exhibit in response to low arterial oxygen levels.

14. Identify the types of clients with fractures who are at an increased risk for developing deep vein thrombosis.
    a. _____
    b. _____
    c. _____
    d. _____

15. Match each of the following fracture complications with its corresponding definition.

    Fracture Complications   **Definitions**
    ___ a. Blood supply to the   1. Delayed union
           bone is disrupted,   2. Fat embolism
           which results in the   3. Fracture blisters
           death of bone tissue   4. Mal-union
           syndrome   5. Avascular necrosis
    ___ b. Incorrect fracture   6. Nonunion
           healing
    ___ c. Fat globules are released from the yellow
           bone marrow into the bloodstream
    ___ d. Incomplete fracture healing
    ___ e. Extensive tissue edema allows fluid to move
           into the weakened space between the epidermis and the dermis
    ___ f. Lack of fracture healing

Answer the following three questions on a separate sheet of paper.

16. Briefly define *crepitation (crepitus)*.

17. Identify five common nursing diagnoses for clients with fractures.

18. Briefly describe the emergency measures taken in an acute trauma situation to assist a client who may have suffered a fracture.

19. Identify the methods used to immobilize fractures.
    a. _____
    b. _____
    c. _____
    d. _____
    e. _____

Answer the following four questions on a separate sheet of paper.

20. The nurse's primary responsibility is to assess the area distal to an immobilization device. Briefly describe what the nurse would be evaluating.

21. Describe nursing interventions used to preserve cast integrity from the time of application to removal.

22. Explain why a nurse may cut a "window" into a cast.

23. Identify complications that may result from cast application.

24. Match each of the following definitions to the corresponding type of traction.

Definitions	**Types of Traction**
____ a. Involves the use of a Velcro boot (Bucks), belt, or halter, which is secured around a body part	1. Plaster traction 2. Brace traction 3. Skin traction 4. Circumferential traction 5. Skeletal traction
____ b. Pins, wires, tongs, or screws are surgically inserted directly into bone	
____ c. Combines skeletal traction and a plaster cast	
____ d. Exerts a pull for correction of alignment deformities	
____ e. Uses a belt around the body	

Answer the following three questions on a separate sheet of paper.

25. Describe the nurse's role in caring for the client in traction.

26. Define the major disadvantage of skin traction.

27. Define the major disadvantages of skeletal traction.

28. Identify the three most common types of medications prescribed for the client with a fracture.
    a. _____
    b. _____
    c. _____

29. Identify alternative (non-drug) nursing interventions that may be used to relieve pain in the client with a fracture.
    a. _____
    b. _____
    c. _____
    d. _____
    e. _____
    f. _____
    g. _____

30. On a separate sheet of paper, explain why open reduction with internal fixation (ORIF) is often the preferred surgical method for older adults.

31. Briefly describe four advantages and one disadvantage of external fixation.
    Advantages:

    Disadvantage:

32. On a separate sheet of paper, prioritize nursing care for the client who has undergone ORIF of the hip.

33. Identify the potential complications related to impaired physical mobility in the client with a fracture.
    a. _____
    b. _____
    c. _____
    d. _____
    e. _____
    f. _____

34. Which of the following mobilization devices is usually preferred for the older client?
    a. Crutches
    b. Cane
    c. Walker
    d. Wheelchair

Answer the following three questions on a separate sheet of paper.

35. Briefly describe an open (guillotine) method amputation.

36. Briefly describe a closed (flap) method amputation.

37. Briefly describe a traumatic amputation and provide examples of such.

38. Identify the complications that may result from an amputation.
    a. _____
    b. _____
    c. _____
    d. _____
    e. _____
    f. _____

39. On a separate sheet of paper, describe the two groups of clients most likely to experience an amputation.

40. Identify two psychosocial manifestations exhibited by the client who experiences an amputation.

41. On a separate sheet of paper, describe the three stages of complex regional pain syndrome (CRPS).

42. Identify the first priority of management in the client with CRPS.

43. Identify three members of the health care team the nurse would collaborate with for management of the client with CRPS.
    a. _____
    b. _____
    c. _____

44. Identify the most common sites of injury to the knee.
    a. _____
    b. _____
    c. _____
    d. _____

45. On a separate sheet of paper, briefly define and describe the McMurray test.

Read the following statements and decide whether each is true or false. Write T for true or F for false in the blanks provided. If the statement is false, correct the statement to make it true.

____ 46. The lateral meniscus is more likely to tear than the medial meniscus.

____ 47. When the anterior cruciate ligament (ACL) is torn, the person may feel a "snap."

____ 48. Complete healing of knee ligaments after surgery only takes 3 to 4 weeks.

____ 49. Rupture of the Achilles tendon is common in older adults.

____ 50. Dislocation is most common in the hip, shoulder, knee, and fingers.

____ 51. A strain is excessive stretching of a ligament.

____ 52. Management of a strain usually involves cold and heat applications.

____ 53. Sprains are usually precipitated by twisting motions from a fall or sports injury.

____ 54. Clients with a torn rotator cuff have shoulder pain and cannot initiate or maintain adduction of the arm at the shoulder (drop arm test).

55. Match each of the following terms related to musculoskeletal injuries with the corresponding definition.

Definitions	Types of Musculoskeletal Injuries
____ a. Incomplete joint surface separation	1. Dislocation
____ b. Injury to ligament	2. Sprain
____ c. Joint surfaces not approximated	3. Strain
____ d. Excessive stretching of muscle or tendon	4. Subluxation

Simon. *Case Study: The Client with Traumatic Amputation*

A 25-year-old carpenter comes running into the emergency department where you are working with a blood-soaked rag over his right hand. He states that while working on a house he was building, he sawed off his right index finger. He has the finger in his pocket. You put on gloves and apply pressure with sterile gauze to the amputated area. You find out during your assessment, that he has a history of depression and takes medication for it. You have identified during your assessment that he has no significant medical history other than depression.

Answer the following questions on a separate sheet of paper:

1. Identify the type of amputation that would be considered for this client.

2. Identify the top nursing priority in dealing with the client's amputated finger.

3. What would you do with the client's finger?

4. Identify two appropriate nursing diagnoses for this client.

5. Identify the type of shock for which this client is at risk.

6. Considering this client's history, what recommendations would you make?

UNIT 12 PROBLEMS OF DIGESTION, NUTRITION, AND ELIMINATION: GI SYSTEM ■ Core Concepts Grid

Anatomy	Physiology	Pathophysiology	History	Physical Exam	Diagnostic Tests	Interventions	Pharmacology
• Oropharynx • Esophagus • Stomach • Small intestine • Large intestine • Liver • Gallbladder • Pancreas • Rectum • Anus	• Absorption • Specialized secretions • Digestion Hydrochloric acid Lipase Amylase • Phagocytosis • Coagulation • Synthesis of Proteins Carbohydrates Fat Vitamins • Detoxification	• Inflammation • Infection • Obstruction • Hemorrhage • Perforation • Dumping syndrome • Erosion • Ascites	• Client history of Past problems Pain • Family history of digestive system problems • Social history Alcohol Drugs Stress management Occupation Age Race Gender • Bowel habits • Diet	• Mouth • Skin Striae Cullen's sign Grey-Turner's sign Color • Peristalsis • Bowel sounds • Bruits • Tympany • Masses • Abdominal distention • Swallowing • Intake • Vital signs	• Upper/lower GI series • Endoscopy • Esophagastroduodenoscopy (EGD) • Endoscopic retrograde cholangiopancreatography (ERCP) • Ultrasonography • CAT scan • Liver biopsy • Gastric analysis • Fecal analysis • Serum bilirubin • Aspartate aminotransferase (AST) • Alanine aminotransferase (ALT) • Lactate dehydrogenase (LDH) • Amylase • Lipase • Culture *Helicobacter pylori*	• Therapeutic diets • Saline lavage • Sclerotherapy • Tamponade • Extracorporeal shock wave lithotripsy (ESWL) • Rest • Tube Blakemore Nasogastric Nasoenteric Gastrostomy • Ostomies Colostomy Ileostomy • Postoperative care • Rest • Fluid replacement • Blood transfusion • Health teaching	• Antacids • Histamine blockers • Vasocontrictors • Corticosteroids • Anticholinergics • Chenodeoxycholic acid • Urodeoxycholic acid • Immune serum globulin • Hepatitis A vaccine (HAV) • Hepatitis B vaccine (HBV) • Bowel stimulants • Antidiarrheals • Antibiotics • Lactulose • Chemotherapeutic agents

Unit 12 (Chapters 53-61)

Problems of Digestion, Nutrition, and Elimination: Management of Clients with Problems of the Gastrointestinal System

Learning Plan

Chapter 53: *Assessment of the Gastrointestinal System*

Learning Outcomes	Learning Activities	Supplemental Resources

1. Recall the anatomy and physiology of the gastrointestinal system.
2. Perform a gastrointestinal assessment using Gordon's functional health patterns.
3. Evaluate important assessment findings in a client with a gastrointestinal health problem.
4. Explain the use of laboratory testing for a client with a gastrointestinal health problem.
5. Identify the use of radiography in diagnosing gastrointestinal health problems.
6. Plan a follow-up care for clients having endoscopic procedures.
	1. Prior to completing the study guide exercises in this chapter, review the following:
	  • Anatomy and physiology of the gastrointestinal system
	  • Effect of central and autonomic nervous systems on the gastrointestinal organs
	  • Normal nutrition, including the essential vitamins, minerals, and foods in the recommended food groups
	  • Special diets (such as low salt, high or low protein, high carbohydrate, high or low fiber, low fat, bland, liquid, and pureed) for clients with gastrointestinal organ disorders
	  • Parameters of a complete gastrointestinal assessment
	  • Principles of enema administration
	  • Normal fluid and electrolyte values
	
	2. Review the **boldfaced** Key Terms and their definitions in Chapter 53 to enhance your understanding of the content.
	
	3. Go Study Guide Number 12.53 on the following pages and complete the learning exercises for this chapter.
		1. Textbook—Chapter 53
		2. Other resources:
		  • Any anatomy and physiology textbook
		  • Any laboratory and diagnostic test manual
		  • Any pathophysiology textbook
		  • Any physical assessment textbook
		  • Butler, M. (1996). Preparing patients for endoscopic tests. *Practice Nurse, 11*(10), 707-712.
		  • Dammel, T. (1997). Fecal occult blood testing: Looking for hidden danger. *Nursing 97, 27*(7), 44-45.
		  • Gitnick, C. (Ed.). (1992). *Current gastroenterology* (Vol. 12). St. Louis: Mosby.
		  • Kirton, C. (1997). Assessing bowel sounds. *Nursing 97, 27*(3), 64.

Chapter 54: Interventions for Clients with Oral Cavity Problems

Learning Outcomes	Learning Activities	Supplemental Resources
1. Develop a teaching plan for clients who have stomatitis. 2. Explain the common causes of malignant oral tumors. 3. Identify common nursing diagnoses for clients with oral cancer. 4. Prioritize postoperative care for clients undergoing surgery for oral cancer. 5. Develop a teaching plan for community-based care of clients with oral cancer.	1. Prior to completing the study guide exercises in this chapter, review the following: • Anatomy and physiology of the oral cavity • Special diets (such as bland, liquid, and pureed) for clients with oral cavity disorders • Parameters of a complete oral assessment • Principles of oral hygiene • Care of nasogastric tubes • Normal fluid and electrolyte values • Principles of perioperative and postoperative nursing management • Concepts of body image and self-esteem • Concepts of grief, loss, death, and dying 2. Review the **boldfaced** Key Terms and their definitions in Chapter 54 to enhance your understanding of the content. 3. Go to Study Guide Number 12.54 on the following pages and complete the learning exercises for this chapter.	1. Textbook—Chapter 53 (Assessment of the Gastrointestinal System) 2. Textbook—Chapter 54 3. Other resources: • Any anatomy and physiology textbook • Any laboratory and diagnostic test manual • Any pathophysiology textbook • Any physical assessment textbook • Dose, A. (1995). The symptom experience of mucositis, stomatitis, and xerostomia. *Seminars in Oncology Nursing, 11*(4), 248-255. • Eilers, J. (1997). Stomatitis as a side effect of cancer treatment. *Quality of Life: A Nursing Challenge, 5*(3), 68-74. • Kretzschmar, J.L. & Kretzschmar, D.P. (1996). Common oral conditions. *American Family Physician, 54*(1), 225-234. • McEwen, D. & Sanchez, M. (1997). A guide to salivary gland disorders. *AORN Journal, 65*(3), 554-566. • National Oral Health Information Clearinghouse: 1 NOHIC Way, Bethesda, MD 20892-3500; telephone: (301) 402-7364.

Chapter 55: Interventions for Clients with Esophageal Problems

Learning Outcomes	Learning Activities	Supplemental Resources
1. Explain the pathophysiology of gastroesophageal reflux disease (GERD). 2. Assess the client who is experiencing GERD. 3. Plan the nursing care for clients with GERD. 4. Develop a postoperative teaching plan for the client having a hiatal hernia repair. 5. Identify the differences in the incidence of esophageal cancer among cultural groups. 6. Describe the risk factors for esophageal cancer.	1. Prior to completing the study guide exercises in this chapter, review the following: • Anatomy and physiology of the gastrointestinal system • Anatomy and physiology of the esophagus • Assessment of the gastrointestinal system • Care of nasogastric (NG) and nasointestinal tubes • Care of feeding tubes and preparation of tube-feeding formulas	1. Textbook—Chapter 53 (Assessment of the Gastrointestinal System) 2. Textbook—Chapter 55 3. Other resources: • American Cancer Society: 1599 Clifton Road NE, Atlanta, GA 30329 • Any anatomy and physiology textbook • Any laboratory and diagnostic test manual • Any pathophysiology book

- Any physical assessment textbook
- Eckardt, V.F., et al. (1997). Complications and their impact after pneumatic dilation for achalasia: Prospective long-term follow-up study. *Gastrointestinal Endoscopy, 45*(5), 349-353.
- Larsen, R.R. (1997). Gastroesophageal reflux disease: Gaining control over heartburn. *Postgraduate Medicine, 101*(2), 181-182.
- Miyata, K. & Kitamura, H. (1997). Accessory nerve damage and impaired shoulder movement after neck dissections. *American Journal of Otolaryngology, 18*(3), 197-201.
- Weant, C. (1995). Easing the pain of esophageal surgery. *RN,* August, 26-31.

- Principles of total parenteral nutrition (TPN) and care of peripheral and central line catheter
- Normal fluid and electrolyte values
- Perioperative nursing management
- Postoperative nursing management
- Concepts of grief, loss, death, and dying
- Concepts of body image and self-esteem

2. Review the **boldfaced** Key Terms and their definitions in Chapter 55 to enhance your understanding of the content.

3. Go to Study Guide Number 12.55 on the following pages and complete the learning exercises for this chapter.

7. Analyze assessment data to determine common nursing diagnoses for the client with esophageal cancer.
8. Discuss the priorities for postoperative care of the client undergoing surgery for esophageal cancer.
9. Plan community-based care for clients diagnosed with esophageal cancer.

Chapter 56: *Interventions for Clients with Stomach Disorders*

Learning Outcomes

1. Compare etiologies and assessment findings of acute and chronic gastritis.
2. Describe the key components of collaborative management for clients with gastritis.
3. Compare and contrast assessment findings associated with gastric and duodenal ulcers.
4. Identify the most common medical complications that can result from peptic ulcer disease (PUD).
5. Analyze assessment data to determine common nursing diagnoses associated with PUD.
6. Develop a teaching plan related to drug therapy for clients experiencing PUD.
7. Prioritize interventions for clients with upper gastrointestinal bleeding.
8. Plan preoperative and postoperative care for the client undergoing gastric surgery.
9. Develop a community-based plan of care for clients who have undergone gastric surgery.
10. Evaluate outcomes for clients with PUD.

Learning Activities

1. Prior to completing the study guide exercises in this chapter, review the following:
- Anatomy and physiology of the stomach
- Assessment of the abdomen
- Effect of the central and autonomic nervous systems on the stomach
- Special diets (such as bland, liquid, and pureed) for clients with stomach disorders
- Care of nasogastric tubes
- Care of feeding tubes and preparation of tube-feeding formulas
- Principles of total parenteral and central line catheters
- Normal fluid and electrolyte values
- Perioperative nursing management
- Concepts of body image and self-esteem
- Concepts of grief, loss, death, and dying

Supplemental Resources

1. Textbook—Chapter 53 (Assessment of the Gastrointestinal System)
2. Textbook—Chapter 56
3. Other resources:
- American Digestive Disease Society: 7720 Wisconsin Ave., Bethesda, MD 20014
- American Gastroenterological Association: 6900 Grove Road, Thorofare, NJ 08086
- Any anatomy and physiology textbook
- Any laboratory and diagnostic test manual
- Any pathophysiology textbook
- Any physical assessment textbook
- Belcaster, A. (1996). Reviewing Zollinger-Ellison syndrome—from A to ZES. *Nursing 96, 26*(3), 32C-32D.
- Brozenac, S.A. (1996). Ulcer therapy update. *RN, 59*(9) 48-50.

Learning Outcomes	Learning Activities	Supplemental Resources
11. Explain Zollinger-Ellison syndrome and its associated clinical manifestations. 12. Analyze risk factors for gastric carcinoma, including cultural considerations. 13. Plan postoperative care for clients who have undergone surgery for gastric cancer. 14. Discuss the psychologic and emotional concerns of clients with gastric cancer.	2. Review the **boldfaced** Key Terms and their definitions in Chapter 56 to enhance your understanding of the content. 3. Go to Study Guide Number 12.56 on the following pages and complete the learning exercises for this chapter.	• Lazzaroni, M., et al. (1997). Triple therapy with ranitidine lansoprazole in the treatment of *Helicobacter pylori* associated with duodenal ulcer. *American Journal of Gastroenterology, 92*(4), 649-651. • Owen, D.A. (1997). The morphology of gastritis. *Yale Journal of Biology and Medicine, 69*(1), 51-60. • Rush, C. (1995). Gastrointestinal bleeding. *Nursing 95, 25*(8), 33.

Chapter 57: *Interventions for Clients with Noninflammatory Intestinal Disorders*

Learning Outcomes	Learning Activities	Supplemental Resources
1. Explain the risk factors for irritable bowel syndrome (IBS) and cancer of the colon. 2. Develop a teaching-learning plan for clients with irritable bowel syndrome. 3. Differentiate the most common types of hernias. 4. Develop a plan of care for a client undergoing hernia repair. 5. Interpret diagnostic assessments for clients with colon cancer. 6. Discuss the psychosocial aspects associated with colon cancer and related surgeries. 7. Explain the role of the nurse in managing the client with colon cancer. 8. Develop a perioperative plan of care for a client undergoing a colon resection and colostomy. 9. Construct a community-based teaching-learning plan for clients requiring colostomy care. 10. Identify community-based resources for clients with colon cancer. 11. Analyze the differences between small-bowel and large-bowel obstructions. 12. Describe assessment findings associated with mechanical and nonmechanical obstructions. 13. Explain the role of the nurse when caring for clients with nasogastric tubes. 14. Develop a plan of care for a client experiencing intestinal obstruction. 15. Prioritize nursing care for the client with abdominal trauma.	1. Prior to completing the study guide exercises in this chapter, review the following: • Anatomy and physiology of the small bowel and large intestine, including the rectum and anus • Assessment of the gastrointestinal system • Effect of the central and autonomic nervous systems on the gastrointestinal organs • Normal nutrition, including essential vitamins, minerals, and recommended food groups • Special diets (such as low protein, high carbohydrate, low fiber, liquid, and pureed) for clients with gastrointestinal organ disorders • Care of nasogastric and nasointestinal tubes • Principles of TPN and care of peripheral and central line catheters • Perioperative and postoperative nursing care • Concepts of body image • Concepts of grief, loss, death, and dying 2. Review the **boldfaced** Key Terms and their definitions in Chapter 57 to enhance your understanding of the content.	1. Textbook—Chapter 53 (Assessment of the Gastrointestinal System) 2. Textbook—Chapter 57 3. Other resources: • Any anatomy and physiology textbook • Any laboratory and diagnostic test manual • Any physical assessment textbook • Any pathophysiology textbook • Black, P. (1996). Stoma appliances: What's new. *Community Nurse, 2*(3), 48-49. • Bond, J. (1997). Screening for colorectal cancer. *Hospital Practice, 32*(1), 59-78. • Bryant, R. & Hampton, B. (1992). *Ostomies and continent diversions: Nursing management.* Baltimore, MD: Mosby. • Cerda, J., et al. (1996). Effective, compassionate management of IBS. *Patient Care, 30*(1), 131-144. • Digestive Disease National Coalition: 711 2nd Street NE, Suite 200, Washington, DC 20002.

3. Go to Study Guide Number 12.57 on the following pages and complete the learning exercises for this chapter.

- Wound, Ostomy, and Continence Nurses Society: 2755 Bristol Street, Suite 110, Costa Mesa, CA 92626.

Chapter 58: *Interventions for Clients with Inflammatory Intestinal Disorders*

Learning Outcomes	Learning Activities	Supplemental Resources

1. Compare and contrast the typical physical assessment finding associated with appendicitis and peritonitis.
2. Prioritize nursing care needs for the client who has peritonitis.
3. Discuss the common causes of gastroenteritis.
4. Compare and contrast the pathophysiology and clinical manifestations of ulcerative colitis and Crohn's disease.
5. Analyze priority nursing diagnoses and collaborative problems for clients with chronic inflammatory bowel disease (IBD).
6. Explain the purpose of and nursing implications related to drug therapy for clients with IBD.
7. Formulate a postoperative plan of care for a client undergoing a colon resection/colectomy and colostomy or ileostomy.
8. Develop a teaching plan for a client needing community-based care for a new ostomy.
9. Identify expected outcomes for clients with chronic IBD.
10. Explain the role of diet therapy in managing the client with diverticular disease.
11. Describe the comfort measures that the nurse can use for the client with an anal abscess, fissure, or fistula.
12. Discuss ways that helminthic infestation, parasitic infection, and food poisoning can be prevented.
	1. Prior to completing the study guide exercises in this chapter, review the following:
	  • Anatomy and physiology of the small bowel, large intestine, rectum, and anus
	  • Effect of the central and autonomic nervous systems on the gastrointestinal organs
	  • Assessment of the gastrointestinal system
	  • Normal nutrition, including essential vitamins, minerals, and recommended food groups as well as special diets (such as high protein, high carbohydrate, low fiber, liquid, bland, and pureed) for clients with gastrointestinal disorders
	  • Perioperative nursing management
	  • Principles of NG, TPN, and peripheral and central line catheters
	  • Principles of infection control
	  • Principles of enema administration
	  • Concepts of body image
	  • Concepts of grief, loss, death, and dying
	2. Review the **boldfaced** Key Terms and their definitions in Chapter 58 to enhance your understanding of the content.
	3. Go to Study Guide Number 12.58 on the following pages and complete the learning exercises for this chapter.
		1. Textbook—Chapter 53 (Assessment of the Gastrointestinal System)
		2. Textbook—Chapter 58
		3. Other resources:
		  • Any anatomy and physiology textbook
		  • Any physical assessment textbook
		  • Any pathophysiology textbook
		  • Any laboratory and diagnostic test manual
		  • Cerda, J., et al. (1997). Diverticulitis: Cure and management strategies. *Patient Care, 33*, 170-186.
		  • Crohn's and Colitis Foundation of America (CCFA): 386 Park Avenue South, 17th Floor, New York, NY 10016-8804; telephone: (212) 685-3440; http://www.ccfa.org
		  • Kirsner, J. & Shorter, R. (1995). *Inflammatory bowel disease.* Philadelphia: Williams and Wilkins.
		  • Mead, M. (1996b). Detecting appendicitis. *Practice Nurse, 11(7),* 486-487.
		  • Sachar, D.B. (1996). Maintenance strategies in Crohn's disease. *Hospital Practice, 31,* 99.
		  • United Ostomy Association (UOA): 19772 MacArthur Blvd, Suite 200, Irvine, CA 92612-2405; telephone: (800) 826-0826; http://www.uoa.org

Chapter 59: *Interventions for Clients with Liver Problems*

Learning Outcomes	Learning Activities	Supplemental Resources
1. Describe the pathophysiology and complications associated with cirrhosis of the liver. 2. Interpret laboratory test findings commonly seen in clients with cirrhosis. 3. Analyze assessment data from clients with cirrhosis to determine priority nursing diagnoses and collaborative problems. 4. Formulate a collaborative plan of care for the client with severe late-stage cirrhosis. 5. Identify emergency interventions for the client with bleeding esophagea varices. 6. Evaluate care for clients with cirrhosis. 7. Develop a community-based teaching plan for the client with cirrhosis of the liver. 8. Compare and contrast the transmission of hepatitis A, B, and C viral infections. 9. Explain ways in which each type of hepatitis can be prevented. 10. Discuss the primary concerns about the increasing incidence of hepatitis C in the United States. 11. Identify treatment options for clients with cancer of the liver. 12. Describe the typical complications that result from liver transplantation.	1. Prior to completing the study guide exercises in this chapter, review the following: • Anatomy and physiology of the liver • Normal F & E levels • Principles of infection control (universal, body substance precautions) • Principles of blood and blood product administration • Perioperative nursing management • Postoperative nursing management • Principles of TPN and care of peripheral and central line catheters • Special diets (such as low fat, low protein, high protein, high carbohydrate, and liquid) for clients with liver disorders • Concepts of body image and self-esteem • Concepts of grief, loss, death, and dying 2. Review the **boldfaced** Key Terms and their definitions in Chapter 59 to enhance your understanding of the content. 3. Go to Study Guide Number 12.59 on the following pages and complete the learning exercises for this chapter.	1. Textbook—Chapter 53 (Assessment of the Gastrointestinal System) 2. Textbook—Chapter 59 3. Other resources: • American Liver Foundation: 1425 Pompton Ave., Cedar Grove, NJ 07009; telephone: (800) 465-4387; http://www.liverfoundation.org • Any anatomy and physiology textbook • Any laboratory and diagnostic test manual • Any pathophysiology textbook • Any physical assessment textbook • Fried, M.W. (1996). Therapy of chronic viral hepatitis. *Medical Clinics of North America, 80*(5), 957-972. • Huston, C.J. (1996). Ruptured esophageal varices. *American Journal of Nursing, 96*(4), 43. • Johnson, C.D. & Hathaway, D.K. (1996). The lived experience of end-stage liver failure and liver transplantation. *Journal of Transplant Coordination, 6*(3), 130-133. • Korpan, N.N. (1997). Hepatic cryosurgery for liver metastases. *Annals of Surgery, 225*(2), 193-201. • Patel, N.H., Chalasani, N., & Jindahl, R.M. (1998). Current status of transjugular intrahepatic portosystemic shunts. *Postgraduate Medical Journal, 74*(878), 716-720.

Chapter 60: *Interventions for Clients with Problems of the Gallbladder and Pancreas*

Learning Outcomes	Learning Activities	Supplemental Resources
1. Identify the common causes of cholecystitis and cholelithiasis (gallbladder disease).	1. Prior to completing the study guide exercises for this chapter, review the following:	1. Textbook—Chapter 53 (Assessment of the Gastrointestinal System)
2. Explain the role of testing in diagnosis of gallbladder disease.	• Anatomy and physiology of the gallbladder and pancreas	2. Textbook—Chapter 60
3. Compare postoperative care of clients undergoing a traditional cholecystectomy with that of clients undergoing a laparoscopic cholecystectomy.	• Special diets (such as low fat, low protein, high protein, high carbohydrate, and liquid) for clients with disorders of the gallbladder and pancreas	3. Other resources: • Ammann, R.W. (1997). A clinically based classification system for alcoholic chronic pancreatitis: Summary of an international workshop on chronic pancreatitis. *Pancreas, 15*(4), 402–408.
4. Develop a community-based teaching plan for clients with gallbladder disease, including care of a T-tube.	• Principles of TPN and care of peripheral and central line catheters	• Any anatomy and physiology textbook
5. Compare and contrast the pathophysiology of acute and chronic pancreatitis.	• Principles of administration of blood and blood products	• Any laboratory and diagnostic test manual
6. Interpret common assessment findings associated with acute pancreatitis and those associated with chronic pancreatitis.	• Perioperative nursing management	• Any pathophysiology textbook
7. Prioritize nursing care needs for clients with acute pancreatitis and clients with chronic pancreatitis.	• Postoperative nursing management	• Any physical assessment textbook
8. Explain the use and adverse effects of drug therapy for clients with chronic pancreatitis.	• Normal F & E values	• Attili, A., DeSantis, A., Capri, R., et al. (1995). The natural history of gallstones: The GREPCO experience. *Hepatology, 21*(3), 655.
9. Develop a postoperative plan of care for clients undergoing a Whipple procedure.	• Care of NG and nasointestinal tubes and care of feeding tubes and preparation of tube-feeding formulas	• Barie, P., & Fischer, E. (1995). Acute acalculous cholecystitis. *Journal of the American College of Surgery, 180*(2), 232.
10. Construct a discharge plan for care of clients with pancreatic cancer in the community.	• Concepts of body image and self-esteem • Concepts of grief, loss, death, and dying	• Berci, G., & Cuschieri, A. (Eds.) (1997). *Bile duct and bile duct stones.* Philadelphia: W.B. Saunders.
11. Discuss the psychosocial needs of the client with pancreatic cancer and the associated nursing interventions.	2. Review the **boldfaced** Key Terms and their definitions in Chapter 60 to enhance your understanding of the content.	• Coyne, P.J. (1998). Assessing and treating the pain of pancreatitis. *American Journal of Nursing, 98*(11), 14, 16.
	3. Go to Study Guide Number 12.60 on the following pages and complete the learning exercises for this chapter.	• National Council on Alcoholism and Drug Dependence: 12 W. 21st Street, New York, NY 10010; telephone: (800) NCA-CALL; http://www.ncadd.org

Chapter 61: *Interventions for Clients with Malnutrition and Obesity*

Learning Outcomes	Learning Activities	Supplemental Resources
1. Identify three anthropometric measurements that the nurse can use to evaluate a client's nutritional status.	1. Prior to completing the study guide exercises for this chapter, review the following: • Anatomy and physiology of the gastrointestinal system	1. Textbook—Chapter 53 (Assessment of the Gastrointestinal System)
2. Explain the potential consequences and complications associated with malnutrition.	• Effect of the central and autonomic nervous systems on the gastrointestinal organs	1. Textbook—Chapter 61
3. Describe the risk factors for malnutrition, especially for older adults.	• Normal nutrition, including the essential vitamins, minerals, and foods in the recommended food groups	2. Other resources: • Any anatomy and physiology textbook • Any physical assessment textbook • Any pathophysiology textbook • Any diagnostic laboratory and test manual
4. Discuss the role of laboratory testing in the diagnosis of malnutrition.		
5. Analyze assessment data to determine common nursing diagnoses for the client with malnutrition.	• Care and management of NG tubes, feeding tubes, and preparation of tube-feeding formulas	• Brolin, R.E. (1996). Update: NIH consensus conference: Gastrointestinal surgery for severe obesity. *Nutrition, 12*(6), 403-404.
6. Identify expected outcomes for clients who are malnourished.	• Perioperative and postoperative nursing management	
7. Describe the nursing care of clients receiving total enteral nutrition.	• Principles of TPN, TEN, and care of peripheral and central line catheters	• Dubin, S. (1996). Geriatric assessment. *American Journal of Nursing,* May (5 Nurse Pract Extra Ed), 50.
8. Identify complications associated with total parenteral nutrition.	• Normal fluid and electrolyte balance	• Dudek, S.G. (1997) *Nutrition handbook for nursing practice* (2nd ed.). Philadelphia: Lippincott-Raven.
9. Prioritize nursing care needs for clients receiving total parenteral nutrition.	• Concepts of body image and self-esteem	
10. Explain the potential consequences and complications associated with obesity.	2. Review the **boldfaced** Key Terms and their definitions in Chapter 61 to enhance your understanding of the content.	• Fried, M., & Peskova, M. (1997). Gastric binding in the treatment of morbid obesity. *Hepatogastroenterology, 44*(14), 582-587.
11. Discuss the role of culture and gender as factors in the prevalence of obesity.		• National Institutes of Health Consensus Development Conference Statement. (1992). Gastrointestinal surgery for severe obesity. *American Journal of Clinical Nutrition, 55*(Suppl 2), 615S-619S.
12. Identify the role of drug therapy in the management of obesity.	3. Go to Study Guide Number 12.61 on the following pages and complete the learning exercises for this chapter.	
13. Develop a postoperative teaching plan for clients having a gastroplasty or intestinal bypass.		• Nutrition Screening Initiative: P.O. Box 753, Waldorf, MD 20604; telephone: (202) 625-1662; http://www.aafp.org/nsi/

STUDY GUIDE NUMBER 12.53

Assessment of the Gastrointestinal System

Study/Review Questions

1. Identify the layers of the gastrointestinal (GI) tract and describe the composition of each.

    a. _____
    _____

    b. _____
    _____

    c. _____
    _____

2. Identify the four major functions of the GI tract.

    a. _____
    _____

    b. _____
    _____

    c. _____
    _____

    d. _____
    _____

3. On a separate sheet of paper, briefly describe the process of digestion.

4. Innervation of the GI tract occurs in two ways. On a separate sheet of paper, identify them and briefly describe their purpose.

5. The blood supply to the GI tract originates from the _____ and then branches to many arteries.

6. The venous system that carries absorbed nutrients away from the lumen of the GI tract drains into the _____.

7. This blood (referred to in Question 6) then circulates through the _____ to the _____ _____ and returns to the _____ via the _____.

8. The oral cavity includes the _____, _____, _____, _____, _____, _____, and _____.

9. Define *mastication*.

10. Identify the three major salivary glands and describe their purpose.

    a. _____
    b. _____
    c. _____
    Purpose: _____
    _____

11. Match the following terms associated with the GI system with their corresponding definitions.

Definitions	GI Terms
____ a. Organ with both exocrine and endocrine functions	1. Bile
	2. Chyme
	3. Duodenum
____ b. Last 8 to 12 feet of the small intestine	4. Elimination
	5. Esophagus
____ c. Finger-like projections into the small intestine	6. Gallbladder
	7. Ileum
	8. Jejunum
____ d. Oral secretion that softens food	9. Large intestine
	10. Liver
____ e. Thick, liquid mass of partially digested food	11. Lobule
	12. Mouth
	13. Mucosa
____ f. Temporary reservoir for food	14. Pancreas
	15. Plicae circulates
____ g. Intestinal hormone that inhibits acid secretion and decreases gastric motility	16. Saliva
	17. Secretin
	18. Stomach
	19. Submucosa
	20. Villi
____ h. Epithelial cell layer lining GI tract	
____ i. Process of expelling feces	
____ j. Central part of small intestine	
____ k. Organ where water absorption occurs	
____ l. Conduit for food from mouth to stomach	
____ m. First 10 inches of small intestine	
____ n. Connective tissue layer of GI lumen	
____ o. Functional unit of liver	

___ p. Liver secretion essential to fat emulsifica-
tion

___ q. Largest abdominal organ with numerous
functions

___ r. Organ that concentrates and stores bile

___ s. Circular folds of mucosa projecting into the
GI lumen

___ t. Beginning pathway for digestion

12. On a separate sheet of paper, list the assessment
data (both subjective and objective) you would
include when performing a GI assessment on your
client.

13. What is the correct sequence of examination procedures for abdominal assessment? Briefly explain
why the sequence used for assessing the abdomen is
different than the sequence that is used to examine
other body systems.

*Explain what each of the following assessment findings may be
indicative of when performing an assessment of your client.*

14. Fruity breath smell

15. Asymmetry in the upper quadrants of the abdomen

16. Asymmetry in the lower quadrants of the abdomen

17. The presence of ecchymosis around the umbilicus
(Cullen's sign)

18. A bruit heard over the abdominal aorta

19. Diminished or absent bowel sounds

20. Loud, gurgling bowel sounds

21. Laboratory values for the client with liver disease
would show:
a. Decreased prothrombin time.
b. Increased aspartate aminotransferase (AST) and
alanine aminotransferase (ALT).
c. Increased albumin values.
d. Decreased ammonia levels.

22. Laboratory values for the client with acute pancreatitis may show decreased:
a. Calcium levels.
b. Serum amylase.
c. Serum lipase.
d. Urine amylase.

23. State what the fecal occult blood test (FOBT) measures and identify a common finding associated
with it.

24. Match the following diagnostic studies with the corresponding descriptions.

Descriptions

___ a. Useful in evaluat-
ing hepatocellular
disease. IV injec-
tion of radioactive
colloid is used.

___ b. X-ray study of the
gallbladder and
biliary ducts. IV
injection of con-
trast material is
given and films
are taken at 20-
minute intervals
for 1 hour (or until
the biliary ducts
are visualized).

___ c. Visualizes organs
in the abdomen.
May reveal masses, tumors, strictures or
obstructions. Patterns of bowel gas appear
light on the film. Jewelry and belts should
be removed before the test.

___ d. Cross-sectional x-ray that detects tissue
densities and abnormalities in the abdomen,
liver, spleen, pancreas, and biliary tract.
Client will be instructed to lie still and hold
breath when asked; client is confined in a
rather enclosed space inside the machine.

___ e. A radiographic visualization of the large
intestine; usually ordered for the client with
blood or mucus in the stool or a change in
bowel habits.

___ f. Visualization of the gallbladder after oral
ingestion of radiopaque, iodine-based contrast medium. The day before the test, the
client eats a fat-free or low-fat meal and
takes six radiopaque iodine tablets approximately 2 hours after the meal. Client is NPO
from midnight on the night before the test.

___ g. X-ray study of the biliary duct system using
instillation of an iodinated dye into the
liver.

___ h. Visualization from the oral part of the pharynx to the duodenojejunal junction. Used to
detect disorders of structure or function of
the esophagus, stomach, or duodenum.

___ i. An extension of the upper GI series; this
test continues to trace the barium through
the small intestine, up to and including the
ileocecal junction, to detect disorders of the
jejunum or ileum.

Diagnostic Studies
1. Flat plate film of
the abdomen
2. Upper GI radio-
graphic series
3. Small bowel series
(SBFT)
4. Barium enema
5. Percutaneous
transhepatic
cholangiography
6. Gallbladder radio-
graphic series
7. Intravenous
cholangiography
8. Computed
tomography
9. Liver-spleen scan

25. Match the following endoscopic procedures to the appropriate follow-up care.

Follow-up Care

Endoscopic Procedures

___ a. The client is informed that mild gas pain and flatulence may be experienced as a result of air instilled into the rectum during the examination. If a biopsy is obtained, a small amount of bleeding may be observed.

___ b. Vital signs must be checked every 15 minutes until the client is stable. Side rails are kept up until sedation wears off. Observe for signs of perforation or hemorrhage. The nurse instructs the client that a feeling of "fullness," cramping, and passage of flatus can be expected for several hours after the

1. Esophagogastro-duodenoscopy (EGD)
2. Endoscopic retro-grade cholangiopan-creatography (ERCP)
3. Colonoscopy
4. Proctosigmoidoscopy

test. A small amount of blood may be in the first stool after the test if a biopsy is taken or a polypectomy is performed. Excessive bleeding should be reported immediately.

___ c. Vital signs assessed frequently until the client is stable. Observe for cholangitis, perforation, sepsis, and pancreatitis (these problems may not occur immediately after the procedure and may take several hours to 2 days to develop). The client is instructed to report abdominal pain, fever, nausea, or vomiting that fails to resolve. The client is on NPO status until the gag reflex returns.

___ d. Vitals checked frequently (usually every 30 minutes) and side rails are up until sedation wears off. Client remains NPO until the gag reflex returns. Monitor for signs of perforation, such as pain, bleeding, or fever. Client is instructed not to drive for 12 hours after the test. A hoarse voice and sore throat may persist for several days; throat lozenges may be used to relieve the discomfort.

STUDY GUIDE NUMBER 12.54

Interventions for Clients with Oral Cavity Problems

Study/Review Questions

1. Identify five etiologic factors associated with stomatitis.
   a. _____
   _____
   b. _____
   _____
   c. _____
   _____
   d. _____
   _____
   e. _____
   _____

2. On a separate sheet of paper, differentiate between primary and secondary stomatitis.

3. Match each of the following descriptions of primary stomatitis with the corresponding type.

Descriptions

Types of Primary Stomatitis

___ a. Erythema, ulceration, and necrosis of gingival margins

___ b. Uniformly sized vesicles on tongue, palate, and buccal mucosa

___ c. Development at the site of an injury

___ d. Shallow, painful ulcerations covered by a yellow-gray ulcer pseudomembrane and exterior erythematous ring

1. Aphthous stomatitis
2. Herpetic stomatitis
3. Vincent's stomatitis
4. Traumatic stomatitis

Read the following statements and decide whether each is true or false. Write T for true or F for false in the blanks provided. If the statement is false, correct the statement to make it true.

___ 4. Lichen planus is an inflammatory mucocutaneous disease involving both the skin and the oral mucous membranes.

___ 5. Nonsymmetric yellow lesions of various patterns appear on the tongue and buccal mucosa in the client with lichen planus.

___ 6. Oral lichen planus may be associated with hepatitis C infection.

___ 7. In oral candidiasis, uniform white ulcerations appear on the tongue, palate, pharynx, and buccal mucosa.

___ 8. Candidiasis is a bacterial infection resulting from an infection elsewhere in the body.

___ 9. Candidiasis is very common among HIV-infected individuals.

10. Oral care for the client with stomatitis includes:
    a. Hard-bristled toothbrush to thoroughly clean the oral cavity.
    b. Rinsing the mouth out with a commercial mouthwash.
    c. Frequent rinsing of the mouth with warm saline, hydrogen peroxide solution, or sodium bicarbonate solution.
    d. Frequent rinsing of the mouth with cold tap water and vinegar solution.

11. Chlorhexidine, an oral rinse, can be beneficial in preventing infection. The nurse must inform the client that it may cause stinging and burning and also causes a discoloration of the teeth (which can be removed with abrasives). This discoloration would be:
    a. Pink.
    b. Brown.
    c. Blue.
    d. Green.

12. For clients with oral candidal infection, an antifungal agent is prescribed, such as nystatin oral suspension. On a separate sheet of paper, explain how the nurse would instruct the client to take this solution the proper way.

13. On a separate sheet of paper, identify the client data (both subjective and objective) you would include for your nursing assessment of a client with stomatitis.

14. Identify four measures that may be used to prevent stomatitis.
    a. _____
    _____
    b. _____
    _____
    c. _____
    _____
    d. _____
    _____

15. On a separate sheet of paper, develop a teaching plan for clients who have stomatitis.

16. Match the following types of oral cavity tumors with their corresponding descriptions.

Descriptions	**Types of Oral Cavity Tumors**
___ a. Painless, raised purple nodule or plaque on the hard palate	1. Leukoplakia
	2. Erythroplakia
	3. Squamous cell carcinoma
___ b. Red, raised, eroded areas on the lips, tongue, buccal mucosa, and oropharynx	4. Basal cell carcinoma
	5. Kaposi's sarcoma
___ c. Thickened, white, firmly attached patches in the oral mucosa, lips, or tongue	
___ d. Raised scab, primarily on the lips, lesion evolves to an ulcer with a raised pearly border	
___ e. Red, velvety lesion on the tongue, palate, floor of the mouth or mandibular mucosa	

17. Identify eight common causes and risk factors of malignant oral tumors.
    a. _____
    _____
    b. _____
    _____
    c. _____
    _____
    d. _____
    _____
    e. _____
    _____
    f. _____
    _____
    g. _____
    _____
    h. _____
    _____

18. On a separate sheet of paper, list the client data (both subjective and objective) that you would include in your nursing assessment of the client with oral cavity tumors.

19. On a separate sheet of paper, identify common nursing diagnoses and interventions for clients with oral cancer.

20. Briefly describe seven preoperative teaching instructions the nurse would provide to the client about to undergo a large surgical resection for oral cancer.

    a. _____

    b. _____

    c. _____

    d. _____

    e. _____

    f. _____

    g. _____

21. Briefly define a *glossectomy*.

22. On a separate sheet of paper, prioritize postoperative care for clients undergoing surgery for oral cancer.

23. To maintain a patent airway in the client after extensive excision or resection (from oral cancer surgery), frequent _____, using sterile technique, may be required for excessive secretions.

24. To protect the operative area (after oral cancer surgery), the nurse would elevate the head of the bed to at least _____ degrees to assist in decreasing edema by gravity.

25. Clients who have undergone surgery for oral carcinomas often describe their pain as _____ or _____.

26. The initial postoperative pain medication given to clients who have had surgery for oral carcinomas is usually _____.

27. Identify three assessments the nurse would make when a client resumes oral liquids after oral surgery.

    a. _____

    b. _____

    c. _____

28. On a separate sheet of paper, develop a teaching plan for community-based care of clients with oral cancer.

29. Identify four expected outcomes, based on the evaluation of care, for the client with a tumor of the oral cavity.

    a. _____

    b. _____

    c. _____

    d. _____

30. Identify three common disorders of the salivary glands.

    a. _____

    b. _____

    c. _____

31. Identify three common causes of acute sialadenitis.

    a. _____

    b. _____

    c. _____

32. Describe five nursing interventions the nurse would include in an attempt to help treat the underlying cause and increase the flow of saliva in the client with acute sialadenitis.

    a. _____

    b. _____

    c. _____

    d. _____

    e. _____

33. Briefly describe *xerostomia*.

34. When facial nerves are involved with tumors of the salivary glands, this can result in _____ _____ _____.

35. Identify the relevant data the nurse would collect while performing an assessment of the client's facial nerve.
    a. _____ _____
    b. _____ _____

c. _____ _____

d. _____ _____

e. _____ _____

f. _____ _____

g. _____ _____ _____

36. Briefly define *parotidectomy*.

STUDY GUIDE NUMBER 12.55

Interventions for Clients with Esophageal Problems

Study/Review Questions

1. Esophageal reflux is defined as _____ _____ _____.

2. Identify the physiologic factors that contribute to gastroesophageal reflux disease (GERD).
   a. _____ _____
   b. _____ _____
   c. _____ _____
   d. _____ _____

Answer the following two questions on a separate sheet of paper.

3. Identify two anatomic factors that support the normal function of the lower esophageal sphincter (LES).

4. Briefly describe Barrett's epithelium.

5. The degree of esophageal inflammation is:
   a. Inversely related to the acid concentration of refluxed stomach contents.
   b. Directly dependent on the number of reflux episodes of stomach contents.

   c. Primarily determined by the duration of exposure to irritating material.
   d. A result of increased peristaltic activity as irritants return to the stomach.

6. On a separate sheet of paper, briefly describe the relationship that nighttime reflux has to GERD.

7. Match each of the following definitions of GERD-associated symptoms with the corresponding term.

Definitions	GERD-Associated Symptoms
____ a. Pain described as a substernal or retrosternal burning sensation that tends to move up and down the chest in a wavelike fashion	1. Dyspepsia 2. Regurgitation 3. Water brash 4. Dysphagia 5. Odynophagia
____ b. Difficulty in swallowing	
____ c. Occurrence of warm fluid traveling up the throat with a sour or bitter taste	
____ d. Painful swallowing	
____ e. Reflex salivary hypersecretion in response to reflux	

8. On a separate sheet of paper, list the client data (subjective and objective) you would include when performing a nursing assessment of a client with GERD.

9. On a separate sheet of paper, briefly describe the Bernstein's test.

10. In regard to dietary modifications, the nurse would counsel an adult client with GERD to do all of the following *except*:
   a. Eat four to six small meals a day.
   b. Avoid spicy and acidic foods.
   c. Avoid carbonated beverages.
   d. Include evening snacks, particularly 1 to 2 hours before going to bed.

11. The lifestyle adjustment a client may have to make to best control GERD would be to:
   a. Sleep in the Trendelenburg position.
   b. Attain and maintain his ideal body weight.
   c. Wear snug-fitting belts and waistbands.
   d. Engage in strenuous exercise such as weightlifting.

12. The physician has prescribed Maalox for a client with GERD. The nurse instructs him to take the antacid _____ hour(s) before and _____ hour(s) after each meal.

13. Histamine blockers such as famotidine (Pepcid), ranitidine (Zantac), and cimetidine (Tagamet) act by inhibiting _____.

14. The primary action of metoclopramide is to _____ _____.

Answer the following three questions on a separate sheet of paper.

15. Differentiate between *sliding hernia* and *rolling hernia*, two types of hiatal hernias.

16. List the client data (subjective and objective) you would include when performing a nursing assessment of the client with a hiatal hernia.

17. Briefly describe a fundoplication.

Read the following interventions for the client who has had a fundoplication procedure and decide whether each is true or false. Write T for true or F for false in the blanks provided. If the statement is false, correct the statement to make it true.

___ 18. The nurse elevates the head of the client's bed 10 degrees to lower the diaphragm and facilitate lung expansion.

___ 19. Incentive spirometry and deep breathing are routinely used after surgery to maintain patency of the airways.

___ 20. Nasogastric drainage is initially dark brown with old blood but should become normal yellowish-green within the first 48 hours after surgery.

___ 21. The nurse explains to the client that meals consumed will need to be much larger and less frequent than before.

___ 22. The nurse teaches the client to avoid drinking carbonated beverages, eating gas-producing foods, chewing gum, and drinking with a straw.

___ 23. The client is taught to inspect the healing incision daily. The nurse explains that if swelling, redness, tenderness, discharge, or fever occur, the client should not worry because these are all common responses to the procedure.

24. Briefly describe achalasia.

25. Identify four complications that can result from achalasia.
   a. _____
   _____
   b. _____
   _____
   c. _____
   _____
   d. _____
   _____

26. Following esophageal dilation of a client, the nurse:
   a. Monitors the client for subcutaneous emphysema, hemoptysis, fever, and signs of perforation.
   b. Encourages the client to consume a small meal immediately after the procedure.
   c. Massages the client's shoulder when he or she complains of shoulder pain.
   d. Teaches the client to swallow any oral secretions that accumulate.

27. Which of the following statements about esophageal tumors is false?
   a. Esophageal tumors exhibit rapid local growth.
   b. Esophageal tumors can protrude into the esophageal lumen and cause thickening.
   c. Leiomyomas are malignant tumors and are almost always fatal.
   d. Most malignant esophageal tumors arise from the epithelium.

28. Identify six risk factors associated with esophageal cancer.

    a. _____

    b. _____

    c. _____

    d. _____

    e. _____

    f. _____

29. The greatest incidence of adenocarcinoma of the esophagus can be found in _____.

30. The incidence of squamous cell cancer of the esophagus has greatly increased in the United States over the past several decades, particularly among _____.

31. The incidence of esophageal cancer is extremely high in areas of the Transeki region of southern Africa, the Caspian Sea (around Russia and Iran), Japan, and _____.

32. Identify the two primary clinical manifestations in clients with esophageal cancer.

    a. _____
    b. _____

Answer the following three questions on a separate sheet of paper.

33. Identify the relevant assessment data (subjective and objective) the nurse would collect and analyze to determine appropriate nursing diagnoses for the client with esophageal cancer.

34. Identify the priority nursing diagnosis for clients with cancer of the esophagus.

35. Formulate additional nursing diagnoses based on your assessment in Question 33.

36. Identify treatment options available for the client with cancer of the esophagus that can assist in both disease management and nutrition management.

    a. _____
    b. _____
    c. _____
    d. _____
    e. _____
    f. _____
    g. _____

Read the following seven statements related to treatment options for esophageal cancer and decide whether each is true or false. Write T for true or F for false in the blanks provided. If the statement is false, correct the statement to make it true.

____ 37. The nurse encourages the client to consume semi-soft foods and thickened liquids because they are easier to swallow.

____ 38. When performing swallowing therapy for a client, the nurse would assist the client in positioning the head in hyperextension and placing the food in the front of the mouth in preparation for swallowing.

____ 39. For clients receiving radiation therapy, frequent gentle mouth care is important because the client is at risk for monilial esophagitis.

____ 40. Immediately after photodynamic therapy, the client is instructed to sunbathe as often as possible.

____ 41. Esophageal dilation provides permanent relief for dysphagia.

____ 42. Chemotherapy appears to be more effective when given in combination with radiation.

____ 43. Radical surgery represents the only definitive treatment for esophageal cancer and is the preferred treatment for clients in advanced disease stages.

44. The preferred surgical procedure for the client with esophageal cancer is _____.

45. The client who has had surgery for esophageal cancer requires meticulous postoperative care and is at risk for multiple serious complications. In prioritizing your nursing care for the client, care of what would be your highest priority?

46. Postoperative pulmonary complications include _____ and _____.

47. Once the client is extubated, the nurse begins _____ breathing, _____, and _____ routines with the client.

48. The nurse assesses the client for decreased breath sounds and shortness of breath at least every _____ to _____ hours.

49. The nurse keeps the client in a _____ or _____ position to support ventilation and prevent _____.

50. The nurse ensures patency of the water seal drainage system for _____ and monitors for changes in the _____ or _____ of the drainage.

51. The nurse monitors the client for signs and symptoms of fluid volume _____, particularly in clients who have undergone _____ dissection.

52. The nurse assesses for _____, crackles in the lungs, and increased _____.

53. The nurse does/does not *(Select one.)* independently irrigate or reposition the NG tube in clients who have undergone esophageal surgery.

Answer the following three questions on a separate sheet of paper.

54. Develop a teaching plan for community-based care for clients diagnosed with esophageal cancer.

55. Briefly define *diverticula*.

56. Identify the two most common ways in which diagnosis of esophageal diverticula is made.

57. Identify the two major interventions for controlling symptoms related to diverticula.
   a. _____
   b. _____

58. Trauma to the esophagus can result from:
   a. _____
   b. _____
   c. _____
   d. _____
   e. _____

59. The nurse assesses the client with trauma to the esophagus for:
   a. _____
   b. _____
   c. _____
   d. _____
   e. _____

60. Nonsurgical management for the client with trauma to the esophagus may include which of the following? *Check all that apply.*
   ____ a. Total parental nutrition (TPN)
   ____ b. Broad-spectrum antibiotics
   ____ c. Opioid and non-opioid analgesics
   ____ d. High-dose corticosteroids

STUDY GUIDE NUMBER 12.56

Interventions for Clients with Stomach Disorders

Study/Review Questions

Answer the following four questions on a separate sheet of paper.

1. Briefly define *gastritis*.

2. Identify the function of the mucosal barrier.

3. Describe the early pathologic manifestation of gastritis.

4. Briefly differentiate between acute and chronic gastritis.

5. Match each of the following etiologic factors with the corresponding type of gastritis. *Answers may be used more than once.*

Etiologic Factors	Types of Gastritis
____ a. Long-term alcohol use	1. Acute gastritis
____ b. NSAIDs	2. Chronic gastritis
____ c. Ingestion of corrosive substances	
____ d. Pernicious anemia	
____ e. A client who is NPO	
____ f. History of smoking	
____ g. Physiologic stress	

6. Identify six assessment findings relevant to acute gastritis.
   a. _____
   b. _____
   c. _____
   d. _____
   e. _____
   f. _____

7. Identify six assessment findings relevant to chronic gastritis.
   a. _____
   b. _____
   c. _____
   d. _____
   e. _____
   f. _____

8. What diagnostic test is used most commonly to diagnose gastritis?

9. Management of gastritis is directed toward supportive care for _____ and _____ of discomfort.

10. Match the following commonly used drugs for the client with gastritis to their primary mode of action.

Drug Action	Drugs Used to Treat Gastritis
a. ___ Antacids used as buffering agents	1. H_2-receptor antagonists
b. ___ Prevention or treatment of pernicious anemia	2. Sucralfate
	3. Maalox, Mylanta
c. ___ Blocks gastric secretions	4. Vitamin B_{12}
d. ___ A mucosal barrier fortifier	

11. Collaborative management of gastritis includes all of the following *except*:
   a. Instructing the client to limit intake of any foods and spices that cause distress.
   b. Encouraging client to engage in stress reduction techniques (relaxation therapy, imagery, etc.).
   c. Instructing the client to avoid medications such as aspirin and ibuprofen.
   d. Introducing new foods into the diet several at a time.

12. Define *peptic ulcer disease* (PUD).

13. List the three types of ulcers and give their common locations.
   a. _____
   b. _____
   c. _____

14. Identify the four most common medical complications that can result from PUD.
   a. _____
   b. _____
   c. _____
   d. _____

15. Match each of the following assessment findings in the client with PUD to its corresponding complication. *Answers may be used more than once.*

Assessment Findings	Complications of PUD
___ a. Melena (occult blood in a tarry stool)	1. Hemorrhage
	2. Pyloric obstruction
	3. Perforation
___ b. Tender, rigid, board-like abdomen	4. Intractable disease
___ c. Abdominal bloating, nausea, and vomiting	
___ d. Recurrent pain and discomfort despite treatment	
___ e. Hypokalemia	
___ f. Sudden, sharp pain beginning at mid-epigastric region spreading to entire abdomen	
___ g. Vomiting of bright red blood	
___ h. Metabolic alkalosis	
___ i. Granular dark vomitus with a coffee-ground appearance	
___ j. No longer responding to conservative management	
___ k. Assumes a knee-chest position	

Answer the following three questions on a separate sheet of paper.

16. Identify the data (subject and objective) you would include when performing an assessment on the client with PUD.

17. Formulate common nursing diagnoses for the client with PUD.

18. What is the major diagnostic test for PUD?

19. Identify the four primary goals of drug therapy in the treatment of PUD.
   a. _____
   b. _____
   c. _____
   d. _____

Provide the appropriate teaching plan related to each of the following drug therapies used for the client experiencing PUD. Use a separate sheet of paper for your answers as needed.

20. Antisecretory agents

21. H_2-receptor antagonists

22. Prostaglandin analogs

23. Antacids

24. Mucosal barrier fortifiers

25. The purpose of interventions to reduce bleeding is to limit the amount of blood _____ from the _____ and _____ GI tract resulting from _____ related to PUD.

Answer the following two questions on a separate sheet of paper.

26. The nurse monitors the client for signs and symptoms indicating GI bleeding. Describe the assessment findings you would expect for the following clients.
    a. The client with mild bleeding (less than 500 mL)
    b. The client with blood loss exceeding 1 L/24 hours

27. What type of therapy may be required to replace blood loss?

28. Identify the goals of therapeutic intervention for bleeding secondary to PUD.
    a. _____
    b. _____

29. Identify the four therapeutic, nonsurgical interventions used to control acute bleeding and prevent recurrent bleeding.
    a. _____
    b. _____
    c. _____
    d. _____

30. Briefly describe the three primary methods of endoscopic therapy that may be effective for an acute bleeding episode.
    a. _____
    b. _____
    c. _____

Answer the following three questions of a separate sheet of paper.

31. In planning preoperative care for the client with PUD, explain why the nurse inserts an NG tube and connects it to suction to remove secretions and empty the client's stomach.

32. Provide a rationale for why the NG tube would remain in place postoperatively for the client who undergoes gastric surgery.

33. Identify and describe the most commonly performed surgical procedures for the client with PUD.

Read the following three statements related to postoperative nursing care and decide whether each is true or false. Write T for true or F for false in the blanks provided. If the statement is false, correct the statement to make it true.

____ 34. The nurse monitors the NG tube for patency and carefully secures the tube to prevent dislodgement.

____ 35. The nurse routinely irrigates and repositions the NG tube after gastric surgery.

____ 36. Acute gastric dilation is manifested by vertigo, sweating, and confusion.

37. Signs and symptoms of dumping syndrome include:
    a. Severe pain.
    b. Bradycardia.
    c. Profuse vomiting.
    d. Vertigo.

38. In teaching the client to manage dumping syndrome, which of the following instructions by the nurse would be appropriate?
    a. Consume a low-protein, high-fat, high-carbohydrate diet.
    b. Consume a high-protein, high-fat, low-carbohydrate diet.
    c. Increase liquid intake with meals.
    d. Increase the amount of food taken in at one meal.

39. Develop a community-based plan of care for clients who have undergone gastric surgery. *Use a separate sheet of paper for your answer.*

40. Identify the expected outcomes for clients with PUD.
    a. _____
    b. _____
    c. _____
    d. _____
    e. _____
    f. _____
    g. _____
    h. _____
    i. _____

Answer the following four questions on a separate sheet of paper.

41. Briefly describe Zollinger-Ellison syndrome (ZES).

42. What is steatorrhea?

43. What is the goal of medical therapy for the client with ZES?

44. Briefly describe the methods of gastric carcinoma extension.

45. Identify 13 risk factors associated with the development of gastric carcinoma.

    a. _____
    b. _____
    c. _____
    d. _____
    e. _____
    f. _____
    g. _____
    h. _____
    i. _____
    j. _____
    k. _____
    l. _____
    m. _____

46. Which three cultural groups are two times as likely to develop gastric cancer as compared with whites?

    a. _____
    b. _____
    c. _____

47. What are the two most common symptoms in the client with early gastric carcinoma?

    a. _____
    b. _____

48. Which of the following statements about the management of gastric cancer is correct?
    a. Combination chemotherapy for advanced disease is less effective than single-agent therapy.
    b. The response to combination chemotherapy is unaffected by radiation therapy.
    c. Combining chemotherapy and radiation therapy after surgery has proven to be effective and is preferred.
    d. High-dose radiation therapy is the recommended adjuvant therapy to surgical treatment.

49. Which of the following statements about surgical interventions for gastric cancer is true?
    a. Surgery has the lowest cure rate for early gastric cancer.
    b. Neoplasm location in the stomach determines the type of surgical procedure.
    c. Palliative resection can help the cure rate for clients with advanced disease.
    d. The primary surgical procedure for the treatment of gastric cancer is gastroenterostomy.

50. Identify the specific complications that may follow gastric surgery.

    a. _____
    b. _____
    c. _____
    d. _____
    e. _____
    f. _____
    g. _____
    h. _____
    i. _____
    j. _____

51. Which of the following statements about postoperative nursing care is false?
    a. Auscultate the lungs for adventitious sounds.
    b. Auscultate the abdomen for return of bowel sounds.
    c. Inspect the operative site every day for the presence of redness, swelling, or drainage.
    d. Ensure proper positioning of the client to prevent aspiration from reflux.

52. Anemia, vitamin B_{12}, and folate deficiency can result after a gastrectomy. Oral _____ and _____ replacement and _____ injections can help correct these deficiencies.

Answer the following two questions on a separate sheet of paper.

53. Briefly discuss the indications for placing a client on total parenteral nutrition (TPN) after gastric surgery.

54. Briefly describe the psychologic and emotional concerns of clients with gastric cancer.

STUDY GUIDE NUMBER 12.57

Interventions for Clients with Noninflammatory Intestinal Disorders

Study/Review Questions

1. Briefly describe irritable bowel syndrome (IBS).

2. Briefly explain why IBS is *not* a true colitis.

3. Identify three factors that may contribute to IBS.
   a. _____
   b. _____
   c. _____

4. IBS is commonly characterized by:
   a. Chronic constipation.
   b. Chronic diarrhea.
   c. Alternating diarrhea and constipation.
   d. Normal bowel habits with flatulence.

5. Which of the following statements about IBS is true?
   a. Individual lifestyle is relatively unaffected.
   b. Most clients can identify factors that precipitate exacerbations.
   c. IBS is estimated to occur in less than 5% of the population in the United States.
   d. IBS has not been associated with the use of analgesics.

6. On a separate sheet of paper, identify the assessment data (both subjective and objective) you would include relevant to the client with IBS.

Read the following five statements related to client education for IBS and decide whether each is true or false. Write T for true or F for false in the blanks provided. If the statement is false, correct the statement to make it true.

___ 7. Information would be provided to the client regarding what constitutes normal bowel function and laxative abuse.

___ 8. The client is advised to increase caffeine intake but limit alcohol use.

___ 9. Fiber supplements are never recommended because they may cause more constipation.

___ 10. The client is advised to limit fluid intake.

___ 11. Bentyl and Pro-Banthine can help relieve abdominal cramping and intestinal spasm.

12. Which of the following statements indicates that the client with IBS understands his or her home maintenance regimen?
    a. "I enjoy having a glass or two of wine with my dinner."
    b. "I understand that I am lactose intolerant; therefore I can continue to eat my cheese sandwiches."
    c. "When I feel the urge to have a bowel movement, I should wait for 1 to 2 hours and then go."
    d. "I will enroll in a stress management workshop."

13. Identify six causes of increased intra-abdominal pressure that can lead to a hernia.
    a. _____
    b. _____
    c. _____
    d. _____
    e. _____
    f. _____

14. Match each of the following types of hernias with the corresponding description.

Descriptions

Types of Hernias

1. Femoral
2. Incarcerated
3. Indirect
4. Reducible
5. Strangulated
6. Umbilical
7. Ventral

____ a. Contents of the sac can be replaced into the abdominal cavity
____ b. Occurs when the canal enlarges, allowing peritoneum through
____ c. Occurs in the region of the navel
____ d. Hernia pushes downward at an angle in the inguinal canal
____ e. Cannot be replaced back into the abdominal cavity
____ f. Blood supply to the herniated bowel segment is cut off
____ g. Occurring at the site of a prior surgical incision

15. Which of the following statements about hernias is correct?
    a. Direct hernias are the most common type.
    b. Umbilical hernias are more common in the elderly.
    c. Indirect inguinal hernias occur most often in men.
    d. Incisional hernias are common in obese people.

16. On a separate sheet of paper, list the client data (subjective and objective) you would include relevant to hernias for your nursing assessment.

17. Interventions for the client who uses a truss for a hernia include:
    a. Using a surgical binder to hold the truss in place.
    b. Inspecting the skin under the truss several times a week.
    c. Applying the truss while sitting on the edge of the bed.
    d. Applying powder to the skin under the truss daily.

18. Identify and briefly describe the two common types of hernia repair.
    a. _____
    b. _____

19. To promote lung expansion in the client who undergoes surgery for hernia repair, the nurse encourages deep breathing and frequent turning but instructs the client to avoid _____.

20. Postoperative measures for the male client who has had an inguinal herniorrhaphy include:
    a. Applying a warm pack to the scrotum.
    b. Elevating the scrotum on a pillow.
    c. Encouraging use of a bedpan to void.
    d. Decreasing fluid intake to decrease bladder emptying.

21. Number the following steps describing the growth and spread of an intestinal tumor in sequential order.
    ____ a. Enlargement into the bowel lumen
    ____ b. Presence of a polyp in the bowel
    ____ c. Malignant cells found in the liver
    ____ d. Malignant cells line the bowel wall
    ____ e. Local invasion into layers of the bowel wall
    ____ f. Spread via the lymphatic system or circulatory system

22. Identify five sites where intestinal tumors can metastasize.
    a. _____
    b. _____
    c. _____
    d. _____
    e. _____

23. Identify four risk factors that are involved in the development of colorectal cancer.
    a. _____
    b. _____
    c. _____
    d. _____

24. On a separate sheet of paper, list the client data (subjective and objective) you would include in your assessment relevant to intestinal cancer.

Read the following statements related to diagnostic assessments and decide whether each is true or false. Write T for true or F for false in the blanks provided. If the statement is false, correct the statement to make it true.

____ 25. Hemoglobin and hematocrit values are usually increased as a result of the intermittent bleeding associated with the tumor.

____ 26. A negative test result for occult blood in the stool confirms bleeding in the GI tract.

____ 27. Colonoscopy is the definitive test for the diagnosis of colon cancer.

____ 28. A liver scan is used to remove polyps.

29. Identify four psychosocial implications associated with colon cancer.
    a. _____
    b. _____
    c. _____
    d. _____

30. Briefly describe a *hemicolectomy*.

31. Briefly describe a *colostomy*.

32. Why would the nurse caring for a client who is about to undergo a hemicolectomy and colostomy consult an enterostomal therapist?

33. What training is required for one to be an enterostomal therapist (ET)?

34. On a separate sheet of paper, develop a perioperative plan of care for the client undergoing a colon resection and colostomy.

35. After colostomy surgery, the nurse:
    a. Covers the stoma with a dry, sterile dressing.
    b. Applies a pouch system as soon as possible.
    c. Makes a hole in the pouch for gas to escape.
    d. Watches for the colostomy to start functioning on day one.

36. The nurse reports immediately all of the following signs and symptoms related to the colostomy to the surgeon *except*:
    a. Liquid stool immediately postoperatively.
    b. Unusual bleeding.
    c. Signs of ischemia and necrosis.
    d. Mucocutaneous separation.

37. Which of the following should the client who has a perineal wound and cavity be instructed to report to the physician immediately?
    a. Serosanguineous drainage from the wound
    b. Sensations of having a bowel movement
    c. Constant perineal odor and pain
    d. Occasional perineal pain and itching

38. A food that the client with a colostomy may want to avoid would be:
    a. Yogurt.
    b. Peas.
    c. Toast.
    d. Buttermilk.

39. Identify and discuss community-based resources for the client with colon cancer. *Use a separate sheet of paper for your answer.*

40. Match each of the following terms related to intestinal obstruction with the corresponding definition.

Definitions	Terms Related to Intestinal Obstruction
____ a. Blockage of the bowel lumen resulting from internal or external factors	1. Adhesions
	2. Complete obstruction
	3. Mechanical obstruction
____ b. Incomplete blockage of intestine	4. Nonmechanical obstruction
	5. Partial obstruction
____ c. Blockage of bowel lumen caused by decreased intestinal activity	6. Strangulated obstruction
____ d. Total blockage of intestinal lumen	
____ e. Blockage with compromised blood flow	
____ f. Bands of scar tissue encircling intestine and constricting lumen	

41. Identify five of the common causes of mechanical obstructions: two of the small intestine and three of the large bowel.
    Small intestine:
    a. _____
    b. _____
    Large bowel:
    a. _____
    b. _____
    c. _____

42. Match the following metabolic disturbances with their levels of bowel obstruction.

Level of Bowel Obstruction	Metabolic Disturbances
____ a. High in the small intestine	1. Insignificant imbalance
____ b. Below the duodenum but above the large bowel	2. Metabolic acidosis
	3. Metabolic alkalosis
____ c. Below the terminal ileum	

43. On a separate sheet of paper, briefly describe assessment findings associated with mechanical and nonmechanical obstructions.

44. Nursing care of the client with a newly inserted nasointestinal tube includes:
    a. Anchoring the tube firmly to the client's cheek.
    b. Irrigating with 30 mL of sterile saline PRN.
    c. Changing the client's position every 2 hours.
    d. Setting the tube to low continuous suction.

45. Which of the following NG tubes would be connected to low intermittent suction?
    a. Salem sump
    b. Levin
    c. Anderson
    d. Carney

46. At least every _____ hours, the nurse assesses the client with an NG tube for _____ of the tube, tube _____, and _____.

47. _____ girth is measured at the _____ point each day.

48. The client is assessed for _____, vomiting, _____ abdominal distention, and _____ of the tube.

49. Interventions for clients with Fluid Volume Deficit related to an intestinal obstruction include:
    a. Frequent mouth care with lemon glycerin swabs.
    b. Ice chips to suck on before surgery.
    c. A small glass of water.
    d. Assessing for edema from third spacing.

50. Which of the following observations of the client with an intestinal obstruction should the nurse report immediately?
    a. A urinary output of 1000 mL in an 8-hour period
    b. The client's request for something to drink
    c. Abdominal pain changing from colicky to constant discomfort
    d. The client who is changing positions frequently

51. Discharge instructions for the client who has had an intestinal obstruction caused by fecal impaction include:
    a. Encouragement to report abdominal distention, nausea or vomiting, and constipation.
    b. Providing a written description of a low-fiber diet.
    c. Reminding the client to limit activity.
    d. Reminding the client to decrease fluid intake.

52. Identify the two major categories of abdominal injury and identify examples of each.
    a. _____
    b. _____

53. Identify the three main issues health care providers focus on in the emergency phase of treatment for abdominal injury.
    a. _____
    b. _____
    c. _____

54. Identify the two priority nursing assessments for client with abdominal injury.
    a. _____
    b. _____

55. To assess the abdomen for possible trauma, the nurse:
    a. Exposes only the area from the xiphoid process to the symphysis pubis.
    b. Immediately removes antishock trousers.
    c. Palpates deeply over the abdominal wall for masses and areas of tenderness.
    d. Inspects for symmetry, abrasions, lacerations, ecchymosis, and penetrating wounds.

56. Ecchymosis following abdominal trauma may signify what?

57. Describe how the nurse would assess for Ballance's sign and identify its significance.
    a. Assessment

    b. Significance

Answer the following two questions on a separate sheet of paper.

58. Briefly discuss why the nurse would place at least two large-bore IV catheters in the client with abdominal trauma.

59. Briefly explain why serial hemoglobin and hematocrit levels are assessed for the client with abdominal injury.

60. If the client has an open abdominal wound or evisceration, the nurse would cover it with a _____ _____ unless the physician orders otherwise.

61. Identify two reasons why the nurse would insert an NG tube in the client with abdominal trauma.
    a. _____
    b. _____

62. On a separate sheet of paper, briefly explain why all clients who have suffered abdominal trauma are taught the signs and symptoms to report, regardless of whether they have had surgery or not.

63. Are the following statements about intestinal polyps true or false? *Write* T *for true or* F *for false in the blanks provided.*
    ___ a. Most polyps are malignant.
    ___ b. Polyps of certain tissue types are more likely to become malignant.
    ___ c. Most intestinal polyps are attached to the surface of the intestine.
    ___ d. Hyperplastic polyps are always malignant.
    ___ e. Villous adenomas tend to be benign.
    ___ f. Pedunculated polyps are stalklike.
    ___ g. Sessile polyps become elongated as peristalsis pulls them into the lumen of the intestine.
    ___ h. Familial polyposis is characterized by progressive development of colorectal adenomas.
    ___ i. Polyps frequently cause pain and rectal bleeding.
    ___ j. A polypectomy can be done during a colonoscopy.

64. Which of the following would *not* be included in the nurse's care of the client who has had a colorectal polypectomy?
    a. Examining all stools for blood or mucopurulent drainage
    b. Monitoring the client for abdominal distention and pain
    c. Reassuring the client that recurrence is unlikely
    d. Encouraging follow-up examinations

65. What are the two most common symptoms of hemorrhoids?
    a. _____
    b. _____

66. Which of the following interventions is contraindicated in the nonsurgical management of hemorrhoids?
    a. Encouraging diets low in fiber and fluids
    b. Witch hazel soaks for pain
    c. Warm sitz baths three or four times a day
    d. Cleansing the anal area with moistened cleaning tissues

67. Identify three potential postoperative complications that may occur after a hemorrhoidectomy.
    a. _____
    b. _____
    c. _____

68. Identify the types of disorders that may result in malabsorption, and provide an example of which nutrients are not absorbed in each disorder.
    a. _____
    b. _____
    c. _____
    d. _____
    e. _____
    f. _____

69. What is the classic symptom of malabsorption?

70. Identify eight clinical manifestations relevant to malabsorption.
    a. _____
    b. _____
    c. _____
    d. _____
    e. _____
    f. _____
    g. _____
    h. _____

71. Interventions for most malabsorption syndromes focus on:
    a. _____
    b. _____

72. Which of the following drugs would be used to treat tropical sprue?
    a. Bentyl
    b. Lomotil
    c. Steroids
    d. Bactrim

Case Study: The Client with a Bowel Obstruction

You are working in the emergency room of the hospital when a 47-year-old man comes in complaining of acute upper to mid-abdominal, sporadic pain and cramping. Upon assessment you observe abdominal distention and high-pitched bowel sounds. The physician has ordered flat plate and upright abdominal x-rays that have came back showing distention of loops of intestine, with fluid and gas in the small intestine in conjunction with absence of gas in the colon. The physician has diagnosed this client with a bowel obstruction.

Answer the following questions on a separate sheet of paper:

1. Based on the findings, identify which type of bowel obstruction this client most likely has and why.

2. What other signs and symptoms would you observe this client for?

3. Identify the most likely interventions for this client, based on his type of bowel obstruction.

4. It is found that the client has a small fecal impaction. Identify how fecal impaction usually resolves.

STUDY GUIDE NUMBER 12.58

Interventions for Clients with Inflammatory Intestinal Disorders

Study/Review Questions

1. Describe the function of the appendix.

2. Number the following events related to appendicitis in sequential order.
   ___ a. Infection causes more swelling
   ___ b. Gangrene from hypoxia or perforation
   ___ c. Blood flow to the appendix is restricted
   ___ d. Peritonitis
   ___ e. Mucosa continues to secrete fluid
   ___ f. Lumen of appendix becomes obstructed
   ___ g. Further reduction of blood flow to the appendix
   ___ h. Pressure within the lumen exceeds venous pressure
   ___ i. Bacteria invade the wall of the appendix

3. On a separate sheet of paper, briefly define *fecalith* and its relationship to obstruction of the appendix.

4. Which of the following statements about appendicitis is correct?
   a. The peak incidence is between the ages of 20 and 30 years.
   b. The peak incidence is between the ages of 15 and 25 years.
   c. Appendicitis affects more women than men.
   d. Appendicitis affects more women than men before the age of 25.

5. On a separate sheet of paper, list the client data (both subjective and objective) you would include relevant to appendicitis for your nursing assessment.

6. Identify three complications of appendicitis that may result from Altered Tissue Perfusion.
   a. _____
   b. _____
   c. _____

7. A 25-year-old carpenter has just been admitted to your unit with acute appendicitis. He began to experience periumbilical pain, fever of 100.2° F, and nausea and vomiting while working on a house. Currently his pain is constant and located to the right lower quadrant. He is requesting that you bring him a heating pad to relieve his pain. His WBC count is 15,000 with a "shift to the left." His appendectomy is scheduled for today. Use this information and the information presented in your textbook to develop rationales for the following interventions that have been selected for this client.
   a. Explain to client why you cannot give him the heating pad.
   b. Position client in a semi-Fowler's position.
   c. Maintain client's NPO status.
   d. Administer IV fluids as ordered.
   e. Do not administer a laxative or enema.

8. Which of the following interventions regarding postoperative nursing care for a client who has had an appendectomy is incorrect?
   a. Administering IV antibiotics as ordered.
   b. Monitoring output of any drains that may be present.
   c. Observing for and reporting any unusual bleeding immediately.
   d. Encouraging client to get back to work the next day.

9. On a separate sheet of paper, briefly describe primary peritonitis and secondary peritonitis.

10. The fluid shift that occurs in peritonitis results in:
    a. Intracellular fluid moving into the peritoneal cavity.
    b. A significant increase in circulatory volume.
    c. Eventual renal failure and electrolyte imbalance.
    d. Increased bowel motility caused by increased fluid volume.

11. The respiratory problems that may accompany peritonitis are a result of:
    a. Associated pain interfering with ventilation.
    b. Decreased pressure against the diaphragm.
    c. Fluid shifts to the thoracic cavity.
    d. Decreased oxygen demands related to the infectious process.

12. On a separate sheet of paper, list the client data (subjective and objective) you would include relevant to peritonitis for your nursing assessment.

13. Which of the following is *not* an expected assessment finding in the client with generalized peritonitis?
    a. Abdominal wall rigidity
    b. High urine output
    c. High fever
    d. Tachycardia

14. Which of the following would *not* be nonsurgical management for the client with peritonitis?
    a. Monitoring of daily weight and intake and output.
    b. Insertion of an NG tube to decompress the stomach.
    c. Ordering a breakfast tray because the client is hungry.
    d. Administering morphine sulfate IV for pain.

15. Interventions following abdominal surgery for peritonitis include:
    a. Maintaining the client in a supine position.
    b. Using clean technique for peritoneal irrigation.
    c. Ambulating client on day one.
    d. Monitoring level of consciousness at least hourly initially after surgery.

16. Briefly define *gastroenteritis*.

17. What are the two types of organisms responsible for gastroenteritis?
    a. _____
    b. _____

18. Identify three circumstances in which invading organisms can infect a person and result in gastroenteritis.
    a. _____
    b. _____
    c. _____

19. Identify the three organisms most commonly responsible for bacterial gastroenteritis.
    a. _____
    b. _____
    c. _____

Answer the following three questions on a separate sheet of paper.

20. Briefly describe the primary route of transmission for invading organisms causing gastroenteritis.

21. Identify four ways in which to avoid contamination and prevent the spread of gastroenteritis.

22. Briefly describe the pathophysiology of ulcerative colitis.

23. Identify the complications associated with ulcerative colitis.
    a. _____
    b. _____
    c. _____
    d. _____
    e. _____
    f. _____
    g. _____
    h. _____

24. Identify the client data (both subjective and objective) relevant to ulcerative colitis for your nursing assessment. *Use a separate sheet of paper for your answer.*

25. Before an invasive diagnostic workup is performed on a client, the client's stools are examined for _____ blood, _____, and _____, and specimens for _____ are obtained. This is done because _____ can cause symptoms similar to those of ulcerative colitis, and other problems must be ruled out before a definitive diagnosis is made.

26. Nonsurgical management of ulcerative colitis includes:
    a. A high-fiber, high-roughage diet.
    b. Antidiarrheal agents.
    c. Regular exercise.
    d. All clients being on NPO status.

27. On a separate sheet of paper, identify and analyze priority nursing diagnoses and collaborative problems for the client with ulcerative colitis.

28. Match each of the following descriptions of common medications used for ulcerative colitis to the corresponding drug category. *Answers may be used more than once.*

    Descriptions
    ___ a. As single agents, these drugs are not effective in the treatment of ulcerative colitis.
    ___ b. Administered orally or rectally to reduce inflammation
    ___ c. Oral or IV therapy may be prescribed during exacerbations.
    ___ d. Take with a full glass of water and with meals to prevent GI discomfort.
    ___ e. These drugs can precipitate colonic dilation and toxic megacolon.
    ___ f. The nurse observes for side effects, some of which may include thrombocytopenia,, leukopenia, anemia, and renal failure.
    ___ g. Long-term adverse effects of this drug can include hyperglycemia, osteoporosis, PUD, and increased risk for infection.

    Drug Category
    1. Salicylate compounds
    2. Corticosteroids
    3. Immunosuppressive drugs
    4. Antidiarrheal drugs

29. A client who has had a total proctocolectomy with a traditional permanent ileostomy would most likely have the stoma placed where?

30. A client who has had a total colectomy with a continent ileostomy would have the pouch located where?

31. On a separate sheet of paper, explain to the client how they would drain the pouch with a Koch's ileostomy.

32. The nurse teaches the client with an ileostomy to include adequate amounts of _____ and _____ in their diets because the ileostomy promotes the _____ of these elements.

33. On a separate sheet of paper, formulate a post-operative plan of care for the client with a colon resection/colectomy, colostomy, and ileostomy.

34. Identify the expected outcomes for the client with ulcerative colitis.
    a. _____
    b. _____
    c. _____
    d. _____
    e. _____
    f. _____
    g. _____

35. Briefly describe Crohn's disease.

36. Identify two common complications of Crohn's disease.
    a. _____
    b. _____

37. On a separate sheet of paper, briefly discuss the implications that a fistula has for the client with Crohn's disease.

38. Crohn's disease is different from ulcerative colitis in that:
    a. The stools may show evidence of blood.
    b. The etiology is unknown.
    c. Hemorrhage may occur.
    d. Severe malabsorption by the small intestine is more common.

39. Which of the following statements about Crohn's disease is correct?
    a. The peak incidence is in the 15- to 40-year age group.
    b. There is a decreased incidence of Crohn's disease in the Jewish population.
    c. The incidence is 20% greater in men than in women.
    d. No known familial link correlates with its incidence.

40. Identify the client data (both subjective and objective) relevant to Crohn's disease you would include for your nursing assessment. *Use a separate sheet of paper for your answer.*

41. Differentiate between Crohn's disease and ulcerative colitis by matching each of the following characteristics to its corresponding chronic disease. *Answers may be used more than once.*

Characteristics	Chronic Diseases
___ a. Slowly progressive	1. Chrohn's disease
	2. Ulcerative colitis
___ b. Begins in the rectum and proceeds in a continuous manner to cecum	3. Both Crohn's and ulcerative colitis
___ c. Remissions and exacerbations	
___ d. Patchy involvement, all layers of the bowel	
___ e. Hemorrhage more common	
___ f. Etiology is unknown	
___ g. Can have 10 to 20 liquid, bloody stools per day	
___ h. Terminal ileum, site most affected	

42. Sepsis can result from abscesses or fistulas that may be present with Crohn's disease. Identify the category of drugs that can mask the symptoms of infection, thus making it essential that the nurse monitors the client vigilantly for signs and symptoms of infection.

43. Treatment of the client with a fistula is multidimensional and includes _____ and _____ therapy, _____ care, and prevention of _____.

44. On a separate sheet of paper, identify and analyze priority nursing diagnoses and collaborative problems for clients with Crohn's disease.

45. Identify the nursing diagnoses related to a serious life-threatening complication seen in Crohn's disease that does not normally occur in ulcerative colitis.

46. Develop a teaching plan for a client needing community-based care for a new ostomy. *Use a separate sheet of paper for your answer.*

47. Briefly describe diverticula.

48. Which of the following statements about diverticular disease is correct?
   a. Most diverticula occur in the descending colon.
   b. Diverticula are uncomfortable even when not inflamed.
   c. High-fiber diets contribute to diverticula occurrence.
   d. Diverticula form where intestinal wall muscles are weak.

49. Preventive measures for diverticular disease include:
   a. Excluding whole-grain breads from the diet.
   b. Avoiding fresh apples, broccoli, and lettuce.
   c. Taking bulk agents such as psyllium hydrophilic mucilloid.
   d. Taking routine anticholinergics to reduce bowel spasm.

50. Briefly explain why invasive radiographs or diagnostic tests are *not* done for the client with acute diverticulitis.

51. Identify the complications that would indicate that a client with diverticulitis will need surgery.
   a. _____
   b. _____
   c. _____
   d. _____
   e. _____
   f. _____

52. Which of the following types of stomas will the client with diverticulitis most likely have postoperatively?
   a. Ileostomy
   b. Kock pouch
   c. Colostomy
   d. Cecostomy

53. All clients with diverticular disease require education regarding a _____ diet.

54. On a separate sheet of paper, develop a teaching plan explaining the role of diet therapy for the client with diverticular disease.

55. Match each of the following anorectal problems with the corresponding descriptions.

Descriptions	Anorectal Problems
___ a. Duct obstruction and infection	1. Anal fissure
	2. Anal fistula
___ b. Perianal laceration, superficial erosion	3. Anorectal abcess
___ c. Communicating tract	

56. The nurse focuses on comfort measures that can be used for the client with anorectal problems. Identify four such measures for helping the client maintain comfort.

    a. _____

    b. _____

    c. _____

    d. _____

57. On a separate sheet of paper, describe the significance of warm sitz-baths as an intervention in managing anorectal problems.

58. Identify the most common route of transmission of parasitic infection.

Answer the following four questions on a separate sheet of paper.

59. Briefly explain why other household members and sexual partners of the infected clients should also be examined for parasites.

60. Which type of food poisoning is the most life-threatening and why?

61. Complete the following table by comparing and contrasting food poisoning and gastroenteritis.

Characteristic	Food Poisoning	Gastroenteritis
Communicability		
Incubation period		
Immunity status after recovery		
Diarrhea		
Nausea and vomiting		

62. Describe ways that parasitic infection, helminthic infestation, and food poisoning could be prevented.

Case Study: The Client with Diverticulitis

An 18-year-old body-builder has just come into your office complaining of left lower quadrant abdominal pain, temperature of 100.8° F, constipation, and blood-streaked stool. On examination of the abdomen, you observe slight distention and tenderness on palpation, especially in the left lower quadrant. This client has an elevated white blood cell count and his stool for occult blood is positive. He has been diagnosed with diverticulitis.

Answer the following questions on a separate sheet of paper:

1. Identify key findings noted in the examination and indicate the significance.

2. The client tells you, "Oh, I'll just go home and take a laxative or an enema and I'll be fine." Explain why these should be avoided.

3. Nonsurgical management has been selected for this client, and he may return home after receiving special instructions. Identify a key factor, based on your assessment, that you would need to instruct him on.

4. Provide this client with discharge instructions.

STUDY GUIDE NUMBER 12.59

Interventions for Clients with Liver Problems

Study/Review Questions

1. Match each of the following descriptions with the corresponding type of liver cirrhosis. *Answers may be used more than once.*

Descriptions
___ a. Viral induced
___ b. Vascular congestion
___ c. Hobnailed capsule
___ d. Associated with bile stasis
___ e. Fatty infiltration of hepatocytes
___ f. Chemical hepatotoxin-induced
___ g. Alcohol-induced
___ h. Liver anoxia
___ i. Massive hepatocyte death
___ j. Severe obstructive jaundice
___ k. Increased hepatic volume
___ l. Diffuse hepatic fibrosis

Types of Liver Cirrhosis
1. Laënnec's cirrhosis
2. Postnecrotic cirrhosis
3. Biliary cirrhosis
4. Cardiac cirrhosis

2. Match each of the following descriptions of pathophysiology with the corresponding complication of liver cirrhosis.

Pathophysiology
___ a. Bilirubin not excreted
___ b. Vitamin K deficiency
___ c. Backflow of blood to liver and spleen
___ d. Impaired ammonia metabolism
___ e. Plasma leaking into peritoneal cavity
___ f. Kidneys unable to excrete solutes
___ g. Thin-walled distended veins

Complications of Liver Cirrhosis
1. Portal hypertension
2. Ascites
3. Bleeding
4. Esophageal varices
5. Jaundice
6. Encephalopathy
7. Hepatorenal syndrome

Answer the following four questions on a separate sheet of paper.

3. Identify the most common form of cirrhosis in the United States and discuss how it can be prevented.

4. The cause of cirrhosis varies with the type. Identify the top cause of cirrhosis in the world.

5. List the client data (both subjective and objective) relevant to cirrhosis of the liver for your nursing assessment.

6. Analyze your assessment data and identify priority nursing diagnoses and collaborative problems for the client with cirrhosis.

7. Match each of the following abnormal laboratory findings in the cirrhotic client with the corresponding cause. *Answers may be used more than once.*

Abnormal Laboratory Findings
___ a. Serum aspartate aminotransferase elevates
___ b. Globulins elevate
___ c. Total proteins decrease
___ d. Ammonia increases
___ e. Serum alanine aminotransferase elevates
___ f. Prothrombin time prolongs
___ g. Total serum bilirubin increases
___ h. Albumin decreases
___ i. Lactate dehydrogenase elevates
___ j. Alkaline phosphatase elevates

Causes
1. Hepatocyte death
2. Biliary obstruction
3. Decreased liver synthesis
4. Increased immune response
5. Decreased conversion

8. A cirrhotic client has been admitted to your unit with ascites. Use the information presented in your textbook as a basis for developing appropriate rationales for the following interventions that have been selected for this client. *Write your answers on a separate sheet of paper.*
   a. Placing her on a low-sodium diet
   b. Placing her on fluid restriction
   c. Vitamin supplements added to her IV fluids
   d. Administering a diuretic
   e. Assessing intake and output
   f. Weighing her daily
   g. Measuring her abdominal girth
   h. Monitoring electrolyte balance
   i. Administering potassium supplements
   j. Administering low-sodium antacid therapy
   k. Elevating her head of bed at least 30 degrees

9. Which of the following would indicate the need for the physician to perform a paracentesis?
   a. Client discomfort
   b. Decreased blood pressure
   c. Fetor hepaticus
   d. Respiratory distress

Answer the following two questions on a separate sheet of paper.

10. Briefly explain why the cirrhotic client with medically unmanageable ascites is a poor surgical risk for a shunting procedure.

11. Briefly explain the purpose of a peritoneovenous shunt.

12. Because the client with cirrhosis has many underlying medical problems, an optimal physical state is desired before surgery is performed. Before surgery for a peritoneovenous shunt, electrolyte _____ are corrected, and abnormal coagulation is treated with the administration of fresh _____ and vitamin _____. Packed _____ cells are made available for transfusion, because these clients have _____ tendencies.

13. An adult client has come to your emergency department with bleeding esophageal varices, and emergency interventions must be initiated to control rapid blood loss. Identify six methods the emergency team could institute in an attempt to control the bleeding in this client.
   a. _____
   b. _____
   c. _____
   d. _____
   e. _____
   f. _____

14. Nursing responsibilities related to esophagogastric balloon tamponade include:
   a. Identifying and labeling each lumen after the tamponade tube is inserted.
   b. Attaching the esophageal and gastric drainage lumens to low continuous suction.
   c. Ensuring that balloon pressures are kept at levels needed to control bleeding.
   d. Repositioning the tube if it migrates upward and causes airway obstruction.

15. Identify the types of intravenous products that the nurse may need to administer in cases of massive esophageal hemorrhage.
   a. _____
   b. _____
   c. _____
   d. _____

16. Vasopressin (Pitressin) therapy results in:
   a. Improved blood flow in the portal system.
   b. Relaxation of vascular bed smooth muscle.
   c. Effective long-term control of variceal bleeding.
   d. Decreased blood flow to the abdominal organs.

17. Identify the nonsurgical procedure that is considered a last-resort intervention for clients with portal hypertension and esophageal varices.

18. After shunting procedures clients are susceptible to oliguria and often become hypovolemic. The nurse administers the ordered fluid volume and assesses the effects of the volume by monitoring for:
   a. _____
   b. _____
   c. _____

19. For the client with portal-systemic encephalopathy, identify what food group may be totally eliminated from the diet as the client's mental status deteriorates.

20. Which of the following drugs is usually contraindicated for the client with portal-systemic encephalopathy?
   a. Levodopa (Dopar)
   b. Diazepam (Valium)
   c. Lactulose (Cephulac)
   d. Neomycin sulfate (Mycifradin sulfate)

Answer the following two questions on a separate sheet of paper.

21. Formulate a collaborative plan of care for the client with severe late-stage cirrhosis.

22. Develop a community-based teaching plan for the client with cirrhosis of the liver.

23. Identify six expected outcomes based on the nursing diagnoses and collaborative problems for the client with cirrhosis of the liver.
    a. _____
    b. _____
    c. _____
    d. _____
    e. _____
    f. _____

24. On a separate sheet of paper, briefly describe *hepatitis*.

25. Number in chronologic order the following steps describing the pathologic changes that occur in hepatitis.
    ___ a. Intrahepatic jaundice results from edema of bile channels
    ___ b. Liver enlargement and congestion resulting from inflammatory cells, edema, and lymphocytes
    ___ c. Portal circulation impaired because of distorted lobular pattern
    ___ d. Eventual regeneration of liver cells
    ___ e. Widespread inflammation, necrosis, and hepatocellular regeneration
    ___ f. Exposure to causative agents occurs
    ___ g. Active phagocytosis and enzyme activity remove damaged cells

26. Identify the types of viral hepatitis.
    a. _____
    b. _____
    c. _____
    d. _____
    e. _____

27. Identify the type of viral hepatitis that is of most concern to health care workers.

28. Match each of the following descriptions with its corresponding type of hepatitis. *Answers may be used more than once.*

Descriptions	**Types of Hepatitis**
___ a. Occurs only in the presence of hepatitis B virus	1. Hepatitis A
	2. Hepatitis B
	3. Hepatitis C
___ b. Rarely life-threatening	4. Delta hepatitis (hepatitis D)
___ c. Does not lead to chronic infection	5. Hepatitis E

___ d. Often goes unrecognized
___ e. Spread by contaminated water, shellfish
___ f. Transmitted from mother to fetus
___ g. Leading cause of cirrhosis worldwide
___ h. Low concentrations of virus are found in semen and saliva
___ i. Approximately one half of liver transplants in United States are for end stage (of this virus)
___ j. Spread by sexual contact with multiple partners
___ k. Rarely transmitted sexually or mother to fetus

29. Identify two ways in which hepatitis A, B, and C could be prevented.
    a. Hepatitis A _____
    _____
    _____
    b. Hepatitis B _____
    _____
    _____
    c. Hepatitis C _____
    _____
    _____

30. On a separate sheet of paper, briefly explain the primary concerns about the increasing incidence of hepatitis C in the United States.

31. Match the following complications of viral hepatitis with their descriptions.

    Descriptions
    ___ a. Chronic active hepatitis
    ___ b. Chronic persistent hepatitis
    ___ c. Fulminant hepatitis

    Complications of Viral Hepatitis
    1. Non-progressive liver damage
    2. Progressive liver damage with necrosis, inflammation, and fibrosis
    3. Severe and often fatal, failure of liver cells to regenerate

32. Jaundice in hepatitis results from intrahepatic _____ and is caused by _____ of the liver's _____.

33. Which of the following drugs is contraindicated for managing nausea in the client with viral hepatitis?
    a. Trimethobenzamide hydrochloride (Tigan)
    b. Prochlorperazine maleate (Compazine)
    c. Dimenhydrinate (Dramamine)
    d. Ranitidine (Zantac)

34. Instructions for the client with viral hepatitis would include all of the following *except*:
    a. Avoid sharing bathroom towels with family members.
    b. Avoid alcohol, sedatives, and acetaminophen (Tylenol).
    c. Begin an exercise program at the local health spa.
    d. Eat small, frequent meals with a high-carbohy-drate, low-fat content.

35. Match each of the following descriptions with the corresponding liver disorder. *Answers may be used more than once.*

    Descriptions
    ___ a. Bacterial invasion
    ___ b. Result of faulty metabolism
    ___ c. Penetrating or blunt injury
    ___ d. Sudden onset of symptoms
    ___ e. Hemorrhagic shock
    ___ f. Confirmed by liver biopsy
    ___ g. Hepatomegaly
    ___ h. Right shoulder pain
    ___ i. Associated with chronic alcoholism
    ___ j. Anorexia, weight loss
    ___ k. Multiple blood products

    Liver Disorders
    1. Fatty liver
    2. Hepatic abscess
    3. Liver trauma

36. The liver is a common site for metastasis from what sources?
    a. _____
    b. _____

37. Identify the possible causes of liver cancer.
    a. _____
    b. _____
    c. _____
    d. _____
    e. _____
    f. _____
    g. _____

38. Identify five treatment options for clients with cancer of the liver.
    a. _____
    b. _____
    c. _____
    d. _____
    e. _____

Answer the following two questions on a separate sheet of paper.

39. Describe the type of client who would be a potential candidate for liver transplantation.

40. Describe the type of client who would not be considered a candidate for liver transplantation.

41. Donor livers are obtained primarily from what source?

42. Identify the complications that may result from liver transplantation.
    a. _____
    b. _____
    c. _____
    d. _____
    e. _____
    f. _____
    g. _____
    h. _____
    i. _____

43. When is organ rejection most likely to occur following liver transplantation?

44. Identify four clinical manifestations the nurse would observe for when assessing the client who may be experiencing acute rejection after liver transplantation.
    a. _____
    b. _____
    c. _____
    d. _____

45. Identify the drug therapy used to prevent organ rejection in the client who has had a liver transplantation.
    a. _____
    b. _____
    c. _____
    d. _____

Case Study: The Client with Cirrhosis and Esophageal Bleeding

A recently retired locomotive engineer is looking forward to his retirement so that he and his wife "can finally enjoy" their lives together. He states he feels he has maintained sobriety quite well, but occasionally "sneaks a little drink now and then," and unfortunately his cirrhotic liver has never fully recovered from 25 years of fairly heavy drinking. Periodically, and through the years, he still has symptoms of residual effects. For the past several days he states he has been coughing on and off. His wife states that this morning he coughed up "bright red blood" and that is why she made him come to the hospital. As for now, he is not coughing or bleeding but has been admitted for observation. As you are doing your rounds, his wife comes out of his room hysterical; you enter his room and observe blood all over his gown and bed linens. He appears terrified.

Answer the following questions on a separate sheet of paper:

1. What would you need to do immediately?

2. The physician enters the room to perform an esophagogastric balloon tamponade. Before the physician inserts the tube, (a) identify your priority nursing intervention and what measures you would take to ensure it. (b) What would your responsibility be in assisting the physician before insertion of the tube?

3. After insertion of the tube and placement has been verified, explain how you would assist the physician with securing the tube and applying traction.

STUDY GUIDE NUMBER 12.60

Interventions for Clients with Problems of the Gallbladder and Pancreas

Study/Review Questions

1. On a separate sheet of paper, briefly differentiate between acute and chronic cholecystitis.

2. Cholecystitis can be caused by the formation of gallbladder calculi. Identify other possible causes.
   a. _____
   b. _____
   c. _____
   d. _____
   e. _____
   f. _____
   g. _____
   h. _____
   i. _____
   j. _____
   k. _____

3. Obstructive jaundice can result in all of the following except:
   a. Pruritus.
   b. Dark and foamy urine.
   c. Pink discoloration of sclera.
   d. Clay-colored stools.

4. Identify the common underlying factor that contributes to the etiology of acute cholecystitis.

5. A high incidence of biliary tract disease and cholecystitis is associated with:
   a. Leading an active lifestyle.
   b. Having a familial tendency.
   c. Being slightly underweight.
   d. Having non-insulin-dependent diabetes.

Answer the following two questions on a separate sheet of paper.

6. Identify the client data (both subjective and objective) relevant to biliary disorders for your nursing assessment.

7. Because there is no specific laboratory test for gallbladder disease, explain the course of action taken in determining a diagnosis for gallbladder disease.

8. What is the best diagnostic test for cholecystitis?

9. Which of the following medications is usually *not* given to clients for pain management in gallbladder disease?
   a. Morphine
   b. Lomine
   c. Bentyl
   d. Demerol

10. What is the usual surgical treatment for clients with cholecystitis?

11. Preoperatively for the client about to undergo a traditional cholecystectomy, the nurse reinforces teaching methods to prevent respiratory complications. The nurse would demonstrate _____ methods, using a _____ or folded _____ to minimize abdominal/incisional _____ during coughing, _____, and _____.

12. Postoperatively the nurse cares for the _____, the surgical _____, and the _____.

13. The client's T-tube can remain in place for how long?

14. Management of a T-tube in a client who has had gallbladder surgery includes:
   a. Routinely irrigating the tube with 30 mL of normal saline every shift.
   b. Keeping the client in a supine position.
   c. Giving synthetic bile salts as ordered.
   d. Keeping the drainage system above the level of the gallbladder.

15. After the removal of the gallbladder, the client's dietary intake of fat should be:
   a. Eliminated completely.
   b. Adjusted according to individual tolerance.
   c. Limited to less than 10% of the diet.
   d. Increased to more than 50% of the diet.

16. Laparoscopic cholecystectomy is commonly done on an _____ care basis in a _____ surgery suite.

17. Postoperatively with laparoscopic procedures, some clients have a problem with "free air pain." The nurse would teach the client about the importance of _____ ambulation to promote _____ of the carbon _____.

18. With a laparoscopic procedure the client is usually discharged from the surgery center _____ _____. *(How long?)*

19. After having a laparoscopic procedure done, most clients are able to resume usual activities after how long?

20. Identify the most common cause of inflammation in clients with cholelithiasis.

21. Match the following terms related to gallbladder disorders with their definitions.

Definitions	Terms Associated with Gallbladder Disorders
____ a. Common bile duct stones	1. Ascending cholangitis
____ b. Gallbladder stones	2. Cholangitis
____ c. Inflammation of bile ducts (involves infection)	3. Choledocholithiasis
____ d. Inflammation of biliary tree	4. Cholelithiasis

22. Identify the substances that are normally found in gallstones.
   a. _____
   b. _____
   c. _____
   d. _____
   e. _____

23. What examination permits radiographic visualization of the common bile duct, pancreas, pancreatic ducts, and biliary tree and permits the physician to pinpoint the nature of a biliary obstruction?

24. Pruritis resulting from obstructive jaundice is treated with:
   a. Cholestyramine.
   b. Meperidine.
   c. Ursodiol.
   d. Dicyclomine hydrochloride.

25. Match the following procedures with their definitions.

Definitions
___ a. Powerful shock waves shatter gallstones
___ b. Incision into common bile duct for stone removal
___ c. Removal of gallbladder
___ d. Direct visualization of biliary tract
___ e. Opening into the gallbladder

Procedures
1. Cholecystectomy
2. Cholecystotomy
3. Choledocholithotomy
4. Choledochoscopy
5. Extracorporeal shock wave lithotripsy

Answer the following three questions on a separate sheet of paper.

26. Develop a community-based teaching plan for clients with gallbladder disease, including care of a T-tube.

27. Identify and briefly describe the four major pathophysiologic processes that occur in acute pancreatitis.

28. Briefly define *autodigestion*.

29. Identify the theories that attempt to explain the triggering mechanisms leading to enzyme activation in acute pancreatitis.
   a. _____
   b. _____
   c. _____
   d. _____

30. Match the following complications of pancreatitis with their pathophysiologies.

Pathophysiology
___ a. Disruption of alveolar-capillary membrane results in edema
___ b. Release of glucagon and damaged islet cell
___ c. Consumption of clotting factors and microthrombi formation
___ d. Head of pancreas swells and restricts bile flow through common bile duct
___ e. Seepage of digested proteins and lipids into mesentery
___ f. Pancreatic exudate migrates via transdiaphragmatic coagulation lymphatics

Complications of Pancreatitis
1. Peritoneal irritation
2. Jaundice
3. Transient hyperglycemia
4. Pleural effusion
5. Adult respiratory distress syndrome (ARDS)
6. Disseminated intravascular coagulation (DIC)

31. Identify the two most common factors that cause injury to the pancreas.
   a. _____
   b. _____

32. On a separate sheet of paper, list the client data (both subjective and objective) relevant to acute pancreatitis for your assessment.

33. Identify the two serum studies that are considered the "cardinal" diagnostic signs important in the diagnosis of pancreatitis.
   a. _____
   b. _____

Read the following seven statements and decide whether each is true or false. Write T for true or F for false in the blanks provided. If the statement is false, correct the statement to make it true.

___ 34. Abdominal pain is the prominent symptom of pancreatitis.

___ 35. Anticholinergics are given to increase vagal stimulation, increase GI motility, and inhibit pancreatic enzyme and bicarbonate volume and concentration.

___ 36. Pain management for acute pancreatitis should begin with rapid infusion of opioids by means of patient-controlled analgesia (PCA).

___ 37. Helping the client to assume a cross-legged position may decrease the abdominal pain of pancreatitis.

___ 38. Surgical intervention for acute pancreatitis is usually not indicated.

___ 39. The client in the early stages of acute pancreatitis is usually maintained on NPO status.

___ 40. If total parenteral nutrition (TPN) is used for nutritional support, the nurse assesses for glucose intolerance by monitoring for decreased blood glucose levels.

41. Prioritize nursing care needs for clients with acute pancreatitis. *Use a separate sheet of paper for your answer.*

42. Briefly describe chronic pancreatitis.

43. On a separate sheet of paper, differentiate between chronic calcifying pancreatitis and chronic obstructive pancreatitis.

44. Match each of the following complications of chronic pancreatitis with the related cause. *Answers may be used more than once.*

    Complications of
    Chronic Pancreatitis   **Causes**
    ___ a. Steatorrhea   1. Loss of endocrine
    ___ b. Decrease in   function
           muscle mass   2. Loss of exocrine
    ___ c. Ketoacidosis   function
    ___ d. Peripheral edema
    ___ e. Hyperglycemia

45. The only definitive diagnostic test for chronic pancreatitis is the identification of _____ of pancreatic _____ in a _____ specimen.

46. Identify the significant serum laboratory findings most commonly associated with chronic pancreatitis.
    a. _____
    b. _____
    c. _____
    d. _____

47. On a separate sheet of paper, list the client data (both subjective and objective) relevant to chronic pancreatitis for your nursing assessment.

48. On a separate sheet of paper, discuss problems the nurse may encounter with pain management for the client with chronic pancreatitis.

Read the following seven statements related to chronic pancreatitis and decide whether each is true or false. Write T for true or F for false in the blanks provided. If the statement is false, correct the statement to make it true.

____49. Pancreatic enzymes are essential dietary supplements.

____50. Pancreatic enzymes are given on an empty stomach.

____51. The nurse mixes the powdered form of pancreatic enzymes in milk.

____52. Enzyme preparation should be mixed with foods containing protein.

____53. After administration of the enzyme preparation, the nurse advises the client to wipe the lips with a dry napkin.

____54. Glucose levels for the client should be checked daily, particularly for the client on TPN.

____55. The health care provider may prescribe Zantac to increase gastric acid.

56. Discharge planning for the client with chronic pancreatitis includes:
    a. Renting a commode for bedside use.
    b. Gradually tapering off the dosage of the pancreatic enzymes.
    c. Asking a member of Alcoholics Anonymous to visit.
    d. Encouraging the client to consume high-fat large meals.

57. Prioritize nursing care needs for clients with chronic pancreatitis. *Use a separate sheet of paper for your answer.*

58. Identify the primary sources of tumors that metastasize to the pancreas.
    a. _____
    b. _____
    c. _____
    d. _____
    e. _____

59. Briefly explain why cancer of the pancreas has a poor prognosis.

60. Tumors in the head of the pancreas:
    a. Are usually large and invade the entire organ.
    b. Frequently cause jaundice and gallbladder distention.
    c. Spread more extensively than tumors in the tail.
    d. Are the least common of the pancreatic cancers.

61. A common complication of pancreatic carcinoma is:
    a. Seizures.
    b. Pneumonia.
    c. Thrombophlebitis.
    d. Uncontrolled bleeding.

62. Identify the test that is the most diagnostic for cancer of the pancreas.

63. The Whipple procedure is used to treat cancer of the _____ and of the _____.

64. What is the most common and most serious postoperative complication of the Whipple procedure?

65. A client had a Whipple procedure. On a separate sheet of paper, identify the rationales for the following postoperative nursing interventions.
    a. Monitoring of wound drainage and drainage tubes
    b. Maintaining patency of NG tube
    c. Protecting the skin from wound drainage
    d. Positioning in a semi-Fowler's position
    e. Monitoring vital signs
    f. Administering ordered IV fluids
    g. Measuring hourly urinary output
    h. Checking serum glucose levels
    i. Monitoring the Swan-Ganz catheter

66. On a separate sheet of paper, develop a discharge plan for care of clients with end-stage pancreatic cancer in the community.

For Questions 67 to 72 regarding pancreatic cancer, fill in the blanks to correctly complete the sentences.

67. When the client with pancreatic cancer is discharged to home, many of the care measures are _____ and aimed at providing relief of _____ such as _____.

68. In many cases, the _____ of pancreatic _____ is made a _____ before _____ occurs.

69. For clients with end-stage pancreatic cancer, the nurse helps the _____ identify what needs to be _____ to prepare for _____.

70. The above client may want to write a _____ or see _____ and _____ whom he or she has not seen recently.

71. The above client needs to make specific _____ for the _____ or memorial _____ known to family members or _____.

72. These actions help the client prepare for death in a _____ manner.

73. Identify and explain psychosocial needs for the client with pancreatic cancer and associated nursing interventions. *Use a separate sheet of paper for your answer.*

STUDY GUIDE NUMBER 12.61

Interventions for Clients with Malnutrition and Obesity

Study/Review Questions

1. Identify the four nutritional components the Recommended Dietary Allowance (RDA) has established as recommendations for a healthy population.
   a. _____
   b. _____
   c. _____
   d. _____

2. Recommended Dietary Allowance (RDA) is a:
   a. Standard for determining malnutrition.
   b. Guide for selecting daily food choices.
   c. Standard for evaluation of nutritional problems.
   d. Guide for estimating the adequacy of nutrient intake over time.

3. On a separate sheet of paper, briefly describe the lacto-vegetarian diet.

4. What vitamin is lacking in the diet of vegans that can contribute to the development of megaloblastic anemia?

5. What factors affect a person's nutrient requirements?
   a. _____
   b. _____
   c. _____

6. What factors influence a person's nutrient intake?
   a. _____
   b. _____
   c. _____
   d. _____
   e. _____
   f. _____

7. What are the components of a nutritional status assessment?
   a. _____
   b. _____
   c. _____
   d. _____
   e. _____
   f. _____
   g. _____

8. Briefly describe anthropometric measurements.

9. Identify three anthropometric measurements that the nurse can use to evaluate a client's nutritional status.
   a. _____
   b. _____
   c. _____

Read the following statements related to anthropometric measurements and decide whether each is true or false. Write T for true or F for false in the blanks provided. If the statement is false, correct the statement to make it true.

____ 10. The nurse must obtain accurate measurements, because clients who report their own measurements tend to underestimate height and overestimate weight.

____ 11. Clients should be measured and weighed while wearing minimal clothing and shoes.

____ 12. In determining height, the client should stand erect and look straight ahead, with the heels apart and the arms forward.

____ 13. The nurse weighs all clients with an upright balance beam scale.

____ 14. No medical condition the client may have would affect his or her weight.

____ 15. An involuntary weight loss of 10% at any time significantly affects nutritional status.

____ 16. The body mass index is a measure of nutritional status that depends on frame size.

____ 17. Skinfold measurements estimate body fat.

____ 18. The midarm circumference can be obtained to measure muscle mass only.

19. Energy balance refers to the relationship between _____ expended and energy _____.

20. Protein-calorie malnutrition may present in three forms. Identify the three forms and give a brief description of each.
   a. _____
   b. _____
   c. _____

21. In a malnourished client, _____ catabolism exceeds protein _____ and _____, resulting in _____ nitrogen balance, _____ loss, _____ muscle mass, and _____.

22. Identify the complications associated with severe malnutrition.
   a. _____
   b. _____
   c. _____
   d. _____
   e. _____
   f. _____
   g. _____
   h. _____
   i. _____

23. Identify the factors that may influence inadequate nutrient intake.
   a. _____
   b. _____
   c. _____
   d. _____
   e. _____
   f. _____
   g. _____
   h. _____
   i. _____
   j. _____
   k. _____
   l. _____
   m. _____
   n. _____

24. Acute protein-calorie malnutrition (PCM) may develop in clients who were adequately nourished before hospitalization if they experience _____ _____ while in a _____ state resulting from _____, stress, or _____.

25. On a separate sheet of paper, list the client data (both subjective and objective) relevant to malnutrition for your nursing assessment.

26. Older adults are particularly at risk for malnutrition. Identify six factors that have been associated with placing the older adult at risk for malnutrition.
    a. _____
    b. _____
    c. _____
    d. _____
    e. _____
    f. _____

27. Match the following laboratory test values with their indications of nutritional status.

Indications of Nutritional Status	Laboratory Test Values
____ a. Indicates the body's protein status	1. Hemoglobin
	2. Hematocrit
____ b. A sensitive indicator of protein deficiency	3. Serum albumin
	4. Serum transferring
____ c. Assesses immune function	5. Thyroxine-binding prealbumin
____ d. Value below 160 mg/dL could indicate malnutrition, sepsis, and anemia	6. Serum cholesterol
	7. Total lymphocyte count
____ e. Iron deficiency anemia	
____ f. Total iron-binding capacity	
____ g. Indicates iron status (a measure of cell volume)	

28. Identify the most common nursing diagnosis for the client with malnutrition (use your data from Question 25).

29. On a separate sheet of paper, identify additional nursing diagnoses and collaborative problems based on your assessment.

30. Identify three expected outcomes for the client who is malnourished.
    a. _____
    b. _____
    c. _____

31. For the client who has difficulty chewing or is without teeth, the preferred diet would be:
    a. Clear liquid.
    b. Full liquid.
    c. Pureed food.
    d. Regular food.

32. Total enteral nutrition (TEN) would be contraindicated for which of the following clients?
    a. An older adult receiving chemotherapy
    b. A client who has had a stroke and has dysphagia
    c. A client who has had extensive jaw and mouth surgery
    d. A client who had intestinal obstruction that has progressed to diffuse peritonitis

33. Identify the type of feeding tube that is used primarily for clients requiring short-term enteral feedings.

34. Briefly describe a gastrostomy.

35. Match each of the following types of feeding tubes with the corresponding description.

Descriptions	Types of Feeding Tubes
____ a. Small amounts are continually infused over a specified time	1. Bolus feeding tube
	2. Continuous feeding tube
____ b. Infusion is stopped for a specified time	3. Cycle feeding tube
____ c. Intermittent feeding of a specified amount at specified times	

36. What is the most common problem associated with feeding tubes?

37. Identify the most accurate method of confirming the placement of a feeding tube.

38. Clients receiving enteral therapy are at an _____ risk for fluid _____.

39. In clients with inadequate renal and cardiac function who are receiving enteral nutrition, identify the major complication associated with increased osmolarity.

40. If the nurse delivers hyperosmolar enteral preparations too quickly, what might be a possible consequence?

41. Identify the two most common electrolyte imbalances associated with enteral nutrition.
    a. _____
    b. _____

The following descriptions relate to parenteral nutrition. If the phrase refers to partial parenteral nutrition, write PPN in the blank provided; if the phrase refers to total parenteral nutrition, write TPN in the blank provided.

_____ 42. Used when nutritional support is needed less than 2 weeks

_____ 43. Delivered through a cannula in a large distal vein of the arm

_____ 44. Delivered through access to central veins, usually the subclavian or internal jugular

_____ 45. Client should be able to tolerate large fluid volumes

_____ 46. Given when the client requires intensive nutritional support for an extended time

_____ 47. Solutions contain higher concentrations of dextrose and proteins

_____ 48. The two common solutions used are lipid emulsions and amino acid dextrose

49. Clients receiving PPN or TPN are at increased risk for fluid imbalance. Identify the underlying factor that contributes to this risk.

50. The nurse monitors for complications of fluid imbalance by taking daily _____ and by recording accurate _____ and _____ while the client is receiving parenteral nutrition.

51. Identify the three most common electrolyte imbalances associated with parenteral nutrition.
    a. _____
    b. _____
    c. _____

52. Match the following terms related to obesity with their definitions.

Definitions

____ a. Weight that negatively affects health status

____ b. Excessive amount of body fat

____ c. Increase in body weight for height as compared to a standard

Terms Related to Obesity
1. Obesity
2. Overweight
3. Morbid obesity

53. Identify the complications of obesity that can improve with weight loss.
    a. _____
    b. _____
    c. _____
    d. _____
    e. _____
    f. _____
    g. _____
    h. _____
    i. _____

54. Identify the five major causes of obesity, and provide an example for each.
    a. _____
    b. _____
    c. _____
    d. _____
    e. _____

55. Culture appears to be a factor in the prevalence of obesity. The prevalence of obesity among ethnic minorities is substantially _____ than in whites, especially among _____.

56. Identify five medical conditions the overweight female could be at risk for developing.
    a. _____
    b. _____
    c. _____
    d. _____
    e. _____

57. Identify expected outcomes for the client with obesity.
    a. _____
    b. _____
    c. _____

58. Which of the following diets promotes safe weight loss?
    a. Low-energy diet
    b. Liquid formula diet
    c. The grapefruit diet
    d. Short-term fasting

59. Anorectic drugs used for obesity suppress _____ _____.

60. Orlistat inhibits _____ and leads to partial hydrolysis of _____.

61. Identify the major side effects of drugs used to treat obesity.
    a. _____
    b. _____
    c. _____
    d. _____
    e. _____
    f. _____

62. Identify surgical procedures that may be performed to reduce food intake of an obese client; provide a brief description of each.
    a. _____
    b. _____
    c. _____
    d. _____

63. Postoperative care for the client who has undergone a gastroplasty would include never _____ the nasogastric (NG) tube because its movement can disrupt the _____ line.

64. The NG tube would be removed on the third day after intestinal bypass if the client has _____ _____ and is passing _____.

65. The most important features of client education focus on _____-related behavior patterns.

66. Formulate additional postoperative teaching for clients having a gastroplasty or intestinal bypass.

UNIT 13 PROBLEMS OF REGULATION AND METABOLISM: ENDOCRINE SYSTEM ■ Core Concepts Grid

Anatomy	Physiology	Pathophysiology	History	Physical Exam	Diagnostic Tests	Interventions	Pharmacology
• **Glands** Anterior pituitary Posterior pituitary Thyroid Parathyroid Pancreas Adrenal • **Hormones** Antidiuretic hormone (ADH) Thyroid-stimulating hormone (TSH) Adrenocorticotropic hormone (ACTH) Growth hormone (GH) Mineralocorticoids Glucocorticoids Androgens Epinephrine Norepinephrine Thyroxine Thyrocalcitonin Parathormone Insulin Glucagon	• **Neuroregulation** • **Hypothalamus** • **Regulation** Metabolism Fluids/electrolytes Glucose levels Stress response	• **Inflammation** • **Hypersecretion** • **Hyposecretion** • **Infection** • **Diabetic ketoacidosis** • **Hyperglycemic hyperosmolar nonketotic syndrome (HHNKS)** • **Adrenal crisis**	• **Client history** Energy level Elimination pattern Nutrition Reproductive function Libido • **Family history** Endocrine disease • **Social history** Drug/alcohol use Coping skills Age Gender • **Weight change**	• **Appearance** Skin Hair Body fat distribution Muscle mass Bruising Petechiae Edema Face Genitalia • **Size of thyroid** • **Vital signs** • **Weight**	• **Adrenocorticotropic hormone (ACTH) levels** • **Aldosterone assay** • **Antidiuretic hormone (ADH)** • **Blood glucose** • **Catecholamines** Vanillylmandelic acid (VMA) • **Cortisol** • **Glycosolated hemoglobin A$_{1c}$** • **17-hydroxycorticosteroids** • **Ketones** • **Parathyroid hormone level** • **T$_3$/T$_4$** • **Thyroid scan**	• **Hormone replacement** • **Nutrition** • **Fluid management** • **Stress management** • **Client education** Diet Exercise Hormone replacement regimen Overdose Underdose Foot care Signs of complications Need for carrying emergency medical information • **Postoperative care/monitoring for complications** Thyroidectomy Adrenalectomy Pancreas transplantation • **Monitoring for hypoglycemia and hyperglycemia**	• **Glucagon** • **Insulin** • **Oral hypoglycemic agents** • **Thyroid replacement** • **Thyroid inhibitors** • **Pituitary hormone replacements** • **Pituitary hormone inhibitors** • **Parathyroid hormone replacement** • **Parathyroid hormone inhibitors** • **Calcium** • **Adrenal hormone replacements** • **Adrenal hormone inhibitors**

Unit 13 (Chapters 62-65)

Problems of Regulation and Metabolism: Management of Clients with Problems of the Endocrine System

Learning Plan

Chapter 62: *Assessment of the Endocrine System*

Learning Outcomes	Learning Activities	Supplemental Resources

1. Describe the relationship between hormones and receptor sites.
2. Explain negative feedback as a control mechanism for hormone secretion.
3. Discuss the structure and function of the hypothalamus.
4. Discuss the structure and function of the anterior and posterior pituitary glands.
5. Discuss the structure and function of the adrenal glands.
6. Discuss the structure and function of the thyroid and parathyroid glands.
7. Discuss the structure and function of the pancreas.
8. Describe changes in the endocrine system associated with aging.
9. Identify laboratory tests that aid in determining endocrine function and dysfunction.
	1. Prior to completing the study guide exercises for this chapter, review the following:
	  • Anatomy and physiology of the endocrine system
	  • Hormones and their functions
	  • Normal growth and development and the effects of the endocrine system on the aging process
	  • Skills for performing a physical assessment
	  • Gordon's functional health patterns
	2. Review the **boldfaced** Key Terms and their definitions in Chapter 62 to enhance your understanding of the content.
	3. Go to Study Guide Number 13.62 on the following pages and complete the learning exercises for this chapter.
		1. Textbook—Chapter 62
		2. Other resources:
		  • American Association of Clinical Endocrinologists: 1000 Riverside Ave, Suite 205, Jacksonville, FL 32204; http://www.aace.com
		  • Any anatomy and physiology textbook
		  • Any diagnostic and laboratory manual
		  • Any physical assessment textbook that includes changes in assessment findings of the older adult
		  • Endocrine Nurses Society: 2258 SE Darline Ave, Gresham, OR 97080; http://www.endonurses.org/
		  • Gordon, M. (1997). *Manual of nursing diagnosis: 1997-1998.* St. Louis: Mosby.
		  • Hospital/institution policy and procedures
		  • Rusterholtz, A. (1996). Interpretation of diagnostic laboratory tests in selected endocrine disorders. *Nursing Clinics of North America, 31,* 715.
		  • Winger, J. & Hornick, T. (1996). Age-associated changes in the endocrine system. *Nursing Clinics of North America, 31*(4), 827-844.

Chapter 63: *Interventions for Clients with Pituitary and Adrenal Gland Problems*

Learning Outcomes	Learning Activities	Supplemental Resources
1. Compare and contrast the common clinical manifestations associated with pituitary hypofunction and pituitary hyperfunction. 2. Use clinical changes and laboratory data to determine the effectiveness of interventions for pituitary hypofunction. 3. Identify the teaching priorities for the client taking hormone replacement therapy for pituitary hypofunction. 4. Prioritize the nursing care needs of the client immediately after a transsphenoidal hypophysectomy. 5. Use clinical changes and laboratory data to determine the effectiveness of interventions for pituitary hyperfunction. 6. Compare and contrast the problems associated with oversecretion and undersecretion of antidiuretic hormone. 7. Explain the effect of diabetes insipidus on blood and urine volumes and blood and urine osmolarity. 8. Explain the effect of syndrome of inappropriate antidiuretic hormone (SIADH) on blood and urine volumes and blood and urine osmolarity. 9. Use clinical changes and laboratory data to determine the effectiveness of interventions for diabetes insipidus. 10. Identify teaching priorities for the client with diabetes insipidus. 11. Use clinical changes and laboratory data to determine the effectiveness of interventions for SIADH. 12. Identify the teaching priorities for the client with SIADH. 13. Compare and contrast the clinical manifestations of Cushing's syndrome and Addison's disease. 14. Use clinical changes and laboratory data to determine the effectiveness of interventions for Cushing's syndrome. 15. Identify teaching priorities for the client with Cushing's syndrome. 16. Use clinical changes and laboratory data to determine the effectiveness of interventions for Addison's disease. 17. Identify teaching priorities for the client with Addison's disease.	1. Prior to completing the study guide exercises in this chapter, review the following: • Anatomy and physiology of the hypothalamus, pituitary gland, and adrenal glands • Functions of hormones of the pituitary gland and the adrenal glands • Normal growth and development and the effects of the pituitary and adrenal gland hormones on these processes • Normal laboratory values for serum and urine potassium and sodium levels and for urine specific gravity • Principles of fluid and electrolyte balance and acid-base balance • Concepts of human sexuality • Perioperative nursing care • Assessment of the endocrine system 2. Review the **boldfaced** Key Terms and their definitions in Chapter 63 to enhance your understanding of the content. 3. Go to Study Guide Number 13.63 on the following pages and complete the learning exercises for this chapter.	1. Textbook—Chapter 62 (Assessment of the Endocrine System) 2. Textbook—Chapter 63 3. Other resources: • Any anatomy and physiology book • Any diagnostic and laboratory manual • Any pathophysiology book • Any pharmacology book • Any physical assessment text that includes changes in the older adult • Carson, P. (2000). Emergency: Adrenal crisis. *American Journal of Nursing,* 100(7), 49-50. • Clayton, L. & Dilley, K. (1998). Cushing's syndrome. *American Journal of Nursing, 98*(7), 40-41. • Eisenberg, A. & Redick, E. (1999). Caring for a patient after resection of pituitary adenoma. *Nursing 99, 29*(12), 32cc1-32cc6. • Heater, D. (1999). If ADH goes out of balance: Diabetes insipidus. *RN, 62*(7), 44-46. • Heater, D. (1999). If ADH goes out of balance: SIADH. *RN, 62*(7), 47-49.

Chapter 64: Interventions for Clients with Problems of the Thyroid and Parathyroid Glands

Learning Outcomes	Learning Activities	Supplemental Resources
1. Compare and contrast the common clinical manifestations associated with hyperthyroidism and hypothyroidism. 2. Explain the pathophysiology of Graves' disease. 3. Use clinical changes and laboratory data to determine the effectiveness of interventions for hyperthyroidism. 4. Prioritize the nursing care needs for the client during the first 24 hours following a total thyroidectomy. 5. Explain the pathophysiology of Hashimoto's thyroiditis. 6. Identify teaching priorities for the client taking thyroid hormone replacement therapy. 7. Use clinical changes and laboratory data to determine the effectiveness of interventions for hypothyroidism. 8. Compare and contrast the clinical manifestations associated with hyperparathyroidism and hypoparathyroidism. 9. Prioritize the nursing care needs of the client during the first 24 hours following a parathyroidectomy. 10. Use clinical changes and laboratory data to determine the effectiveness of interventions for parathyroid problems.	1. Prior to completing the study guide exercises in this chapter, review the following: • Anatomy and physiology of the thyroid and parathyroid glands • Functions of the hormones of the thyroid and parathyroid glands • Normal growth and development and the effects of aging on the thyroid and parathyroid glands • Sympathetic nervous system • Normal laboratory values for serum and urine sodium, calcium, and phosphorus • Principles of fluid and electrolyte balance and acid-base balance • Perioperative nursing care • Principles of airway management • Concepts of body image and self-esteem • Concepts of fatigue • Assessment of the endocrine system 2. Review the **boldfaced** Key Terms and their definitions in Chapter 64 to enhance your understanding of the content. 3. Go to Study Guide Number 13.64 on the following pages and complete the learning exercises for this chapter.	1. Textbook—Chapter 13 (Interventions with Electrolyte Imbalances) 2. Textbook—Chapter 62 (Assessment of the Endocrine System) 3. Textbook—Chapter 64 4. Other resources: • Any anatomy and physiology textbook • Any diagnostic and laboratory manual • Any fluid and electrolyte textbook • Any pharmacology textbook • Any physical assessment textbook that includes changes in assessment findings of the older adult • Elliott, B. (2000). Diagnosing and treating hypothyroidism. *The Nurse Practitioner, 25*(3), 92-105. • Endocrine Nurses Society: http://www.endonurses.org • Goldsmith, C. (1999). Hypothyroidism. *American Journal of Nursing, 99*(6), 42-43. • Kennedy, L.W. & Caro, J.F. (1996). The ABCs of managing hyperthyroidism in the older patient. *Geriatrics, 51*(5), 22-24, 27, 31, 32. • Trotto, N. (1999). Hypothyroidism, hyperthyroidism, hyperparathyroidism. *Patient Care, 33*(14), 186-188, 191, 195-200. • Winger, J.M. & Hornick T. (1996). Age-associated changes in the endocrine system. *Nursing Clinics of North America, 31,* 827.

Chapter 65: Interventions for Clients with Diabetes Mellitus

Learning Outcomes	Learning Activities	Supplemental Resources
1. Compare and contrast the age of onset, clinical manifestations, and pathologic mechanisms of type 1 and type 2 diabetes mellitus. 2. Identify clients at risk for developing type 2 diabetes mellitus. 3. Explain the effects of insulin on carbohydrate, protein, and fat metabolism. 4. Evaluate the laboratory data to determine whether the client is using the prescribed dietary, medication, and exercise intervention of diabetes. 5. Explain the effect of aerobic exercise on blood glucose levels. 6. Describe the significance of the presence of ketone bodies in the urine of a diabetic client. 7. Use the exchange system to plan a menu for a client with diabetes who is prescribed to eat 1800 calories per day, divided into 3 meals and a snack, with 15% of calories from fat, 20% of calories from protein, and the remaining calories from carbohydrate sources. 8. Compare the mechanisms of action of the sulfonylureas, biguanides, alpha-glucosidase inhibitors, and the thiazolidinediones as antidiuretic agents. 9. Explain the effect of hypertension on the development of diabetic nephropathy and diabetic retinopathy. 10. Identify the clients at risk for development of hypoglycemia. 11. Prioritize nursing interventions for the client with mild to moderate hypoglycemia. 12. Prioritize nursing interventions for the client with moderate to severe hypoglycemia. 13. Identify clients at risk for developing diabetic ketoacidosis (DKA). 14. Prioritize nursing interventions for clients with DKA. 15. Identify clients at risk for developing HHNS or HHNKS. 16. Prioritize nursing interventions for clients with HHNS. 17. Use laboratory data and clinical manifestations to determine the effectiveness of the interventions for DKA and HHNS. 18. Describe the correct technique to use when mixing different types of insulin within the same syringe. 19. Compare and contrast the clinical manifestations of hyperglycemia and hypoglycemia.	1. Prior to completing the study guide exercises for this chapter, review the following: • Anatomy and physiology of the pancreas and kidneys • Function of insulin in the body • Normal laboratory values for serum and urine glucose, osmolarity, and electrolytes • Principles of fluid and electrolyte balance and acid-base balance • Subcutaneous injections • Assessment of the endocrine system 2. Review the **boldfaced** Key Terms and their definitions in Chapter 65 to enhance your understanding of the content. 3. Go to Study Guide Number 13.65 on the following pages and complete the learning exercises for this chapter.	1. Textbook—Chapter 62 (Assessment of the Endocrine System) 2. Textbook—Chapter 65 3. Other resources: • Arezzo, J.C. (1999). New developments in the diagnosis of diabetic neuropathy. *American Journal of Medicine, 107*(2B), 9S-16S. • Bennett, G.A. (1998). Neuropathetic pain: New insights, new interventions. *Hospital Practice, 33*(10), 95-114. • Bichler, L.M. (1999). Foot ulcers in diabetes. *Advance for Nurse Practitioners, 7*(1), 49-52. • Brenner, Z.R. (1999). Preventing postoperative complications. *Nursing 99, 29*(10), 34-39. • Chase, S. (1997). Oral hypoglycemics. *RN,* (Dec), 45-50. • Cleary, M.E. (Ed.). (1994). *Diabetes and visual impairment: An educator's resource guide.* Chicago: American Association of Diabetes Educators. • Consensus Development Conference on Diabetic Foot Wound Care. (1999). *Ostomy/Wound Management, 45*(9), 32-47. • Consult a diabetes clinical nurse specialist regarding the role of the nurse in the care of clients with diabetes. • Contact the American Diabetes Association for position statements. For example, Position statement: Self-monitoring of blood glucose. • Contact the American Diabetes Association for professional and client information. • Dewey, C.M. & Riley, W.J. (1999). Have diabetes, will travel. *Postgraduate Medicine, 101*(2), 111-126. • *Diabetes Care* • *Diabetes Self Management*

- Dinsmoor, R. (1999). Tools of the trade: New insulins, drugs and devices. *Diabetes Self Management, 16*(6), 46-54.
- Farkas-Hirsh, R. (2000). All about hypoglycemia. *Diabetes Self Management, 17*(1), 21-27.
- Fishman, L.M. (1999). The normal pathophysiology of aging. *The Journal of Long Term Health Care, 1*(2), 114-124.
- Funnell, M. & Barlage, D. (2000). Saying a mouthful about oral diabetes drugs. *Nursing 2000, 30*(11), 34-39.
- Halpin-Landry, J.E. & Goldsmith, S. (1999). Feet first: diabetes care. *American Journal of Nursing, 99*(2), 26-33.
- Hernandez, D. (1998). Microvascular complications of diabetes: Nursing assessment and intervention. *American Journal of Nursing, 98*(6), 26-32.
- Konick-McMahan, J. (1999). Riding out a diabetic emergency. *Nursing 99, 29*(9), 34-40.

STUDY GUIDE NUMBER 13.62

Assessment of the Endocrine System

Study/Review Questions

1. Identify the six glands that make up the endocrine system.
   a. _Ant & Post pituitary_
   b. _Adrenal cortex & medulla_
   c. _Thyroid (alpha, Beta, delta)_
   d. _____
   e. _____
   f. _____

2. The substance that all these glands secrete is called _hormones_

3. These glands are referred to as "ductless" glands. On a separate sheet of paper, explain the meaning of a "ductless" gland.

4. On a separate sheet of paper, briefly describe the structure and function of the hypothalamus and pituitary gland.

5. Match each hormone with the corresponding gland. *Answers can be used more than once.*

   Hormones
   _8_ a. Somatostatin
   _5_ b. Thyrocalcitonin (calcitonin)
   _3_ c. Cortisol
   _4_ d. Epinephrine and norepinephrine
   _1_ e. Growth hormone, somatotropin
   _6_ f. Glucagon
   _9_ g. PTH
   _3_ h. Aldosterone
   _5_ i. Triiodothyronine (T$_3$)
   _10_ j. Estrogens and androgens
   _7_ k. Insulin
   _6_ l. Glucagon
   _2_ m. Antidiuretic hormone (ADH)
   _2_ n. Oxytocin
   _5_ o. Thyroxin (T$_4$)
   _1_ p. Thyroid-stimulating hormone (TSH) _Ant_
   _1_ q. ACTH _Ant_

   Glands
   1. Anterior pituitary
   2. Posterior pituitary
   3. Adrenal cortex
   4. Adrenal medulla
   5. Thyroid gland
   6. Alpha cells— Islets of Langerhans
   7. Beta cells— Islets of Langerhans
   8. Delta cells— Islets of Langerhans
   9. Parathyroid
   10. Gonads— ovaries and testes

6. Hormones work on a negative feedback mechanism. On a separate sheet of paper, briefly explain how that works in the body.

7. True or False? *Write* T *for true or* F *for false in the blank provided.*
   _T_ In addition to insulin, two other examples of the negative feedback mechanism are hormones secreted by the adrenal cortex and thyroid gland.

8. Read the following statements related to hormones and the endocrine system and decide whether each is true or false. *If the statement is true, write* T *in the blank provided. If it is false, correct the statement to make it true.*
   _T_ a. A low concentration of hormone is all that is needed to have an effect on the body.

   _F_ b. When hormones are secreted, the duration of effect is long. _(short)_

   _F_ c. Hormones must be bound to a plasma protein in order to be connected with a receptor site. _(must be free)_

   _F_ d. All hormones are stored for when there is a need. _(2 as exception)_

   _T_ e. Hormones must be able to attach themselves to a receptor site in order to be used by the body. _(attach Not bound)_

   _T_ f. The body uses all the hormones, which are then cleared from the body by other systems.

   _T_ g. _balance_ Homeostasis involves the endocrine system working together with the nervous system for good hormone function.

   _T_ h. Circulating blood hormones bind to specific receptor sites that result in changes in target tissue activity.

Exercise continued on next page

T i. There are specific levels of each of the hormones.

T j. Hormones are regulated in the body by negative feedback system.

T k. More than one hormone can be stimulated before the target tissue is affected.

F l. Only the hypothalamus has releasing and inhibiting factors that affect specific hormone production.

9. Identify the two hormones that are *not* stored in the body.
   a. Epinephrine and norepinephrine
   b. Glucogon and insulin
   c. Thyroid and adrenal medullary hormones
   d. Parathyroid and thyroid

10. Name the gland that is often called the "master gland" because it controls many functions of the endocrine system. pituitary gland

11. The release of epinephrine into the bloodstream is an example of which of following endocrine processes?
    a. "Lock and key" manner
    b. Neuroendocrine regulation
    c. Positive feedback mechanism
    d. Stimulus-response theory

12. The hypothalamus has a major role in regulating the endocrine function because it:
    a. Has only very specific endocrine functions.
    b. Has two distinct lobes that function independently.
    c. Is the connection with the central nervous system.
    d. Produces hormones that affect the posterior pituitary.

13. Identify the hormones that would be secreted for each of the following endocrine glands.

Endocrine Glands	Principle Hormones Secreted
a. Anterior pituitary	GH, THS, ACTH
b. Posterior pituitary	ADH, oxytocin
c. Thyroid	T3, T4) Thyrocalcitonin
d. Parathyroid	PTH Calcitonin
e. Adrenal cortex	Cortisol, Aldosterone
f. Pancreas	insulin
g. Ovaries	
h. Testes	Estrogens E androgens

14. Which of the following statements is correct about the pituitary gland?
    a. The main role of the posterior pituitary is to secrete tropic hormones.
    b. The posterior pituitary gland stores hormones produced by the hypothalamus.
    c. The anterior pituitary is connected to the thalamus gland.
    d. The anterior pituitary releases stored hormones produced by the hypothalamus.

15. The anterior pituitary gland secretes tropic hormones in response to which of the following hormones from the hypothalamus?
    a. Releasing hormones
    b. Target tissue hormones
    c. Growth hormones and prolactin
    d. Demand hormones

16. Which of the following statements about pituitary hormones is correct?
    a. The adrenocorticotropic hormone (ACTH) acts on the adrenal medulla.
    b. Follicle-stimulating hormone stimulates sperm production in men.
    c. Growth hormone promotes protein catabolism.
    d. Vasopressin decreases systolic blood pressure.

17. Which of the following statements about the gonads is correct?
    a. Ovaries and testes develop from the same embryonic tissue.
    b. The function of the hormones begins at birth in low, undetectable levels.
    c. The placenta secretes testosterone for the development of male external genitalia.
    d. External genitalia maturation is stimulated by gonadotropins in late adolescence.

18. Which of the following statements about the adrenal glands is correct?
    a. The cortex secretes androgens in women.
    b. Catecholamines are secreted from the cortex.
    c. Glucocorticoids are secreted by the medulla.
    d. The medulla secretes hormones essential for life.

19. Which of the following is an assessment finding in women with an excess of androgens secreted by the adrenal cortex?
    a. Increase in adipose tissue
    b. Thinning of hair
    c. Excessive facial hair
    d. Fluid retention

20. Which of the following is the major function of the hormones produced by the adrenal cortex?
    a. "Fight or flight" response
    b. Control of sugar, salt, and sex hormones
    c. Energy and steroid production
    d. Calcium regulation, stress regulation

21. Which of the following are hormones that are also neurotransmitters from the sympathetic nervous system?
    a. Norepinephrine and epinephrine
    b. Cortisol and glucocorticoids
    c. Aldosterone and renin
    d. ACTH and epinephrine

22. True or False? *If the following statements regarding the hormone cortisol that is secreted by the adrenal cortex are true, write* T *in the blank provided. If it is false, change the statement to make make it correct.*
    __F__ a. It affects only carbohydrate production. *protein, fat, mito sodium*
    __T__ b. It is needed for other physiologic processes, such as secretion of insulin, to occur.
    __F__ c. It is regulated by ACTH from the posterior pituitary and CRH. *from Ant pituitary* NO
    __F__ d. Peaks occur late in the day, with lowest points 12 hours before and after. *morning*

23. Stress causes an increase in the production of cortisol from the adrenal cortex. This may cause an increase in susceptibility to which of the following, and why?
    a. Cold or flu
    b. Fractures
    c. Sexual dysfunction
    d. Fluid retention
    Reason: _____
    _____
    _____

24. Lab values indicate a decrease in serum sodium and elevated serum potassium. Which of the following hormones would be secreted by the body that would affect the regulation of these electrolytes?
    a. Aldosterone from the adrenal cortex
    b. Cortisol from the adrenal medulla
    c. ADH from the posterior pituitary
    d. Calcitonin from the thyroid gland

25. Identify assessment findings a nurse would monitor in response to catecholamines released by the adrenal medulla.
    a. _____
    b. _____
    c. _____
    d. _____
    e. _____
    f. _____

26. True or False? *If the following statements about the thyroid gland and its hormones are true, write* T *in the blank provided. If they are false, change the statements to make them correct.*
    ____ a. The gland is located posteriorly in the neck directly below the cricoid cartilage.
    ____ b. Thyroid hormone production depends on sufficient iodine and protein intake.
    ____ c. The gland has four distinct lobes joined by a thin isthmus.
    ____ d. Oxygen consumption decreases in response to thyroid hormones.

27. Which of the following is the hormone that responds to a low serum calcium by increasing bone resorption?
    a. Parathyroid hormone
    b. Thyroxine (T_4)
    c. Triiodothyronine (T_3)
    d. Calcitonin

28. Which of the following is the hormone that responds to elevated serum calcium by decreasing bone and kidney resorption?
    a. Parathyroid hormone
    b. Thyroxine (T_4)
    c. Triiodothyronine (T_3)
    d. Calcitonin

29. Which of the following statements is correct regarding T_3 and T_4 hormones? *Check all that are correct.*
    ____ a. Affects the basal metabolic rate.
    ____ b. Hypothalamus is stimulated by cold and stress to secrete TRH.
    ____ c. These hormones need intake of protein and iodine for production.
    ____ d. Circulating hormone in the blood affects the production of TSH.

30. Identify the target organs of parathyroid hormone in the regulation of calcium and phosphorus.
    a. _____
    b. _____
    c. _____

31. Which of following statements about the pancreas is correct?
    a. Endocrine functions of the pancreas include secretion of digestive enzymes.
    b. Exocrine functions of the pancreas include secretion of glucagon and insulin.
    c. The islets of Langerhans are the only source of somatostatin secretion.
    d. Somatostatin inhibits pancreatic secretion of glucagon and insulin.

32. Which of the following statements is correct about glucagon secretion?
    a. It is stimulated by an increase in blood glucose levels.
    b. It is stimulated by a decrease in amino acid levels.
    c. It exerts its primary effect on the pancreas.
    d. It acts to increase blood glucose levels.

33. Which of the following statements about insulin secretion is correct?
    a. Insulin drops sharply following the ingestion of a meal.
    b. Insulin is stimulated primarily by fat ingestion.
    c. Basal levels are secreted with increases in glucose intake.
    d. Glycogenolysis and gluconeogenesis processes are promoted.

34. In addition to the pancreas that secretes insulin, another gland that secretes hormones that affect protein, carbohydrate, and fat metabolism is/are the:
    a. Adrenal medulla
    b. Thyroid gland
    c. Gonads
    d. Parathyroid

35. The bloodstream delivers glucose to the cells for energy production. The hormone that controls the cells' use of glucose is:
    a. T_4.
    b. Growth hormone.
    c. Adrenal steroids.
    d. Insulin.

36. Which of the following diseases involves a disorder of the islets of Langerhans?
    a. Diabetes insipidus
    b. Diabetes mellitus
    c. Addison's disease
    d. Cushing's disease

37. On a separate sheet of paper, identify what subjective data a nurse would obtain when performing an assessment of the endocrine system.

38. What objective data would a nurse obtain when performing an assessment of the endocrine system? *Use a separate sheet of paper for your answer.*

39. Which of the following statements is true about age-related changes in older adults and the endocrine system?
    a. All hormone levels are elevated.
    b. Thyroid hormone levels decrease.
    c. Adrenal glands enlarge.
    d. There is enlargement of the thyroid gland.

40. For each of the following structures, identify a physiologic change in the endocrine system associated with aging and name the cause of each change.
    a. Gonad:
    b. Pancreas:
    c. Posterior pituitary gland:
    d. Thyroid:

41. An older adult complains of a lack of energy and not being able to do the usual daily activities without several naps. These symptoms could indicate which of the following problems that is often seen in the older client?
    a. Hypothyroidism
    b. Hyperparathyroidism
    c. Overproduction of cortisol
    d. Underproduction of glucagon

42. Which of the following are changes in hair and nails that reflect normal age-related changes in the older adult and are unrelated to endocrine disorders?
    a. Increased body hair
    b. Thick yellow nails
    c. "Paper-thin" skin
    d. Increased skin turgor

43. A nurse is performing a physical assessment of the endocrine system. Which of the following glands can be palpated?
    a. Pancreas
    b. Thyroid
    c. Adrenal glands
    d. Parathyroids

44. Which of the following statements is correct about performing a physical assessment of the thyroid gland?
    a. The thyroid gland is easily palpated in all clients.
    b. The client is instructed to swallow to aid palpation.
    c. The anterior approach is preferred for thyroid palpation.
    d. The thumbs are used to palpate the thyroid lobes.

45. A client is to have a suppression/stimulation test completed. On a separate sheet of paper, briefly explain the purpose of this test.

46. If a routine urine specimen cannot be sent immediately to the laboratory, the nurse should:
    a. Store the specimen at room temperature.
    b. Discard the specimen and collect a new specimen at a later time.
    c. Refrigerate the specimen until it can be transported.
    d. Refrigerate the specimen for no more than 6 hours, then discard.

47. Which of the following nursing interventions is most appropriate when collecting a 24-hour urine specimen for endocrine studies?
    a. Recording the client's intake and output for the duration
    b. Checking whether any preservatives are needed
    c. Placing the collection container on ice for the 24 hours
    d. Weighing the client before beginning the collection

48. Which of the following instructions should be included in teaching a client about urine collection for endocrine studies? *Check all answers that are correct.*
    ___ a. Fast before starting the urine collection.
    ___ b. Measure the urine in mL rather than ounces.
    ___ c. Empty the bladder completely then start timing.
    ___ d. Time the test for exactly 24 hours.
    ___ e. Notify the lab of all medications.
    ___ f. Remember that medications can interfere with lab results.

49. Identify the types of radiographic tests that may be used for an endocrine assessment.
    a. _____
    b. _____
    c. _____
    d. _____
    e. _____

50. A client is suspected of having pituitary tumor. Which radiographic test would aid in determining this diagnosis?
    a. Skull x-rays
    b. CT /MRI
    c. Angiography
    d. Ultrasound

51. A thyroid nodule is palpated on physical examination. To determine whether the nodule is cystic or a solid tumor, a client would undergo which of the following tests?
    a. CT scan
    b. MRI
    c. Ultrasound
    d. Needle biopsy

52. After the ultrasound of the thyroid gland, which of the following diagnostic tests would determine the need for surgical intervention?
    a. CT scan
    b. MRI
    c. Angiography
    d. Needle biopsy

53. For each of the following Gordon's functional health patterns, identify one or more assessment finding(s) that may indicate an actual or potential endocrine problem.
    a. Nutritional-metabolic pattern: _____
       _____
    b. Elimination pattern: _____
       _____
    c. Sleep-rest pattern: _____
       _____
    d. Sexuality-reproduction pattern: _____
       _____
    e. Activity-exercise pattern: _____
       _____

54. The nursing diagnosis *Risk for Falls Related to the Effect of Pathologic Fractures as a Result of Bone Demineralization* is pertinent to which of the following endocrine problems?
    a. Underproduction of parathyroid hormone
    b. Overproduction of parathyroid hormone
    c. Underproduction of thyroid hormone
    d. Overproduction of thyroid hormone

55. Calcium metabolism is regulated by the parathyroid hormone. Which of the following vitamins is directly involved in this metabolic process?
    a. Vitamin K
    b. Vitamin C
    c. Vitamin B complex
    d. Vitamin D

56. For thyroid hormones to be produced, a client needs to have sufficient intake of which type of food?
    a. Protein and iodine
    b. Protein and carbohydrates
    c. Calcium and protein
    d. Calcium and iodine

57. On physical assessment of a client with possible excess of adrenocortical hormones, the nurse notices reddish-purple "stretch marks" on the breasts and abdomen. The nurse would document these findings as:
    a. Vitiligo.
    b. Hirsutism.
    c. Striae.
    d. Depigmentation.

58. When performing a nursing assessment of the endocrine system, a key piece of subjective data to obtain is information about the client's:
    a. Sexual functions.
    b. Intake of daily supplemental vitamins.
    c. Energy level and fatigue.
    d. Lifestyle changes.

59. In performing a nursing assessment, which of the following are common nonspecific assessment findings that could signal the nurse of a potential endocrine problem and the need for further testing?
    a. Protruding eyeballs and jugular vein distention
    b. Complaints of thirst, increased urination, and hunger
    c. Weight loss, feeling tired, and difficulty coping
    d. Enlarged gland and infertility

60. In addition to weight loss, feeling tired, and difficulty coping, identify other subtle assessment findings that would indicate to the nurse possible endocrine dysfunction. *Use a separate sheet of paper for your answer.*

STUDY GUIDE NUMBER 13.63

Interventions for Clients with Pituitary and Adrenal Gland Problems

Study/Review Questions

1. Differentiate primary and secondary pituitary dysfunction and the end results that occur.
    a. Primary:_____
    _____
    b. Secondary: _____
    _____

2. Identify the most common and least common pituitary tumors:
    Most common: _____
    Least common: _____

3. Identify the six hormones that are produced and secreted by the anterior pituitary gland.
   a. _____
   b. _____
   c. _____
   d. _____
   e. _____
   f. _____

4. Identify the two hormones that are produced by the hypothalamus then stored and secreted by the posterior pituitary gland.
   a. _____
   b. _____

5. A malfunctioning anterior or posterior pituitary gland can result in which of the following disorders?
   a. Pituitary hypofunction
   b. Pituitary hyperfunction
   c. Both

6. The assessment findings of a male client with anterior pituitary tumor include complaints of changes in secondary sex characteristics, such as episodes of impotence and decreased libido. The nurse explains to the client that these findings are a result of overproduction of which hormone? Identify a nursing diagnosis for this client.
   a. Gonadotropins inhibiting prolactin (PRL)
   b. Thyroid hormone inhibiting prolactin (PRL)
   c. Prolactin (PRL) inhibiting secretion of gonadotropins
   d. Steroids inhibiting production of sex hormones
   Nursing diagnosis: _____

7. A client with prolactin-secreting tumor would more than likely be treated with which of the following medications?
   a. Bromocriptine
   b. Octrotide
   c. Steroids
   d. Growth hormone

8. Interventions for the drug bromocriptine mesylate (Parlodel) include:
   a. Advising the client to get up slowly from a lying position.
   b. Instructing the client to take medication on an empty stomach.
   c. Taking daily for purposes of raising GH levels to reduce symptom of acromegaly.
   d. Teaching the client to begin with a maintenance level dose.

9. Clients diagnosed with an anterior pituitary tumor can result in having symptoms of acromegaly or gigantism. These symptoms are a result of overproduction of which hormone?
   a. Growth hormone (GH)
   b. Prolactin
   c. ACTH
   d. Gonatropins

10. Upon performing an assessment of a client with acromegaley, the nurse would expect to find:
    a. Extremely long arms and legs.
    b. Significant changes in facial features and oily, coarse skin.
    c. Changes in menses with infertility.
    d. Rough, extremely dry skin.

11. On a separate sheet of paper, describe characteristic findings for acromegaly and gigantism. Identify a nursing diagnosis for these clients.

12. When analyzing lab values, the nurse would expect to find which of the following as a direct result of overproduction of growth hormone, and why?
    a. Hyperglycemia
    b. Hyperphosphatemia
    c. Hypocalemia
    d. Hypercalemia

Answer the following two questions on a separate sheet of paper.

13. Describe the type of pain a client may have with excessively high growth hormone levels.

14. Describe assessment findings a nurse could expect with *deficient* growth hormone from a hypofunction pituitary. Identify a nursing diagnosis related to these findings.

15. A laboratory value report shows a decreased TSH level and a decreased thyroid hormone level. Identify the thyroid disorder and the findings a nurse would expect on assessment. Also, identify a nursing diagnosis for this client.
    Thyroid disorder: _____
    Assessment findings: *Check all that apply.*
    ____ a. Weight gain
    ____ b. Heat intolerance
    ____ c. Inability to concentrate, impaired memory
    ____ d. Increased libido
    ____ e. Alopecia
    ____ f. Fine tremors
    ____ g. Lack of energy
    ____ h. Weight loss
    ____ i. Increased GI motility
    Nursing diagnoses: _____

16. For anterior pituitary function, identify hormone assays that can be performed to determine basal levels of target organ hormones.
    a. _____
    b. _____
    c. _____
    d. _____

17. Which of the following statements about the etiology of hypopituitarism is correct?
    a. Secondary dysfunction can result from radiation treatment to the pituitary gland.
    b. Primary dysfunction can result from infection or a congenital defect.
    c. Postpartum hemorrhage is the most common cause of pituitary trauma.
    d. Severe malnutrition and body fat depletion can depress pituitary gland function.

18. An intervention for a client with hypothyroidism includes:
    a. Relating to the client according to physical appearance.
    b. Encouraging the client to express feelings and concerns.
    c. Suggesting the client purchase an elevated toilet seat.
    d. Recommending clothing stores that stock adolescent sizes.

19. Which of the following statements about hormone replacement therapy for hypopituitarism is correct?
    a. Somatotropin (Humatrope) is given after closure of the epiphyses.
    b. Therapy usually corrects physiologic and psychologic problems.
    c. Testosterone replacement therapy does not produce male fertility.
    d. Clomiphene citrate (Clomid) is used to suppress ovulation in women.

20. Female clients receiving hormone replacement therapy should be instructed to:
    a. Report any recurrence of symptoms, such as decreased libido, between injections.
    b. Monitor blood pressure at least weekly for potential hypotension.
    c. Treat leg pain, especially in the calves, with gentle muscle stretching.
    d. Schedule periodic gynecologic and breast examinations with the physician.

21. The onset of menopause is related to which of the following?
    a. Underproduction of FSH
    b. Overproduction of FSH

22. On a separate sheet of paper, identify at least one preoperative teaching point regarding each of the following topics for a client going for a transsphenoidal hypophysectomy.
    a. Body image changes
    b. Nasal dressing and packing
    c. Preventive measures
    d. Bacteria cultures
    e. Postoperative hospital routines
    f. Hormone replacement

23. Following a hypophysectomy, the client would more than likely need instruction on hormone replacement for which of the following hormones? *Check all that apply.*
    ___✓_ a. Cortisol
    ___✓_ b. Thyroid
    ___✓_ c. Gonadal
    ___✓_ d. Vasopressin

24. Following a hypophysectomy, home care monitoring by the nurse would include assessing for which of the following? *Check all those that apply.*
    ____ a. SIADH
    ____ b. CSF leaks
    ___✓_ c. Bowel habits
    ___✓_ d. Signs and symptoms of increased intracranial pressure
    ___✓_ e. 24-hour intake of fluids and urine output
    ___✓_ f. 24-hour diet recall
    ___✓_ g. Activity level

25. Postoperative care for the client who has had a transsphenoidal hypophysectomy includes:
    a. Encouraging coughing and deep breathing to decrease pulmonary complications.
    b. Testing nasal drainage for glucose to determine whether it contains cerebrospinal fluid.
    c. Keeping the bed flat to decrease central cerebrospinal fluid leakage.
    d. Assisting the client with brushing his teeth to decrease halitosis.

26. The nurse notices a "halo sign" on the dressing of a client with a hypophysectomy. The nurse would notify the physician, because this is a sign of

    _____.

27. Which of the following forms an *incorrect* statement about postoperative instructions for a client
with diabetes who has had a hypophysectomy? For
the remainder of her lifetime, the client will:
a. Be unable to have any children.
b. Have to take cortisol replacement medication.
c. Have to take thyroxine replacement medication.
d. Require a larger dose of insulin than she did preoperatively.

28. A client with a hypophysectomy can postoperatively
experience transient diabetes insipidus. The nurse
would signal this problem by assessing:
a. The output is much greater than intake.
b. A change in mental status indicating confusion.
c. Lab results indicating hyponatremia.
d. Nonpitting edema.

29. The action of antidiuretic hormone (ADH) influences normal kidney function by stimulating the:
a. Glomerulus to control the filtration rate.
b. Proximal nephron tubules to reabsorb water.
c. Distal nephron tubules to reabsorb water.
d. Glomerulus to prevent loss of protein in urine.

30. The disorder that results from a deficiency of vasopressin (antidiuretic hormone ADH) from the posterior pituitary gland is called:
a. Syndrome of inappropriate antidiuretic hormone
(SIADH).
b. Diabetes insipidus.
c. Cushing's syndrome.
d. Addison's disease.

31. Read the following statements related to diabetes
insipidus (ADH deficiency) and decide whether
each is true or false. *If the statement is true, write* T
*in the blank provided. If it is false, correct the state-
ment to make it true.*
   T a. The level of injury to the hypophyseal tract
determines the extent of ADH deficiency.

   F b. The primary indication of diabetes insipidus is the client's complaint of urinary *No*
retention and thirst.

   T c. The primary complications of diabetes
insipidus are hypovolemia and shock.

   F d. A diagnostic test of diabetes insipidus is
urine specific gravity greater than 1.005.

   T e. Urine output of greater than 4 L/24 hours is
the first diagnostic indication of diabetes
insipidus.

   T f. Laboratory findings in cases of diabetes
insipidus include serum osmolality within
normal limits, if the patient is taking fluids.

32. Clients with permanent diabetes insipidus must be
instructed to:
a. Continue vasopressin therapy until symptoms
disappear.
b. Monitor for recurrence of polydipsia and
polyuria.
c. Monitor and record their weight twice a week.
d. Check urine-specific gravity three times a week.

33. A client uses desmopressin actate metered dose
spray as a replacement hormone for ADH. Which of
the following is an indication for another dose?
Check all that apply.
   ✓ a. Excessive urination
   ✓ b. Specific gravity of 1.003
   ___ c. Dark concentrated urine
   ___ d. Edema in the legs

34. A client is undergoing a fluid deprivation test for
diabetes insipidus. Which of the following statements are true regarding this test? *Check all that
apply.*
   ✓ a. Teach the client that fluid restriction must
be maintained for accurate results.
   ___ b. Administer a normal water load followed by
IV dextrose.
   ✓ c. A positive result of a fluid deprivation test
is an increase in urine osmolality and specific gravity.
   ___ d. Five units of aqueous vasopressin are given
for this test.

35. Which of the following oral medications is not used
to treat mild diabetes insipidus, and why? On a separate sheet of paper, identify at least one nursing
intervention for each of the correct answers.
a. Diabinese
b. Atromid-S
c. Lithium
d. Novo-Pramine

36. Upon taking a history, which of the following
clients would be associated with the development of
SIADH or diabetes insipidus?
a. A 27-year-old client on high-dose steroids
b. A 47-year-old hospitalized adult client with acute
renal failure
c. A 58-year-old with metastatic lung or breast cancer
d. An older adult with history of a stroke within the
last year

37. On a separate sheet of paper, briefly compare diabetes insipdus (DI) with the syndrome of inappropriate antidiuretic hormone (SIADH).

38. Which of the following statements about the pathophysiology of SIADH is correct?
    a. ADH secretion is inhibited in the presence of low plasma osmolality.
    b. Water retention results in dilutional hyponatremia and expanded extracellular fluid (ECF) volume.
    c. The glomerulus is unable to increase its filtration rate to reduce the excess plasma volume.
    d. Renin and aldosterone are released and help to decrease the loss of urinary sodium.

39. Which of the following statements about the etiology and incidence of SIADH is correct?
    a. Malignant cells act on the posterior pituitary gland to decrease ADH release.
    b. Clofibrate (Atromid-S) can potentiate the action of vasopressin.
    c. Ectopic ADH production can result from benign gastrointestinal polyps.
    d. SIADH that results from vasopressin overdose in DI is irreversible.

40. The effect of increased ADH in the blood results in which of the following effects on the kidney?
    a. Urine concentration tends to decrease.
    b. Glomerular filtration tends to decrease.
    c. Tubular reabsorption of sodium and water increases.
    d. Tubular reabsorption of potassium and water increases.

41. In SIADH, as a result of water retention from excess ADH, which of the following laboratory values would the nurse expect to find? *Check all that apply.*
    ___ a. Increased urine osmolality (increased sodium in urine)
    ___ b. Elevated serum sodium level
    ___ c. Increased specific gravity (concentrated urine)
    ___ d. Decreased serum osmolarity
    ___ e. Decreased urine osmolaity (decreased sodium in urine)

42. Which of the following is a priority nursing intervention of a client with SIADH?
    a. Measure intake and output. Encourage fluid intake to prevent dehydration.
    b. Monitor the neurologic status at least every 2 hours.
    c. Weigh daily to monitor for severe weight loss.
    d. Monitor urine tests for decreased sodium levels and low specific gravity.

43. Which of the following is the type of intravenous fluids that a nurse uses to treat a client with SIADH, and why?
    a. D5 1/2 NS
    b. D5/W
    c. 3% NS
    d. NS

44. In addition to intravenous fluids, the client is on a fluid restriction as low as 500 to 600 mL/24 hours. Indicate the serum and urine results that would demonstrate effectiveness of this treatment. *Choose increases or decreases for each of the following.*
    a. Specific gravity results (increases or decreases)
    b. Serum sodium results (increases or decreases)
    c. Urine output (decreases or increases)

45. Which of the following statements is correct about pheochromocytoma?
    a. It is most often malignant.
    b. It is a catecholamine-producing tumor.
    c. It is found only in the adrenal medulla.
    d. It is manifested by hypotension.

46. A client in the emergency room is diagnosed with possible pheochromocytoma. A priority nursing intervention for this client is to:
    a. Monitor the client's intake and output and the specific gravity.
    b. Monitor blood pressure for severe hypertension.
    c. Monitor blood pressure for severe hypotension.
    d. Administer medication to increase cardiac output.

47. The nurse would expect to perform which of the following diagnostic tests for pheochromocytoma?
    a. 24-hour urine collection for sodium, potassium, and glucose
    b. Catecholamine stimulation test
    c. Administration of beta-adrenergic blocking agent and monitor results
    d. 24-hour urine collection for vanilylmandelic acid (VMA)

48. Interventions for the client with pheochromocytoma include:
    a. Assisting the client to sit in a chair for blood pressure monitoring.
    b. Instructing the client to get up slowly from a sitting position.
    c. Encouraging the client to maintain an active exercise schedule including activity such as running.
    d. Advising the client that there are no special dietary restrictions to follow.

49. Which of the following diuretics is ordered by the physician to treat hyperaldosteronism, and why?
    a. Furosemide (Lasix)
    b. Ethacrynic acid (Edecrin)
    c. Bumetanide (Bumex) 24-hour urine collection for vanilylmandelic acid (VMA)
    d. Spironolactone (Aldactone)

50. Which of the following statements about hyperaldosteronism is correct?
    a. Peripheral edema due to hypernatremia is common.
    b. It occurs more often in men than in women.
    c. It is a common cause of hypertension in the population.
    d. Fluid and electrolyte disturbances are resultant effects.

51. Identify two types of tests and the findings that are diagnostic for clients suspected of having hyperaldosteronism.
    a. _____
    b. _____

52. When diagnosed with Cushing's syndrome, the manifestations are most likely related to an *excess production* of which of the following hormones?
    a. Insulin from the pancreas
    b. ADH from posterior pituitary gland
    c. Prolactin from anterior pituitary gland
    d. Cortisol from the adrenal cortex

53. The most common cause of hypercortisolism, or Cushing's syndrome, is:
    a. Pituitary hypoplasia.
    b. Insufficient ACTH production.
    c. Adrenocortical hormone deficiency.
    d. Hyperplasia of the adrenal cortex.

54. A classic physical finding of Cushing's syndrome is:
    a. A "moon-faced" appearance.
    b. Decreased amount of body hair.
    c. Barrel chest.
    d. Coarse facial features.

55. In addition to a "moon face," identify other key findings of a client with Cushing's syndrome. *Use a separate sheet of paper for your answer.*

56. When assessing the client with Cushing's syndrome, the nurse would expect to find:
    a. Signs of dehydration.
    b. Pitting edema.
    c. Hypertension.
    d. Muscle atrophy.

57. On a separate sheet of paper, explain why samples of plasma cortisol levels should always be taken at the same time each day.

58. A client suspected of a diagnosis of Cushing's syndrome is scheduled for various 24-hour urine testing. What does a nurse include in client education for these tests? *Use a separate sheet of paper for your answer.*

59. The positive urine tests for Cushing's syndrome would show _____.

60. A nurse selects "Risk for Injury Related to Effects of Demineralization of Bone" as a nursing diagnosis for a client with Cushing's disease. On a separate sheet of paper, identify the nursing interventions for this client.

61. A female client with Cushing's syndrome expresses concern to the nurse about the changes in her general appearance. The nurse determines a nursing diagnosis of Disturbed Body Image. The desired outcome for this client would be for the client to:
    a. Verbalize an understanding that many of the physical appearance changes will be eliminated once there is a drop in excess cortisol.
    b. Ventilate about the frustration of these lifelong physical changes.
    c. Verbalize ways to cope with the changes such as joining a support group or changing style of dress.

62. Match each of the following drugs with the corresponding clinical use for hypercortisolism.

    Medications
    ____ a. Mitotane (Lysodren)
    ____ b. Aminoglutethimide (Cytadren)
    ____ c. Trilostane (Modrastane)
    ____ d. Cyproheptadine (Periactin)

    Clinical Uses
    1. Adrenal enzyme inhibitor used in combination with other antiadrenal agents
    2. Adrenal cytotoxic agent used for inoperable adrenal tumors
    3. Used to treat adrenal hyperfunction resulting from pituitary disease
    4. Adrenal enzyme inhibitor that decreases cortisol production

63. Indicate the two surgical procedures for adrenocortical hypersecretion.
    a. _____
    b. _____

64. A client is scheduled for bilateral adrenalectomy. Prior to surgery, steroids are to be given. Identify the reason why this medication is administered and identify the name of the medication.
    a. To promote glycogen storage by the liver for body energy reserves
    b. To compensate for sudden lack of adrenal hormones following surgery
    c. To increase the body's inflammatory response to promote scar formation
    d. To enhance urinary excretion of salt and water following surgery
    Name of medication: _____

65. What is the rationale for using strict aseptic technique for a client about to undergo adrenalectomy?

66. Discharge teaching about medications for the client following bilateral adrenalectomy includes emphasizing that:
    a. The dosage of steroid replacement medications will be consistent throughout the client's lifetime.
    b. The steroid medications should be taken in the evening so as not to interfere with sleep.
    c. The client should take the medication on an empty stomach.
    d. The client should learn how to give himself an intramuscular injection of hydrocortisone.

67. On a separate sheet of paper, discuss how you would explain the significance of wearing a medical alert tag to a client who has had a bilateral adrenalectomy.

68. Which of the following statements is correct regarding a client with hyperaldosteronism following a successful unilateral adrenalectomy?
    a. The low-sodium diet must be continued postoperatively.
    b. Glucocorticoid replacement therapy is temporary.
    c. Spironolactone (Aldactone) must be taken for life.
    d. Additional measures are needed to control hypertension.

69. Identify the three reasons for the decreased production of adrenocortical steroids.
    a. _____
    b. _____
    c. _____

70. Which of the following clients are at risk for developing Addison's disease, and why?
    a. A client who suddenly stops taking high-dose steroid therapy
    b. A client who tapers the dosages of steroid therapy
    c. A client who is deficient in ADH
    d. A client with an adrenal tumor causing excessive secretion of ACTH

71. On a separate sheet of paper, identify the functions of the following adrenal hormones and their effects on laboratory values.
    a. Cortisol
    b. Aldosterone
    c. Androgens

72. On a separate sheet of paper, briefly discuss Addisonian crisis.

73. A client in the emergency room complaining of lethargy, muscle weakness, nausea, vomiting, and weight loss over the past weeks is diagnosed with Addisonian crisis (acute adrenal insufficiency). The nurse would expect to administer which of the following?
    a. Beta blocker to control the hypertension and arrythmias
    b. Solu-Cortef IV along with IM injections of hydrocortisone
    c. IV fluids of D5 NS with KCl for dehydration
    d. Lasix for reducing pitting edema and pulmonary edema

74. The nurse would determine that the administration of hydrocortisone for Addisonian crisis was effective when the nurse assesses which of the following?
    a. Increased urine output
    b. No signs of pitting edema
    c. Blood pressure resuming normal range
    d. Lethargy improving, client is alert and oriented

75. Complete the chart by comparing the clinical findings in Addison's disease with those in Cushing's syndrome. *Indicate by + for increase or − for decrease. Insert a checkmark if normal value.*

Clinical Finding	Addison's Disease	Cushing's Syndrome
a. Serum sodium level		
b. Serum potassium level		
c. ECF volume		
d. Blood pressure		
e. Serum glucose level		
f. Serum calcium		
g. Cortisol level		
h. Leukocyte count		
i. Lymphocyte count		

76. A client with a diagnosis of chronic adrenal insufficiency is admitted to a nursing unit. Which of the following room assignments is contraindicated?
    a. A double room with an older client who has had a cerebrovascular accident
    b. A double room with a middle-aged client who has bacterial pneumonia
    c. A private room that is away from the nurses' station but within view
    d. A double room next to a teenager who has a fractured leg and is in traction

77. Preventive measures for adrenocortical insufficiency include:
    a. Maintaining the client on long-term, high-dose glucocorticoid therapy.
    b. Vaccinating clients at increased risk for contracting tuberculosis and acquired immunodeficiency syndrome (AIDS).
    c. Tapering glucocorticoid doses quickly and discontinuing the drug as soon as possible.
    d. Decreasing glucocorticoid doses gradually, permitting pituitary and adrenal function to return.

78. A client with adrenal hypofunction reports weakness and dizziness on arising in the morning. The nurse explains to the client that this is most likely related to:
    a. Postural hypertension.
    b. A potassium deficiency.
    c. A hypoglycemic reaction.
    d. Salt and fluid retention.

79. A client's laboratory results indicate that she has Addison's disease. The nurse plans to discuss the need for:
    a. A special low-salt diet.
    b. Using an alcohol-based skin cleaner.
    c. Physical activity restrictions.
    d. Lifelong hormone replacement therapy.

80. In teaching the client with adrenal hypofunction about diet, the nurse advises the client to:
    a. Add a little extra salt to food at the table.
    b. Limit the daily intake of fluids to 1500 mL.
    c. Restrict the daily intake of calories to 1200.
    d. Decrease protein intake to 20 to 30 g/day.

81. The client on prolonged cortisone therapy should be instructed to observe for and report signs of:
    a. Anuria and hypoglycemia.
    b. Weight gain and moon face.
    c. Anorexia and muscle twitches.
    d. Hypotension and fluid loss.

82. A female client with Addison's disease has been on cortisone therapy for several months and expresses concern that she is beginning to look more masculine. The nurse should tell the client:
    a. That the changes are a sign of the disease's progression.
    b. Not to worry because the changes are only temporary.
    c. That the changes are related to the cortisone therapy.
    d. That the changes are a minor inconvenience compared to dying.

83. When observing the client for excessive drug therapy of cortisone, the nurse should be alert for:
    a. Cold intolerance.
    b. Rapid weight gain.
    c. Hypoglycemia.
    d. Severe weight loss.

84. Complete this chart comparing endocrine disorders.
Use a separate sheet of paper if necessary.

Categories	Pituitary Disorder		Adrenal Disorder	
	Excess	Deficit	Excess	Deficit
Common abnormal diagnostic lab test values				
Common abnormal radiologic tests				
Common clinical manifestations				
Common therapeutic drug regimen				
Diet therapy				

STUDY GUIDE NUMBER 13.64

Interventions for Clients with Problems of the Thyroid and Parathyroid Glands

Study/Review Questions

1. When performing a physical exam of the thyroid gland, precautions are taken in performing the correct technique because palpation can result in:
   a. Damage to the esophagus, causing gastric reflux.
   b. An obstruction of the carotid arteries causing a stroke.
   c. Pressure on the trachea and laryngeal nerve causing hoarseness.
   d. An exacerbation of symptoms by releasing additional thyroid hormone.

2. Thyroid hormones affect the basal metabolic rate. On a separate sheet of paper, briefly describe the effect of excessive and inadequate thyroid hormone production on the basal metabolic rate and the resulting thyroid disorder.

3. Differentiate the general assessment findings by matching them with the corresponding type of thyroid deficiency. *Answers may be used more than once.*

Assessment Findings

Thyroid Deficiency
1. Hyperthyroidism
2. Hypothyroidism

____ a. Weight loss with increased appetite
____ b. Constipation
____ c. Increased heart rate, palpitations
____ d. Fatigue
____ e. Depression
____ f. Decreased libido
____ g. Dyspnea with or without exertion
____ h. Insomnia
____ i. Cold intolerance
____ j. Diarrhea
____ k. Ophthalmopathy
____ l. Severe fatigue, increased sleeping
____ m. Increased irritability with depression
____ n. Impaired attention span and memory
____ o. Fine, soft, silky hair
____ p. Apathetic demeanor
____ q. Increased libido
____ r. Heat intolerance, warm skin
____ s. Weight gain
____ t. Generalized weakness, muscle aches
____ u. Diaphoresis
____ v. Tremors

4. The hallmark assessment finding that is often reported by a client signifying hyperthyroidism is:
   a. Weight loss.
   b. Increased libido.
   c. Heat intolerance.
   d. Diarrhea.

5. The hallmark assessment finding that is often reported by a client signifying hypothyroidism is:
   a. Irritability.
   b. Cold intolerance.
   c. Constipation.
   d. Fatigue.

6. One of the first signals of hyperthyroidism that is often noticed by a client is:
   a. Eyelid or globe lag.
   b. Vision changes or tiring of the eyes.
   c. Protruding eyes.
   d. Photophobia.

7. Which of the following laboratory results is consistent with hyperthyroidism?
   a. Decreased serum triiodothyronine (T_3) and thyroxine (T_4) levels
   b. Elevated serum thyrotropin-releasing hormone (TRH) level
   c. Decreased radioactive iodine uptake
   d. Increased free T_3 and T_4

8. The laboratory results for a 53-year-old client indicate a low T_3 level and elevated TSH. These lab values indicate:
   a. Hyperthyroidism.
   b. Hypothyroidism.
   c. Malfunctioning pituitary gland.
   d. Normal lab values for this age.

9. The clinical manifestation resulting from an increase in thyroid hormone production is known as:
   a. Thyrotoxicosis.
   b. Euthyroid function.
   c. Graves' disease.
   d. Hypermetabolism.

10. The most common cause of hyperthyroidism is:
    a. Radiation to thyroid.
    b. Graves' disease.
    c. Thyroid cancer.
    d. Thyroiditis.

11. Identify clinical manifestations of Graves' diseases that distinguish it from other causes of hyperthyroidism.
    a. _____
    b. _____
    c. _____
    d. _____
    e. _____

12. On a separate sheet of paper, describe each of the following assessment findings that are associated with hyperthyroidism and Graves' disease.
    a. Exophthalmos
    b. Pretibial edema
    c. Eyelid retraction (eyelid lag)
    d. Globe (eyeball) lag

13. Graves' disease and Hashimoto's disease are autoimmune disorders of the thyroid. On a separate sheet of paper, briefly describe the cause and pathophysiology of each disease.

14. Read the following statements regarding hypothyroidism and hyperthyroidism. *If the statement is true, write T in the blank provided. If it is false, correct the statement to make it true.*

___ a. Exophathalmos only occurs in hyperthyroidism resulting from Graves' disease.

___ b. Graves' disease is hereditary.

___ c. A decreased metabolic rate results in TSH binding to thyroid cells, causing an enlarged thyroid.

___ d. Hypothyroidism can occur anytime throughout the life span.

___ e. Hypothyroidism and hyperthyroidism occur more frequently in women than men.

___ f. Simple goiter associated with hypothyroidism is usually due to insufficient iodine intake.

___ g. Hashimoto's disease is a type of hypothyroidism.

___ h. The effect of antithyroid medication can be delayed due to storage and release of large amounts of thyroid hormone.

___ i. Hypothyroidism causes elevated systolic pressure, wide pulse pressure, tachycardia, and dysrhythmias.

___ j. Thyroid storm following surgical intervention for hyperthyroidism is rare because of pretreatment with medications.

___ k. Euthyroid is defined as near normal thyroid function.

___ l. Radiation precautions are required with treatment of I_{131} for hyperthyroidism.

___ m. Nonsurgical treatment is the preferred treatment for hyperthyroidism.

15. A client has been diagnosed with having a thyroid goiter. On a separate sheet of paper, briefly define thyroid goiter and how it differs from thyroid nodule.

16. Laboratory findings of elevated T_3 and T_4, decreased TSH, and high thyrotropin receptor antibody titer indicates:
   a. A multinodular goiter.
   b. Hyperthyroidism related to overmedication.
   c. A pituitary tumor suppressing TSH.
   d. Graves' disease.

Answer the following two questions on a separate sheet of paper.

17. A client with hypothyroidism and a simple goiter asked the physician about possible causes of this disorder. Briefly explain the four causes of a simple goiter.

18. A client who has been diagnosed with hypothyroidism has problems with constipation and dry, rough skin. What interventions can the nurse teach the client to perform in order to help relieve these problems?

19. After a visit to the physician's office, a client is diagnosed with a thyroid nodule and elevated thyroid hormone level. This would be an indication of:
   a. Hyperthyroidism and goiter.
   b. Hypothyroidism and goiter.
   c. Nodules on the parathyroid gland.
   d. Thyroid or parathyroid cancer.

20. A newly diagnosed client with hypothyroidism is at risk for which of the following health problems? (This problem causes damage to the heart muscle resulting in decreased cardiac output and perfusion to the brain, hypothermia, hypoglycemia, and hyponatremia.)
   a. An endemic goiter
   b. Myxedema coma
   c. A toxic multinodular goiter
   d. Thyroiditis

21. A client with exophthalmos from hyperthyroidism complains of dry eyes, especially in the morning. The nurse teaches the client to perform which of the following interventions to help correct this problem?
   a. Wear sunglasses at all times when outside in the bright sun.
   b. Use cool compresses to the eye four times a day.
   c. Hold the eyes closed at night; tape or cover the eyelids.
   d. There is nothing that can be done to relieve this problem.

22. A client was admitted to the hospital from the emergency room with a diagnosis of thyroid storm (crisis). On a separate sheet of paper, define *thyroid storm,* what triggers it, and the clinical manifestations that a nurse would expect to find on assessment.

23. A client has the following assessment findings: elevated TSH level, low T_3 and T_4 level, difficulty with memory, lethargy, and muscle stiffness. These are clinical manifestations of:
    a. Hypothyroidism.
    b. Hyperthyroidism.
    c. Hypoparathyroidism.
    d. Hyperparathyroidism.

24. With correction of hypothyroidism with thyroid hormone, the client can expect improvement in mental awareness within:
    a. A few days.
    b. 2 weeks.
    c. 1 month.
    d. 3 months.

25. On a separate sheet of paper, briefly describe interventions a nurse would perform for a client with a diagnosis of thyroid storm.

26. Management of the client with hyperthyroidism focuses on: *Check all that apply.*
    ___ a. Blocking the effects of excessive thyroid secretion.
    ___ b. Treating the signs and symptoms the client experiences.
    ___ c. Establishing euthyroid function.
    ___ d. Preventing spread of the disease.

27. Match each of the following characteristics with the corresponding intervention for hyperthyroidism. *Answers may be used more than once. Chose all answers that apply to each characteristic.*

Characteristics	Interventions for Hyperthyroidism
___ a. Discontinue if sore throat, fever, headache, or skin eruptions occur	1. Antithyroid drug Tapazole 2. Antithyroid drug PTU

___ b. Use includes preoperative treatment to obtain euthyroid
___ c. Action decreases the production of thyroid hormone
___ d. Works to control symptoms related to sympathetic nervous system of tachycardia, palpations, anxiety, and diaphoresis
___ e. Requires lifelong thyroid replacement
___ f. Limited use due to side effects
___ g. Causes GI disturbance; take with food
___ h. Monitor for hypothyroidism over time
___ i. Contraindicated in pregnancy; crosses placenta barrier
___ j. Administer around the clock
___ k. May require antithyroid medication for up to 8 weeks past treatment
___ l. Acts to decrease blood flow to reduce hormone production with results in 2 to 6 weeks
___ m. Treatment works by damaging thyroid gland
___ n. Removal of all of the thyroid gland
___ o. Treatment for thyroid cancer
___ p. No medications or treatments with iodine before intervention

3. Iodine preparations
4. Lithium carbonate
5. Beta-blocking agents (Inderal, Tenormin)
6. Radioactive iodine (I_{131})
7. Subtotal thyroidectomy
8. Total thyroidectomy

28. Preoperative instructions for clients having thyroid surgery would include which of the following? *Check all those that apply. Make changes to the incorrect answers to make them correct.*
    ___ a. Teach postoperative restrictions such as no cough and deep breathing exercises to prevent strain on the suture line.

    ___ b. Teach moving and turning technique of manually supporting the head and avoiding neck extension to minimize strain on the suture line.

    ___ c. Inform the client that hoarseness for a few days after surgery is usually the result of a breathing tube (endotracheal tube) used during surgery but will be monitored with respiration and weakness of voice.

    ___ d. Humidification of air maybe helpful to promote expectoration of secretions. Suctioning may also be used.

____ e. Clarify any questions regarding placement of incision, complications, and postoperative care.

____ f. Supine position and lying flat will be maintained postoperatively to avoid strain on suture line.

____ g. Teach the client to immediately report any respiratory difficulty, tingling around lips or fingers, or muscular twitching.

____ h. A drain may be present in the incision. All drainage and dressings will be monitored closely for 24 hours.

29. A nurse is preparing to receive a client on the postoperative unit following thyroid surgery. Explain the purpose of each of the following items that should be available for this client. What assessment findings would indicate immediate notification of the physician and potential use of these items?
    a. Tracheostomy equipment
    b. Calcium gluconate or calcium chloride for IV administration
    c. Oxygen and suction equipment

30. Following a thyroidectomy, a client complains of tingling around the mouth and muscle twitching. These assessment findings indicate to the nurse which of the following complications?
    a. Hemorrhage
    b. Respiratory distress
    c. Thyroid storm
    d. Hypocalemia, parathyroid gland injury

Answer the following three questions on a separate sheet of paper.

31. Postoperatively, the nurse monitors the client for the complication of laryngeal nerve damage. Identify assessment findings that may indicate this problem. What can you tell the client about these findings?

32. Identify the three common nursing diagnoses for a client with hypothyroidism. Also, briefly describe both the rationale for your selection and the related nursing interventions.

33. Describe the monitoring and teaching nursing interventions related to a client receiving thyroid hormone replacement therapy.

34. Following hospitalization for myxedema, a client is prescribed thyroid replacement medication. Which of the following statements would demonstrate the client's understanding of this therapy?
    a. " I will be taking this medication until my symptoms are completely resolved."
    b. " I will be taking thyroid medication for the rest of my life."
    c. " Now that I am feeling better, no changes in my medication will be necessary."
    d. " I am taking this medication to prevent symptoms of an 'overactive thyroid gland.'"

35. Match each characteristic with the corresponding thyroid disorder. *Answers may be used more than once, and more than one disorder may apply to each characteristic. Choose all that apply.*

Characteristic	Thyroid Disorder
____ a. Defined as inflammation of the thyroid gland	1. Thyroiditis
____ b. "Chronic thyroiditis"	2. Hashimoto's disease
____ c. Common age range 30s to 50s	3. Acute thyroiditis
____ d. Caused by viral infection of thyroid gland after an upper respiratory infection	4. Subacute thyroiditis
____ e. Bacterial infection of thyroid gland	
____ f. Subtotal thyroidectomy is a form of treatment	
____ g. Treated symptomatically	
____ h. Treated with thyroid replacement hormone	
____ i. Diagnosed by circulating antithyroid antibodies and needle biopsy	
____ j. Most uncommon thyroid disorder	

36. Serum calcium levels are maintained by which of the following two hormones? *Select two answers.*
    a. Cortisol
    b. Calcitonin
    c. ADH
    d. PTH

37. On a separate sheet of paper, briefly explain how parathyroid hormone (PTH) and calcitonin maintain the serum calcium levels.

38. Match each hormone with the corresponding effect on the serum calcium levels.

    Hormone
    ___ a. Parathyroid hormone production
    ___ b. Calcitonin production

    Effect
    1. Raises levels
    2. Lowers levels

39. Bone changes in the older adult are often seen with endocrine dysfunction and increased secretion of:
    a. Parathyroid hormone.
    b. Calcitonin.
    c. Insulin.
    d. Testosterone.

40. In addition to regulation of calcium levels, parathyroid hormone and calcitonin regulate the circulating blood levels of:
    a. Potassium.
    b. Sodium.
    c. Phosphate.
    d. Chloride.

41. On a separate sheet of paper, briefly explain how the parathyroid hormone and calcitonin maintain phosphate balance.

42. A client has a positive Trousseau's or Chvostek's sign resulting from hypoparathyroidism. This assessment finding indicates:
    a. Hypercalemia.
    b. Hypocalemia.
    c. Hyperphosphatemia.
    d. Hypophosphatemia.

43. Chvostek's sign and Trousseau's sign are late signs for which of the following problems?
    a. Cardiac arrhythmias
    b. Tetany
    c. Vitamin D deficiency
    d. Parathyroid cancer

44. A client in the emergency room who had continuous spasm of the muscles was diagnosed with hypoparathryoidism. The muscle spasms are a clinical manifestation of:
    a. Nerve damage.
    b. Seizures.
    c. Tetany.
    d. Decreased potassium.

45. Match the following causes with the parathyroid disorder. *Answers may be used more than once.*

    Cause
    ___ a. Chronic renal disease
    ___ b. Vitamin D deficiency
    ___ c. Removal of the thyroid gland
    ___ d. Radiation to the neck
    ___ e. Carcinoma of the lung, kidney, or GI tract producing PTH-like substance
    ___ f. Parathyroidectomy

    Parathyroid disorder
    1. Hypoparathyroidism
    2. Hyperparathyroidism

46. When interpreting laboratory values, what would the nurse expect to find in relationship to hypoparathyroidism and hyperparathyroidism? *Indicate an increase (+) or decrease (−) in the adult normal range for the following laboratory tests.*

Laboratory Test	Hyper-parathyroidism (+/−)	Hypo-parathyroidism (+/−)
a. Serum calcium		
b. Serum phosphate		
c. Serum parathyroid hormone (PTH)		
d. Urinary cAMP		

47. The priority nursing intervention for a client with hyperparathyroidism and high levels of serum calcium is to:
    a. Force fluids (IV or PO) and administer Lasix.
    b. Administer calcitonin.
    c. Administer oral phosphates.
    d. Administer mithramycin.

48. Postoperative nursing care for parathyroidectomy is similar to that of thyroid surgery with emphasis on monitoring and providing emergency intervention for:
    a. Hypercalemia.
    b. Hypocalemia.
    c. Intake and output.
    d. Vitamin D deficiency.

49. On a separate sheet of paper, identify the signs and symptoms of hypocalcemia.

50. Identify the four medications that are frequently used to treat hypoparathyroidism.
    a. _____
    b. _____
    c. _____
    d. _____

51. Discharge planning for a client who has chronic hypoparathyroidism should include:
    a. Reinforcing that the prescribed medications must be taken for the client's entire life.
    b. Teaching client to eat foods low in vitamin D and foods high in phosphates.
    c. After several weeks, medications can be discontinued.
    d. Kidney stones are no longer a risk to the client.

52. In older adults, assessment findings of fatigue, altered thought processes, dry skin, and constipation are often mistaken for signs of aging rather than assessment findings for the endocrine disorder of:
    a. Hyperthyroidism.
    b. Hypothyroidism.
    c. Hyperparathyroidism.
    d. Hypoparathyroidism.

53. Complete the following chart comparing endocrine disorders. *Use a separate sheet of paper if necessary.*

	Thyroid Disorder		Parathyroid Disorder	
Categories	**Excess**	**Deficit**	**Excess**	**Deficit**
Common abnormal diagnostic lab test values				
Common abnormal radiologic tests				
Common clinical manifestations				
Common therapeutic drug regimen				
Diet therapy				

54. Complete the following chart comparing endocrine emergencies. *Use a separate sheet of paper if necessary.*

Categories	**Myxedema**	**Thyroid storm**
Events that precipitate the crisis		
Common abnormal lab and other diagnostic tests		
Priority emergency interventions		

STUDY GUIDE NUMBER 13.65

Interventions for Clients with Diabetes Mellitus

Study/Review Questions

1. On a separate sheet of paper, briefly describe the syndrome of diabetes mellitus.

2. Identify the four classifications of diabetes mellitus.
    a. _____
    b. _____
    c. _____
    d. _____

3. Which of the following statements is correct about insulin?
    a. It is secreted by alpha cells in the islets of Langerhans.
    b. It is a catabolic hormone that builds up glucagon reserves.
    c. It is necessary for glucose transport across cell membranes.
    d. It is stored in muscles and converted to fat for storage.

4. Glucose is vital to the body's cells because it:
    a. Is used to build cell membranes.
    b. Is used by cells to extract energy.
    c. Affects the process of protein metabolism.
    d. Provides nutrients for genetic material.

5. Identify the counter-regulatory hormones released during episodes of hyperglycemia.
    a. _____
    b. _____
    c. _____
    d. _____
    e. _____

Match the following terms with their correct definitions. On a separate sheet of paper, briefly describe the pathophysiology that causes these classic symptoms.

____ 6. Polydipsia   a. Frequent urination
____ 7. Polyphagia   b. Frequent fluid intake
____ 8. Polyuria   c. Frequent eating

9. Which of the following individuals is at greatest risk for developing diabetes mellitus?
    a. An African-American woman, age 25 years
    b. An African-American man, age 36 years
    c. A Hispanic woman, age 56 years
    d. A Hispanic man, age 42 years

10. Which of the following four laboratory findings is most diagnostic of diabetes mellitus?
    a. Fasting blood sugar = 80 mg/dL
    b. 2-hour postparandial blood sugar = 110 mg/dL
    c. 1-hour glucose tolerance blood sugar = 110 mg/dL
    d. 2-hour glucose tolerance blood sugar = 140 mg/dL

11. On a separate sheet of paper, compare and contrast insulin-dependent diabetes mellitus (type 1; IDDM) and non–insulin-dependent diabetes mellitus (type 2; NIDDM). Underline similarities and highlight differences.

12. Untreated hyperglycemia results in:
    a. Respiratory acidosis.
    b. Metabolic alkalosis.
    c. Respiratory alkalosis.
    d. Metabolic acidosis.

13. The respiratory pattern of the client with untreated hyperglycemia is:
    a. Rapid and shallow (tachypneic).
    b. Deep and labored (Cheyne-Stokes respiration).
    c. Rapid and deep (Kussmaul's respiration).
    d. Shallow and labored (Biot's respiration).

14. The electrolyte most affected by hyperglycemia is:
    a. Sodium.
    b. Chloride.
    c. Potassium.
    d. Magnesium.

15. Identify the three emergencies for clients with diabetes mellitus and their causes:

   a. _____

   b. _____

   c. _____

16. In determining whether a client is hypoglycemic, a characteristic to consider is:

   a. Nausea.
   b. Irritability.
   c. Rapid pulse.
   d. Moist skin.

17. The primary difference between diabetic ketoacidosis (DKA) and hyperglycemic hyperosmolar nonketotic coma (HHNC) is the:

   a. Level of hyperglycemia.
   b. Amount of ketones produced.
   c. Level of hyperosmolarity.
   d. Amount of volume depletion.

18. A client is admitted with a blood glucose level of 900 mg/dL. Intravenous fluids and insulin are administered. Two hours after treatment is initiated, the blood glucose level is 400 mg/dL. Which of the following complications is the client most at risk for developing?

   a. Hypoglycemia
   b. Cerebral edema
   c. Renal shutdown
   d. Pulmonary edema

19. The type of insulin used in the emergency treatment of DKA and HHNC is:

   a. NPH.
   b. Lente.
   c. Regular.
   d. Protamine zinc.

20. Early treatment of DKA and HHNC includes intravenous:

   a. Glucagon.
   b. Potassium.
   c. Bicarbonate.
   d. Normal saline.

21. Which of the following cells is capable of using glucose in the absence of insulin?

   a. Cardiac cells
   b. Brain cells
   c. Kidney cells
   d. Pancreatic cells

22. Glucagon is used primarily to treat the client with:

   a. DKA.
   b. Idiosyncratic reaction to insulin.
   c. Insulin-induced hypoglycemia.
   d. HHNC.

23. Glucagon is given in a dextrose solution because dextrose:

   a. Promotes more storage of glucose in the liver.
   b. Stimulates the pancreas to produce more insulin.
   c. Increases blood sugar levels at a controlled rate.
   d. Inhibits glycogenesis, gluconeogenesis, and lipolysis.

24. When glucagon is administered, it:

   a. Competes for insulin at the receptor sites.
   b. Frees glucose from hepatic stores of glycogen.
   c. Supplies glycogen directly to the vital tissues.
   d. Provides a glucose substitute for rapid replacement.

Match each of the following etiologic factors with the corresponding type of diabetes mellitus. Answers may be used more than once.

Etiologic Factor	Type of Diabetes Mellitus
____ 25. Aging process	a. IDDM
____ 26. Autoimmune process	b. NIDDM
____ 27. Remission period	
____ 28. Obesity	
____ 29. Heredity	
____ 30. Viral infection	
____ 31. Decreased physical activity	

32. Preventive measures for diabetes mellitus include:

   a. Controlling hypertension.
   b. Prenatal care beginning the third trimester of pregnancy.
   c. Working in a high-stress environment.
   d. Maintaining ideal body weight.

33. A diabetic client is scheduled to have a blood glucose test the next morning. Which of the following should the nurse tell the client to do before coming in for the test?

   a. Eat the usual diet but have nothing after midnight.
   b. Take the usual oral hypoglycemic tablet in the morning.
   c. Eat a clear liquid breakfast in the morning.
   d. Follow the usual diet and medication regime.

34. The frequency with which a client should monitor capillary blood glucose levels depends on levels of:
    a. Urine glucose.
    b. Serum ketones.
    c. Serum glucose.
    d. Urine ketones.

Answer the following three questions on a separate sheet of paper.

35. Briefly discuss the rationale for determining blood urea nitrogen (BUN) and creatinine levels in the diabetic client.

36. Discuss the concept of renal threshold and its significance for using measurement of urine glucose levels to manage diabetes mellitus.

37. Identify the problems of using urine tests for monitoring glucose levels.

38. The nurse should instruct the client who is taking the oral hypoglycemic agents that:
    a. Dietary restrictions can be relaxed while taking the medication.
    b. The exercise program should be changed to include more intensive aerobic exercise.
    c. There are no particular restrictions for taking over-the-counter medications.
    d. Drinking alcoholic beverages will cause nausea and a "hot flash" feeling.

Match each of the following oral hypoglycemic medications with the corresponding nursing intervention.

Medication	Nursing Intervention
___ 39. Metformin (Glucophage)	a. Give drug with first bite of food.
___ 40. Acarbose (Precose)	b. Hold drug for 48 hours if having x-ray with IV contrast dye (renal).
___ 41. Glipizide (Glucotrol)	c. Give drug 30 minutes before meals.

42. Identify the two most common side effects of administering oral hypoglycemic agents.
    a. _____
    b. _____

43. When giving oral hypoglycemic agents, the nurse should demonstrate caution with clients who are known to have what four types of body system breakdowns?
    a. _____
    b. _____
    c. _____
    d. _____

44. Which of the following statements is correct about insulin?
    a. Exogenous insulin is necessary for management of all cases of type 2 diabetes.
    b. Insulin's effectiveness depends on the individual client's absorption of the drug.
    c. Insulin doses should be regulated according to self-monitoring urine glucose levels.
    d. Insulin administered in multiple doses per day decreases the flexibility of a client's lifestyle.

45. Which of the following statements is correct about insulin administration?
    a. Insulin may be given either orally, intravenously, or subcutaneously.
    b. Insulin injections should be spaced no closer than ½ inch apart.
    c. Rotating injection sites improves absorption and prevents lipodystrophy.
    d. In a mixed-dose protocol, the longer-acting insulin should be withdrawn first.

46. A diabetic is on a mixed-dose insulin protocol of 8 units regular insulin and 12 units NPH insulin at 7 a.m. At 10:30 a.m., the client reports feeling uneasy, shaky, and complains of a headache. Which is the probable explanation for this?
    a. The NPH insulin's action is peaking, and there is an insufficient blood glucose level.
    b. The regular insulin's action is peaking, and there is an insufficient blood glucose level.
    c. The client consumed too many calories at breakfast, and now has an elevated blood glucose level.
    d. The symptoms are unrelated to the insulin administered in the early morning or diet taken in at lunchtime.

47. A client has orders for 40 units of insulin zinc suspension (Lente insulin) and 10 units of regular insulin every morning. Explain how these drugs should be prepared for administration. What should the client be told about these actions and the side effects of these medications? *Use a separate sheet of paper for your answer.*

48. Describe three problems with blood glucose levels that may occur during the night if a client is on insulin therapy.
    a. _____
    b. _____
    c. _____

49. The client who is to use an external insulin pump should be told that:
   a. Self-monitoring of blood glucose levels can be done only twice a day.
   b. The insulin supply must be replaced every 2 to 4 weeks.
   c. The pump's battery should be checked on a regular weekly schedule.
   d. The needle site must be changed every 1 to 3 days.

50. A 47-year-old client with a history of type 2 diabetes mellitus and emphysema who reports smoking three packs per day is admitted to the hospital with a diagnosis of acute pneumonia. The client is placed on his regular oral hypoglycemic agents, sliding scale insulin, and antibiotic medications. On day two of hospitalization, the doctor orders prednisone therapy. The nurse would expect the blood glucose to:
   a. Decrease.
   b. Stay the same.
   c. Increase.
   d. Return to normal.

51. Identify the laboratory test that is the best indicator of the client's average blood glucose level and/or compliance to the diabetes mellitus regimen over the last 3 months.
   a. Postparandial test
   b. Oral glucose tolerance test (OGTT)
   c. Casual blood glucose test
   d. Glycosylated hemoglobin (HbA1c)

52. Identify the earliest clinical sign of nephropathy.
   a. Proteinuria
   b. Ketonuria
   c. Glucosuria
   d. Microalbuminuria

53. The client's blood glucose level obtained from a fingerstick AccuCheck machine reads 20 mg/dL. Determine the next three priority nursing interventions.
   a. _____
   b. _____
   c. _____

54. A diabetic client has just returned from surgery with stable blood sugars between 120 to 180 mg/dL. Identify the appropriate IV solution to promote adequate hydration and normoglycemia.
   a. D5 ½ NS at 125 mL/hr
   b. D5W at 125 mL/hr
   c. 0.45 % NSS at 100 mL/hr
   d. 0.9% NSS at 100 mL/hr

55. A client with type 2 diabetes mellitus, usually controlled with a sulfonylurea, develops a urinary tract infection. Due to the stress of the infection, she must be treated with insulin. She should be instructed that:
   a. The sulfonylurea must be discontinued and insulin taken until the infection clears.
   b. Insulin will now be necessary to control the client's diabetes for life.
   c. The sulfonylurea dose must be reduced until the infection clears.
   d. The insulin is necessary to supplement the sulfonylurea until the infection clears.

Match each of the following diabetic complications with the corresponding pathophysiology. Answers may be used more than once.

Complications	Pathophysiologies
___ 56. Neovascularization	a. Nephropathy
___ 57. End-stage renal	b. Neuropathy
disease	c. Retinopathy
___ 58. Muscle atrophy	
___ 59. Proteinuria	
___ 60. Hemorrhage into vitreous cavity	
___ 61. Pain or numbness	
___ 62. Hard exudates on fundus	
___ 63. Permanent blindness	

64. Identify lower extremity complications that may result from compromised circulation in a diabetic client.
   a. _____
   b. _____
   c. _____

65. According to the Diabetes Control and Complication Trial (DCCT) study of type 1 diabetes mellitus clients and the United Kingdom Prospective Diabetes Study (UKPDS) of type 2 diabetes mellitus clients, intensive therapy with good glucose control resulted in what types of health benefits? *Use a separate sheet of paper for your answer.*

66. On a separate sheet of paper, develop a concept map relevant to diabetes mellitus. Consider physiologic, psychosocial, and developmental factors. Identify data that are subjective and data that are objective. Include significant laboratory and other diagnostic tests.

67. Identify the factors that should be considered when developing an individualized meal plan for the diabetic client.
   a. _____
   b. _____
   c. _____
   d. _____

68. Basic principles of meal planning for the diabetic client include:
    a. Five small meals per day plus a bedtime snack.
    b. Providing a favorite sweet dessert once a day.
    c. High-protein, low-carbohydrate, and low-fiber foods.
    d. Considering the action time of the client's insulin.

69. Identify the food groups in the exchange system of diabetic meal planning.
    a. _____
    b. _____
    c. _____
    d. _____
    e. _____
    f. _____

70. Which of the following food exchange examples is *not* equivalent?
    a. 1 teaspoon butter = 1 strip bacon
    b. 1 tablespoon peanut butter = 1 ounce ground beef
    c. 1 cup milk = 1 cup yogurt
    d. ½ cup carrots = ½ cup broccoli

71. Which of the following statements is correct about the diet a diabetic client should follow?
    a. Alcoholic beverage consumption is unrestricted.
    b. Dietetic foods may contain more fat than regular foods.
    c. Sweeteners should be avoided because of the side effects.
    d. Both soluble and insoluble fiber foods should be limited.

72. The recommended protocol for most diabetic clients who must lose weight is to:
    a. Participate in aerobic program twice a week for 20 minutes each session.
    b. Slowly increase insulin dosage until mild hypoglycemia occurs.
    c. Reduce calorie intake and walk briskly for 30 minutes daily.
    d. Reduce daily calorie intake to 1200 calories and monitor for ketones.

73. The recommended calorie reduction for the diabetic client who must lose weight is:
    a. 500 calories/week.
    b. 1500 calories/week.
    c. 2500 calories/week.
    d. 3500 calories/week.

74. Identify the eating disorders that the diabetic client may develop if food becomes an unhealthy focus of attention.
    a. _____
    b. _____

75. The diabetic who swims for exercise should be advised to administer insulin, prior to exercising, in the:
    a. Abdomen
    b. Thighs
    c. Arms
    d. Hips

76. On a separate sheet of paper, discuss the purpose of having a supply of simple sugar available for the diabetic client when he or she is exercising.

77. Diabetic foot care includes:
    a. Using rubbing alcohol to toughen the skin on the soles of the feet.
    b. Wearing open-toed shoes or sandals in warm weather to prevent perspiration.
    c. Applying lanolin lotion to moisturize the skin and keep it smooth and supple.
    d. Using cool water for bathing feet to prevent inadvertent thermal injury.

78. A 25-year-old female client with diabetic nephropathy tells the nurse, "I have two kidneys and I'm still young. I expect to be around for a long time, so why should I worry about my blood sugar?" Which of the following is the nurse's best reply?
    a. "You have little to worry about as long as your kidneys keep making urine."
    b. "You should discuss this with your physician because you are being unrealistic."
    c. "You would be correct if your diabetes could be managed with insulin."
    d. "Unsafe blood sugars affect both kidneys, even with insulin management."

79. Which of the following statements best describes education for diabetic clients?
    a. General education promotes a sense of well-being because it helps the client feel that he or she has control over the disease.
    b. Survival education includes assisting the client to adapt self-care practices to meet his or her needs.
    c. Home management education includes information about when to call the physician.
    d. Lifestyle improvement education includes emphasis on daily care such as hygiene.

80. The best time to begin teaching a newly diagnosed diabetic client is when:
    a. Blood sugars range between 220 to 350 mg/dL.
    b. An arthritis flare up is beginning to calm down.
    c. Fever decreases to 101.0° F in a client with a foot infection.
    d. Blood sugars range between 120 to 160 mg/dL.

81. Which of the following statements about sexual intercourse for diabetic clients is correct?
    a. The incidence of sexual dysfunction is lower in men than women.
    b. Retrograde ejaculation does not interfere with male fertility.
    c. Impotence is associated with diabetes mellitus in male clients.
    d. Sexual dysfunction in female clients includes inability to attain orgasm.

82. Identify the fears related to the condition most common among diabetic clients.
    a. _____
    b. _____
    c. _____
    d. _____

83. An insulin-dependent diabetic client is planning to travel by air and asks the nurse about preparations for the trip. The nurse should tell the client to:
    a. Pack insulin and syringes in a labeled, crush-proof kit in the checked luggage.
    b. Carry all necessary diabetic supplies in a clearly identified pack aboard the plane.
    c. Ask the flight attendant to put the insulin in the galley refrigerator once on the plane.
    d. Take only minimal supplies and get the prescription filled at his or her destination.

84. Which of the following statements reflects that the diabetic client understands the principles of self-care?
    a. "I don't like the idea of sticking myself so often to measure my sugar."
    b. "I plan to measure the sugar in my urine at least four times a day."
    c. "I plan to get my spouse to exercise with me to keep me company."
    d. "If I get a cold, I can take my regular cough medication until I feel better."

85. After a 2-hour glucose challenge, impaired glucose tolerance is present when the values are between _____ and _____ mg/dL.

86. A 50-year-old client was seen in the emergency room for complaints of nausea, vomiting, and dehydration. When admitted to the hospital, the fasting blood glucose was over 500. A blood gas showed a pH of 7.38. He was diagnosed with diabetes and treated with insulin and fluids. What does this situation tell you about this client?
    a. He will require insulin injections for the rest of his life.
    b. He will only require insulin when he is stressed or ill.
    c. His pancreas is producing enough insulin to prevent ketoacidosis.
    d. His diabetes is temporary.

Answer the following two questions on a separate sheet of paper.

87. Briefly explain the importance of adequate glucose and insulin during exercise.

88. What is the primary reason for using an insulin pump instead of injections?

89. A client with type 2 diabetes often has which of the following laboratory values?
    a. Elevated thyroid studies
    b. Elevated triglycerides
    c. Ketones in the urine
    d. Low hemoglobin

Answer the following three questions on a separate sheet of paper.

90. A newly diagnosed client with diabetes is being seen for instruction regarding insulin administration. Identify points of emphasis in teaching this client.

91. A client with type 1 diabetes takes two shots a day of mixed NPH and regular insulin. The client takes one shot in the morning and one in the evening. What instruction would you give this client regarding a meal regimen?

92. A client with type 1 diabetes notifies the physician of flu-like symptoms with nausea. What do you tell this client about sick day rules?

93. Hypovolemic shock can be a complication of DKA or HHNK. _____ is a key indication of hypovolemic shock in these clients.

Answer the following two questions on a separate sheet of paper.

94. What are the signs and symptoms of hypoglycemia?

95. Discuss tight glucose control and the older adult.

96. A client with type 1 diabetes is taking a mixture of NPH and regular insulin at home. He is now NPO after midnight and scheduled for surgery the next day.
    A. On the day of surgery, what action would the nurse take regarding the morning dose of insulin?
       1. Administer the dose that is routinely prescribed at home since he has type 1 diabetes and needs the insulin.
       2. Administer half the dose since the client is NPO.
       3. Hold the insulin with all the other medications since the client is NPO and there is no need for insulin.
       4. Contact the physician for a physician's order regarding the insulin because a client with type 1 diabetes must have exogenous insulin.
       5. Administer just the NPH since it is the long-acting insulin and should have good coverage for the day.
       6. Administer just the regular insulin since he will be going to surgery.

    B. Which of the above actions would the nurse take if the client has type 2 diabetes?

97. A client with diabetes has signs and symptoms of hypoglycemia. The client is alert and oriented with a blood glucose of 56.
    A. The nurse would administer:
       1. A glass of orange juice with two packets of sugar and continue to monitor the client.
       2. A glass of orange or other type of juice and continue to monitor the client.
       3. A glass of orange or other type of juice, followed by a complex carbohydrate, and monitor the client.
       4. D50 IV push and give the client something to eat.

    B. Which of the above actions would the nurse take if the client was not alert and oriented or unable to take PO fluids?

98. Nurses must know the onset, peak, and duration of the types of insulins in order to monitor the effectiveness of the medication and monitor for side effects. As students, read and study this information from the text or your pharmacology book. Have this information on a reference card and use it in clinical setting. Memorize this information in order to give safe nursing care.

99. Compare the common endocrine emergencies using the chart below. *Use a separate sheet of paper for your answer.*

	Myxedema	Thyroid Storm	Diabetic Keto-acidosis	Hyper-glycemia	Hypogly-cemia	Hyperos-molar Nonketotic Coma
Events that precipitate the crisis						
Common abnormal lab and other diagnostic tests						
Priority emergency interventions						

Case Study: The Client with Diabetes Mellitus

Your client is a 48-year-old woman who is admitted to the emergency department, and she is unconscious. She has a known history of insulin-dependent diabetes mellitus. Her daughter accompanies her and tells the staff that her mother has had the "flu" and has been unable to eat or drink very much. The daughter is uncertain whether her mother has taken her insulin in the past 24 hours. The client's vitals signs are temperature 101.8° F; pulse 120, weak and irregular; respiration, 22, deep and fruity odor; and blood pressure, 80/42. Blood specimens and arterial blood gases are drawn and an intravenous infusion begun.

Answer the following questions on a separate sheet of paper:

1. Based on this client's history, give the probable changes in laboratory results for serum glucose, serum osmolarity, serum acetone, BUN, arterial pH, and arterial Pco_2. What medical emergency do these data indicate?

2. What type of intravenous solutions should the nurse be prepared to administer to this client? What drugs should the nurse be prepared to give? Explain your answers.

3. Identify the relevant nursing diagnoses for this client based on the above assessments.

4. A large-bore intravenous needle is inserted, and the client is placed on continuous cardiac monitoring. What is the rationale for these interventions?

5. During the first 24 hours, what complications should the nurse monitor for in this client? Why?

6. The client eventually becomes normoglycemic, regains consciousness, and begins a 1500-calorie diabetic diet. Develop a teaching-learning plan for her about this diet.

7. Prior to this emergency, this client had been monitoring urine glucose and ketones for self-care and insulin administration. Her physician prescribes blood glucose monitoring instead of urine testing. What is the rationale for this change?

8. Which aspect of diabetic self-care should the nurse discuss with this client prior to her discharge?

9. The client is to be discharged on a mixed-dose protocol for insulin. She is to receive 10 units regular insulin and 18 units NPH insulin before breakfast and another 5 units regular insulin and 12 units NPH at dinner time. Develop a teaching-learning plan for these medications.

10. What should the nurse discuss with this client about diabetes, insulin, and illness?

11. What can this client do to prevent future emergency episodes? Consider "Instructions for Sick Day" rules.

Case Study: The Client with Diabetes Mellitus and Visual Impairment

Your adult male client has had diabetes mellitus for several years. He takes 30 units of NPH with 10 units of regular insulin in the morning before breakfast and 20 units of NPH before the evening meal. He has recently undergone laser therapy for treatment of diabetic retinopathy. He wants to be independent in insulin administration, and your assessment indicates that he has the intellectual ability to learn the needed skills.

Answer the following questions on a separate sheet of paper:

1. List three methods for preventing both hypoglycemia and hyperglycemia that you would stress during your teaching sessions.

2. Discuss four ways of altering the environment to aid in the measurement of accurate insulin doses.

3. List five critical points that would be included in a teaching session on adaptive devices for use with insulin syringes.

UNIT 14   PROBLEMS OF PROTECTION: SKIN, HAIR, AND NAILS ■ Core Concepts Grid

Anatomy	Physiology	Pathophysiology	History	Physical Exam	Diagnostic Tests	Interventions	Pharmacology
• **Skin** Subcutaneous fat Epidermis Dermis • **Hair** • **Nails** • **Glands**	• **Protection** • **Regulation** Fluid balance Electrolyte balance Temperature • **Vitamin** **synthesis**	• **Inflammation** • **Infection** • **Tumors** • **Burns** Thermal Chemical Electrical	• **Client history** Dermatologic problems Medications Liver, gallbladder, renal disease • **Family history** Chronic skin prob- lems • **Social history** Occupation Nutritional status Sun exposure Age Race • **Risk for pressure** **ulcers**	• **Skin** Color Lesions Moisture Vascular markings Edema Intactness Tattoos Temperature Texture Turgor Depth (stage) of wound Drainage • **Hair/nails** Shape Distribution Texture	• **Cultures** • **Skin tests** Patch Scratch • **Biopsy**	• **Burn wound** **assessment** Depth Area Rule of Nines • **Burn fluid** **replacement** **formulas** • **Graft care** • **Care of burn** **wounds** • **Hypertrophy** • **Precautions for** **itching** • **Emotional** **support** • **Debridement** • **Wound dressings** • **Nutrition** • **Prevention of** **pressure ulcers** • **Skin/wound** **ongoing** **assessment**	• **Topical** **antibiotics** • **Topical anti-** **inflammatories** • **Keratolytic** **agents** • **Antipsoriasis** **agents** • **Debriding** **agents** • **Systemic** **antibiotics**

Unit 14 (Chapters 66-68)

Problems of Protection: Management of Clients with Problems of the Skin, Hair, and Nails

Learning Plan

Chapter 66: Assessment of the Skin, Hair, and Nails

Learning Outcomes	Learning Activities	Supplemental Resources
1. Compare the structures and functions of the dermis with those of the epidermis. 2. Describe the integumentary changes associated with aging. 3. Use proper terminology to describe different skin lesions. 4. Describe the technique to assess skin changes in clients with dark skin. 5. Distinguish between normal variations and abnormal skin manifestations with regard to skin color, texture, warmth, and moisture. 6. Explain the role of the melanocytes in determining skin color. 7. Describe the ABCD method of assessing skin lesions for cancer. 8. Prioritize educational needs for the client undergoing an excisional biopsy for a skin lesion.	1. Prior to completing the study guide exercises for this chapter, review the following: • Anatomy and physiology of the skin and its appendages • Principles of fluid and electrolyte balance • Principles of infection control • Concepts of body image and self-esteem 2. Review the **boldfaced** Key Terms and their definitions in Chapter 66 to enhance your understanding of the content. 3. Go to Study Guide Number 14.66 on the following pages and complete the learning exercises for this chapter.	1. Textbook—Chapter 66 2. Other resources: • Contact a nurse practitioner and assist in examinations of skin, hair, and nails in a variety of clients to enhance your assessment skills. • Ebersole, P. & Hess, P. (1998). *Toward healthy aging* (5th ed.) (pp.87-89). St. Louis: Mosby.

Chapter 67: Interventions for Clients with Problems of the Skin and Nails

Learning Outcomes	Learning Activities	Supplemental Resources
1. Prioritize the nursing care needs for clients with dry skin. 2. Compare and contrast wound healing by first, second, and third intention. 3. Identify clients at risk for pressure ulcer development. 4. Plan an individualized strategy for pressure ulcer prevention for a specific client at increased risk. 5. Differentiate the clinical manifestations for stage I through stage IV pressure ulcers. 6. Prioritize the nursing interventions for a client with a stage III ulcer. 7. Evaluate the effectiveness of interventions for pressure ulcer management.	1. Prior to completing the study guide exercises for this chapter, review the following: • Anatomy and physiology of the skin and its appendages • Principles of fluid and electrolyte balance • Principles of infection control • Concepts of body image and self-esteem • Pain management • Principles of wound healing and wound care • Principles of general nutrition	1. Textbook—Chapter 66 (Assessment of the Skin, Hair, and Nails) 2. Textbook—Chapter 67 3. Other resources: • Contact a medical supply company to become familiar with products for pressure ulcer prevention. • Peters, J. (2000). Toxic epidermal necrolysis. *Nursing Times, 96*(36), 43-44.

2. Review the **boldfaced** Key Terms and their definitions in Chapter 67 to enhance your understanding of the content.
3. Go to Study Guide Number 14.67 on the following pages and complete the learning exercises for this chapter.

• Visit a nursing home and discuss current practices of preventing and caring for pressure ulcers.

8. Compare the clinical manifestations and modes of transmission for bacterial, viral, and fungal skin infections.
9. Prioritize nursing care and education needs for clients who have parasitic skin infections.
10. Explain the rationale for drug therapy for psoriasis.
11. Explain the rationale for ultraviolet therapy for psoriasis.
12. Identify interventions for the prevention of cancer.
13. Describe the clinical manifestations of melanoma.

Chapter 68: Interventions for Clients with Burns

Learning Outcomes

1. Identify clients with burns who are at risk for inhalation injury.
2. Compare and contrast the clinical manifestations of superficial, partial-thickness, and full-thickness injuries.
3. Explain the expected clinical manifestations of neural and hormonal compensation during the emergent phase of burn injury.
4. Calculate the total body surface area involved in a burn injury.
5. Prioritize the nursing care needs for a client during the emergent phase of burn injury.
6. Use laboratory data and clinical manifestations to determine the effectiveness of fluid resuscitation during the emergent phase of burn injury.
7. Use the Parkland formula to establish the correct rate and timing of fluid replacement.
8. Prioritize the nursing care needs for a client during the acute phase of burn injury.
9. Explain the alteration of nutritional needs for the burn client during the acute phase of burn injury.
10. Evaluate wound healing in a client during the acute phase of burn injury.
11. Compare and contrast pain management strategies for clients in the emergent and acute phases of burn injury.
12. Describe the characteristics of infected burns.
13. Explain the positioning and range of motion interventions for prevention of mobility problems in the client with burns.
14. Prioritize nursing care needs for the client during the rehabilitation phase of burn injury.
15. Discuss the potential psychosocial problems associated with burn injury.

Learning Activities

1. Prior to completing the study guide exercises for this chapter, review the following:
   • Anatomy and physiology of the skin and its appendages
   • Principles of fluid and electrolyte balance
   • Principles of acid-base balance
   • Principles of infection control
   • Concepts of body image and self-esteem
   • Pain management
   • Principles of wound healing and wound care
   • Perioperative care
   • Principles of general nutrition
   • Procedure for application of topical medications
   • Concepts of human sexuality
   • Concepts of loss, grief, death, and dying
   • The principles of airway management
2. Review the **boldfaced** Key Terms and their definitions in Chapter 68 to enhance your understanding of the content.
3. Go to Study Guide Number 14.68 on the following pages and complete the learning exercises for this chapter.

Supplemental Resources

1. Textbook—Chapter 66 (Assessment of the Skin, Hair, and Nails)
2. Textbook—Chapter 68
3. Other resources:
   • Atkins, S. (1999). Burns assessment and initial management. *Nursing Times, 95*(35), 46-48.
   • Covington, D., Wainwright, D., & Parks, D. (1996). Prognostic indicators in the elderly patient with burns. *Journal of Burn Care and Rehabilitation, 17*(3) 222-230.
   • Flynn, M. (1999). Identifying and treating inhalation injuries in fire victims. *DCCN: Dimensions of Critical Care Nursing, 18*(4), 18-23.
   • Kraft, P. (2000). The osmotic shift. *Journal of Intravenous Nursing, 23*(4), 220-224.
   • Nagy, S. (1999). Strategies used by burn nurses to cope with infliction of pain on patients. *Journal of Advanced Nursing, 29*(6), 1427-1433.
   • Visit a burn center and focus on the nursing methods of coping with these critically ill patients during management of the client with burns.
   • Winfree, J. & Barillo, D. (1997). Nonthermal injuries. *Nursing Clinics of North America, 32*(2), 275-296

STUDY GUIDE NUMBER 14.66

Assessment of the Skin, Hair, and Nails

Study/Review Questions

1. Match each of the following properties with the appropriate layer of skin.

   Properties
   ___ a. Contains elastin
   ___ b. Serves as insulator
   ___ c. Contains no cells
   ___ d. Collagen is main component
   ___ e. Does not have a separate blood supply
   ___ f. Provides padding
   ___ g. Innermost layer of skin
   ___ h. Rich in sensory nerves
   ___ i. Synthesis of vitamin D
   ___ j. Melanin production

   Layers of Skin
   1. Fat
   2. Dermis
   3. Epidermis

2. A clinical example of a secondary lesion is/are:
   a. Cysts.
   b. Acne.
   c. Psoriasis.
   d. Hives.

3. What is the most significant factor leading to the degeneration of the skin components?
   a. Systemic disease
   b. Genetic background
   c. Sun exposure
   d. Hormonal changes

4. In regulating body temperature, evaporative water loss can be as much as:
   a. 600 mL/day.
   b. 10 to 12 L/day.
   c. 2 L/day.
   d. 900 mL/day.

5. Which of the following statements are true about integumentary changes in older adults? *Check all that apply.*
   ___ a. Decreased thickness in the epidermal layer results in increased skin transparency and fragility replacement.
   ___ b. Thinning of the fat layer decreases the susceptibility to hypothermia.
   ___ c. Increased blood flow to the nail bed increases longitudinal nail ridges.
   ___ d. Decreased number of Langerhans cells increases cutaneous inflammatory response.
   ___ e. Decreased eccrine and apocrine gland activity increases susceptibility to dry skin.

6. Identify two characteristics for each of the following primary and secondary lesions.
   a. Nodules:
   b. Papules:
   c. Wheals:

7. Match the terminology with the corresponding definitions.

   Terms
   ___ a. Serpiginous
   ___ b. Circinate
   ___ c. Diffuse
   ___ d. Coalesced
   ___ e. Annular

   Definitions
   1. Lesions merging with each other
   2. Widespread
   3. Ring-like with raised borders around flat, clear centers of normal skin
   4. Having wavy borders
   5. Circular

8. Pallor in dark-skinned clients may be detected by:
   a. Ash-gray color of mucous membranes.
   b. Reddish pink color of the skin.
   c. Whitish color of the skin.
   d. Bluish tinge of the nail beds.

9. In a dark-skinned clients, a color change of the
   _____ is the best indicator of jaundice.
   a. Conjunctiva and sclera
   b. Palms of the hands
   c. Soles of the feet
   d. Oral mucosa

10. On a separate sheet of paper, describe the ABCD
    method of assessing skin lesions for cancer.

11. To differentiate between color changes in the nail
    bed related to vascular supply and those from pig-
    ment disposition, the nurse should:
    a. Examine the nail plate under a Wood's light.
    b. Assess for thickness.
    c. Blanch the nail bed.
    d. Evaluate for lesions.

12. On a separate sheet of paper, identify the probable
    causes for each skin manifestation identified below:
    a. Increased body hair growth on the face in a
       female client
    b. Drumstick appearance of nail shape
    c. Decreased skin turgor
    d. "Heaped up" appearance on a older adult's toe-
       nail

13. Your adult client is scheduled for an excisional
    biopsy and is very apprehensive about pain. On a
    separate sheet of paper, describe what the nurse
    does to reassure this client.

STUDY GUIDE NUMBER 14.67

Interventions for Clients with Problems of the Skin and Nails

Study/Review Questions

1. The most common symptom of pruritus is:
   a. Blisters.
   b. Itching.
   c. Flaking.
   d. Tenderness.

2. In assessing clients, what is it important that a nurse
   know about pruritus?
   a. It can be associated with a systemic disease
      rather than skin disease.
   b. It is worse at night.
   c. It is caused by the stimulation of itch-specific
      nerve fibers.
   d. Rubbing the skin may further stimulate itching.

3. To facilitate rehydration of the skin, creams or
   lotions should be applied:
   a. Within 2 to 3 minutes after bathing.
   b. With vigorous and circular motions.
   c. To completely dry skin.
   d. After the first sign of flakiness appears.

4. Which of the following statements about xerosis are
   true? *Check all that apply.*
   ___ a. It is worse in dry climates.
   ___ b. Wind, cold, and sunlight contribute to the
          problem.
   ___ c. Frequent bathing with deodorant soap and
          hot water relieve the problem.
   ___ d. Using a dehumidifier during humid days
          decreases the risk of getting xerosis.
   ___ e. Avoiding caffeine and alcohol ingestion is
          helpful in preventing this condition.

5. Management of urticaria includes: *Check all that
   apply.*
   ___ a. Avoiding overexertion and warm environ-
          ments.
   ___ b. Using antihistamines as the drug of choice.
   ___ c. Restricting alcohol consumption.
   ___ d. Avoid scratching and touching the lesions.

6. A client is complaining about painful sunburn. On a separate sheet of paper, describe what treatment information the nurse would share.

7. In wound healing, which of the following statements is healing by second intention?
   a. There is minimal tissue destruction with no open areas or dead spaces.
   b. The wound is closed surgically after it was open for several days.
   c. The chronic wound is allowed to heal from the inside out.
   d. The wound is surgically made and has minimal tissue reaction.

8. The degree to which epithelialization and contraction can restore wound integrity depends on the _____ of the injury and extent of _____ loss.

9. Partial-thickness wound healing by epithelialization takes:
   a. 2 to 3 days.
   b. 5 to 7 days.
   c. 24 hours.
   d. 12 to 14 days.

10. A full-thickness wound: *Check all that apply.*
    ___ a. Requires necrotic tissue to be removed for healing to occur.
    ___ b. Results in unstable epithelial surface.
    ___ c. Heals by primary intention.
    ___ d. Is typically a burn.

11. Identify three reasons why older adults are at risk for pressure ulcers.
    a. _____
    b. _____
    c. _____

12. An 89-year-old nursing home client is now bedridden and has been losing weight steadily. The dietitian is working with her family to improve her diet and encourage her eating. She is at high risk, but what interventions can prevent her from getting a pressure ulcer? *Use a separate sheet of paper for your answer.*

13. It was noted that this client (Question 12) has developed a pressure ulcer from friction of the sheets. It is described as an intact blister on her left heel that is 6 cm long and 5 cm wide with no signs of cellulitis. This is a stage _____ pressure ulcer.

14. This client is complaining of discomfort from a pressure ulcer. Which nursing diagnosis would be appropriate?

15. Complete the following statements.
    a. A _____ dressing material is beneficial when the wound is relatively free of drainage.
    b. To prevent maceration with a draining wound, a _____ dressing is used.

16. For a successful skin graft, the graft area must: *Check all that apply.*
    ___ a. Have an adequate blood supply.
    ___ b. Be free of infection.
    ___ c. Be completely immobilized.
    ___ d. Be irrigated frequently.

17. Herpes zoster (shingles) is a varicella-zoster viral infection related to chicken pox and:
    a. Is manifested by pain, itching, and tenderness.
    b. Usually causes a larger, single lesion.
    c. Is painless.
    d. Lasts 1 to 2 days.

18. Match each tinea infection with the corresponding location.

Location	Infection
___ a. Feet	1. Tinea capitis
___ b. Hands	2. Tinea manus
___ c. Groin (jock itch)	3. Tinea barbae
___ d. Scalp	4. Tinea pedis
___ e. Beard	5. Tinea corporis
___ f. Smooth skin surfaces	6. Tinea cruris

19. Pediculosis capitis is typically:
    a. Not treated with chemical agents.
    b. Not contagious through bed linens and hats.
    c. Seen in adults.
    d. Self-limiting.

20. A client who complains of intense itching at night may have:
    a. Tinea corporis.
    b. Scabies.
    c. Furuncles.
    d. Contact dermatitis.

21. Determine the type of skin infection based on each description of the clinical manifestations.
    a. Cracks and fissures at the corners of the mouth with creamy white plaques: _____
    b. Fever, redness, warmth, lymphadenopathy: _____
    c. Group of blisters on anterior trunk, painful, itching: _____

22. Psoriasis is an inflammatory dermatosis that:
    a. Can be cured with proper management of systemic drugs and topical agents.
    b. Is a scaling disorder with underlying dermal inflammation.
    c. Slows the rate of shedding at the outermost stratum corneum.
    d. Is infected with *Staphylococcus aureus*.

23. The characteristic lesions of psoriasis are:
    a. Plaques surmounted by silvery-white scales.
    b. Circular areas of redness.
    c. Multiple blisters with a yellowish crust.
    d. Patches of tender raised areas limited to extremities.

24. Treatment for psoriasis can include:
    a. UV light therapy.
    b. Dovonex topical cream.
    c. Methotrexate.
    d. Ciprofloxacin.

25. The most common type of benign tumor is a:
    a. Wart.
    b. Nevus.
    c. Hemangioma.
    d. Hematoma.

26. Melanoma is a cancer that:
    a. Is highly metastatic.
    b. Is the most lethal form of skin cancer.
    c. Originates in the melanin-producing cells of the epidermis.
    d. Is likely to have a favorable prognosis.

27. Identify four ways to prevent skin cancer.
    a. _____
    b. _____
    c. _____
    d. _____

28. You have a 25-year-old client who has recently had a rhinoplasty. He is swallowing repeatedly and belching. What is this an indication of?

29. Accutane is a systemic medication that:
    a. Is used for severe cases of acne.
    b. Has no side effects.
    c. Requires strict birth control measures.
    d. Is the first choice.

30. Nursing care for a client with toxic epidermal necrolysis (TEN) should include:
    a. Assessment of input and output.
    b. Monitoring fluid and electrolyte balance.
    c. Monitoring for hyperthermia.
    d. Managing nausea with medication.

31. Rewarming frostbite tissue is done:
    a. Slowly to avoid more damage.
    b. In a water bath at 90° F to 107° F.
    c. With warm water compresses of normal saline applied directly to the area.
    d. After the blisters are punctured to facilitate healing.

32. Leprosy (Hansen's disease) is a contagious disease for which the exact mechanism of transmission to a susceptible host is unknown. However, clinical manifestations are directly related to the _____ of the individual's _____ to mycobacteria.

STUDY GUIDE NUMBER 14.68

Interventions for Clients with Burns

Study/Review Questions

1. Tissue destruction caused by a burn injury causes local and systemic problems. Identify six of these potential problems.

   a. _____

   b. _____

   c. _____

   d. _____

   e. _____

   f. _____

2. Match each of the following terms with the corresponding definitions.

   ____ a. Dermal appendages
   ____ b. Anesthetic
   ____ c. Vesicle
   ____ d. Eschar
   ____ e. Desquamation
   ____ f. Fasciotomy
   ____ g. Viable
   ____ h. Hyperkalemia
   ____ i. Hyponatremia
   ____ j. Hemoconcentration
   ____ k. Catabolism

   1. Decreased sodium levels
   2. Peeling of dead skin
   3. Living
   4. Sweat, oil, and hair follicles
   5. Burn crust
   6. Elevated potassium levels
   7. Blister
   8. Incision through the eschar and fascia
   9. Does not transmit sensation
   10. Fat breakdown
   11. Elevated blood osmolarity

3. When a burn injury occurs, the skin can regenerate as long as:
   a. The basement membrane is present.
   b. The "true skin" has function elements of the skin.
   c. The dermis layer has blood vessels, sensory nerves, hair follicles, lymph vessels, sebaceous glands, and sweat glands.
   d. All of the above

4. Which of the following statements are true? *Check all that apply.*
   ____ a. The depth of dermal appendages is equal across body areas.
   ____ b. Full-thickness burn is identified by the total destruction of the dermis.
   ____ c. Full-thickness burn results in loss of excretory ability.
   ____ d. All burn injuries are painful.
   ____ e. The skin can tolerate temperatures of 158° F.
   ____ f. The magnitude of the injury is based on the depth and extent of the total body surface burn.
   ____ g. Blood transfusions are critical in the first 24 hours for all burns.

5. Complete the following table on the classification by burn thickness.

Classification	Color	Healing Time	Examples
Superficial			
Partial-thickness superficial			
Partial-thickness deep			
Full-thickness			
Deep full thickness			

6. Partial thickness wounds can convert to full thickness when:
   a. Scar formation is large.
   b. Tissue damage increases with ischemia.
   c. Blisters are present.
   d. Skin integrity is impaired.

7. Before a full-thickness wound heals:
   a. Edema must be reduced by diuretics.
   b. Eschar must be removed.
   c. Blisters must be opened to prevent immunosuppression.
   d. There must be a decrease in tissue perfusion.

8. Third spacing or capillary leak syndrome in a client with severe burns:
   a. Usually happens in the first 36 to 48 hours.
   b. Is a leak of plasma fluids into the interstitial space.
   c. Is present even in unburned tissues when greater than 5% to 10% total body surface area.
   d. Can usually be prevented.

9. As a result of this fluid shift, during the acute phase, imbalances occur such as:
   a. Hyperkalemia.
   b. Hypernatremia.
   c. Hypokalemia.
   d. Hypercalcemia.

10. Because of the fluid shifts in burns, cardiac output:
    a. May be depressed until 36 hours after the burn.
    b. Is not affected.
    c. Is improved with fluid restriction.
    d. Responds to diuretics.

11. Pulmonary complications cause or contribute to death in _____ of clients with combined inhalation and cutaneous burn injury.
    a. 24%
    b. 18%
    c. 77%
    d. 33%

12. A serious gastrointestinal disorder that can occur with a major burn is:
    a. Increased motility.
    b. Increased flow of blood to the area.
    c. Decreased secretion of catecholamines.
    d. Paralytic ileus.

13. The hypermetabolic state with a significant burn causes: *Check all that apply.*
    ____ a. Fat breakdown and the rapid use of use of glucose and calories.
    ____ b. A decrease in the secretion of catecholamines.
    ____ c. An increase in caloric needs.
    ____ d. An increase in core temperature.

14. Fluid remobilization is: *Check all that apply.*
    ____ a. A result of the decreasing inflammatory response.
    ____ b. The plasma shifting into the interstitial space.
    ____ c. The cause of hyponatremia.
    ____ d. The cause of hyperkalemia.

15. Tissue injury is a threat to homeostasis. The two compensatory responses are:
    a. _____
    b. _____

16. Identify the sources of burn injuries.
    a. _____
    b. _____
    c. _____
    d. _____
    e. _____
    f. _____

17. Resistance to electricity varies in different parts of the body. Which of the following has the least resistance?
    a. Tendons, fat, and bone
    b. Skin
    c. Dry, callused areas
    d. Nerve, muscle, and blood vessels

Answer the following two questions on a separate sheet of paper.

18. Identify the age-related changes that increase morbidity and mortality in the older adult.

19. Identify information that should be included in a history.

20. Indications of a possible inhalation injury could be: *Check all that apply.*
    ____ a. Black carbon particles in the mouth.
    ____ b. Burns of the ears, face, and lips.
    ____ c. Edema of the septum.
    ____ d. Black carbon particles in the nares.

21. Which of following laboratory results would *not* be expected during the emergent period?
    a. Potassium level of 3.2 mEq/L
    b. Glucose level of 180 mg/dL
    c. Hematocrit of 45%/dL
    d. pH of 7.20

22. Which of the following statements are true about carbon monoxide poisoning? *Check all that apply.*
    ____ a. It causes "cherry-red" color in burn clients.
    ____ b. The partial pressure of oxygen (Pao_2) dissolved in the arterial blood is reduced.
    ____ c. Carbon monoxide binds to the hemoglobin molecule 250 times more tightly then oxygen.
    ____ d. It has a high mortality rate.

23. What should a nurse assess relevant to the cardio-vascular system for the client with severe burns? *Check all that apply.*
    ___ a. Presence and strength of peripheral and central pulses
    ___ b. Capillary refill
    ___ c. Presence of edema
    ___ d. Blood pressure

24. Renal function is assessed accurately by:
    a. Measuring urine output and comparing this value with fluid intake.
    b. Weighing the client.
    c. Noting the amount of edema.
    d. Measuring abdominal girth.

Answer the following two questions on a separate sheet of paper.

25. Why it is important to be accurate when evaluating the size of the burn injury?

26. For an African-American client with a burn injury, an additional blood test may be appropriate. Which test and why?

27. Hypovolemic shock occurs in burned clients as a result of:
    a. Erratic lymphatic drainage.
    b. Altered osmotic pressure in vessels.
    c. Albumin trapped in the interstitial spaces.
    d. A marked increase in capillary permeability.

A 70-kg woman with 50% TBSA with 50% TBSA burn arrived at 11 a.m. and was burned at 9 a.m., according to her family. Answer the following four questions relating to this client.

28. Using the Parkland (Baxter) formula, calculate the fluids needed for the first 8 hours after injury.

29. What time does the first 8-hour period end?

30. How much fluid is required for the 24 hours?

31. Hourly urine output is adjusted to _____ mL/kg.

32. Which of the following statements are true about escharotomies and fasciotomies?
    a. They are frequently done under general anesthesia.
    b. No anesthesia is required.
    c. Sedation and analgesia are commonly given to reduce anxiety.
    d. They are often done at the bedside.

33. Airway maintenance for a client with a burn injury and respiratory involvement includes:
    a. Monitoring for signs and symptoms of upper airway edema during fluid resuscitation.
    b. Inserting a naso- or oropharyngeal airway when the client's airway is completely obstructed.
    c. Securing loose dressing with a rib binder instead of tape.
    d. Weighing the client three times a week for fluid overload.

34. Fluid remobilization occurs:
    a. Within the first 4 hours after the burns were sustained.
    b. After the scar tissue is formed and fluids are no longer being lost.
    c. After 48 hours, when the fluid is reabsorbed from the interstitial tissue.
    d. Immediately after the burns occur.

35. Which of the following statements is true about pain associated with burn injuries?
    a. The pain is both chronic and acute.
    b. The preferred route of administration of narcotics in the emergent state is intravenous.
    c. Massaging nonburn areas may reduce pain.
    d. Maintaining a warm room temperature prevents shivering and stimulates a relaxation response.

36. The acute stage of burn injury:
    a. Begins at 24 hours and lasts until the wound closure is complete.
    b. Is when the client is at a high risk for infection.
    c. Is when caloric requirements are decreased.
    d. Is when chances of pneumonia have minimized.

37. Débridement involves: *Check all that apply.*
    ___ a. Removing eschar and other cellular debris from the wound.
    ___ b. Both mechanical and enzymatic actions.
    ___ c. Removing nonviable tissue during hydrotherapy.
    ___ d. Opening larger blisters.

38. A biologic dressing that uses skin from a cadaver provided from a skin bank is called a(n):
    a. Heterograft.
    b. Xenograft.
    c. Allograft.
    d. Autograft.

39. What type of wound is crated in the typical donor site?
    a. First degree
    b. Deep partial-thickness
    c. Superficial partial-thickness
    d. Full-thickness, deep dermal

40. Drug therapy to reduce the risk of wound infection in the burn client includes:
    a. Tetanus toxoid given IM prophylactically once early in the hospitalization.
    b. Silver nitrate solution covered by dry dressings applied every 4 hours.
    c. Silver sulfadiazine (Sulfadine) on full-thickness injuries every 4 hours.
    d. Large doses of broad-spectrum antibiotics.

41. Early detection of wound infection is important. The wound should be examined for which signs of infection?
    a. _____
    b. _____
    c. _____
    d. _____
    e. _____
    f. _____

42. Nutritional requirements for a client with a relatively large burn area can exceed:
    a. 1500 kcal/day.
    b. 2000 kcal/day.
    c. 3000 kcal/day.
    d. 5000 kcal/day.

43. After a dressing is applied to a client's ankle, the ankle is placed in a position of:
    a. Dorsiflexion.
    b. Adduction.
    c. External rotation.
    d. Hyperextension.

44. The client with severe burns progresses through typical stages and exhibits feelings such as: *Check all that apply.*
    ___ a. Denial.
    ___ b. Regression.
    ___ c. Anger.
    ___ d. Suicidal tendencies.

45. Which of the following interventions best promotes a positive image in a burn client?
    a. The physician discusses future scar revision with the client.
    b. The dietitian helps the client select choices from the menus.
    c. The spouse plays cards with the client.
    d. The nurse applies the pressure garment upon discharge.

46. A 28-year-old male client sustained second- and third-degree burns on his legs (30%) when his clothing caught fire while he was burning leaves. He was hosed down by his friend and has arrived at the burn center in severe discomfort. Identify the priority nursing diagnosis for this client at this time.
    a. Acute Pain Related to Damaged or Exposed Nerve Endings
    b. Deficient Fluid Volume Related to Electrolyte Imbalance
    c. Risk for Pulmonary Edema
    d. Disturbed Body Image related to the appearance of legs

47. After his stay at the center, this client is discharged but has some minimal wound areas remaining open. Describe what kinds of needs should be addressed before he is discharged.

UNIT 15   PROBLEMS OF EXCRETION: RENAL/URINARY SYSTEM ■ Core Concepts Grid

Anatomy	Physiology	Pathophysiology	History	Physical Exam	Diagnostic Tests	Interventions	Pharmacology
• **Macro-structures** Kidneys Ureters Bladder Urethra • **Micro-structures** Cortex Medulla Pelvis Glomerulus Nephron	• **Regulation** Water balance Waste products Acid-base balance • **Synthesis of hor-mones** Erythropoietin Renin Activated vitamin D • **Glomerular filtration**	• **Obstruction** • **Inflammation** • **Infection** • **Trauma** • **Tumors** • **Metabolic acidosis**	• **Client history** Past renal problems Difficulty with urination Change in urinary elimination pattern Pain Hypertension • **Family history** Diabetes mellitus Hypertension • **Social history** Alcohol/drug use Occupation Age	• **Skin** Color/turgor Moisture • **Eyes** Conjunctiva • **Mouth** Moisture/color Ulceration • **Chest** Shape Pulsation • **Periphery** Color Hair distribu-tion Striae/edema Pulses/rashes • **Abdomen** Striae/tender-ness over kidney Bruits over renal artery	• **Urinalysis** • **Specific gravity** • **Sediment** • **Serum creatinine** • **Blood urea nitrogen (BUN)** • **Uric acid** • **Scans** • **Renal arteriogram** • **Kidney, ureter, and bladder (KUB)** • **Sonograms** • **Intravenous pyelography (IVP)** • **Biopsy** • **Creatinine clearance** • **Serum pH** • **Cystoscopy**	• **Fluid regulation** • **Dialysis** Hemodialysis Peritoneal dialysis Continuous ambulatory peritoneal dialysis (CAPD) • **Renal transplantation** • **Extracorporeal shock wave lithotripsy (ESWL)** • **AV fistula** • **AV shunt** • **Therapeutic diet** • **Fluids, as appropriate** • **Lithotripsy** • **Health teaching** • **Bladder training** • **Skin care** • **Urinary catherter care**	• **Diuretics** • **Anti-inflammatories** • **Antibiotics** • **Immunosup-pressive agents** • **Calcium replacement agents** • **Hormone replacement agents** • **Chelating agents** • **Phosphorus-binding agents** • **Anticholiner-gics** • **Skin barrier topical agents**

Unit 15 (Chapters 69-72)

Problems of Excretion: Management of Clients with Problems of the Renal/Urinary System

Learning Plan

Chapter 69: *Assessment of the Renal/Urinary System*

Learning Outcomes	Learning Activities	Supplemental Resources
1. Compare and contrast kidney function with functions of the ureter, bladder, and urethra. 2. Describe the roles of the afferent and efferent arterioles in glomerular filtration. 3. Explain the influence of antidiuretic hormone and aldosterone on urine formation and composition. 4. Describe age-related changes in the renal/urinary system. 5. Use laboratory data to distinguish between dehydration and renal impairment. 6. Describe how to obtain a sterile urine specimen from a patient with a Foley catheter. 7. Identify teaching priorities for a client who needs to obtain a 24-hour urine specimen. 8. Identify teaching priorities for a client who needs to obtain a "clean catch" urine specimen. 9. Describe the correct techniques to use in physically assessing the renal system. 10. Prioritize nursing care for the client during the first 24 hours following a renal arteriogram.	1. Prior to completing the study guide exercises in this chapter, review the following: • Anatomy and physiology of the renal system • Process of excretion • Procedures for obtaining urine specimens 2. Review the **boldfaced** Key Terms and their definitions in Chapter 69 to enhance your understanding of the content. 3. Go to Study Guide Number 15.69 on the following pages to complete the learning exercises for this chapter.	1. Textbook—Chapter 69 2. Other resources: • Any anatomy and physiology textbook • Any laboratory resource textbook • Any physical assessment textbook that includes changes of the older adult • Beck, L.H. (1998). Changes in renal function with aging. *Clinics in Geriatric Medicine, 14*(2), 199-209. • Guyton, A.C. & Hall, J.E. (2000). *Textbook of medical physiology* (10th ed.). Philadelphia: W.B. Saunders. • Pagana, K. & Pagana, T. (1999). *Diagnostic testing and nursing implications: A case study approach.* St. Louis: Mosby. • School audiovisual materials • School laboratory instructor • Shinopulos, N. (2000). Bedside urodynamic studies: Simple urine testing for urinary incontinence. *The Nurse Practitioner, 25*(6), 19-20, 22, 25-26, 28, 33-34, 37.

Chapter 70: *Interventions for Clients with Urinary Problems*

Learning Outcomes	Learning Activities	Supplemental Resources
1. Describe the clinical manifestations of cystitis. 2. Prioritize educational needs of a person at risk for cystitis. 3. Compare and contrast the pathophysiology and manifestations of stress incontinence, urge incontinence, overflow incontinence, mixed incontinence, and functional incontinence.	1. Prior to completing the study guide exercises in this chapter, review the following: • Anatomy and physiology of the renal and urinary tract systems • Process of excretion • Intake and output procedure	1. Textbook—Chapter 69 (Assessment of the Renal/Urinary System) 2. Textbook—Chapter 70 3. Other resources:

Supplemental Resources

- Adams, D.H. & Abernathy, B.B. (1996). Laser ureterolithotripsy for cystine calculi. *AORN Journal, 64*(6), 924, 926-927, 929-930.
- American Cancer Society. (2000). *Cancer facts and figures, 1998* (Report No. 00-300M-No.5008.00). Atlanta, GA: American Cancer Society.
- Any anatomy and physiology textbook
- Any laboratory rescue textbook
- Any physical assessment textbook
- Balaji, K.C. & Menon. M. (1997). Mechanism of stone formation. *The Urologic Clinics of North America, 24*(1), 1-11.
- Duffield, P. (1997). Urinary tract infections in the elderly. *ADVANCE for Nurse Practitioners, 5*(4), 30-32.
- Hruska, K. (1996). Renal calculi. In J.C. Bennett & G. Plum (Eds.). *Cecil textbook of medicine.* Philadelphia: W.B. Saunders.

- Fluid and electrolyte balance
- Assessment of renal and urinary tract
- Infusion therapy
- Normal renal lab values

2. Review the **boldfaced** Key Terms and their definitions in Chapter 70 to enhance your understanding of the content.
3. Go to Study Guide Number 15.70 on the following pages to complete the learning exercises for this chapter.

Learning Outcomes (continued)

4. Prioritize educational needs for the client taking sulfonamide antibiotics for a urinary tract infection.
5. Describe the techniques used to assess pelvic floor strength in a client who is experiencing some incontinence.
6. Explain the proper application of exercises to strengthen pelvic floor muscles.
7. Explain the drug therapy for different types of incontinence.
8. Prioritize nursing care for a client with renal colic.
9. Describe the common clinical manifestations of bladder cancer.
10. Develop a teaching plan for a client who has had urinary diversion for bladder cancer.

Chapter 71: *Interventions for Clients with Renal Disorders*

Learning Outcomes

1. Prioritize nursing care needs for the client with polycystic kidney disease.
2. Describe the clinical manifestations of hydronephrosis.
3. Identify clients at risk for pyelonephritis.
4. Use laboratory data and clinical manifestations to determine the effectiveness of therapy for pyelonephritis.
5. Compare and contrast the pathophysiology and clinical manifestations of acute glomerular nephritis and nephrotic syndrome.
6. Prioritize nursing care for the client during the first 24 hours after a nephrectomy.
7. Explain how diabetic nephropathy can affect glucose metabolism and control in the client with diabetes mellitus.
8. Develop a teaching plan for the client who has had a nephrectomy for renal cell carcinoma.

Learning Activities

1. Prior to completing the study guide exercises in this chapter, review the following:
   - Anatomy and physiology of the renal system
   - Normal renal laboratory values
   - Assessment of the renal and urinary system
   - Acid-base balance
   - Intake and output
   - Infusion therapy
   - Fluid and electrolytes
2. Review the **boldfaced** Key Terms and their definitions in Chapter 71 to enhance your understanding of the content.

Supplemental Resources

1. Textbook—Chapter 69 (Assessment of the Renal/Urinary System)
2. Textbook—Chapter 71
3. Other resources:
   - Any anatomy and physiology textbook
   - Any physical assessment textbook
   - Anver, E.D., Woychik, R.P., Dell, K.M., Sweeney, W.E. (1999). Cellular pathophysiology of cystic kidney disease: Insight into future therapies. *International Journal of Developmental Biology, 43*(5 Spec No), 457-461.

- Bonsib, S.M. (1999). Risk and prognosis in renal neoplasms: A pathologist's perspective. *Urologic Clinics of North America, 26*(3), 643-660,viii.
- Crook, E.D. (1999). The role of hypertension, obesity, and diabetes in causing renal vascular disease. *American Journal of Medical Science, 27*(3), 183-188.
- Gonzalez, R.P., Falimirski, M., Holevar, M.R., & Evankovich, C. (1999). Surgical management of renal trauma: Is vascular control necessary? *Journal of Trauma, 47*(6), 1039-1042, discussion 1042-1044.
- Little, C. (2000). Renovascular hypertension. *American Journal of Nursing, 100*(2), 46-51.
- Roberts, J.A. (1999). Management of pyelonephritis and upper urinary tract infections. *Urology Clinics of North America, 26*(4), 753-763.
- Torres, R. (1999). Autosomal dominant polycystic kidney disease type 2 (PDK2 disease). *Advances in Nephrology Necker Hospital, 29*(11), 277-287.

3. Go to Study Guide Number 15.71 on the following pages to complete the learning exercises for this chapter.

Chapter 72: Interventions for Clients with Chronic and Acute Renal Failure

Learning Outcomes	Learning Activities	Supplemental Resources

1. Compare and contrast the pathophysiology and causes of chronic renal failure (CRF) and acute renal failure (ARF).
2. Identify clients at risk for development of ARF.
3. Identify clients at risk for development of CRF.
4. Use laboratory data and clinical assessment to determine the effectiveness of therapy for renal failure.
5. Discuss interventions to prevent ARF.
6. Prioritize nursing care for the client with ARF.
7. Compare the clinical manifestations of stage I, stage II, and stage III CRF.
8. Discuss the mechanisms of peritoneal dialysis (PD) and hemodialysis (HD) as renal replacement therapies.
9. Prioritize nursing care for the client with end-stage renal disease.
10. Prioritize teaching needs for the client using continuous ambulatory PD.
11. Prioritize teaching needs for the client with a permanent vascular access for long-term HD.
12. Compare and contrast the dietary modifications needed for the client undergoing HD with those for the client undergoing PD.
13. Plan prevention strategies for the complications of PD.
14. Discuss the criteria for kidney donation.
15. Prioritize nursing care needs for the client during the first 24 hours after kidney transplantation.
	1. Prior to completing the study guide exercises in this chapter, review the following:
	  • Anatomy and physiology of the renal system
	  • Assessment of the renal and urinary systems
	  • Normal renal lab values
	  • Intake and output
	  • Fluid and electrolyte
	  • Infusion therapy
	  • Diuretics
	2. Review the **boldfaced** Key Terms and their definitions in Chapter 72 to enhance your understanding of the content.
	3. Go to Study Guide Number 15.72 on the following pages to complete the learning exercises for this chapter.
		1. Textbook—Chapter 69 (Assessment of the Renal/Urinary System)
		2. Textbook—Chapter 72
		3. Other resources:
		  • Any anatomy and physiology textbook
		  • Any physical assessment textbook
		  • Bartucci, M.R. (1999). Kidney transplantation: State of the art. *AACN Clinical Issues. Advanced Practice in Acute and Critical Care, 10*(2), 153-163.
		  • Giuliano, K. & Sims, T.W (1999). Transplant issues: Infections and immunosuppressant drugs. *Dimensions of Critical Care Nursing, 18*(2)m 16-19.
		  • Hayes, D. (2000). Caring for your patient with a permanent renal dialysis access. *Nursing 2000, 30*(3), 41-46.
		  • Kellum, J. (2000). An evaluation of pharmacological strategies for the prevention and treatment of acute renal failure. *Drugs, 59*(1), 79-91.
		  • King, B. (2000). Meds and the dialysis patient. *RN, 63*(7), 54-59.
		  • Ray, T. (2000). Chronic and acute renal failure: Primary care issues. *Advance for Nurse Practitioners, 8*(8), 69-72.
		  • Tran, M. & Rutechi, G. (2000). Renal disease: Tips on prevention and early recognition. *Consultant, 40*(2), 222-229.

STUDY GUIDE NUMBER 15.69

Assessment of the Renal/Urinary System

Study/Review Questions

Answer the following three questions on a separate sheet of paper.

1. Identify the six ways the kidneys contribute to health.

2. Identify the parts of the renal system.

3. Define the retroperitoneal space where the kidney is located.

4. An ultrasound of the kidney that reveals a larger or smaller kidney is indicative of which possible problem?
   a. Renal obstruction
   b. Polycystic disease
   c. Chronic renal disease
   d. All of the above

5. The outer surface of the kidney is the renal capsule that covers the kidney, *except* at the:
   a. Renal artery.
   b. Hilum.
   c. Ureters.
   d. Veins.

6. Which of the following is the functional renal tissue in the kidneys? *Check all that apply.*
   ___ a. Renal cortex
   ___ b. Medulla with pyramids
   ___ c. Columns
   ___ d. Papilla

7. The path of urine flows from:
   a. Papilla to the calyx that merge to form the renal pelvis and become the ureter.
   b. Papilla to the calyx to the renal pelvis and into the ureter.
   c. Calyx to the papilla to the renal pelvis and into the ureter.
   d. Calyx to the papilla that merge to form the renal pelvis and become the ureter.

8. On a separate sheet of paper, construct a diagram and trace the blood supply to the kidney.

9. The kidneys receive _____% of the cardiac output.

True or False? Write T for true and F for false in the blank provided.

___ 10. Venous blood drains into the veins and eventually into the inferior vena cava.

___ 11. The nephron removes the urine from the blood.

12. The glomerulus is a series of specialized capillary loops that filters the blood to make urine, and the excess blood exits:
   a. Afferent arterioles.
   b. Peritubular capillaries.
   c. Efferent arterioles.
   d. Vas recta.

13. The hormone renin regulates: *Check all that apply.*
   ___ a. Blood flow to the kidneys.
   ___ b. Glomerular filtration rate (GFR).
   ___ c. Systemic blood pressure.
   ___ d. Cardiac rate and rhythm.

14. True or False? *Write T for true and F for false in the blank provided.*
   ___ Changes in blood volume and pressure are sensed by macula densa and will cause the excretion of renin.

15. When the body's blood pressure or sodium level is low, renin does which of the following?
   a. Converts angiotensinogen to angiotensin I to secrete aldosterone
   b. Converts aldosterone to angiotensinogen to secrete angiotensin I
   c. Converts angiotensin I to angiotensinogen to secrete aldosterone
   d. Converts angiotensin I to angiotensin II to secrete angiotensin III

16. The kidneys have both regulatory and hormonal functions. Identify which process each of the following involves. Use R for regulatory and H for hormonal.
   ___ a.   Controls fluid
   ___ b.   Vitamin D activation
   ___ c.   Blood pressure
   ___ d.   Acid-base balance
   ___ e.   Controls electrolytes
   ___ f.   Controls RBC formation

17. Identify the part of the kidney in which the filtrate is made.
   a. Endothelium
   b. Epithelium
   c. Glomerular capillary wall
   d. Loop of Henle

18. When albumin, globulin, and RBC are seen in a urinalysis, the cells are too large to go through the:
   a. Glomerular filtration system.
   b. Tubular filtrate in the glomerular filtration system.
   c. Afferent arterioles.
   d. Efferent arterioles.

19. The part(s) of the kidney that help regulate the blood pressure (except when the blood pressure is below 75 mm Hg) is/are the:
   a. Nephron.
   b. Afferent arterioles.
   c. Efferent arterioles.
   d. Medullary capsule.

20. During water reabsorption, the membrane of the distal convoluted tubule is more permeable to water due to the influence of which hormones?
   a. Renin and aldosterone
   b. Aldosterone and antidiuretic hormone (ADH)
   c. Antidiuretic hormone (ADH) and renin
   d. Calcitonin and renin.

21. The proximal convoluted tubule is the area that reabsorbs:
   a. Na, Cl, water, 20% to 40% K, bicarbonate, and phosphates.
   b. Na, Cl, urine, and renin.
   c. Na, Cl, water, renin, and K.
   d. Na, K, phosphates, and glucose.

22. The calcium level is controlled by:
   a. Calcitonin.
   b. Renin.
   c. Parathormone.
   d. Secretin.

True or False? Write T for true and F for false in the blank provided.

___ 23. The renal threshold for glucose is 220 mg/dL; when it is greater, glucose appears in the urine.

___ 24. Although 50% of all urea in glomerular filtrate is reabsorbed, creatinine is not.

25. In the kidney, tubular secretion continues filtration and regulates:
   a. Hormones.
   b. Electrolytes and pH.
   c. Blood pressure.
   d. Heart rate.

Answer the following two questions on a separate sheet of paper.

26. Identify the hormonal functions of kidneys.

27. Describe the effects of the release of renin.

28. Prostaglandin produced in the kidney:
   a. Regulates glomerular filtration and promotes excretion of Na and water.
   b. Regulates kidney vascular resistance and decreases membrane permeability.
   c. Regulates renin production.
   d. Inhibits ADH secretion.

29. In the kidney, the release of bradykinin is regulated by angiotensin II, prostaglandin, and ADH, which:
   a. Dilates afferent arterioles and increases capillary permeability.
   b. Dilates efferent arterioles and increases capillary permeability.
   c. Increases tubular function.

True or False? Write T for true and F for false in the blank provided.

___ 30. Erythropoietin production is stimulated by decreased O_2 tension in the renal blood supply, which stimulates RBC production in the bone marrow.

___ 31. Activated vitamin D is a hormone needed to absorb Ca+, which is absorbed through the skin from ultraviolet light and converted in the liver.

32. Using the text and Figure 69-9, draw and label the structures of urinary system from the kidneys on a separate sheet of paper.

33. Identify the three areas the ureter narrow on your drawing.

34. What is the length of each ureter?
    a. 12 to 18 cm
    b. 12 to 18 in
    c. 3 to 6 cm
    d. 3 to 6 in

35. Which of the following are layers of the ureters? *Check all that apply.*
    ___ a. Urothelium
    ___ b. Smooth muscle fibers
    ___ c. Scar tissue
    ___ d. Fibrous tissue

36. Urine is moved through the ureter by:
    a. Peristalsis.
    b. Gravity.
    c. Force.
    d. Backflow.

37. The bladder is a muscular sac located directly behind the:
    a. Pubis symphysis and, in women, in front of the rectum.
    b. Pubis symphysis and, in men, in front of rectum.
    c. Pubis symphysis and, in women, in front of the vagina.
    d. All of the above

38. Which of the following are parts of the bladder?
    a. Sac, bladder neck, internal and external sphincter
    b. Body, bladder neck, internal sphincter
    c. Body, bladder neck, external sphincter
    d. Body, bladder, internal and external sphincter

39. The pudendal nerve's function is to control the:
    a. External sphincter located at the base of the bladder in women.
    b. External sphincter located at the base of prostate gland in men.
    c. External sphincter located at the base of the bladder.
    d. All of the above

40. On a separate sheet of paper, identify the renal changes and effects seen with aging.

41. Impairment in the thirst mechanism of older adults increases the incidence of:
    a. Dehydration.
    b. Hypercalcemia.
    c. Hypokalemia.
    d. Hyperkalemia.

42. Sodium retention problems are more prominent among:
    a. Chinese people.
    b. African Americans.
    c. Japanese people.
    d. Germans.

43. 1) For women, changes in the bladder result in:
    a. Dysuria.
    b. Incontinence.
    c. Hematuria.
    d. Retention.

    2) But for men, changes in the bladder are related to:
    a. Prolapsed bladder.
    b. Enlarged prostate.
    c. Dehydration.
    d. Rectocele.

44. One primary indicator of kidney disease is:
    a. Hypernatremia.
    b. Sudden onset of hypertension.
    c. Dehydration.
    d. Hypokalemia.

45. 1) ESRD has an increased incidence rate in which culture? *Check all that apply.*
    ___ a. Chinese
    ___ b. African-American
    ___ c. Japanese
    ___ d. Indian

    2) The above cultural differences are due to a high incidence of:
    a. Hypertension.
    b. Diabetes mellitus.
    c. Liver disease.
    d. Bowel disease.

46. On a separate sheet of paper, identify the 10 areas the nurse should cover when taking a history of a client with renal disease.

47. Renal failure causes an increase in nitrogenous waste products that can cause which of the following changes? *Check all that apply.*
    ___ a. Anorexia
    ___ b. Alteration in taste acuity
    ___ c. Inability to discriminate tastes
    ___ d. Halitosis

48. Renal calculi can be caused by: *Check all that apply.*
    ___ a. Hypercalcemia.
    ___ b. Insufficient fluid intake.
    ___ c. Fluid overload.
    ___ d. Hyperkalemia.

49. Which of these changes should a client report to the nurse during an assessment for urologic problems? *Check all that apply.*
    ___ a. Hypertension
    ___ b. Changes in color, odor, clarity
    ___ c. Urinary pattern
    ___ d. Ability to initiate voiding
    ___ e. Ability to control urination
    ___ f. Burning
    ___ g. Tinnitus

50. A client with renal colic presents with:
    a. Severe spasmodic pain.
    b. Diaphoresis.
    c. Possible hypotension and pallor.
    d. All of the above

51. The symptoms of uremia include: *Check all that apply.*
    ___ a. Anorexia, nausea, and vomiting.
    ___ b. Increased energy.
    ___ c. Muscle cramp and pruritus.
    ___ d. Jaundiced skin.

52. In renal disorders, edema can be found in:
    a. Presacral tissues and around the eyes.
    b. Pretibial and pedal edema.
    c. *a* and *b*
    d. None of the above

53. When the nurse listens over the renal arteries for a bruit, she expects:
    a. A quiet pulsating sound.
    b. A swishing sound.
    c. A faint wheezing.
    d. No sound at all.

54. On a separate sheet of paper, describe how to percuss the abdomen to determine whether there is a distended bladder present.

55. A report of dysuria by the client should lead the nurse to suspect:
    a. Urethral irritation.
    b. Increased urine.
    c. Less voiding.
    d. Nocturia.

56. An excellent indicator of kidney function is:
    a. Electrolytes.
    b. Serum creatinine.
    c. pH.
    d. Color of urine.

57. The serum creatinine level is closely monitored by the nurse and doctor because:
    a. The level does not change until 50% of renal function is lost.
    b. The level does not change until 25% of renal function is lost.
    c. The level changes suddenly.
    d. The level changes slowly.

58. The blood urea nitrogen (BUN) test measures the:
    a. Renal excretion of nitrogen.
    b. Nitrogenous waste.
    c. Creatinine clearance.
    d. Urine output.

59. High BUN can be masked as other problems, including:
    a. Infection causing cell destruction.
    b. Steroid therapy.
    c. Liver disorders.
    d. All of the above
    e. *a* and *b*

60. In the client with dehydration, the lab tests would show:
    a. BUN and creatinine ratio stay the same.
    b. BUN will rise faster than creatinine level.
    c. Creatinine will rise faster than BUN.
    d. BUN and creatine have a direct relationship.

61. Match each urine specimen finding with the corresponding characteristic.

Findings
___ a. Color
___ b. Odor
___ c. Turbidity
___ d. Specific gravity
___ e. pH
___ f. Glucose
___ g. Ketone bodies
___ h. Protein
___ i. Microalbuminuria
___ j. Sediment
___ k. Cells
___ l. Cast
___ m. Crystals
___ n. Bacteria

Characteristics
1. Less than 7 acidic, greater than 7 alkaline
2. Byproduct of fatty usually acid, not seen in urine
3. Only identified by microscopic exam for protein
4. Structure found around cell, bacteria, protein, and clumps
5. Urine is normally sterile; these multiply and grow
6. Urochrome pigment
7. 1.000 to 1.35
8. Not normally in the urine, albumin
9. Cells, casts, crystals, and bacteria
10. Various salts
11. Epithelial cells, RBC, WBC, tubular cells
12. Not seen in urine until blood sugar above 220
13. Clear urine
14. Faint ammonia

STUDY GUIDE NUMBER 15.70

Interventions for Clients with Urinary Problems

Study/Review Questions

1. On a separate sheet of paper, develop and complete the following chart. Use Chapter 70 text, tables, and charts.

Diagnosis	Pathology and Symptoms	Treatment	Medications	Complications	Nursing Diagnosis
Urethritis					
Cystitis					
Prostatitis					
Urosepsis					
Urethral strictures					

2. The effects of urinary disorders affect the quality of life in many:
   a. Functional areas.
   b. Physical areas.
   c. Psychologic areas.
   d. All of the above

3. Nursing interventions are directed toward: *Check all that apply.*
   ___ a. Prevention.
   ___ b. Detection.
   ___ c. Medical management.
   ___ d. Cure.

4. To determine treatment for urinary tract infection, which of the following two actions must be taken?
   ___ a. Site of infection must be determined
   ___ b. Identification of bacteria
   ___ c. Increased fluid intake
   ___ d. Prophylactic antibiotic therapy

5. Asymptomatic bacteriuria is a condition that is:
   a. Cancer.
   b. Benign.
   c. Infectious.
   d. Contagious.

6. Inserting a catheter into the bladder will typically cause a urinary tract infection (UTI) in:
   a. 25% of clients.
   b. 50% of clients.
   c. 75% of clients.
   d. None of the clients.

7. A UTI related to *Candida* can be caused from: *Check all that apply.*
   ___ a. Being on long-term antibiotics.
   ___ b. Being immunocompromised.
   ___ c. Receiving long-term glucocorticosteroids.
   ___ d. Taking chemotherapeutic agents.
   ___ e. Receiving long-term antihypertensive agents.

8. How is a microorganism in the urine usually treated if it is commonly found in the vagina?

9. Causes of noninfectious cystitis include: *Check all that apply.*
   ___ a. Cyclophosmed.
   ___ b. Long-term radiation.
   ___ c. Immunologic response to systemic lupus erythematosus.
   ___ d. Cytoxin.

10. Interstitial cystitis is a chronic inflammation of the bladder that:
    a. Is very common.
    b. Has the same symptoms as UTI, only more intense.
    c. Affects mostly men.
    d. Does not require treatment.

11. For women older than 80 years, the cause of UTI is most commonly due to:
    a. Lack of estrogen.
    b. Changes in the skin and mucous membranes.
    c. Decreased fluid intake.
    d. Normal changes of aging.

12. A vesicoureteral reflex is diagnosed by a _____ _____.

13. A cystoscope can identify the following bladder problems:
    a. _____
    b. _____
    c. _____
    d. _____
    e. _____

14. The most common treatment for a fungal urinary tract infection is:
    a. Sulfa drugs.
    b. Antibiotics.
    c. Amphotericin B.
    d. Quinolones.

15. Daily fluid intake to prevent a bladder infection should include:
    a. 2 to 3 L of water.
    b. Cranberry juice.
    c. Coffee.
    d. Orange juice.

16. When instructing clients about medication for UTI, be sure to tell them: *Check all that apply.*
    ___ a. To take all of the medication as ordered.
    ___ b. That it could possibly change the color of the urine.
    ___ c. To wear cotton underwear only.
    ___ d. To drink plenty of fluids.

17. Pyelonephritis in pregnant women can cause _____ and can affect the _____.

18. Treatment for a urethral stricture often includes:
    a. Dilatation.
    b. Antibiotic therapy.
    c. Fluid restriction.
    d. Radiation.

19. Urinary incontinence is: *Check all that apply.*
    ___ a. One of the most under-reported health problems.
    ___ b. Caused by aging and childbirth.
    ___ c. A cause of social and hygiene problems.
    ___ d. Usually caused by bladder cancer.

20. Identify which reasons are given for urinary incontinence in older adults. *Check all that apply.*
    ___ a. Decreased mobility
    ___ b. Neurologic dysfunction
    ___ c. Musculoskeletal degeneration
    ___ d. Diuretics and multiple medication
    ___ e. Vision and hearing impairment

21. Define *cystocele.*

22. A rectal exam may reveal which of the following about the urinary tract? *Check all that apply.*
    ___ a. Position of the bladder
    ___ b. Presence of an enlarged prostate
    ___ c. Occurrence of fecal impaction
    ___ d. Patency of ureters

23. Identify the tests that can be done on the urinary tract prior to surgical interventions.
    a. _____
    b. _____
    c. _____
    d. _____
    e. _____
    f. _____
    g. _____
    h. _____

24. Your client has been performing Kegel exercises for 2 months. How will you and your client know whether the exercises are working?
    a. Incontinence still present, but client states that it is less.
    b. Client is able to stop urinary stream.
    c. No complaints of urgency from the client.
    d. Client still needs clothing protection.

25. After a bladder suspension, a suprapubic catheter is typically maintained for how long?
    a. 24 hours postoperatively
    b. 48 hours postoperatively
    c. Until client is able void on her own
    d. Until client is able to void and residual is below 50 mL

26. Use your textbook, charts, and tables to complete the chart below on types of incontinence. *Use a separate sheet of paper for your answer.*

27. As the nurse, your care plan for teaching the client with incontinence problems should include:
    a. _____
    b. _____
    c. _____
    d. _____
    e. _____
    f. _____
    g. _____
    h. _____
    i. _____

28. Define the following terms related to how stones are formed in the urinary system:
    a. Urolithiasis: _____
    b. Nephrolithiasis: _____
    c. Ureterolithiasis: _____

Diagnoses	Pathology and Symptoms	Medications	Treatment	Nursing Diagnosis	Test
Stress incontinence					
Urge incontinence					
Overflow incontinence					
Functional incontinence					

29. Everyone excretes small amounts of crystals. Which problem is presented when the body excretes too many crystals? *Check all that apply.*
    ___ a. Slow in the urine flow
    ___ b. Damage to the lining
    ___ c. Decreased inhibitor substance that prevents supersaturation and aggregation
    ___ d. High acidity or alkalinity

30. Your client appears in the emergency department with a complaint of severe sporadic pain radiating into the groin; the client is pale and hypotensive. You would suspect the client has:
    a. A severe UTI.
    b. Renal calculi.
    c. Bladder cancer.
    d. Urosepsis.

31. True or False? *Write T for true or F for false in the blank provided.*
    ___ Stones can be identified on KUB (x-ray of kidney, ureters, and bladder).

32. The nurse would expect to observe which of the following signs or symptoms with a stat urinalysis that is performed on a client with a possible stone? *Check all that apply.*
    ___ a. Blood in the urine
    ___ b. Mucus in the urine
    ___ c. Clear urine
    ___ d. Odorous urine

Answer the following two questions on a separate sheet of paper.

33. Complete the following chart with necessary interventions for a client with calculi.

Pain Relief Measures	Nonsurgical Management	Complementary/ Alternative Therapies	Lithotripsy	Surgical Management	Postoperative Management

34. Complete the following chart regarding the different types of stones found in the kidney system and interventions for treatment.

Types of Stone	Description	Medications and Effect	Dietary Intervention	Health Teaching

35. Most urothelial cancer tumors are located in the:
    a. Bladder.
    b. Kidney pelvis.
    c. Urethra.
    d. Ureters.

36. Cancer in situ of the bladder:
    a. Is a flat tumor.
    b. Invades the submucosa.
    c. Invades perivesical fat.
    d. Is not located in the bladder.

37. The only early symptom of bladder cancer is:
    a. Cloudy urine.
    b. Pain.
    c. Hematuria.
    d. Glycosuria.

38. Nonsurgical management of bladder cancer includes: *Check all that apply.*
    ___ a. Radiation.
    ___ b. Instillation of the bacille Calmette-Guérin.
    ___ c. Intravesical chemotherapy.
    ___ d. Antibiotic therapy.

39. For bladder cancer, the surgical option(s) are:
    a. Partial cystectomy.
    b. Transurethral resection of tumor.
    c. Complete cystectomy with ileal conduit.
    d. All of the above

40. An ileoconduit involves:
    a. Surgical implantation of the ureters in a portion of the ileum.
    b. Surgical implantation of the ureters to the abdominal wall.
    c. Implantation of the ureters on either side of the abdomen.
    d. Implantation of the ureters together on the abdomen.

41. How does a urinary diversion usually affect a client?
    a. _____
    b. _____
    c. _____
    d. _____

42. The nurse should instruct the client with a urinary diversion regarding: *Check all that apply.*
    ___ a. Medications.
    ___ b. Diet.
    ___ c. Pouching.
    ___ d. Catheterization if applicable.
    ___ e. Fluid intake.

43. Bladder trauma is usually caused by:
    a. _____
    b. _____
    c. _____
    d. _____

STUDY GUIDE NUMBER 15.71

Interventions for Clients with Renal Disorders

Study/Review Questions

1. The causes of renal disorders may include: *Check all that apply.*
   ___ a. Congenital.
   ___ b. Obstructive.
   ___ c. Infections.
   ___ d. Glomerular degeneration.

2. Polycystic kidney disease (PKD) is the most common:
   a. Inherited disease of African Americans.
   b. Inherited disease of whites.
   c. Acquired disease of African Americans.
   d. Acquired disease of whites.

3. True or False? *Write T for true or F for false in the blank provided.*
   ___ Genetic counseling and early intervention to slow renal involvement are the treatment for polycystic kidney disease (PKD).

4. Clients with PKD have much discomfort due to: *Check all that apply.*
   ___ a. Pressure from enlargement.
   ___ b. Infection.
   ___ c. Rupture of cysts.
   ___ d. Weight gain.

5. In a client with PKD, hypertension and renal ischemia are due to:
   a. Compressed blood flow.
   b. Decreased renal flow.
   c. Both of the above
   d. None of the above

6. The effect on the renin-angiotensin system in the kidney in PKD results in:
   a. Increased blood pressure.
   b. Decreased blood pressure.
   c. Decreased renal flow.
   d. Increased renal flow.

7. True or False? *Write* T *for true or* F *for false in the blank provided.*

   ___ Cysts from PKD can form in other organs and cause harm.

8. Clients with PKD often have all of the following *except:*
   a. Berry aneurysms.
   b. Gastric ulcers.
   c. Kidney stones.
   d. Heart valve abnormalities.

9. True or False? *Write* T *for true or* F *for false in the blank provided.*

   ___ Men and women have equal chances of inheriting either form of PKD.

10. Match each characteristic of clients with polycystic disease to the corresponding gene trait. *Answers may be used more than once.*

Characteristic	Gene Trait
___ a. About 40 years old	1. Autosomal
___ b. Death in childhood	recessive
___ c. Affects 5% to 10%	2. Autosomal
nephrons early in life	dominant
___ d. Cysts develop every-where and get larger	
___ e. Present at birth	
___ f. Kidneys are like bunches of grapes	
___ g. Slow cystic rate	
___ h. Progressive renal failure	

11. A client presenting with PKD typically has: *Check all that apply.*
    ___ a. Complaints of abdominal or flank pain.
    ___ b. Hypertension.
    ___ c. Edema.
    ___ d. Nocturia.

12. Sharp pain followed by blood in the urine in the client with PKD is usually caused by:
    a. Infection.
    b. A ruptured cyst.
    c. Increased kidney size.
    d. Increased tumor growth.

13. As PKD becomes more severe, symptoms from berry aneurysms can include:
    a. Severe headache.
    b. Pruritus.
    c. Edema.
    d. Fatigue.

14. Nocturia in clients with PKD is due to:
    a. Increased fluid intake in the evening.
    b. Increased hypertension.
    c. Decreased renal concentrating ability.
    d. Release of renin.

15. Clients diagnosed with PKD may need a nursing diagnosis of Impaired Coping because they:
    a. Know other family members who are being treated or have died.
    b. Have feelings of anger, resentment, hostility, futility, sadness, or anxiety.
    c. Have feelings of guilt and concerns for own children.
    d. All of the above

16. A urinalysis on a client with PKD may show all of the following *except*:
    a. Proteinuria.
    b. Glucosuria.
    c. Hematuria.
    d. Bacteria.

17. Blood studies on a deteriorating client with PKD will result in all of the following *except*:
    a. Increased BUN and serum creatinine.
    b. Sodium loss or retention.
    c. Potassium loss.
    d. Decreased creatinine clearance.

18. Of the following diagnostic studies, which can show PKD with minimal risk?
    a. MRI
    b. CT
    c. Renal sonography
    d. X-ray

19. For the client with PKD, the best strategy for pain management is:
    a. Pharmacologic.
    b. Physical.
    c. Integrative approaches.
    d. A combination of all above.

20. To relieve discomfort, the client with PKD may need which of the following? *Check all that apply.*
    ___ a. Moist heat to abdominal or flank
    ___ b. Lipid-soluble antibiotics
    ___ c. Percutaneous needle aspiration and drainage of cysts
    ___ d. Aspirin-containing compounds

21. The client with PKD usually experiences constipation; the nurse should provide instruction on: *Check all that apply.*
    ___ a. Stool softener.
    ___ b. Decreased dietary fiber.
    ___ c. Increased fluids.
    ___ d. Bulk-forming agents.

22. The client with PKD has nocturia and needs to:
    a. Drink 2 L of fluid daily.
    b. Restrict fluid in the evening.
    c. Only drink 1000 mL/24 hours.
    d. Take diuretics as ordered.

23. To control hypertension in a client with PKD, the best choice of medications is:
    a. ACE inhibitors.
    b. Calcium channel blockers.
    c. Beta blockers.
    d. Vasodilators.

24. On a separate sheet of paper, identify priority nursing care needs for clients with polycystic kidney disease.

25. After the nurse instructs a client with PKD on his home care, the client should know to contact the physician immediately when:
    a. The blood pressure rises a little.
    b. There is a sudden weight gain (3 to 5 pounds within 3 days).
    c. The laxative needs to be increased.
    d. Fluid intake has been excessive.

26. Hydronephrosis, hydroureter, and urethral stricture have much in common because they are all forms of:
    a. Tumors.
    b. Obstructions.
    c. Stones.
    d. Congenital deformities.

27. What do hydronephrosis and hydroureter have in common?
    a. Both cause severe damage to the renal system.
    b. Structures of renal system do not stop working during either.
    c. Both are caused by tumors, stones, and congenital deformities.
    d. All of the above

28. A decrease in the glomerular filtration rate will result in: *Check all that apply.*
    ___ a. Decreased serum creatinine and BUN.
    ___ b. Hyperphosphatemia and hypocalcemia.
    ___ c. A bicarbonate deficit causing metabolic acidosis.
    ___ d. Hyperkalemia.

29. Chronic pyelonephritis has several causes, but acute pyelonephritis is usually caused from:
    a. Repeated UTI.
    b. Bacteria.
    c. Vesicoureteral reflux.
    d. Obstruction.

30. Identify clients at risk for pyelonephritis.

31. In acute pyelonephritis, acute inflammation is followed by:
    a. Tubular cell necrosis and abscess formation.
    b. Abscesses in capsule, cortex, and medulla.
    c. Fibrosis forms.
    d. *a* then *b* then *c*

32. Vesicoureteral and intrarenal reflux are: *Check all that apply.*
    ___ a. Described as the urine running backward.
    ___ b. Major causes of acute pyelonephritis.
    ___ c. Refluxing papillae in upper and lower poles of the kidney.
    ___ d. Normal changes associated with aging.

33. Those who develop chronic pyelonephritis as an adult may have: *Check all that apply.*
    ___ a. Spinal cord injury.
    ___ b. Bladder tumor.
    ___ c. Prostatic hypertrophy.
    ___ d. Chronic renal calculi.
    ___ e. Diabetes with bladder atony.

34. The two most common causes of pyelonephritis are which of the following gastrointestinal tract organisms?
    a. *Escherichia coli* and *Enterococcus faecalis*
    b. *Proteus mirabilis* and *Klebsiella* species
    c. *Pseudomonas aeruginosa* and *Klebsiella* species
    d. *Staphylococcus aureus, Salmonella* species, and *Candida* species

35. Screening a client for pyelonephritis testing would include:
    a. Urinalysis.
    b. KUB and intravenous urography.
    c. Gallium scan.
    d. All of the above

36. Nonsurgical management of pyelonephritis could include: *Check all that apply.*
    ___ a. Shock wave lithotripsy.
    ___ b. Percutaneous ultrasonic pyelolithotomy.
    ___ c. Diet and fluid therapy.
    ___ d. Medication.

37. Preserving the kidney is the priority in surgery for pyelonephritis; therefore, which of these surgeries may be performed?
    a. Nephrectomy
    b. Ureteral diversion, or reimplantation
    c. Ureteroplasty
    d. Pyelolithotomy

38. Which of the following is the main nursing diagnosis for a client with pyelonephritis?
    a. Deficient Knowledge
    b. Fear
    c. Pain
    d. Activity Intolerance

39. Postoperative instruction for a client with pyelonephritis is important and will include all of the following *except*:
    a. Controlling the blood pressure.
    b. Fluid restriction.
    c. Protein restriction.
    d. Ingesting at least 2 L of fluid per day.

40. Which is the most important for a client with pyelonephritis to do?
    a. Complete all antibiotic regimens
    b. Report any problems with medications to the doctor
    c. Stop taking the antibiotic when pain is relieved
    d. Notify physician of any over-the-counter drugs

41. As an outcome for a client with pyelonephritis, you would expect all of the following *except*:
    a. Comfort with pain management.
    b. Following the dietary plan.
    c. Deficient knowledge of disease process.
    d. Compliance with antibiotics.

42. Renal abscess can occur in the:
    a. Renal parenchyma.
    b. Gerota's fascia.
    c. Flank.
    d. All of the above

43. Renal abscess can be identified on a: *Check all that apply.*
    ___ a. Sonography.
    ___ b. Computed tomography (CT).
    ___ c. MRI.
    ___ d. Cystoscopy.

44. Treatment for a renal abscess may include: *Check all that apply.*
    ___ a. Surgical incision or needle aspiration.
    ___ b. Ureteral diversion.
    ___ c. Antibiotics.
    ___ d. Cystectomy.

45. The treatment for renal tuberculosis includes: *Check all that apply.*
    ___ a. Antibiotics.
    ___ b. Vitamin therapy.
    ___ c. Antitubercular therapy.
    ___ d. Narcotics.

46. Acute glomerulonephritis has which of the following causes?
    a. Immunologic basis
    b. Underlying genetic basis
    c. Systemic disease
    d. Bacterial infections

47. In glomerulonephritis, the glomeruli are injured and the symptoms may include: *Check all that apply.*
    ___ a. Edema.
    ___ b. Proteinuria and hematuria.
    ___ c. Nocturia and hematuria.
    ___ d. Hypotension.

48. Glomerulonephritis is caused by:
    a. Genetic and familial tendencies.
    b. Antibodies in the bloodstream.
    c. Bacteria and viruses.
    d. Immune complexes deposited in glomeruli.

49. Acute glomerulonephritis can have: *Check all that apply.*
    ___ a. An onset of about 2 days.
    ___ b. A quick recovery.
    ___ c. Multiple causes.
    ___ d. A grave prognosis.

50. Upon physical assessment, the client with acute glomerulonephritis may tell the nurse:
    a. The urine has been smoky or cola-colored.
    b. The urine has been clear.
    c. That nocturia has been a problem.
    d. That diaphoresis has been present at night.

51. Which of the following diagnostic tests and results would you expect in acute glomerulonephritis? *Check all that apply.*
    ___ a. UA reveals hematuria
    ___ b. UA reveals proteinuria
    ___ c. Microscopic red blood cell casts
    ___ d. Sediment not present in UA
    ___ e. 24-hour urine for creatinine clearance decreased
    ___ f. Serum nitrogen level decreased
    ___ g. Serum albumin levels decreased
    ___ h. Antistreptolysin-O titers increased
    ___ i. Type III cryoglobulin present

52. Which of the following statements is true regarding treatment of a client with late-stage chronic glomerulonephritis?
    a. The appropriate anti-infective medication is used for treatment.
    b. Dialysis of transplantation are used.
    c. The client is treated with radiation.
    d. Immunosuppressive agents are used.

53. To prevent complications from acute glomerulonephritis, which interventions are typically implemented? *Check all that apply.*
    ___ a. Diuretic and antihypertensive drugs
    ___ b. Fluid restriction
    ___ c. Protein restriction
    ___ d. Potassium restriction

54. To relieve stress in a client with acute glomerulonephritis, the nurse:
    a. Promotes rest and a stress-free environment.
    b. Instructs the client if dialysis becomes a temporary need.
    c. Teaches care of peritoneal or vascular access device.
    d. All of the above

55. Rapidly progressive glomerulonephritis is related to:
    a. Previous multisystem disease.
    b. Tuberculosis.
    c. Urinary tract infection.
    d. Pyelonephritis.

56. Chronic glomerulonephritis may involve all of the following *except*:
    a. An onset at 20 to 30 years of age, with a possible history of infection.
    b. HTN, proteinuria, hematuria, and edema.
    c. Decreased BUN, reduced GFR, and abnormal electrolytes.
    d. Confusion and irritability.

57. Nephrotic syndrome has all of the following characteristics *except:*
    a. Massive proteinuria and edema.
    b. Altered liver activity.
    c. Nocturia with urgency.
    d. Renal vein thrombosis.

58. Immunologic, interstitial, and tubulointerstitial disorders may be:
    a. Immunologically mediated.
    b. Acute or chronic.
    c. Drug-induced problems.
    d. All of the above

59. Nephrosclerosis involves changes in nephron blood vessels that:
    a. Reduce blood flow, and the tissue is hypoxic, followed by ischemia and fibrosis.
    b. Is associated with HTN, atherosclerosis, and diabetes mellitus.
    c. Requires dialysis or transplant.
    d. All of the above

60. Renovascular disease affects the renal arteries by stenosis or thrombosis and which of the following characteristics?
    a. Sudden onset of hypertension after 50 years of age
    b. Can be from arteriosclerosis or atherosclerosis
    c. May have thrombosis or renal aneurysms
    d. All of the above

61. Treatment for renal artery stenosis includes all of the following *except*:
    a. Renal transplant.
    b. Control hypertension.
    c. Percutaneous transluminal balloon angioplasty.
    d. Renal bypass surgery.

62. Diabetic nephropathy is related to all of the following *except*:
    a. Atherosclerosis and HTN autonomic neuropathy.
    b. Immunologic response mechanisms.
    c. Glomerular malfunction.
    d. Both type 1 and type 2 diabetes.

63. In the client with diabetic nephropathy, what area correlates with damage to renal microvascular changes?
    a. Heart
    b. Retina
    c. Oral mucosa
    d. Skin

64. True or False? *Write* T *for true and* F *for false in the blank provided.*
    ___ Since the nephropathy client may no longer need insulin or antihyperglycemic drugs, the client's diabetes is improved.

65. Renal cell carcinoma is referred to as *adenocarcinoma of the kidney.* Which of the following symptoms are present in this condition? *Check all that apply.*
    ___ a. Urinary tract infection
    ___ b. Erythrocytosis
    ___ c. Hypercalcemia
    ___ d. Liver dysfunction
    ___ e. Increased sedimentation rate
    ___ f. Elevated BUN
    ___ g. Anemia
    ___ h. Hypertension

66. True or False? *Write* T *for true and* F *for false in the blank provided.*
    ___ The parathyroid hormone produced by the tumor cells may cause the hypercalcemia.

67. Renal tumors are classed into four stages and can cause which of the following complications? *Check all that apply.*
    ___ a. Obstruction in the urinary tract
    ___ b. Metastasis to distant tissues
    ___ c. Bowel obstruction
    ___ d. Paralytic ileus

68. The client with renal cell carcinoma typically presents with:
    a. Flank pain, gross hematuria, palpable renal mass, and renal bruit.
    b. Gross hematuria, hypertension (HTN), diabetes, and renal bruit.
    c. UTI, flank pain, and real mass.
    d. Gross hematuria, HTN, and UTI.

69. The best treatment for renal cancer is:
    a. Chemotherapy.
    b. Surgical removal.
    c. Interferon.
    d. Tumor necrosis factors.

70. True or False? *Write* T *for true and* F *for false in the blank provided.*
    ___ A radial nephrectomy means the periaortic lymph nodes are also removed.

71. A decrease in blood pressure in the postoperative nephrectomy client means:
    a. Hypertension has been corrected.
    b. There is a possibility of internal hemorrhage.
    c. The other kidney is failing.
    d. The client is responsive to medication.

72. Postoperative urine flow in the client following nephrectomy should be:
    a. 10 to 30 mL/hr.
    b. 30 to 50 mL/hr.
    c. 40 to 60 mL/hr.
    d. 50 to 70 mL/hr.

73. Due to the type of surgery (see Question 72) and the major muscles being cut that relate to breathing, pain medication should be:
    a. Limited because they slow respiration.
    b. An oral analgesic.
    c. Given parenterally prn for 3 to 5 days.
    d. Given parenterally on a schedule.

74. Of the levels of renal trauma, which one needs immediate repair?
    a. Major
    b. Minor
    c. Pedicle
    d. Palliative

75. For a client with pedicle injury, the best diagnostic test is:
    a. Urinalysis.
    b. Renal arteriography.
    c. CT.
    d. Intravenous urography.

76. The client with renal trauma needs to be observed for:
    a. Hemodynamic instability.
    b. Hemorrhage.
    c. Hypertension.
    d. Renal failure.

77. True or False? *Write* T *for true and* F *for false in the blank provided.*
    ___ When a renal repair is done by removing the kidney and repairing and replacing, it is called *bench surgery,* or *autotransplantation.*

STUDY GUIDE NUMBER 15.72

Interventions for Clients with Chronic and Acute Renal Failure

Study/Review Questions

1. True or False? *Write* T *for true and* F *for false in the blank provided.*
   ____ The most common cause of renal failure is poorly controlled diabetes.

2. Chronic renal function deteriorates the kidney slowly; significant failure is not seen until what percent of the nephrons are destroyed?
   a. 30% to 50%
   b. 50% to 60%
   c. 60% to 75%
   d. 90% to 95%

3. Acute renal failure may occur with only what percent of nephrons functioning?
   a. 30%
   b. 50%
   c. 75%
   d. 90%

4. True or False? *Write* T *for true and* F *for false in the blank provided.*
   ____ Acute renal failure affects all of the body systems, while chronic failure affects some of the body systems.

Answer the following three questions on a separate sheet of paper.

5. Compare and contrast the pathophysiology and causes of chronic renal failure and acute renal failure. Use the textbook and Tables 72-2, 72-6, and 72-7.

6. Identify clients at risk to develop acute renal failure (ARF).

7. Discuss intervention to prevent ARF.

True or False? *Write* T *for true and* F *for false in the blanks provided.*

____ 8. Hypofusion is an autoregulatory response, which causes increased blood volume and improved renal perfusion responsible for oliguria.

____ 9. Injury to the tubular cells of the kidney will occur because of hypoperfusion.

10. Renal failure is present when:
    a. The BUN and creatinine levels rise and remain constant.
    b. The BUN rises faster than creatinine level.
    c. The BUN is lower than creatinine level.
    d. Both BUN and creatine levels decrease.

11. Match each cause to the corresponding urologic change. *Answers may be used more than once.*

Causes	Urologic Changes
____ a. Urethral cancer	1. Prerenal
____ b. CHF	2. Intrarenal
____ c. Vasculitis	3. Postrenal
____ d. Sepsis	
____ e. Exposure to nephrotoxins	
____ f. Renal calculi	
____ g. Atony of bladder	
____ h. Renal artery stenosis or thrombosis	
____ i. Shock	

12. Two types of nephrotoxic drugs are:
    a. Aspirin and NSAIDs.
    b. Antibiotics and aspirin.
    c. Antibiotics and NSAIDs.
    d. Antihypertensives and antibiotics.

13. True or False? *Write* T *for true and* F *for false in the blank provided.*
    ____ With prompt attention, prerenal azotemia can be reversed.

14. When the vascular volume is depleted, the nurse can expect the signs of:
    a. Decreased urine output, postural hypotension, and tachycardia.
    b. Increased urine output, postural hypotension, and tachycardia.
    c. Tachycardia, hypertension, and decreased urine output.
    d. Tachycardia, hypertension, and increased urine output.

15. An early sign of renal tubular damage is:
    a. Elevated BUN.
    b. Decreased urine specific gravity.
    c. Low electrolytes.
    d. Oliguria.

16. When a client is taking a nephrotoxic drug, the nurse should monitor:
    a. BUN and creatinine.
    b. Electrolytes.
    c. Drug peak and trough.
    d. All of the above

17. When taking a history of a client with prerenal failure, the nurse notes: *Check all that apply.*
    ___ a. Exposure to nephrotoxins or recent surgery.
    ___ b. Use of anti-infectives, antibiotics, NSAIDs, or ACE inhibitors.
    ___ c. Any systemic diseases.
    ___ d. Trauma or transfusions.

18. True or False? *Write T for true and F for false in the blank provided.*
    ___ The symptoms of a client with prerenal azotemia mimic those of a client with heart failure or dehydration.

19. Identify the symptoms of prerenal azotemia.
    a. _____
    b. _____
    c. _____
    d. _____
    e. _____
    f. _____

20. Identify the symptoms of intrarenal acute renal failure that are different from those of prerenal azotemia.
    a. _____
    b. _____
    c. _____
    d. _____
    e. _____
    f. _____

g. _____
h. _____
i. _____

21. A flat plate x-ray could reveal which of the following about the kidneys?
    a. Decreased glomerular function
    b. Enlargement due to hydronephrosis
    c. Renal calculi
    d. Hypoperfusion of the kidneys

22. True or False? *Write T for true and F for false in the blank provided.*
    ___ An ultrasonography and a CT scan without contrast can diagnose any obstructions.

23. On a separate sheet of paper, identify priorities for care of clients with acute renal failure.

24. For clients in prerenal azotemia, a fluid challenge is done to promote renal perfusion by:
    a. Administering normal saline 500 to 1000 mL infused over 1 hour.
    b. Expectorating urine production.
    c. Having a diuretic ordered.
    d. All of the above

25. True or False? *Write T for true and F for false in the blank provided.*
    ___ Low-dose dopamine may enhance renal perfusion or elevate blood pressure.

26. In the client with acute renal failure, calcium channel blockers are used to:
    a. Prevent buildups of calcium in the kidneys.
    b. Prevent buildups of vitamin D in the kidneys.
    c. Increase diuresis.
    d. Maintain cell integrity and improve GFR.

27. Clients in acute renal failure have a high rate of catabolism that is related to:
    a. Increased levels of catecholamines, cortisol, and glucagon.
    b. Breakdown of muscle for protein.
    c. Stress of critical illness.
    d. All of the above

28. When the client with acute renal failure is anorexic:
    a. Give normal saline to prevent dehydration.
    b. The dietitian will prescribe a calculated diet.
    c. Total parental nutrition (TPN) can be ordered if lab results are monitored.
    d. Fat emulsion can be added to TPN.

29. The goal of TPN is to:
   a. Preserve lean body mass.
   b. Restore or maintain fluid balance.
   c. Preserve renal function.
   d. All of the above

30. On a separate sheet of paper, identify the indications for dialysis in the client with acute renal failure.

True or False? Write T for true and F for false in the blank provided.

___ 31. An HD catheter has two lumens separating the outflow and inflow of blood because it prevents the mixing of undialyzed blood with dialyzed blood.

___ 32. Peritoneal dialysis is not used on a client on a ventilator because such clients are unable to assist the nurse.

33. Continuous arteriovenous hemodialysis and filtration (CAVH) is used on clients that are: *Check all that apply.*
   ___ a. Fluid volume overloaded.
   ___ b. Resistant to diuretics.
   ___ c. Hemodynamically unstable.
   ___ d. Hypertensive.

34. True or False? *Write T for true and F for false in the blank provided.*
   ___ CAVH uses a pump to make rate of filtration more reliable.

35. Match each characteristic with the corresponding device. *Answers may be used more than once.*

Characteristic	Device
___ a. Requires placement of arterial and venous catheter	1. CAVH
	2. CAVHD
	3. CVVH
___ b. Requires a double-lumen venous catheter	
___ c. Uses pump	
___ d. Arterial pressure of at least 60 mm Hg	
___ e. Removes plasma and electrolytes	
___ f. Risk of air embolus	
___ g. Uses dialysate to remove nitrogenous waste	

36. On a separate sheet of paper, prioritize teaching needs for the client using continuous ambulatory peritoneal dialysis (CAPD).

37. On a separate sheet of paper, identify each of the following terms and abbreviations:
   ESRD
   Uremia
   Uremic syndrome
   Azotemia
   CRF
   Hyposthenuria
   Isosthenuria
   Polyuria
   GFR
   HTN

38. Match each characteristic with the corresponding stage of renal failure. *Answers may be used more than once.*

Characteristics	Stages
___ a. Excessive waste products	1. Diminished renal reserve
___ b. Increased BUN and creatinine	2. Renal insufficiency
___ c. Dialysis	3. End-stage renal disease (ESRD)
___ d. Reduced function	
___ e. Nephrons compensation	
___ f. Hypertension (HTN)	
___ g. Stress of illness can compromise this stage fast	
___ h. Medical management very important	
___ i. Severe fluid overload	
___ j. Electrolyte and acid-base imbalances	
___ k. Renal osteodystrophy	

39. The GFR functions can maintain kidney function until only 20% of the nephrons are left, and then nephrons:
   a. Become edematous.
   b. Decrease water absorption.
   c. Increase water absorption.
   d. Begin to atrophy.

40. As the client with end-stage renal disease experiences hyposthenuria, polyuria, and then isosthenuria, the nurse needs to be alert for:
   a. The diuretic stage.
   b. Fluid volume overload.
   c. Dehydration.
   d. Acid-base imbalance.

41. The creatinine levels stay pretty constant *except* when there is a decrease in renal function because it:
    a. Is excreted in the urine.
    b. Is excreted in renal tubules, elevating the serum creatinine.
    c. Is excreted in renal tubules, decreasing the serum creatinine.
    d. Varies with protein intake.

True or False? Write T for true and F for false in the blanks provided.

____ 42. An effective way to monitor kidney function is to monitor the creatinine clearance values.

____ 43. Sodium depletion is seen in early chronic renal failure (CRF), which is caused by a necessary loss in the kidneys and a diminishing number of nephrons to reabsorb sodium.

____ 44. As the nephrons are being lost, the remaining nephrons increase their production of acid excretion. This deficit is a bicarbonate deficit or metabolic alkalosis.

45. Which of the following is a result of kidney failure? Excessive hydrogen ions:
    a. Cannot be excreted.
    b. Are counteracted by ammonia.
    c. Are balanced by excessive bicarbonate.
    d. Cause metabolic alkalosis.

46. With acid retention, respiratory compensation is manifested as:
    a. An increased respiratory rate.
    b. An increased depth of breathing to give off carbon dioxide.
    c. Decreased respirations.
    d. Increased arterial carbon dioxide levels.

47. True or False? *Write T for true and F for false in the blank provided.*
    ____ Chronic hypocalcemia results in hyperplasia and hypertrophy of the parathyroid gland, which triggers bone reabsorption of calcium.

48. A client in uremia will have all of the following *except*:
    a. Uremic halitosis or stomatitis.
    b. Hiccups and anorexia.
    c. Anxiety and tremors.
    d. Nausea and vomiting.

49. Identify the two most common causes of CRF.
    a. _____
    b. _____

50. On a separate sheet of paper, identify clients at risk for the development of CRF.

51. When the nurse is taking a history on a client with CRF, he or she needs to be aware of characteristic symptoms. Review Chart 72-7 and identify effects on each body system.

52. A client with CRF can use many nursing diagnoses as the condition changes daily. Identify the three diagnoses that apply until transplant or death.
    a. _____
    b. _____
    c. _____

True or False? Write T for true and F for false in the blank provided.

____ 53. A client receiving dialysis will need additional protein in the diet due to protein loss during the procedure.

____ 54. A client receiving peritoneal dialysis needs more protein than a client receiving hemodialysis.

55. The nurse should instruct the CRF client to document: *Check all that apply.*
    ____ a. Daily weight.
    ____ b. Accurate intake and output.
    ____ c. Blood pressure.
    ____ d. Respiratory rate.

56. A precaution to prevent infection in the client with CRF is: *Check all that apply.*
    ____ a. Taking antibiotics as ordered.
    ____ b. Monitoring vital signs.
    ____ c. Inspecting vascular access device sites.
    ____ d. Reporting any pain.

57. Review Chart 72-3 and identify drugs typically given to clients with CRF. Note important side effects or toxicities that can result from poor kidney function.

58. Giving recombinant erythropoietin to a client with CRF may have which of the following effects? *Check all that apply.*
    ___ a. Hematocrit of 30% to 35%
    ___ b. Improved appetite
    ___ c. A need for an iron supplement
    ___ d. A need for periodic blood transfusions

59. Pulmonary edema can develop in the alveoli due to injury to the vascular endothelium or alveolar epithelial cells. Signs and symptoms the nurse needs to look for include: *Check all that apply.*
    ___ a. Restlessness and heightened anxiety.
    ___ b. Diaphoresis.
    ___ c. Bradycardia.
    ___ d. Dyspnea.

60. As the nurse with a client suffering from pulmonary edema, you will do all of the following *except*:
    a. Elevate bed to high Fowler's position.
    b. Start oxygen.
    c. Have intravenous access.
    d. Lie the client on the left side.

61. True or False? *Write T for true and F for false in the blank provided.*
    ___ The medications commonly ordered for pulmonary edema include intravenous loop diuretic and morphine sulfate.

62. Hemodialysis is initiated *immediately* for all of the following reasons *except*:
    a. Fluid overload refractory to diuretics, pericarditis, and uncontrolled HTN.
    b. Neurologic manifestations (decreased attention span).
    c. Increased creatinine clearance.
    d. Development of bleeding diathesis.

63. True or False? *Write T for true and F for false in the blank provided.*
    ___ The duration of the survival of a client on hemodialysis is based on renal disease and other pre-existing diseases, as well as the client's stability.

Answer the following three questions on a separate sheet of paper.

64. Compare and contrast dietary modifications needed for a client on hemodialysis with those for a client on peritoneal dialysis. Use Table 72-8.

65. Discuss mechanisms of peritoneal dialysis and hemodialysis as renal replacement therapies.

66. Prioritize teaching for a client using CAPD.

True or False? Write T for true and F for false in the blanks provided.

___ 67. The procedure for dialysis is based on diffusion, accomplished by running the blood and dialysate in opposite directions between a membrane. Waste products, water, potassium, and sodium can move across the membrane.

___ 68. Sterility of the dialysate is *not* an issue because it is made from clear water and chemicals and is free of metabolic waste and drugs. Bacteria and microorganisms are too big to move through it.

69. Heparin is used to prevent the blood from clotting; the nurse must be aware that: *Check all that apply.*
    ___ a. The drug is short-acting but is in the body for 5 to 6 hours.
    ___ b. The dose is adjusted to each client.
    ___ c. Clients receiving erythropoietin may need additional heparin.
    ___ d. Protamine sulfate can be given as an antidote.

70. On a separate sheet of paper, prioritize teaching needs with permanent vascular access device for long-term dialysis.

71. Precautions for a client with AV fistula or AV graft include: *Check all that apply.*
    ___ a. Monitoring for circulation by checking for a bruit or a thrill.
    ___ b. Not taking blood pressure on the arm with the fistula or graft.
    ___ c. Avoiding venipuncture or IV administration on the arm with access device.
    ___ d. Take vital signs every 4 hours.

72. Identify the complications that can occur regardless of type of access for renal replacement therapies.
    a. _____
    b. _____
    c. _____
    d. _____
    e. _____
    f. _____

73. True or False? *Write T for true and F for false in the blank provided.*
    ___ The most common infection in an AV fistula or graft is *Staphylococcus aureus*.

74. Dialysis disequilibrium syndrome is caused by rapid decrease in the BUN levels, which causes cerebral edema and increased intracranial pressure with all of the following symptoms *except*:
    a. Headache, nausea, and vomiting.
    b. Seizures and coma.
    c. High anxiety or fear.
    d. Decreased level of consciousness.

75. Dialysis disequilibrium syndrome is treated with:
    a. A return to dialysis.
    b. Barbiturates and anticonvulsants.
    c. Hypnotic agents.
    d. Antibiotics.

True or False? Write T for true and F for false in the blanks provided.

___ 76. The incidence of hepatitis and HIV have been decreased due to consistent standards of practice, routine screening of blood, and fewer blood transfusions.

___ 77. Peritoneal dialysis is provided through an abdominal access device; the membrane is the peritoneal space to hold the dialysate.

___ 78. Heparin cannot prevent fibrin clot formation in peritoneal dialysis.

79. On a separate sheet of paper, identify the types of peritoneal dialysis and note the difference of each.

80. Peritonitis is the most common major complication identified and is diagnosed by: *Check all that apply.*
    ___ a. Cloudy dialysate.
    ___ b. Immediate culture and sensitivity, Gram stain, and cell count.
    ___ c. Antibiotic therapy.
    ___ d. Client complaints of fever or abdominal pain.

81. True or False? *Write T for true and F for false in the blank provided.*
    ___ Infection in the peritoneal dialysis catheter site or tunnel infections requires that the catheter be removed.

82. Problems with the flow of dialysate in clients with peritoneal dialysis can be caused by:
    a. Constipation.
    b. Positioning.
    c. Migration of the peritoneal tube.
    d. Catheter lumen site.

83. Which of the following are true and about the color of peritoneal dialysis dialysate? *Check all that apply.*
    ___ a. Red or pink indicates possible bleeding.
    ___ b. Brown color indicates there may be a bowel perforation.
    ___ c. A yellow color means there may be a bladder perforation.
    ___ d. Cloudy means there are obvious problems.

84. On a separate sheet of paper, identify the reasons a client may *not* qualify for transplantation.

85. True or False? *Write T for true and F for false in the blank provided.*
    ___ Most donors for kidney transplants are cadaveric donors.

86. On a separate sheet of paper, identify the criteria that living related donors must meet for kidney transplantation.

87. Before a kidney is determined a suitable donor for transplant, the client and kidney undergo what testing?
    a. _____
    b. _____
    c. _____

88. True or False? *Write T for true and F for false in the blank provided.*
    ___ A kidney transplant recipient receives dialysis 24 hours before transplant and a blood transfusion of donor-specific blood to increase graft survival.

89. Postoperatively, the nurse monitors the kidney recipient by means of: *Check all that apply.*
    ___ a. Hourly urine output.
    ___ b. Blood pressure.
    ___ c. Bladder irrigation.
    ___ d. Dialysis therapy.

90. On a separate sheet of paper, prioritize nursing care for the client during the first 24 hours after kidney transplant.

91. Identify the possible complication if the recipient has no urine output.

True or False? Write T for true and F for false in the blanks provided.

___ 92. A recipient of a living donor may develop diuresis and needs to be watched for electrolyte imbalances.

____ 93. To save the transplant when acute tubular necrosis is present, dialysis may be needed as well as re-evaluation of immunosuppression.

94. In a transplant client, a sudden decrease in urine at 2 to 3 days postoperative is a sign of:
   a. Rejection.
   b. Thrombosis.
   c. Stenosis.
   d. Other complications.

95. True or False? *Write* T *for true and* F *for false in the blank provided.*
   ____ Because of the immunosuppressed drugs that must be taken, a kidney recipient is a candidate for fatal viral, fungal, bacterial, or protozoal infections.

Answer the following two questions on a separate sheet of paper.

96. Identify the drugs used for immunosuppression.

97. The nurse is responsible for teaching a client in home care. Use Chart 72-12 to develop a teaching plan for the home care client on dialysis and post transplant. Include the family.

98. Psychosocial support is important for a client on dialysis due to the changing moods of managing the disease process, which includes:
   ____ a. The honeymoon period.
   ____ b. Disillusionment.
   ____ c. Denial.
   ____ d. Acceptance or resolution.

99. The cost of care is astronomical because the kidney transplant client will need: *Check all that apply.*
   ____ a. Help from many types of professionals from various disciplines.
   ____ b. Continuous dialysis.
   ____ c. Require medications.
   ____ d. Require financial aid.

UNIT 16 PROBLEMS OF REPRODUCTION ■ Core Concepts Grid

Anatomy	Physiology	Pathophysiology	History	Physical Exam	Diagnostic Tests	Interventions	Pharmacology
• **Female** Ovaries Fallopian tubes Uterus Vagina • **Male** Penis Scrotum Testes Ducts • **Breasts**	• **Procreation** • **Nurturing** • **Sexual pleasure** • **Urinary elimination**	• **Infection** • **Obstruction** • **Inflammation** • **Tumors**	• **Client history** Past problems Contraceptives Obstetric history Self-examination Breast Testes Difficult/painful urination Menstrual history Erectile dysfunction Renal/endocrine dysfunction Hypertension • **Family history** Cancer Thyroid Diabetes • **Social history** Sexual history Alcohol use Smoking Exposure to sexually transmitted disease (STDs) Age Race	• **Skin/hair distribution** • **Skin ulceration/ rashes/color** • **Discharge** Vagina Penis Nipple • **Hernia** • **Breasts** Size Shape Masses	• **Mammography** • **Ultrasonography** • **Pap smear** • **Estrogen levels** • **Androgen levels** • **Venereal Disease Research Laboratory (VDRL) test** • **Fluorescent Treponemal Antibody Absorption (FTA-ABS) test** • **Gram stain** • **Acid phosphate** • **Prostate-specific antigen (PSA)** • **Carcinoembryonic antigen (CEA)**	• **Radiation therapy** • **Client education** Self-examination Breast Testes Safer sex Hormone replacement therapy (HRT) Kegel exercises • **Bladder irrigations** • **Urinary catheter care** Foley (3-way) Suprapubic • **Penile implants** • **Postoperative care and monitoring for complications (e.g., hemorrhage)** • **Sperm banking** • **Emotional support** • **Health teaching**	• **Antibiotics** • **Antivirals** • **Antiprotozoals** • **Antifungals** • **Hormone replacement therapy** • **Anti-impotence agents** • **Chemotherapeutic agents**

Unit 16 (Chapters 73–77)

Problems of Reproduction: Management of Clients with Problems of the Reproductive System

Learning Plan

Chapter 73: *Assessment of the Reproductive System*

Learning Outcomes	Learning Activities	Supplemental Resources

1. Review the anatomy and physiology of the reproductive system.
2. Discuss components of a health history for reproductive health problems using Gordon's Functional Health Patterns.
3. Interpret common reproductive diagnostic tests.
4. Describe the client preparation for common reproductive diagnostic tests.
5. Develop a teaching plan for clients undergoing endoscopic studies for reproductive health problems.
6. Explain the importance of selected reproductive tests in promoting and maintaining health (e.g., mammogram).
	1. Prior to completing the study guide exercises for this chapter, review the following:
	  • Anatomy and physiology of the male and female reproductive systems
	  • Effect of the endocrine system on genitoreproductive tissue
	  • Concepts of human sexuality
	  • Concepts of body image and self-esteem
	  • Normal growth and development
	2. Review the **boldfaced** Key Terms and their definitions in Chapter 73 to enhance your understanding of the content.
	3. Go to Study Guide Number 16.73 on the following pages and complete the learning exercises for this chapter.
		1. Textbook—Chapter 73
		2. Other resources:
		  • Contact the local chapter of the American Cancer Society {AU: **Did you mean "American *Cancer* Society" here?**} to discover educational programs offered to women about breast self-examinations, latest statistical information on breast and ovarian cancer, and support groups in the area.
		  • Higgins, P. & Smith, P. (1997). Assessing cervical cancer risks. *AWHONN's Lifelines, 1*(6), 43-47.
		  • Jarvis, C. (2000). *Physical examination and health assessment* (3rd ed.). Philadelphia: W.B. Saunders.

Chapter 74: *Interventions for Clients with Breast Disorders*

Learning Outcomes	Learning Activities	Supplemental Resources

1. Describe the three-pronged approach to early detection of breast masses: mammography, clinical breast examination, and breast self-examination (BSE).
2. Teach a client how to do BSE.
3. Explain the options available for a woman at high genetic risk for breast cancer.
4. Compare and contrast assessment findings associated with benign and malignant breast lesions.
5. Analyze assessment data to determine priority nursing diagnosis and collaborative problems for the woman with breast cancer.
6. Develop a plan of care for a client with breast cancer.
	1. Prior to completing the study guide exercises for this chapter, review the following:
	  • Anatomy and physiology of male and female breast
	  • Effect of the endocrine system on breast tissue
	  • Concepts of human sexuality
	  • Concepts of body image and self-esteem
	  • Normal growth and development of breast tissue
	  • Concepts of grief, loss, death, and dying
		1. Textbook—Chapter 73 (Assessment of the Reproductive System)
		2. Textbook—Chapter 74
		3. Other resources:
		  • Contact the local chapter of the American Cancer Society to discover educational programs offered to women about breast self-examinations, latest statistical information on breast and ovarian cancer, and support groups in the area.

- Higgins, P. & Smith, P. (1997). Assessing cervical cancer risks. *AWHONN's Lifelines 1*(6), 43-47.
- Jarvis, C. (2000). *Physical examination and health assessment* (3rd ed.). Philadelphia: W.B. Saunders.

7. Discuss the psychosocial aspects related to having breast cancer and undergoing surgery for breast cancer.
8. Formulate a community-based teaching plan for the client undergoing surgery for breast cancer.

- Care of the patient undergoing chemotherapy and radiation therapy
- Principles of perioperative nursing management
- Assessment of the reproductive system

2. Review the **boldfaced** Key Terms and their definitions in Chapter 74 to enhance your understanding of the content.

3. Go to Study Guide Number 16.74 on the following pages and complete the learning exercises for this chapter.

Chapter 75: *Interventions for Clients with Gynecologic Problems*

Learning Outcomes

1. Compare and contrast common menstrual cycle disorders.
2. Discuss common assessment findings associated with menopause.
3. Develop a teaching plan for a client with a vaginal inflammation or infection.
4. Prioritize postoperative care for the client undergoing an anterior and/or posterior repair.
5. Analyze assessment data for clients with leiomyomas to determine nursing diagnoses and collaborative problems.
6. Formulate a plan of care for a client undergoing a hysterectomy.
7. Identify the risk factors for gynecologic cancers.
8. Discuss the psychosocial issues associated with gynecologic cancers.
9. Explain the purpose of radiation and chemotherapy for clients with gynecologic cancers.
10. Develop a community-based plan of care for clients with gynecologic cancers.

Learning Activities

1. Prior to completing the study guide exercises for this chapter, review the following:
   - Anatomy and physiology of the female reproductive system
   - Effect of the endocrine system on the female reproductive system
   - Concepts of human sexuality
   - Concepts of body image and self-esteem.
   - Normal growth and development
   - Concepts of grief, loss, death, and dying
   - Perineal care
   - Sitz baths
   - Enema administration
   - Care of the patient undergoing chemotherapy and radiation therapy
   - The principles of perioperative nursing management
   - Assessment of the reproductive system

2. Review the **boldfaced** Key Terms and their definitions in Chapter 75 to enhance your understanding of the content.

3. Go to Study Guide Number 16.75 on the following pages and complete the learning exercises for this chapter.

Supplemental Resources

1. Textbook—Chapter 73 (Assessment of the Reproductive System)
2. Textbook—Chapter 75
3. Other resources:
   - Jarvis, C. (2000). *Physical examination and health assessment* (3rd ed.). Philadelphia: W.B. Saunders.
   - Johnson, S. (1998). Menopause and hormone replacement therapy. *Medical Clinics of North America, 82*(2), 297-320.
   - Lessick, M., Wickham, R., & Rehwaldt, M. (1997). Breast and ovarian cancer: Genetic update and implications for nursing. *MEDSURG Nursing, 6*(6), 341-349.
   - Scura, K.W. & Whipple, B. (1997). How to provide better care for the postmenopausal woman. *American Journal of Nursing, 97*(4), 36-44.

Chapter 76: *Interventions for Male Clients with Reproductive Problems*

Learning Outcomes	Learning Activities	Supplemental Resources
1. Describe common physical assessment findings for the client with benign prostatic hyperplasia (BPH).	1. Prior to completing the study guide exercises for this chapter, review the following:	1. Textbook—Chapter 73 (Assessment of the Reproductive System)
2. Discuss options for nonsurgical and surgical management of the client with BPH.	• Anatomy and physiology of the male reproductive system	2. Textbook—Chapter 76
3. Develop a postoperative plan of care for the client undergoing a transurethral resection of the prostate (TURP).	• Effect of the endocrine system on the male reproductive tissue	3. Other resources:
4. Identify the procedures for prostate cancer screening.	• Concepts of human sexuality	• American Cancer Society. (2000). *Cancer facts and figures 1996*. Atlanta, GA: Author.
5. Explain the role of hormonal therapy in treating prostate cancer.	• Concepts of body image and self-esteem	• Miller, K. (1999). Testicular torsion. *American Journal of Nursing, 99*(6), 33.
6. Describe the options for treating erectile dysfunction.	• Normal growth and development	• Tingen, M., et al. (1999). Perceived benefits: A predictor of participation in prostate cancer screening. *Cancer Nursing, 21*(5), 349-357.
7. Discuss the cultural considerations related to male reproductive problems.	• Concepts of grief, loss, death, and dying	
8. Analyze assessment data to determine priority nursing diagnoses and collaborative problems for the man with testicular cancer.	• Perineal care	
9. Develop a plan of care for the client with testicular cancer.	• Sitz baths	
10. Formulate a community-based teaching plan for continuing care of clients with testicular cancer.	• Enema administration	
11. Compare and contrast hydrocele, spermatocele, and varicocele.	• Care of the patient undergoing chemotherapy and radiation therapy	
12. Discuss issues related to sexuality and body impact for a man experiencing male reproductive health problems.	• Principles of perioperative nursing management	
	• Assessment of the reproductive system	
	2. Review the **boldfaced** Key Terms and their definitions in Chapter 76 to enhance your understanding of the content.	
	3. Go to Study Guide Number 16.76 on the following pages and complete the learning exercises for this chapter.	

Chapter 77: Interventions for Clients with Sexually Transmitted Diseases

Learning Outcomes	Learning Activities	Supplemental Resources
1. Explain how sexually transmitted diseases (STDs) can be prevented. 2. Compare and contrast the stages of syphilis. 3. Prioritize nursing care for the client with syphilis at each stage. 4. Identify the role of drug therapy in managing clients with genital herpes. 5. Discuss the psychosocial effects of having an STD. 6. Develop a teaching plan for clients diagnosed with gonorrhea. 7. Describe the assessment findings that are typical in clients with *Chlamydia trachomatis* infection. 8. Analyze assessment data to determine common nursing diagnoses for women with pelvic inflammatory disease (PID). 9. Formulate a collaborative plan of care for the client with PID. 10. Develop a community-based teaching plan for clients with PID. 11. Evaluate care for the client with PID. 12. Identify common causes of vaginal infections.	1. Prior to completing the study guide exercises for this chapter, review the following: 　• Anatomy and physiology of the male and female reproductive system 　• Concepts of human sexuality 　• Perineal care 　• Principles of perioperative nursing management 　• Principles of infection transmission 　• Concepts of body image and self-esteem 　• Assessment of the reproductive system 2. Review the **boldfaced** Key Terms and their definitions in Chapter 77 to enhance your understanding of the content. 3. Go to Study Guide Number 16.77 on the following pages and complete the learning exercises for this chapter.	1. Textbook—Chapter 73 (Assessment of the Reproductive System) 2. Textbook—Chapter 77 3. Other resources: 　• Bob, P.S.S. & Famolare, N.E. (1998). Teaching and communication strategies: Working with the hospitalized adolescent with pelvic inflammatory disease. *Pediatric Nursing 24*(1), 17-20, 29-30. 　• Cohen, C.R. & Brunham, R.C. (1999). Pathogenesis of chlamydia induced pelvic inflammatory disease. *Sexually Transmitted Infections, 75*(1), 21-24. 　• Daley, E.M. (1998). Clinical update on the role of HPV and cervical cancer. *Cancer Nursing, 21*(1), 31-35. 　• Norton, N.J. (1998). Coping with HPV: How the help a patient diagnosed with this sexually transmitted disease. *Nursing 1998, 28*(9), 73-74.

STUDY GUIDE NUMBER 16.73

Assessment of the Reproductive System

Study/Review Questions

1. A mother is very concerned that her 13-year-old son is not showing any physical signs of puberty but her daughter was fully developed and menstruating by the age of 13. The nurse's best response to the mother would be:
   a. "Your son will start his growth spurt by his fourteenth birthday, so I would not worry at this time."
   b. "Boys usually mature physically before girls, so your son needs to see your family doctor."
   c. "Girls usually mature physically about 2 years before boys, so I wouldn't be concerned at this time."
   d. "Boys and girls generally mature at about the same age, so you need to take your son to the doctor immediately."

2. Which order of the phases menstrual cycle is correct?
   a. Proliferative, secretory, sloughing, follicular
   b. Sloughing, proliferative, secretory, ischemic
   c. Follicular, proliferative, sloughing, secretory
   d. Proliferative, secretory, sloughing, ischemic

3. Your client, age 13½, experienced menarche 4 months ago. Her mother is very concerned that her daughter has had very irregular menstrual cycles since then. The nurse's best response to the mother would be that:
   a. Her daughter needs to be examined by a doctor for a pelvic exam.
   b. Her daughter needs to have a pregnancy test done.
   c. Her daughter's irregularity will adjust itself within the next 2 years.
   d. Her daughter's irregularity is normal following the onset of menstruation.

4. The menstrual cycle is regulated by a feedback control system of interrelated cycles. These interrelated cycles are:
   a. Mammary, ovarian, and uterine cycles.
   b. Hypothalamic-pituitary, ovarian, and endometrial cycles.
   c. Ovarian, pituitary, and gonadal cycles.
   d. Hypothalamic-pituitary, mammary, and ovarian cycles.

5. During a sex education class, the nurse is explaining the function of the female breasts to a group of seventh-grade students. The nurse's best statement would be which of the following?
   a. The female breasts have only one main function: serving as a source of sexual pleasure.
   b. The only function of the female breasts is to provide nourishment for the mother's baby.
   c. The main function of the female breasts is to provide nourishment for the mother's baby, but the breasts also function as a source of sexual sensation.
   d. The main function of the female breasts is to allow for passive transfer of antibodies to the baby after birth.

6. What is the normal PH of the vagina necessary to decrease the vagina's susceptibility to infection?
   a. 5.0
   b. 4.5
   c. 4.0
   d. 6.0

7. The inner layer of the uterus that allows for implantation of the fetus and is shed during menses is the:
   a. Myometrium.
   b. Parametrium.
   c. Endometrium.
   d. Peritoneum.

8. Which of the following statements is true concerning artificial menopause?
   a. It is a pseudomenopause.
   b. Estrogen levels usually increase.
   c. It can be surgically corrected.
   d. It can be surgically induced.

9. What part of the internal reproductive system of the male aids in maturation of the sperm?
   a. Vas deferens
   b. Epididymis
   c. Seminal vesicles
   d. Ejaculatory glands

10. What is the main function of the prostate gland in the male reproductive system?
   a. To provide fluid to allow sperm to move through the vas deferens
   b. To provide fluid to increase bulk of the ejaculated semen
   c. To provide fluid to increase the vaginal pH to 6.5
   d. To provide fluid to initiate the first stage of the male orgasm

11. Which of the following factors can have a direct negative effect on reproductive health in both men and women? *Check all that apply.*
   ____ a. Substance abuse
   ____ b. Occupational environment
   ____ c. Ethnicity/race
   ____ d. Lifestyle habits

12. Most visits to the health care provider in relation to problems associated with the reproductive system are the result of all of the following *except*:
   a. Unexplained pain.
   b. Tender lymph nodes.
   c. Abnormal bleeding.
   d. Vaginal or penile discharge.

13. Which of the following statements is true concerning a pelvic exam?
   a. The client needs to douche before the examination to allow for better visualization of the cervix.
   b. The client needs to have a full bladder so it is easier to identify on palpation.
   c. The pelvic exam is indicated on a yearly basis if a client is sexually active.
   d. The pelvic exam can be used to assess for infection or menstrual irregularities.

14. A common occurrence in the client after a pelvic examination is:
   a. Abdominal pain.
   b. Orthostatic hypotension.
   c. Bleeding for 1 to 2 hours.
   d. Nausea or anorexia.

15. Annual digital rectal examinations and prostate gland specific antigen (PSA) blood tests are recommended for all men older than age:
   a. 35.
   b. 40.
   c. 45.
   d. 50.

16. Which of the following statements is true concerning a genitourinary reproductive examination of a male client?
   a. The left and right side of the scrotal sac should be symmetrical.
   b. The epididymis and inguinal hernias cannot be palpated by external exam.
   c. The prostate gland is examined by a digital rectal exam.
   d. Penile discharge can only be assessed by an internal examination.

17. Which test which would best evaluate the presence of a tubal dysfunction?
   a. Hysterosalpingography
   b. Computerized tomography
   c. Urologic studies
   d. Radioimmunoassay

18. Which of the following radiologic assessment tests does *not* require any specific client preparation?
   a. IVP
   b. KUB
   c. Barium enema
   d. Hysterosalpingography

19. Which of the following diagnostic procedures necessitates the performing of a small incision?
   a. Laparoscopy
   b. Hysteroscopy
   c. Colposcopy
   d. Cystoscopy

20. Which of the following biopsies would require the use of a local or general anesthesia?
   a. Cervical biopsy
   b. Excisional biopsy of the breast
   c. Needle aspiration of the prostate
   d. Endometrial biopsy

21. An adult client presents to the clinic for her annual physical exam. She tells the nurse practitioner that she has been performing breast self-examination as directed, but was wondering when to have her first mammogram. The nurse tells the client that a baseline mammogram needs to be performed:
    a. At 40 years.
    b. At 30 years.
    c. Between 50 to 55 years.
    d. Between 35 to 40 years.

22. Your adult client is scheduled to have an endometrial biopsy. The nurse is responsible for teaching her about this test. The nurse will teach this client which of the following?
    a. Abdominal cramping will last 1 to 2 weeks.
    b. Vaginal discharge will be heavy at times but will last only 10 to 14 days.
    c. Sexual activity should be postponed until the vaginal discharge stops.
    d. General anesthesia will be used for the procedure.

23. A client's cytologic test (Papanicolaou [Pap] smear) results were reported as having epithelial cell abnormalities with no evidence of dysplasia. These results are indicative of what classification based on the Papanicolaou scale?
    a. Class I
    b. Class II
    c. Class III
    d. Class IV

24. A bilateral vasectomy functions as a male contraceptive because:
    a. Sperm production is prohibited.
    b. Ejaculation is prevented.
    c. Penile erection is limited.
    d. Passage of sperm to the semen is prevented.

25. Which of the most common cancers in young adult males can be treated effectively if found early?
    a. Prostate
    b. Colon
    c. Penile
    d. Testicular

26. Match each diagnostic test with the corresponding definition.

Diagnostic Tests

____ a. Culture
____ b. Radioimmuno-assay method
____ c. Serologic test
____ d. VDRL
____ e. Pap smear
____ f. FTA-ABS
____ g. Wet smear
____ h. ELISA
____ i. PSA
____ j. 24-hour uring sample

Definitions

1. Test that detects cancerous and precancerous cells of the cervix
2. Test used to screen for prostate cancer
3. More specific test used to detect the causative agent of syphilis
4. Levels of estrogen, progesterone, and testosterone can be detected by this type of test
5. Test used to screen all pregnant women and persons at high risk for syphilis
6. These tests involve the use of a spray on preparation and a glass slide specimen
7. Test used to determine the occurrence of ovulation by levels of estrogen and pregnanediol
8. Test that detects antigen-antibody reactions that have occurred in response to foreign substances
9. Test used to detect the presence of a *Chlamydia* infection
10. Test used to determine appropriate antibiotic therapy

27. Match each etiology with the resulting dysfunction.

Etiologies

____ a. Low levels of body fat or poor nutrition

____ b. Infertility in women

____ c. Substance abuse

____ d. Low Rubella titers in child-bearing women

____ e. Mumps in post-pubertal males

____ f. Endocrine disorders

____ g. Chronic disorders of nervous, respiratory, or cardiovascular system

____ h. Medications such as MAOIs, antihypertensives, antihis-tamines, and opioids

____ i. PID, salpingitis

Dysfunctions

1. Teratogenic effects
2. Vaginal dryness, increased yeast infections or impotence
3. Impaired fertility
4. Ovarian dysfunction
5. Decreased sperma-togenesis, libido, or impotence
6. Increased risk of endometrial cancer
7. Pelvis scarring and adhesions or infertility
8. Altered sexual response
9. Orchitis, sterility

Answer the following two questions on a separate sheet of paper.

28. Describe six of the physical changes that occur in a woman's body during climacteric and include the etiology of the physical change(s).

29. Discuss the difference between the terms *menopause* and *climacteric*.

30. State at least five causes of reproductive system dysfunction common to both males and females.

a. _____

b. _____

c. _____

d. _____

e. _____

31. Identify the different areas to be included in a geni-toreproductive nursing history.

a. _____

b. _____

c. _____

d. _____

e. _____

f. _____

32. State five nursing diagnoses most often associated with diagnostic assessment of the male or female reproductive system.

a. _____

b. _____

c. _____

d. _____

e. _____

STUDY GUIDE NUMBER 16.74

Interventions for Clients with Breast Disorders

Study/Review Questions

1. The nurse is teaching a 24-year-old client about breast self-examination (BSE). The nurse will tell her that BSE needs to be performed:
   a. The day before her menstrual flow is due.
   b. On the third day after her menstrual flow starts.
   c. When ovulation occurs.
   d. 1 week after her menstrual flow starts.

2. Your young female adult client is suspected of hav-ing breast cancer. Based on the nurse's knowledge of types and frequencies of breast cancer, which of the following types is this client most likely to be diagnosed as having?
   a. Adenocystic
   b. Infiltrating ductal carcinoma
   c. Invasive lobular
   d. In situ breast

3. Cancer surveillance in high-risk women involves BSE, clinical breast exam (CBE), and mammography. Cancer surveillance is used to detect cancer in its early stages and is referred to as:
   a. Primary prevention.
   b. Secondary prevention.
   c. Tertiary prevention.
   d. Prophylactic prevention.

4. A female client has returned from surgery for breast reconstruction. She has a Jackson-Pratt drain in place that is patent and draining serosanguineous fluid. The nurse notices that at 8:00 a.m. the drainage container is full. It was last emptied at 6:00 a.m. The total drainage for the last 2 hours is measured at 145 mL. Which of the following would be the priority nursing intervention?
   a. Notify the physician of the amount and type of drainage over the last 2 hours.
   b. Empty the drain every 2 hours so the suction will be more effective.
   c. Chart the type and amount of drainage.
   d. Report to the charge nurse that the night nurse really did not empty the drainage container.

5. Which of the following statements is true concerning fibrocystic breast disease?
   a. 70% of women will have fibrocystic changes sometime during their lives.
   b. A diet of low salt, no caffeine, and the addition of vitamins C, E, and B is recommended.
   c. Fibrocystic disease occurs in several stages, which are characterized by painless, fluid-filled cysts.
   d. Danazol is the drug of choice for treating all types of fibrocystic disease.

6. Current research has identified several risk factors for the development of breast cancer. According to the latest studies, which of the following women has the greatest risk of developing breast cancer?
   a. A physician, age 56, who had her first child at 38
   b. A ballet dancer, age 20, who has a 5-year-old son
   c. A radiation tech, age 24, who had her menarche at age 13
   d. A postmenopausal woman, age 52, who had breast reduction surgery at age 26

7. Which of the following best describes a modified radical mastectomy?
   a. Includes the removal of the involved breast and all of the axillary lymph nodes and chest muscles on the affected side
   b. Includes the removal of the breast tumor, all surrounding breast tissue, and axillary lymph nodes on the affected side
   c. Includes the removal of the breast tumor itself
   d. Includes the removal of the entire breast only on the affected side

8. A client had a partial mastectomy yesterday. The nurse writes on the nursing care plan: "Risk for Anxiety related to removal of breast tissue." The nurse's priority intervention would be to:
   a. Use distraction until the client is better and able to think more clearly.
   b. Encourage the client to have a positive attitude so she will heal faster.
   c. Ensure that the client takes her pain medicine every 4 to 6 ours as ordered.
   d. Encourage the client to discuss her fears and ask questions about her concerns.

9. When teaching a ambulatory surgery client discharge instructions regarding care of the arm on the affected side, the nurse will tell the client to be sure to:
   a. Start her arm exercises as soon as the drains are removed from the incision.
   b. Keep her arm elevated so that the elbow is above the shoulder, and wrist is above the elbow.
   c. Blood pressures cannot be taken in the arm on the affected side for the first 6 months postoperatively.
   d. Push-ups and arm circles are the exercises of choice for a full recovery.

10. A female client has been told that her breast tumor is 3 cm, non-fixed, with axillary metastasis. Based on this information, what stage of breast cancer is the most accurate one for this client?
    a. Stage I
    b. Stage II
    c. Stage III
    d. Stage IV

11. Which of the following factors will result in the least favorable prognosis for the above client?
    a. ER positive status of the cancer cells
    b. Accelerated growth rate of the cancer cells
    c. Well-differentiated tumor
    d. Low alteration of DNA content

12. This client's treatment choice in the above question will be based mainly on which of the following factors?
    a. Her age at the time of diagnosis
    b. Overall health status of client
    c. Her personal choice and type of insurance
    d. Extent and location of metastasis of the breast mass

13. The client's priority preoperative nursing diagnosis (in the above questions) will most probably be:
    a. Deficient Knowledge.
    b. Decisional Conflict.
    c. Fear.
    d. Anxiety.

14. Why is the mammogram the most sensitive screening tool presently available for early detection of breast cancer?
    a. It has a higher compliance rate than BSE because it is less painful.
    b. Radioimmunoassay to identify tumor markers is very expensive.
    c. It is able to reveal masses too small to be palpated manually.
    d. It is able to differentiate between fluid and solid masses.

15. The three-pronged approach to early detection of breast cancer is defined as:
    a. Breast self-examination, annual clinical breast examination, and ultrasound.
    b. Clinical breast examination, mammogram, and ultrasound.
    c. Mammogram, breast self-examination, and clinical breast examination.
    d. Breast self-examination, mammogram, and ultrasound.

16. Which of the following breast changes would the nurse be most likely to see during the physical examination of a client with late-stage breast cancer? *Check all that apply.*
    ____ a. Asymmetrical breast size
    ____ b. Orange-peel appearance of the skin
    ____ c. Skin dimpling with nipple retraction
    ____ d. Edema of the affected breast

17. The most common breast dysfunction found in the male breast is:
    a. Nipple discharge.
    b. Nipple retraction.
    c. Gynecomastia.
    d. Disseminated breast cancer.

18. A round, firm, non-tender, mobile breast mass not attached to breast tissue or the chest wall is usually associated with:
    a. Fibroadenomas.
    b. Fibrocystic disease.
    c. Breast cysts.
    d. Ductal ectasia.

19. The client's treatment plan (in the above question) will most likely include which of the following?
    a. Partial mastectomy
    b. Tamoxifen
    c. Radiotherapy
    d. All of the above

20. Metastasis from breast cancer is most likely to occur in the: *Check all that apply.*
    ____ a. Lungs
    ____ b. Liver
    ____ c. Bone
    ____ d. Brain

21. Which of the following interventions would be the nurse's priority in the nursing care plan for a client after a modified radical mastectomy?
    a. Position the client on the affected side to aid with gravity flow of drainage from the incision site.
    b. Immobilize the arm on the affected side for the first 24 hours postoperatively.
    c. Assess the client for anxiety as it has the possibility of impeding the healing process.
    d. Teach the client signs and symptoms of infection and how to monitor for altered wound healing.

22. Which of the following organizations is a community resource available to women with breast cancer?
    a. Reach to Recovery
    b. Empty Arms
    c. Resolve
    d. Nami

23. A woman's acceptance of her postoperative appearance is most likely to be affected by which of the following?
    a. Preoperative teaching of expected appearance of the scar
    b. Ability to discuss her feeling and concerns
    c. Response of her partner and family to her postoperative appearance
    d. Ability to camouflage her postoperative appearance

Read the following ten statements carefully and change the statements to make them true.

24. The incidence of breast disease is most closely related to weight.

25. Prophylactic mastectomy removes the woman's risk for developing breast cancer.

26. Women who teach themselves breast self-examination in the privacy of their own homes are more compliant with the performance of regular monthly exams.

27. Menopausal women need to perform breast self-exams the first day of every other month.

28. Fibroadenoma is the most common breast problem of women between the ages of 20 and 30.

29. Breast cancer has the highest death rate for women between the ages of 25 and 40 years.

30. *Chemoprevention* is another name for chemotherapy, following a partial mastectomy.

31. Small-breasted women are at an increased risk for fungal infections and backaches.

32. Ductal ectasia is associated with a non-palpable mass and a serosanguineous nipple discharge.

33. The TRAM flap is a frequently used method of reconstructive surgery that involves the use of silicon gel implants.

34. On a separate sheet of paper, compare and contrast a benign breast nodule to a malignant breast nodule on physical examination of the breast.

35. Identify five steps to assessing a breast mass.
    a. _____
    b. _____
    c. _____
    d. _____
    e. _____

Answer the following two questions on a separate sheet of paper.

36. Discuss four aspects of discharge home teaching in relation to physical care necessary for a positive postoperative course after a modified radical mastectomy.

37. Identify six instructions necessary for the nurse to teach a woman before having her demonstrate a breast self-examination.

STUDY GUIDE NUMBER 16.75

Interventions for Clients with Gynecologic Problems

Study/Review Questions

1. One current treatment of primary dysmenorrhea with a therapeutic intervention of medication mainly includes the use of:
   a. MAOIs.
   b. Beta blockers.
   c. NSAIDs.
   d. Prostaglandin stimulators.

2. The woman at greatest risk for having premenstrual syndrome is one who is:
   a. 26 years old with her first child.
   b. 35 years old with no children.
   c. 32 years old whose father died 6 months ago.
   d. A 34-year-old mother of four with a recent postpartum tubal ligation.

3. A female client, age 36, has been having hot flashes, crying spells, and mood swings. Her physician wants to put her on hormone replacement therapy for her perimenopausal symptoms. The nurse realizes that this client's age means that she is experiencing menopause at a(n):
   a. Early onset.
   b. Late onset.
   c. Normal time frame.
   d. Undetermined time.

4. Hormone replacement therapy increases this client's (see the above question) risk of:
   a. Breast cancer.
   b. Heart attack.
   c. Deep vein thrombosis.
   d. Osteoporosis.

5. A client is diagnosed with vaginitis as the cause of her vaginal itching and discharge. The nurse is aware that a primary cause of vaginitis is:
   a. Antibiotics.
   b. Swimming.
   c. Wiping front to back.
   d. Inappropriate clothing.

6. Which of the following is a treatment choice for vulvitis, which is caused by a nonpathologic condition?
   a. Vaginal creams
   b. Analgesics
   c. Sitz baths
   d. Antibiotics

7. The antigenic organism involved in toxic shock syndrome is:
   a. *Escherichia coli.*
   b. *Staphylococcus aureus.*
   c. *Haemophilus influenzae.*
   d. Beta-hemolytic *Streptococcus.*

8. A nurse is teaching a group of teenagers about risk factors and toxic shock syndrome. The nurse will teach the class that women are at an increased risk for toxic shock syndrome if they:
   a. Use tampons that are highly absorbent.
   b. Use tampons that have hard, stiff coverings for insertion.
   c. Use tampons through out their menstrual flow.
   d. All of the above

9. Which of the following symptoms would the nurse expect to observe in a woman with toxic shock syndrome?
   a. Hypertension and rash
   b. Sore throat and swollen lymph nodes
   c. Rash and chills
   d. Headache and constipation

10. The most common complaint reported of women with uterine leiomyomas (fibroids) is which of the following?
    a. Vaginal pressure and fullness
    b. Abnormal bleeding
    c. Intermittent pain
    d. Urinary dysfunction

11. Risk factors associated with cancer of the cervix include:
    a. _____
    b. _____
    c. _____

12. Bartholin's cysts are commonly treated by which of the following procedures? *Check all that apply.*
    ___ a. Incision and drainage
    ___ b. Excision of the glands
    ___ c. Marsupialization
    ___ d. Radiation

13. A woman recovering from repair of a cystocele should be taught which of the following?
    a. To perform perineal floor exercises
    b. To take sitz baths three times a day
    c. To perform povidone-iodine douches every other day
    d. To take bedrest for the first 6 weeks

14. The priority nursing diagnosis commonly seen preoperatively as well as postoperatively in a woman with leiomyomas is:
    a. Risk for Infection.
    b. Acute Pain.
    c. Risk for Altered Tissue Perfusion.
    d. Anxiety.

15. The treatment of choice for a symptomatic postmenopausal woman with recurring uterine leiomyomas would be:
    a. Myomectomy.
    b. Hysterectomy.
    c. Hormone replacement therapy.
    d. Anterior-posterior repair.

16. Discharge teaching for the woman after having a total abdominal hysterectomy includes which of the following?
    a. May resume sexual activity, usually in 2 to 3 weeks if the incision has healed
    b. Pain will decrease in about 2 to 3 days but may last for up to 6 weeks
    c. Daily exercise such as walking is encouraged after the first 6 weeks
    d. Wound care to include showering, but no baths

17. A client reports bleeding between her menstrual periods. This type of bleeding is defined as:
    a. Dysmenorrhea.
    b. Menorrhagia.
    c. Metrorrhagia.
    d. Polyrrhea.

18. A client suffering from postmenopausal vaginal dryness can use _____ to decrease sexual discomfort related to intercourse.
    a. Motrin
    b. Water-soluble gel
    c. Vaseline jelly
    d. Gel spermicide

19. Which is the most common symptom found to occur in women diagnosed as having endometrial cancer?
    a. Pelvic pain
    b. Nausea and anorexia
    c. Dysfunctional uterine bleeding
    d. Vaginal discharge

20. The nurse is giving instructions to a woman who is going to have intracavity radiation therapy (IRT). The nurse's postprocedure instructions should include which of the following?
    a. Bedrest with bathroom privileges only
    b. Maintain Trendelenburg position
    c. No visitors for 2 weeks
    d. Provision of a low-residue diet

21. A woman with complaints of abdominal pain and swelling, along with gastrointestinal disturbances, is generally diagnosed with which type of reproductive cancer?
    a. Endometrial
    b. Cervical
    c. Ovarian
    d. Vaginal

22. Amenorrhea can be the result of several physiologic and pathologic etiologies. Which of the following etiologies is characteristic of a pathologic state which causes unusual hair growth in addition to the amenorrhea?
    a. Anorexia nervosa
    b. Pregnancy with lactation
    c. Menopausal climacteria
    d. Polycystic ovarian disease

Read the following ten statements carefully and change the statements to make them true.

23. The physiologic factor thought to be the etiologic cause of dysmenorrhea is the increased production of gonadotropin-releasing hormone.

24. The major reason for the onset of menopause and resulting atrophy of the vulvar organs is a decrease in the hormonal levels of follicle-stimulating hormone.

25. The most common and most serious cause of postmenopausal bleeding is atrophic vaginitis.

26. Endometriosis is the precursor to endometrial cancer.

27. Dysfunctional uterine bleeding can occur in perimenopausal women and is treated with a hysterectomy.

28. Corpus luteum cysts occur in young menstruating women and do not grow without hormonal influence.

29. Treatment of uterine cancer may be a cystectomy or depression of ovulation.

30. The rarest of all gynecologic cancers, occurring mainly in women over the age of 50, is vaginal cancer.

31. Depression from Altered Body Image, Altered Sexual Functioning, or the diagnosis of advanced cancer, peaks 2 to 3 weeks after surgery.

32. Laser therapy is another treatment for CIN that causes freezing of the tissues and subsequent necrosis.

33. Match each of the following terms to the corresponding definition.

    Terms

    ___ a. Uterine prolapse
    ___ b. Polycystic ovary
    ___ c. Cystocele
    ___ d. Ovarian fibroma
    ___ e. Urethrovaginal
    ___ f. Dermoid cyst
    ___ g. Fibroid
    ___ h. Rectocele
    ___ i. Theca-lutein cyst
    ___ j. Polyp
    ___ k. Chocolate cyst
    ___ l. Bartholin's cyst

    Definitions

    1. Area of endometriosis inside of an ovary
    2. Protrusion of the bladder through the vaginal wall
    3. Results in leakage of urine into the vagina
    4. Ovarian cyst associated with a molar pregnancy
    5. Protrusion of the rectum through the vaginal wall
    6. Most common ovarian cyst of childhood
    7. A common disorder of the vulva
    8. Condition associated with weakened pelvic floor muscles and a full feeling in the vagina
    9. Ovarian cyst which causes endometrial hyperplasia
    10. Most common benign tumor, which can be very large and often occurs in post-menopausal women
    11. Most common slow-growing pelvic tumor
    12. Most common benign neoplastic growth of the cervix

34. On a separate sheet of paper, discuss primary dysmenorrhea, including its etiology and how it differs from secondary dysmenorrhea.

35. State four preventative treatment therapies for primary dysmenorrhea.
    a. _____
    b. _____
    c. _____
    d. _____

36. Identify eight major symptoms associated with premenstrual syndrome.
    a. _____
    b. _____
    c. _____
    d. _____
    e. _____
    f. _____
    g. _____
    h. _____

37. On a separate sheet of paper, compare primary amenorrhea to secondary amenorrhea. Include the etiology and fertility prognosis for both disorders.

38. Identify the most common methods of treating cancer of the reproductive organs.
    a. _____
    b. _____
    c. _____
    d. _____
    e. _____

39. Postoperative nursing diagnoses for cancers of the reproductive tract are similar. Identify eight of these priority nursing diagnoses and collaborative problems.
    a. _____
    b. _____
    c. _____
    d. _____
    e. _____
    f. _____
    g. _____
    h. _____

Case Study: The Client with a Gynecologic Health Problem

Your 32-year-old female client has noticed that she and her husband seem to quarrel more often about a week before her menstrual flow starts. Also, she has increased headaches and weight gain during this time. She is going to see the doctor today because her husband said she was impossible to live with during this time and needed help.

Answer the following questions:

1. Based on the above information, what diagnosis is most appropriate for this client?
   a. Primary dysmenorrhea
   b. Endometriosis
   c. Depression
   d. Premenstrual syndrome

2. Which treatment option would be best for the client at this time to help her deal with the above diagnosis?
   a. Referral to join a support group
   b. Talking to her pastor
   c. Recording a complete diet history
   d. Education on the physiologic basis of her symptoms

3. Which foods will the nurse advise the client to avoid?
   a. Foods with vitamins B_6 and calcium
   b. Coffee and chocolate
   c. Steak and potatoes
   d. Sweet tea and spaghetti

4. What other recommendations would be helpful to the client to eliminate her uncomfortable symptoms?
   a. Mild diuretics
   b. NSAIDs
   c. Progesterone
   d. All of the above

Case Study: The Client with Endometriosis

Your female client is a 26-year-old nullipara who has recently married. One day she wants to have children, but right now she is really worried because sexual intercourse is very painful. She has come to the clinic for a checkup.

Answer the following questions:

1. Which of the following questions is most important for the nurse to ask this client at this time?
   a. Has sexual intercourse always been painful?
   b. Do you have a vaginal discharge?
   c. What other symptoms have you been experiencing?
   d. Is there a history of cancer in your family?

2. The client tells the nurse she is afraid she is not going to be able to get pregnant and she is nervous about the tests. The nurse knows that the key diagnostic test for endometriosis is:
   a. Tissue biopsy.
   b. Ultrasound.
   c. Serology tests.
   d. Pelvic exam.

3. The priority nursing diagnosis for this client at this time would be:
   a. Acute Pain.
   b. Anxiety.
   c. Ineffective Coping.
   d. Sexual Dysfunction.

4. This client is diagnosed with endometriosis. The current choice for nonsurgical treatment of endometriosis is:
   a. Pseudo-pregnancy.
   b. Medical oophorectomy.
   c. Pregnancy.
   d. Ovarian suppression.

STUDY GUIDE NUMBER 16.76

Interventions for Male Clients with Reproductive Problems

Study/Review Questions

1. Which symptom would help in differentiating BPH, an obstructive dysfunction, from infection, a nonobstructive dysfunction?
   a. Hesitancy with voiding
   b. Post-void dribbling
   c. Decreased force of stream
   d. All of the above

2. Factors contributing to the development of prostate cancer are:
   a. Family history, age less than 40, and sexually transmitted diseases (STDs).
   b. Advancing age, diet, and history of cytomegalovirus infections.
   c. History of STDs, chicken pox, and decreasing testosterone levels.
   d. Advancing age, family history, and history of STDs

3. Prostate-specific antigen (PSA) is a glycoprotein produced solely by the prostate. After treatment for prostate cancer, an elevated PSA level can be used to indicate:
   a. Recurrence of the prostate cancer.
   b. Responsiveness to cancer therapy.
   c. Presence of a malignancy elsewhere in the body.
   d. *a* and *b*

4. Which is the most common site for the metastasis of prostate cancer?
   a. Bone
   b. Lungs
   c. Liver
   d. Stomach

5. Clients with metastasis of their prostate cancer to the bone usually have an elevated level of:
   a. Alpha fetoprotein
   b. BUN
   c. Serum alkaline phosphatase
   d. Serum creatinine

6. Inflammation of the testicles associated with the occurrence of mumps in the postpubertal male is:
   a. Prostatitis.
   b. Epididymitis.
   c. Orchitis.
   d. Urethritis.

7. Which clinical manifestation is common to both orchitis and epididymitis?
   a. Scrotal pain and hematuria
   b. Scrotal pain and edema
   c. Scrotal edema and dysuria
   d. Scrotal edema and impotence

8. Your adult male client had a prostatectomy earlier this morning. He has a Foley catheter with a continuous bladder irrigation. The nurse would expect his urinary drainage to be:
   a. Light pink with small clots.
   b. Bright red with small clots.
   c. Dark burgundy with no clots.
   d. No drainage for the first 24 hours.

9. Erectile dysfunction is commonly treated using all of the following *except*:
   a. Oral therapies.
   b. Prostheses.
   c. Vacuum devices.
   d. Anticholinergics.

10. Newly married at age 28, your male client has been performing testicular self-examinations since he was 16. He presents today because of a change in the size of his right testicle. Which of the following statements given to him by the nurse is correct information?
    a. Testicular cancer is always bilateral.
    b. Testicular cancer occurs most often in African-American men over age 25 years.
    c. An elevated alpha-fetoprotein level is used as a tumor marker for testicular cancer.
    d. An elevated alpha-fetoprotein level indicates metastatic disease of the testicular cancer.

11. The nurse would expect a client diagnosed with prostatitis to report which of the following symptoms?
    a. Hematuria and dysuria
    b. Urethral discharge
    c. Fever and chills
    d. All of the above

12. The etiology of testicular cancer is still unknown, but the risk for developing a testicular tumor is reported to be higher in males who have a history of:
    a. Hypospadias.
    b. Recurrent urinary tract infections (UTIs).
    c. Cryptorchidism.
    d. Orchitis.

13. During the first 24 hours after prostatectomy, the nursing care plan would include the priority assessment for:
    a. Hemorrhage.
    b. Risk for infection.
    c. Risk for pneumonia.
    d. Altered level of consciousness.

14. An adult male client had surgery for his benign prostatic hyperplasia. He cannot remember the type of surgery but tells you he has no incision. As a nurse, you know that this client had a:
    a. Suprapubic prostatectomy.
    b. Perineal prostatectomy.
    c. Retropubic prostatectomy.
    d. Transurethral resection.

15. Which of the following nursing interventions can the nurse recommend to a client diagnosed with prostatitis?
    a. Take a stool softener to prevent straining.
    b. Take pain medications to prevent pain as needed.
    c. Use comfort measures to provide pain relief, such as sitz baths.
    d. Use bladder antispasmodics to relieve bladder pain.

Change the word(s) in italics to make the following statements true.

16. Benign prostatic hyperplasia is thought to result primarily from a *local* hormonal alteration in which *diet* is a major contributing factor.

17. The *perineal* approach is the most common type of closed procedure used for a prostatectomy.

18. *Prostatic* cancer is the most common malignancy in men ages 15 to 35 years.

19. A differential diagnosis is made between organic erectile dysfunction and functional erectile dysfunction by the presence of *diurnal* erections.

20. The least used open-surgical approach for a prostatectomy associated with an increased incidence of impotency is a *retropubic* approach.

21. *Prostatic impotence* dysfunction is characterized by a gradual decrease in firmness of the penis and a decrease in the frequency of erections.

22. *Amicar* is ordered to control painful bladder spasms after a prostatectomy.

23. Sexual activity can usually resume postprostatectomy in about *4 to 6* months.

24. Match each of the following terms with the corresponding fact. *One answer will be used more than once.*

Terms	Facts
___ a. Spermatocele	1. Results from a disorder in the lymphatic drainage of the scrotum, causing a mass around the testis
___ b. Orchidopexy	
___ c. Hydrocele	
___ d. Phimosis	
___ e. Varicocele	
___ f. Cryptorchidism	2. Uncontrolled penile erection without sexual desire which is very painful
___ g. Penectomy	
___ h. Circumcision	
___ i. Testicular torsion	
___ j. Scrotal support	3. Surgical implantation of the testicle into the scrotal sac
___ k. Priapism	4. Increased risk of suicide after this procedure
___ l. Prostatitis	
	5. Inflammation can result from a viral or bacterial infection, STD, or a psychosexual problem

6. If not done at birth, requires strict personal hygiene to clean the prepuce
7. Very painful, and is a medical emergency
8. Palpation reveals a "worm-like" mass
9. Usually requires no intervention unless the client reports discomfort
10. Promotes drainage and comfort after surgery
11. Corrected by circumcision
12. Surgery for this condition may reduce the risk of testicular cancer

25. Prostate cancer is diagnosed by a combination of which two tests?
   a. _____
   b. _____

26. State five approaches for the medical treatment of prostate cancer.
   a. _____
   b. _____
   c. _____
   d. _____
   e. _____

27. Identify six common causes of organic erectile dysfunction.
   a. _____
   b. _____
   c. _____
   d. _____
   e. _____
   f. _____

28. Identify four common causes of priapism.
   a. _____
   b. _____
   c. _____
   d. _____

29. State three nursing diagnoses associated with male reproductive dysfunctions.
   a. _____
   b. _____
   c. _____

30. State four effects of benign prostatic hypertrophy on urinary elimination.
   a. _____
   b. _____
   c. _____
   d. _____

STUDY GUIDE NUMBER 16.77

Interventions for Clients with Sexually Transmitted Diseases

Study/Review Questions

1. Which of the following is not a complication associated with sexually transmitted diseases (STDs)?
   a. Infertility
   b. Miscarriage
   c. Cancer
   d. Respiratory infections

2. Syphilis is a disease with several stages. A client with central nervous system involvement, including hearing loss, would be diagnosed with what stage of syphilis?
   a. Primary
   b. Secondary
   c. Late-tertiary
   d. Latent-early

3. The medication of choice for treating any stage of syphilis is:
   a. Penicillin-G.
   b. Glucocorticoids.
   c. Amoxicillin.
   d. Tetracycline.

4. Which of the following would *not* be included in a nursing assessment of the client with symptoms of an STD?
   a. Risk assessment with sexual history
   b. Prior testing or treatment for STDs
   c. Allergies to medications
   d. Reason for last hospitalization

5. Blood tests are often used to diagnose syphilis. Which would be the screening test?
   a. ELISA serum test
   b. VDRL serum test
   c. FTA antibody test
   d. MHA assay test

6. Martha has had genital herpes–HSV-2 for several years. She is at the clinic for her annual Papanicolaou smear and asks about long-term problems. The nurse's best response is based on the knowledge that HSV-2 infection is associated with:
   a. Pelvic inflammatory disease.
   b. Vaginitis.
   c. Cervical cancer.
   d. Fetal infection.

7. After being hospitalized for genital herpes, a female client is repeating discharge instructions to the nurse. The nurse knows that further teaching is necessary when she states:
   a. "I can be contagious even when I do not have any lesions."
   b. "If I get pregnant I need to tell my nurse midwife that I have genital herpes."
   c. "After taking all of my acyclovir, I will not have genital herpes anymore."
   d. "I need to have an annual Pap smear because of my increased risk for cervical cancer."

8. The medication of choice in the treatment of lymphogranuloma venereum is:
   a. Doxycycline.
   b. Penicillin-G.
   c. Gentamycin.
   d. Acyclovir.

9. The medication of choice in the treatment of chancroid is:
   a. Zithromax.
   b. Rocephin.
   c. Erythromycin.
   d. All of the above

10. Many STDs involve genital lesions at the site of inoculation. A definitive diagnosis for granuloma inguinale is made from a cytologic smear from the ulcer and reveals the presence of:
    a. Koplik spots.
    b. Barr bodies.
    c. Janeway lesions.
    d. Donovan bodies.

11. Which of the following statements concerning sexually transmitted genital warts is true?
    a. Biopsy is not necessary for diagnosis because the lesion has a characteristic fern appearance.
    b. Treatment for genital warts must be on an inpatient basis and involves surgical removal of the lesions.
    c. The client must keep the genital area clean and dry and observe for secondary infections.
    d. Repeated treatments are not necessary once the external lesions are healed.

12. Complications of gonorrhea develop more often in women than in men because:
    a. Treatment for the disease can leave women infertile.
    b. The disease is asymptomatic in the early stages.
    c. Estrogen leaves the woman more resistant to antibiotic therapy.
    d. The disease is not curable in women.

13. The incubation period for gonorrhea is usually:
    a. 3 to 10 days.
    b. 10 to 14 days.
    c. 2 to 3 weeks.
    d. 2 to 3 months.

14. Gonorrhea is an STD that involves the mucosal surface. Symptomatic manifestations can include: *Check all that apply.*
    ___ a. Anal irritation and bleeding.
    ___ b. Pharyngeal infections and sore throat.
    ___ c. Vaginal discharge and dysuria.
    ___ d. Chancre-type skin lesions.

15. Which is *not* a clinical manifestation of a chlamydial infection in men?
    a. Dysuria with voiding
    b. Urethritis
    c. Frequency of urination
    d. Thick green discharge

16. When obtaining a complete OB-GYN history, the nurse must also take a sexual history from the client. The nurse's most therapeutic intervention to elicit information would be to:
    a. Use a checklist to ask "yes" and "no" questions.
    b. Ask the client if there is anything she needs to tell you about her sexual history.
    c. Ask directly if the client has ever had an STD.
    d. Ask open-ended questions.

17. In order for the nurse to be an effective clinician when working with clients concerning sexuality, STDs, or other sexual concerns, the nurse must first:
    a. Take a course on sexual relations and counseling.
    b. Know all about his or her client's concerns, problems, or needs.
    c. Be aware of his or her own sexual values, attitudes, and sexuality.
    d. Set up a meeting with the client's sexual partner.

18. A female client has an appointment today with her GYN physician because of a troublesome vaginal discharge. The discharge is diagnosed as trichomoniasis, and the client is given oral medication to treat the infection. The nurse will teach this client which of the following about the medication and her vaginal infection?
    a. The *Trichomonas vaginalis* is self-limiting, but the medicine is needed to treat the vaginal itching.
    b. The client's sexual partner must be treated with the medication if the infection is to be resolved.
    c. The medication should be applied liberally to the external genitalia once a day.
    d. The vaginal infection can cause infertility in childbearing women.

19. An adult female has been admitted to the GYN floor with a diagnosis of pelvic inflammatory disease (PID). The nurse will carefully assess this client for complications because women with PID are at an increased risk for:
    a. Ovarian rupture.
    b. Appendicitis.
    c. Infertility.
    d. STDs.

20. The number one causative agent associated with PID is known to be:
    a. *Neisseria gonorrhea.*
    b. *Escherichia coli.*
    c. *Streptococcus* species.
    d. *Chlamydia* species.

21. The nurse knows that the client's (see Question 19) chief complaint that led her to seek medical health was probably:
    a. Vaginal itching.
    b. Lower abdominal pain.
    c. Malaise with fever.
    d. Abnormal menstrual flow.

22. The activity orders for the above client are for bedrest with bathroom privileges. What position is best for her while on bedrest?
    a. Prone position
    b. Supine position
    c. Side-lying position
    d. Semi-Fowler's position

23. The above client is discharged home on oral antibiotics. The nurse should give her which of the following instructions regarding her monthly menstrual flow?
    a. Use tampons only when your menstrual flow is heavy.
    b. Follow your normal routine for using tampons unless the pain increases.
    c. Use perineal pads until you are fully recovered.
    d. Use tampons in the day and perineal pads at night.

24. When performing discharge teaching about the resumption of sexual relations to a client diagnosed with an STD, the nurse should teach the client which of the following?
    a. Sexual relations may be resumed, but she must douche within 24 hours after vaginal intercourse.
    b. Sexual relations are prohibited for 6 months.
    c. Sexual relations should be postponed until the treatment regimen is completed.
    d. Sexual relations are permitted unless there is an increase in abdominal pain.

Change the following six statements about PID to make them true.

25. The use of vaginal douches decreases a woman's risk for developing PID.

26. A woman diagnosed with PID usually has a brown vaginal discharge.

27. Pain associated with PID is relieved by ambulation.

28. Women at risk for PID are not at risk for STDs.

29. The diagnosis of PID can be made solely on the basis of an elevated WBC.

30. PID is easily diagnosed, but is very hard to treat.

31. Match each of the following STDs with the corresponding definition.

Sexually Transmitted Diseases

___ a. Herpes simplex type 2
___ b. Secondary syphilis
___ c. Lymphogranuloma venereum
___ d. Herpes genitalis
___ e. Genital warts
___ f. Primary syphilis
___ g. Granuloma inguinale
___ h. Gonorrhea
___ i. Chancroid
___ j. Chlamydia
___ k. Hepatitis B
___ l. Candida

Definitions

1. Highly infectious state with the presence of a chancre
2. An infection limited to the vagina; very irritating, but has no long-term sequelae
3. The herpes virus responsible for the majority of genital and perianal lesions
4. Transmitted by direct sexual contact with mucosal surfaces and can be transmitted to the vaginally delivered neonate
5. Transient painless lesion that gives rise to secondary signs of infection as headache, malaise, or anorexia
6. Can lead to chronic disease state; vaccines are given as three injections over a period of 6 months
7. Most common sexually transmitted viral disease caused by the human papillomavirus (HPV)
8. Flu-like symptoms and a generalized rash
9. Nodules that ulcerate, grow together, and become a spreading ulcer, which can become mutilating
10. Most common STD in the United States
11. Genital lesions that are painful and bleed easily; known cofactor for HIV transmission
12. Initial infection causes blisters, which rupture and cause painful lesions

32. State four methods for the transmission of organisms that cause STD.
    a. _____
    b. _____
    c. _____
    d. _____

33. Identify four reasons why women have more health problems associated with STDs than men.
    a. _____
       _____
    b. _____
       _____
    c. _____
       _____
    d. _____
       _____

34. Pregnant women are routinely screened for which STDs that can have devastating effects on the fetus or neonate?
    a. _____
    b. _____
    c. _____
    d. _____

35. On a separate sheet of paper, discuss four important facts about the treatment of gonorrheal infections the client needs to know before being released from treatment.

36. State four goals for the treatment of a client with genital herpes.
    a. _____
    b. _____
    c. _____
    d. _____

37. On a separate sheet of paper, describe six nursing responsibilities associated with the management of a client who is newly diagnosed with an STD.

ANSWER KEY

Critical Thinking in the Role of the Medical-Surgical Nurse

1. Level of knowledge, philosophic theories, and cultural and religious beliefs
2. The holistic view of health considers the body, mind, and spirit to be interrelated parts of a person's being. It focuses on promoting health and preventing illness with an emphasis on personal responsibility to achieve high level of wellness. The sociologic perspective views health as a condition that allows for the pursuit and enjoyment of desired cultural values and includes the ability to carry out normal daily activities.
3. Homeostasis implies an unchanging state and most theorists believe that health is always changing.
4. *Biologic* encompasses the structure of body tissues, organs, biochemical interactions and functions within the body. *Psychologic* includes a person's mood, emotions, and personality. *Sociologic* involves the interaction between a person and environment.
5. Increase quality and years of healthy life and eliminate health disparities among different demographic groups in the United States.
6. • Eating three well-balanced meals a day • Eating in moderation • Regular and moderate exercise • Regular sleep in sufficient quantity • Moderate alcohol consumption • No smoking • Minimal exposure to the sun.
7. a. 2; b. 3; c. 1; d. 1; e. 2; f. 2
8. a. 4; b. 3; c. 2; d. 3; e. 1; f. 6; g. 1; h. 2; i. 1; j. 4; k. 6; l. 5
9. Critical thinking or judgment is an essential competency that all nurses need to provide quality, cost-effective client care. When these judgments are based on standards and research, and not on guess-work, it is evidence-based practice or tradition.
10. Client's willingness to learn, receptiveness, educational level, socioeconomic level, support system, age, and cultural considerations.
11. c
12. She is an African-American female.
13. Hospitals, nursing schools, occupational health settings, community health settings, physician's offices, long-term facilities, self-employment (private duty)
14. Critical care units, intermediate or specialty units, long-term units (including subacute units)
15. c
16. • Assessment • Analysis (nursing diagnosis) • Planning • Implementation • Evaluation
17. a
18. Collaborative problems are physiologic complications that nurses monitor, in collaboration with the primary care provider, to detect onset of or changes in a client's status. A nursing diagnosis identifies actual or potential health problems that are able to be treated.
19. d
20. b
21. • Setting priorities and outcomes • Selecting nursing interventions • Determining resources
22. b
23. a. 3; b. 4; c. 1; d. 2
24. b
25. • The client responded as expected. (No additional nursing actions needed.) • Client behaviors indicate no resolution. Outcomes are accomplished but long-term goal not met. (Re-evaluation will continue.) • Client behaviors are similar to those presented initially, no evidence that problem has resolved. (Reassessment and re-planning are indicated.) • Client behaviors indicate new problem. (Assessment, planning, and implementation of an additional plan of action are needed to resolve the problem.)
26. • Write clearly and legibly. Do not erase or white out any part of a client's record. • Use only standard (facility-approved) abbreviations and symbols. • Document significant information as close as possible to the time it is collected. • Transcribe physician's orders carefully and correctly, time and date each entry. Use only blue or black ink. • State facts objectively, avoiding judgments. • Do not refer to any unusual occurrence or report, if the entry is more than a day late, and then state reason.
27. a. Client will eat 2000 cal/daily and to achieve a weight of 125 pounds.
    b. Client will sleep continuously for 6 hours a night without waking.
    c. Client will be able to swallow food intake without episodes of choking.

Community-Based Care

1. Health promotion, health protection, short-term treatment, and follow-up for existing health problems

2. • Physician's offices • Hospital clinics • Freestanding clinics • Surgicenters • Health maintenance organizations
3. • Client education • Health screening • Comprehensive assessment
4. Increased acceptance by the medical and consumer community, a continued shift from inpatient care to community-based and home care, increased technology, lower cost of home care, the increase in managed care that dictates lower cost alternatives, the older adult population and an increased need for health care for elders, and more involvement of educated consumers.
5. c
6. *Home setting*: Nurse is more autonomous and must know which services are reimbursed and document care accordingly and must know about caring for all types and ages of clients. The setting is controlled by the client and there is limited ability for direct supervision of assistive staff. *Inpatient setting:* Nurse relies heavily on physician directives. This environment is controlled by facility and staff. Nurses commonly care for specific types of clients and can have continuous direct supervision of assistive staff. Reimbursement issues are handled by the hospital business office.
7. a
8. c
9. b
10. a, d, e
11. Immediate access to information, ability to access information from many areas, reduced redundancy in entering data.
12. • Resulted in uniform data to track outcomes • Permits comparison to similar agencies • Provides a method for improving client care
13. Clients are discharged from the hospital "quicker and sicker" and/or have complex care needs.
14. a, c, b, d
15. a, c, e

STUDY GUIDE NUMBER 1.3

Introduction to Managed Care and Case Management

1. a
2. In the fee-for-service arrangement, health care providers were paid based on their charges with the financial risk taken by the insurance companies. In the capitated reimbursement system, providers receive a uniform amount of money for each client, and the providers share in the financial risks.
3. achieve client outcomes while managing health care costs.

4. c
5. b
6. b
7. Certified Case Manager (CCM), Certified Disability Management Specialist, CDMS, Certified Rehabilitation Registered Nurse (CCRN), Certified Occupational Health Nurse, (A-CCC), Certified Vocation Evaluator (CVE), Masters Addiction Counselor (MAC), Certified Life Care Planner (CLCP) *(Answer can be any three of these listed.)*
8. a. Assesses, collects data, conducts case screening, identifies support systems, reviews history and determines current health care needs, obtains approvals for contracts. b. Identifies services and funding options, reviews plan for consensus, advocates for client as need, develops plan of care as indicated. c. Communicates regularly with clients and support systems, coordinates treatment plan, promotes coordinated and efficient care, identifies needs for additional services. d. Assesses benefit value to cost and value to quality of life, reviews plan for continuity of care, evaluates satisfaction and compliance with treatment plan. e. Records services and outcomes, submits reports and other documentation as needed
9. • To provide quality health care along a continuum of care • To decrease fragmentation and duplication of care across many health care settings • To enhance the client's quality of life • To increase cost containment through appropriate use of resources
10. clinical, utilization
11. The purpose is to keep clients with chronic conditions as healthy as possible in the community.
12. Collaborative plan of care (POC); multidisciplinary action plan (MAP)

STUDY GUIDE NUMBER 1.4

Introduction to Complimentary and Alternative Therapies

1. Traditional medicine focuses on the treatment of illness, while complementary and alternative therapies focus on the mind-body-spirit connection.
2. a. 1; b. 4; c. 5; d. 9; e. 2; f. 6; g. 3; h. 8; i. 10; j. 7
3. Spirituality exists as part of all people and gives meaning to a person. Religion is a belief system and worship style that is selected by a person.
4. a, b, d, f
5. • Progressive muscle relaxation • Imagery • Music therapy
6. Your client's cultural and age considerations.
7. b, c, d
8. Herbs can interfere with prescription medications and cause toxic or other adverse reactions.

9. Health professionals need to learn more about complementary therapies as research becomes available and incorporate low-risk therapies into the educational programs.

STUDY GUIDE NUMBER 1.5

Health Care of Older Adults

1. a, b, c
2. • Reorient the client frequently to his or her location • Explain all procedures and routines to the client before they occur • Provide opportunities for the client to assist in decision-making • Encourage the client's family and friends to visit often • Establish a trusting relationship with client as soon as possible
3. a, d, e
4. c
5. • Decreased falls • Increased strength • Reduced arthritis pain • Reduced depression • Increased longevity • Reduced risks for diabetes and coronary artery disease
6. b, c, d
7. • History of falls • Major visual impairments • Generalized weakness or decreased mobility • Confusion or disorientation • Communication impairments
8. b
9. a, d
10. b
11. a. 1; b. 4; c. 2; d. 3
12. • Vomiting • Nausea • Dizziness • Weakness • Diarrhea • Confusion • Constipation • Anorexia • Edema
13. a, b, d
14. • They may not understand the correct way to take their medications. • They may take too much or too little medication because of attitudes or feelings about relying on medications. • They may not remember to take their medications.
15. a
16. a, b, d
17. Dementia is a progressive decline in mental status resulting in impaired orientation, memory and judgment, and intellectual functioning. Depression may be a response to multiple life stresses, or may be a primary behavioral health problem that can be managed effectively if correctly diagnosed. Clients with dementia may also become depressed.
18. a
19. • Increasing expenses • Special housing requirements • Declining financial resources • Rising health costs • Rising food costs
20. a. 3; b. 4; c. 1; d. 2

Case Study

Answers provided on the SIMON website: http://www.wbsaunders.com/SIMON/Iggy/

STUDY GUIDE NUMBER 2.6

Cultural Aspects of Health

1. c
2. d
3. a
4. h
5. f
6. g
7. b
8. e
9. Observation, interview, participation. See text for examples.
10. Any two of the following: trips to local churches, trips to ethnic festivals, observing political rallies, visiting community markets, visiting, and eating a meal in a private home in the community.
11. Disabled individuals, individuals with sexual orientations out of the mainstream.
12. True
13. True
14. False. 27% in 2000. Estimated to be 43.8% by 2050.
15. True
16. False. People will have diverse needs.
17. True
18. False. Manifestations of pain vary greatly among and within cultures.
19. False. Time perspective varies among cultures.
20. b
21. a
22. d
23. Cultural competence
24. Any of the following: arrange visiting for client's support system, have staff members learn key phrases in American Sign Language, recognize that facial expressions are another means of communication

Case Study

Answers provided on the SIMON website: http://www.wbsaunders.com/SIMON/Iggy/

STUDY GUIDE NUMBER 2.7

Pain: The Fifth Vital Sign

1. a. True; b. True; c. False. There have been only slight improvements in pain management. d. True; e. False. It varies from person to person.
2. a. 3; b. 2; c. 3; d. 1; e. 2; f. 2; g. 3; h. 1
3. d. Pain is controlled at the level of the spinal cord (gate) so that for pain to be perceived, the stimulus must first be transmitted to the spinal cord then to the brain. (See Figure 7-1.)
4. nociceptors

5. • Superficial receptors in the skin and subcutaneous tissue • Deep somatic receptors in bone, blood vessels, muscles, and connective tissue • Visceral receptors in body organs

6. a. Pain confined to the site of origin. b. Pain along a specific nerve or nerves c. Diffuse pain around the site of origin that is not well localized.

   d. Pain perceived in an area away from the site of painful stimulation. It occurs because the visceral fibers converge (synapse) in the spinal cord close to the fibers that innervate other subcutaneous tissues. (See Figure 7-2.)

7. Neuropathic pain is perceived pain even though there is no obvious physiologic cause. It is difficult to relieve with analgesics. It can be described as shooting, stabbing, or a burning sensation; painful numbness; or sharp pain that often radiates.

8. a. *A delta fibers* are myelinated fibers that are located primarily in the skin and muscle. They transmit rapid, sharp, pricking or piercing sensations that are well located and intermittent.
   b. *C fibers* are unmyelinated or poorly myelinated fibers that are distributed in muscle, periosteum, and viscera. They transmit dull, burning, or achy sensations that are diffuse and constant.

9. Stimulation of peripheral receptors (nociceptors) is transmitted to the spinal cord (gate) where impulses are conveyed to neurons that cross over to the opposite side of the cord. Impulses then continue up the ascending lateral spinothalamic tract via either the neospinothalamic or the paleospinothalamic pathways to the brain. At the level of the thalamus, synapses relay the impulses to the midbrain where the reticular activating system (RAS) signals the cortex to increase awareness of incoming noxious stimuli. The cortex is responsible for locating the pain stimulus as well as interpreting the stimulus as a painful response (cognitive aspect of the pain experience).

10. *Neurotransmitters* are chemicals that slow down or speed up activity at the postsynaptic cell. Examples are acetylcholine, norepinephrine, epinephrine, and dopamine. *Neuromodulators,* also called endogenous opiates or protein hormones, are found in the brain. These natural opiate-like (similar to morphine) substances play a major role in the biologic response to pain and pain relief (analgesic effect) on certain receptor sites in the brain. The two neuromodulor substances are endorphins and enkephalins. Endorphins are produced by the pituitary gland and the hypothalamus. They have a more prolonged analgesic effect. Knowledge of neuromodulators is important because they affect pain management. These natural substances or opioid medications affect the heart (bradycardia), respira-

tions (respiratory depression), and the central nervous system (sedation, euphoria, physical dependence) and are enhanced by strenuous activity, TENS unit, and antidepressant medications.

11. a. 3; b. 2; c. 1; d. 2

12. *Clients themselves.* They are reluctant to report pain, do not take medication because of fear of or myths related to addiction, dependence, and tolerance, and lack knowledge regarding medications.
    Health care providers. They believe myths such as clients will become addicted; lack knowledge regarding assessment, medications, addiction versus dependence, and treatment modalities of pain; and not believing the client is truly in pain, they are afraid of overdosing the client, are overly concerned about side effects such as respiratory depression. They withhold medication from substance abusers; fail to administer medications on time; and have fears related to licensing issues, to name just a few of the barriers.
    The legal system or government regulatory bodies. The guidelines and laws that are set for prescribing pain medication can sometimes be cumbersome. (See text for more information.)

13. The perception of cutaneous pain may diminish because of age-related changes, but the perception or visceral (organ) pain may increase. Older adults may require lower levels of analgesia to relieve the pain. Older adults tend to not report pain because they often believe that pain is something they must live with, feel that expressing pain is unacceptable or a sign of weakness, labels them as a "bad" client, or signifies a serious illness. They also feel that nurses are too busy to listen to complaints of pain. Health care providers often undermedicate or are reluctant to administer analgesics to the older adult. Pain in anyone can cause anxiety, restlessness, anger or temporary disorientation; therefore when assessing the older adult, do not confuse these behaviors with other problems such as dementia or other cognitive impairments. A careful assessment of these older adults is necessary. (See Chart 7-1 for more key points for assessing an older adult in pain.) Avoid the use of Demerol in the older adult because of potential serious adverse effects. The effects and side effects of all opioid analgesics may be greater for the older adult; therefore less may be needed to reach a desired effect and to minimize the side effects.

14. The following is but one example of each variable and the impact it has on treatment. (For more examples, see the text.) *Age:* (See previous question regarding the older adult.) *Gender:* Women express their pain differently than men. For example, women may be more likely to discuss their pain and dis-

tress. HCP can mistakenly label the client as being unable to effectively deal with the pain and then cause inappropriate treatment for it. *Cultural consideration:* Studies have shown that Mexican-American clients, especially women, cry when they are uncomfortable. This can lead to unfair stereotyping and expectations of certain ethnic groups. If English is not the client's first language, the ability to express pain may be limited and misinterpreted. *Personality, affect/mood states:* Personality traits such as being an introvert or extrovert, anxiety, fatigue, fear, anger, depression, and past experiences all impact the perception of pain and how pain is assessed and then treated.

15. a. Skin and subcutaneous tissue
    b. Organs and the linings of the body cavities
    c. Nerve fibers, spinal cord, and central nervous system
16. d (See Table 7-1 for further information.)
17. a

18.

	Acute Pain	Chronic Pain
Purpose	Serves a biologic purpose–signal for injury and the need of intervention; a warning signal	Serves no biologic purpose
Etiology	Usually an injury or trauma, i.e., inflammaton, burns, lacerations, ischemia, surgery	Associated with a variety of health problems. Cause may be unknown and unable to be determined.
Onset	Sudden onset	Persists or recurs for indefinite periods after the original pain experience, usually for more than 2 months.
Duration	Temporary; subsides with or without treatment	Ongoing—constant or intermittent. Pain remains and becomes a syndrome in itself. Develops long after cause of pain is gone. Seeking help or treatment makes no difference. Rest makes no difference. Nothing to be learned from this type of pain.
Intensity	As the area heals, the quality or sensation of pain changes	Character and quality changes over time.
Localization	Specific, easily localized	Frequently involves deep body structures, is poorly localized, and often is diffuse to permit description of localization.
Characteristics	Depends on source of pain—see types of pain	Often difficult to describe, depends on source or types of pain.
Emotional response/ assessment findings	Behavioral changes include inability to concentrate, restlessness, apprehension, and overall distress.	Immobility or physical inactivity, withdrawal, despair, depression, altered behaviors. Doctor shopping is common. Clients invest an incredible amount of time and energy in the health care system in hope of uncovering a solution for their pain. Focus becomes what they cannot do rather than what they can do. The client's fears and the length of time that chronic pain has persisted affect the client's perception, verbalization, and expression of pain, as well as his or her coping abilities. Creates an impact on family and ability to cope. The length of time that it persists affects the client's perception, verbalization, and expression of pain, as well as ability to cope.
Physiologic response assessment findings	Common occurrence. Similar to fight or flight response, which includes increased heart rate, blood pressure and respiratory rate; dilated pupils, sweating, facial expressions of being in pain.	Normal blood pressure, normal pulse rate; normal respiratory rate; normal pupils; dry skin. May be no outward signs of pain. "Doesn't look like he/she is in pain." There may be an absence or observable physiologic changes to support client's subjective report of pain.
Treatment	Drug therapy—opioids and nonopioids based on type of pain. Nonpharmacologic measures, such as the use of a pillow for splinting an incision and complementary therapies, are also effective. These measures usually are used in conjunction with drug therapy.	Based on type of pain. Medication—opioids and nonopioids, complementary and alternative measures; interdisciplinary pain centers.

19. Precipitating factors; aggravating factors; relieving factors; localization of pain, character, and quality of pain; intensity; duration; chronology (pattern over time); psychosocial factors such as meaning of pain to the individual, feeling of anger, powerlessness, hostility, depression, withdrawal, and fear of death or mutilation. See section on "Essential data for a complete pain history" for types of questions to ask when assessing clients.

20. Client self-rating using analog scales and diagrams to locate, describe, and quantify pain; pattern of pain, intensity of pain, crying; writhing; grimacing; tachycardia; tachypnea; increased blood pressure; diaphoresis; guarding; splinting; restlessness, apprehension. See "Physical assessment/clinical manifestations" for specific details regarding how to assess for location, character, and quality of pain; pattern of pain; and intensity of pain.

21. *Advantages*: simple; understandable; economical; easier to use; improvement over subjective reporting alone; variety of types of scales (word and numerical) available. *Disadvantages*: rate only the intensity of pain; biased against clients with low verbal or visual discrimination abilities related to level of education or interference from severe pain.

22. b

23. Anxiety; Fear; Powerlessness; Ineffective role performance; Ineffective sexuality patterns; Impaired physical mobility; Self-care deficit; Activity intolerance; Ineffective health maintenance; Disturbed sleep pattern.

24. a. Relief of pain
   b. Reduction, relief, or modification of pain and prevention of pain recurrence or worsening
   c. Near or complete pain relief with analgesia and other modalities designed to interrupt the pain cycle

25. *Nonopioid or peripheral-acting agents (aspirin, Tylenol)*. Used for mild pain or in conjunction with an opioid to relieve severe pain. It is also used for treating pain related to inflammation.
   Opioids (morphine, Dilaudid, hydrocodone). Used alone or with other types of pain medication to treat severe pain; best for somatic type of pain.
   Nonsteroidal anti-inflammatory agents (ibuprofen, Indocin). Used for inflammation and relief of mild-to-moderate pain.

26. a and c. See text and Table 7-3 for further details.

27. b, d, e

28. A few pitfalls include undermedication of clients, exacerbation of pain by a delay of achieving effective analgesia; the client not requesting medication in a timely manner, and the nurse not responding to the request promptly.

29. Nonopioids augment the effect of opioids, aid in relieving certain types of pain that are not effective with opioids, or relieve anxiety.

30. Oral (tablets and liquid), sublingual, rectal, intramuscular, intraspinal, intravenous, transdermal, and subcutaneous routes

31. c

32. Monitor vital signs for tachycardia, hypotension and respiratory depression; observe for altered level of consciousness and sedation; assess for bowel sounds and monitor for abdominal distention and constipation; monitor urinary output for signs of retention; observe for rash, and nausea and vomiting.

33. a, b, c, e, f

34. b

35. Little personal experience with pain (cannot relate it to self); lack of appreciation for the degree of pain associated with procedures; expectation that clients with chronic pain will react as clients with acute pain do; expectation that clients with pain will react within a certain behavior pattern; concern that age may affect a client's reaction to prescribed doses of analgesics (undermedication).

36. a. False. It is often confused with addiction. Physical dependence does occur in many people who become addicted; however, it does not define the problem of addiction.
   b. True

37. a. 3; b. 1 and 3; c. 1; d. 2; e. 3; f. 2; g. 2; h. 3; i. 1; j. 3; k. 2

38. c, d, e, f, g

39. PCA delivers a desired amount of an opioid pain medication through an IV route using a locked syringe pump system (Figure 7-5). It is designed for short-term use such as with postoperative pain. The advantage is the client can self-administer the analgesic whenever it is necessary to control the pain, and there is reduced risk of over-medicating. The PCA pump is programmed to deliver a prescribed basal and/or dose on demand with a designated time interval between demand doses. Nursing care of the client includes assessing for pain and pain control, monitoring for side effects of the pain medications, and performing interventions set by the institution regarding the pump, documentation, and routine protocols.

40. True

41. TENS, local heat/cold application, pressure, massage, vibration, therapeutic touch. (See Table 7-5 for details.)

42. It is a trial and error process with unpredictable and variable outcomes. Pain relief may not be sustained when stimulation ceases. Stimulation may aggravate or produce new pain.

43. False. Anyone can have pain and health care providers need to believe clients when they say they are in pain and treat the pain accordingly. Withholding pain medication is not appropriate. Also, if currently a substance abuser, abrupt withdrawal can result in physiologic withdrawal symptoms. Chart 9-2 provides information on pain management for the substance abuser.

44. Use a pain assessment tool and pain scale from the text or another source to complete this exercise. Show your work to your clinical instructor, a member of the pain team, or other experts in pain management.

45. See text for details.

46. d

47. True

48. d

49. a. False. These medications relax the client and thus help relieve pain. b. True

50. Anesthesia and pain control. (See Figure 7-9 for meridians.)

51. Rhizotomy is a neurosurgical procedure at the fifth nerve (trigeminal nerve) and used to control chronic pain. An open rhizotomy necessitates a laminectomy to resect the posterior nerve root before it enters the spinal cord. Cutting the nerve interrupts transmission of pain stimuli from the periphery to the cerebral cortex. A closed rhizotomy achieves similar results without an extensive open surgical procedure; the nerve roots are destroyed with chemicals, coagulation, or cryodestruction. (See Figure 7-8.)

52. a

53. a. 2; b. 4; c. 1; d. 3; e. 1; f. 4; g. 2; h. 1

54. Equianalgesic refers to the dose and route of one drug producing a degree of analgesia similar to the given dose and route of another drug. Examples as to why a change is made are the following: client's request, physician preference, volume of medication, side effects, or change in route of administration. Most commonly, 10 mg of morphine is the standard dose against which other opioids are measured. See Table 7-7 for calculating the dilaudid dose. The answer is about 22.5 mg. Dose modification varies from client to client so that the new opioid should be started at one half of the equianalgesic dose. This starting dose would be about 11 mg.

55. False. A slow tapering or weaning of the drug dosage lessens or alleviates the physical withdrawal symptoms, which include nausea, vomiting, abdominal cramping, muscle twitching, profuse perspiration, delirium, and convulsions.

56. b. Morphine is the drug used most commonly for continuous subcutaneous infusion. A prime nursing responsibility, in addition to maintaining good pain control, is care of the infusion site and changing the site on a routine basis. See text for further nursing responsibilities.

57. Epidural and intrathecal. The purpose is to interrupt pain pathways at the point that the sensory fibers exit from the spinal cord. Implantable devices and epidural catheters are used for administering medications for clients with chronic, intractable pain. See text for further details. Sexual dysfunction is often a problem.

58. a. True
    b. True
    c. True
    d. False. It is not easily titrated and only certain clients are able to use this method.
    e. True
    f. False. It is effective for 72 hours before it has to be changed.
    g. False. A fever can increase absorption and cause side effects such as sedation.
    h. True

59. nerve block. (See text for further details regarding this procedure.)

60. The client will (1) report that acute pain is relieved or reduced; (2) report that chronic pain is relieved or reduced or that pain is not worsened; (3) establish realistic goals given the limitations imposed by chronic pain; (4) perform activities of daily living; and (5) participate in his or her usual daily lifestyle, with modifications as needed.

61. Read and implement the quality improvement program of the given institution.

STUDY GUIDE NUMBER 2.8

Substance Abuse

1. a. *Substance abuse* occurs when a person overindulges in using a chemical substance, such as a drug, and becomes so dependent on the substance that it interferes with daily life. *Addiction* is the uncontrollable, habitual urge to use a chemical substance, such that without the substance the body experiences physical and emotional disturbances.

   b. Stimulants-amphetamines, methamphetamine, cocaine, nicotine. (See textbook for effects of drugs and examples.)
   Hallucinogens and related compounds: lysergic acid, ecstasy, phencyclidine, marijuana. (See textbook.)
   Depressants: benzodiazepines, barbiturates, alcohol. (See textbook.)
   Narcotics: opioids and morphine derivatives.
   Inhalants. (See textbook.)
   Steroids. (See textbook.)

c. See text and tables relating to incidence for details.
2. a. True
   b. False. 1 out of 4
   c. False. An important aspect in developing a plan of care is to understand the client's culture. (See text for details.)
   d. False. Alcohol, steroids, nicotine, and prescription drugs are also abused substances.
   e. False. Substance abuse can occur at any age.
   f. True
   g. True
   h. True
   i. True
3. All statements are true.
4. Amphetamines and methamphetamine
5. Snorting causes deterioration of the mucous membranes of the nose and nasal septum and red, irritated nostrils
6. Cocaine
7. b
8. See textbook for description of signs and symptoms.
9. c
10. Nicotine (Nicotine is both a stimulant and depressant. First, the drug stimulates the body to release epinephrine, causing a sudden release of glucose and other substances. Then after recovery from the stimulant effect, nicotine causes sedation and feelings of depression and fatigue.)
11. All statements are true.
12. MDMA
13. LSD
14. MDMA
15. The action of this drug is affected by the dose, personality and mood of the user, anticipated outcome, and environment at the time of use. The exact mechanism of the drug is unknown.
16. b
17. The assessment findings associated with PCP abuse include flushing, increased perspiration, aggression, and incoherence. The user is unaware of his or her surroundings and may experience feelings of superior physical strength. Coma may also result from PCP abuse.
18. Marijuana
19. Marijuana is a hallucinogenic drug that creates sensations of euphoria, sexual arousal, and relaxation. It can also cause problems with short-term memory, distorted perceptions, and increased anxiety.
20. Barbiturates and benzodiazepines
21. See textbook for drug actions.
22. a. True
   b. False. Dependence can occur in a very short time.
   c. True

d. True
e. True
23. a
24. c
25. • *Minor* alcohol withdrawal is characterized by restlessness, anxiety, insomnia, tachycardia, agitation and tremors, diaphoresis, and increased blood pressure.
   • *Major* withdrawal includes the above findings, plus hallucinations and vomiting.
   • *Life-threatening* withdrawal can include any of the above, plus global confusion, delirium tremens (DTs), and the inability to recognize familiar objects or people.
26. d
27. b
28. a
29. heroin
30. Heroin is a highly addictive drug and has no medical use. The hazards of this drug are very serious and include fatal overdoses and spontaneous abortions. Intravenous use of the drug increases the risk of bloodborne diseases, such as hepatitis and HIV infection.
31. d
32. c
33. b
34. c
35. a. True
   b. True
36. a
37. b
38. d

STUDY GUIDE NUMBER 2.9

End-of-Life Care

1. a. 2; b. 4; c. 1; d. 3
2. Controlling symptoms, promoting meaningful interactions between client and significant others, and facilitating a peaceful death
3. d
4. c
5. c
6. a, c, e, f, g, i, j, m, n, o
7. See Chart 9-2.
8. c.
9. There are various views of the meaning of death and dying and of religious beliefs and practices of healing. (See text and Table 9-1.)
10. See Chart 9-4.
11. d
12. b, c, d, e

13. *Euthanasia* simply means that death is a pleasant or easy experience, and sometimes preferred over life. *Active euthanasia* refers to an act of commission that intentionally shortens a person's life. *Passive euthanasia* refers to an act of omission that allows the life to be shortened, such as withholding an intervention that might prolong life.

14. a

15. Submit the completed exercise to the clinical instructor for evaluation and feedback on a separate sheet of paper. (Also see the textbook for discussion.)

16. This statement has ethical considerations that should be considered.

17. Dysphagia, nausea/vomiting, agitation, pain, constipation, and dyspnea.

18. a. False. Clients should not be forced to eat.
    b. True
    c. True
    d. False. The most feared is pain.
    e. True
    f. True
    g. False. Dyspnea is a subjective experience in which the client experiences an uncomfortable awareness of breathing.
    h. True
    i. True
    j. False. There is no diagnostic testing, only a physical assessment and knowledge of underlying condition.
    k. True
    l. True
    m. False. Nausea and vomiting is often seen in clients with AIDS.
    n. True

19. a

20. a. Opioids, especially morphine, relieve the dyspnea that is common when a person is dying.
    b. Diuretics reduce excessive fluid volume that often causes dyspnea, edema, and heart failure.
    c. Bronchodilators open airways to facilitate air flow and treat bronchospasms.
    d. Anticholinergics decrease secretions that can cause dyspnea.
    e. Oxygen is used for clients with hypoxemia to increase comfort.
    f. Sedatives, such as benzodiazepines, control anxiety associated with respiratory distress and help relieve dyspnea when morphine is not effective.
    g. Nonpharmacologic interventions, such as positioning and promoting rest, help to decrease demand on the respiratory system.

21. See Charts 9-1 and 9-2 and text.

22. b

23. See text discussion under these nursing diagnoses.

STUDY GUIDE NUMBER 2.10

Rehabilitation Concepts for Acute and Chronic Problems

1. See textbook, pp. 119-120.
2. c. Disability is correct because the example relates to the client's functional status. Rehabilitation is a process. Impairment relates to body organ or structure. Handicap represents a disturbance at the societal level.
3. d
4. • Prevention of deterioration and further injury. • Restoration, as much function as possible, of the injured or diseased body part or system to facilitate the client's independence. (See text for details and examples.)
5. a. 5; b. 9; c. 4; d. 4; e. 1; f. 8 and 9; g. 8; h. 2; i. 3; j. 11; k. 13; l. 6; m. 2; n. 5 and 7; o. 2 and 4; p. 2; q. 2; r. 2; s. 5; t. 12
6. a
7. b
8. a. True
   b. True
   c. False. Constipation, not diarrhea, can be a problem related to decreased motility and mobility.
   d. True
   e. True
   f. False. Clients should be turned or positioned more often than every 2 hours.
   g. False. Fluid restriction is necessary.
9. • General background data • Health history with a rehabilitation focus; general data about physical abilities and limitations; functional assessment; psychosocial assessment; and vocational assessment
10. b
11. e
12. a
13. a-i, All areas are to be assessed.
14. a. False; six areas
    b. True
    c. True
    d. True
    e. False. Tool is used for initial and ongoing assessments.
    f. False. Tool can be used for many types of chronic illness where a functional assessment is indicated.
    g. True
15. *Pulses profile* is used to evaluate care and develop data for longitudinal projection of an illness. *Barthel Index* is used to measure functional ability and mobility in the physically impaired. *Level of Rehabilitation Scale* and *Functional Independence Measures* provide a general assessment for program evaluation. (See text for details of each tool.)

16. • Bathing • Dressing • Toileting • Achieving transfers • Level of continence • Feeding. (See description of other tools for comparison of areas to be assessed in text.)
17. History of present condition; current medications; in any current special treatment programs; financial status; occupation; educational level; cultural background; home situation; usual activity patterns with ADL; dietary habits; elimination habits; sexuality habits; sleep history; food preferences and allergies. (See text for details of examples.)
18. See text and Chart 10-1.
19. The purpose of a vocational assessment is to help the client find meaningful training, education, or employment following discharge.
20. b
21. • LOA. It is a trial home visit to determine if everything is ready for the client to be discharged to the home setting. • Predischarge assessment. The health care provider visits the home and makes an assessment as it relates to the client's needs. (See text for further details on home care management, health teaching, and health care resources.)
22. c
23. • How the family responds to the client's disability • How decisions are made • Who the family's spokesperson is • Usual coping style • Structure and roles • Communication patterns • Problem-solving skills • Client's status and role in the family • Economic status • Religious and cultural influences.
24. See text for general outcomes as a guide and submit outcomes for review to your clinical instructor.
25. d
26. b
27. a
28. c
29. All answers are correct.
30. c
31. See text for "Potential Problems with Transfers."
32. d
33. c
34. c
35. b
36. b. Choice *a* results from an upper motor neuron injury and *c* is a result of an injury to the frontal lobe, such as a stroke or head injury. An inhibited bladder is normal.
37. c
38. a. 2; b. 1; c. 2 preferred but can use for checking of residual with 1 and 3; d. 1 and 2; e. 3; f. 2; g. 3; h. 1, 2, 3
39. *a, b,* and *c* are correct; d. Maximum is 8 hours with good hydration; e. Clean not sterile technique is used at home.
40. b

41. Give 1 hour before or 2 hours after meals. Instruct clients to change positions slowly. Give 1 hour before toileting or triggering or facilitating measures. (See Chart 10-5 for interventions of other medications.)
42. a
43. • Dantrolene (Dantrium)—photosensitivity can occur, therefore the client should be taught to avoid prolonged sun exposure and that it may cause drowsiness, fatigue, and muscular weakness. • Baclofen (Lioresal)—avoid alcohol. Alcohol potentiates its effect.
44. b
45. d
46. c
47. a
48. a. Spastic bowel results from an upper motor injury and uninhibited bowel results from brain damage. An inhibited bladder is normal.
49. c. *a* relates to a spastic bowel and *b* relates to the flaccid bowel; *d* is common in clients with irritable bowel syndrome.
50. d

STUDY GUIDE NUMBER 3.11

Fluid and Electrolyte Balance

1. a
2. a. True; b. True; c. True; d. False. It is the largest. e. True; f. True; g. True; h. True
3. a. 1; b. 2; c. 3; d. 4; e. 5
4. Body fluids act as solvents for electrolytes and act as a transport medium for hormones, blood cells, and nutrients.
5. Sodium, potassium, calcium, phosphorous, magnesium, chloride
6. Thirst
7. • Knowledge of standard normal range for the age of client • Changes from the normal range for the client—high or low values • Client trends or changes from previous values • Factors that may influence the value, such as medications or a disease process.
8. Fluid monitoring, fluid management, and oral health restoration. (See text and Chart 12-4 for details.)
9. a. 2; b. 1; c. 3; d. 2; e. 1; f. 3; g. 3; h. 1
10. b
11. • Osmolality of ECF • ECF compartment volumes and pressures • ADH regulation • Aldosterone regulation
12. a. 2; b. 6; c. 6; d. 1; e. 4; f. 1; g. 5; h. 2; i. 2; j. 3; k. 4; l. 4; m. 3; n. 5; o. 5; p. 4
13. Sodium, potassium, and chloride
14. • Solid foods and fluids • Renal excretion • Absorption

15. Imbibed fluids (1500 mL), water in ingested food (800 mL), and cellular oxidation (300 mL)
16. 2600 mL
17. • ECF osmolarity • ECF compartment's volumes and pressures • ADH regulation • Aldosterone regulation
18. b
19. a
20. b. In younger adults, using the back of the hand or arm is used to assess turgor, but these sites cannot be used in the older adult because of loss of elasticity as the client ages.
21. c
22. a. 2; b. 1; c. 1; d. 1; e. 2; f. 2
23. Urine, skin, lungs, and GI tract (See "Routes of fluid loss" in text.)
24. b
25. • Excessive salivation • Fistula and wound drainage • GI suction • Fever • Hot/dry weather • Diaphoresis • Diarrhea • Hypermetabolic state, such as occurs with trauma, burns, or stress
26. a. (soy sauce); c. butter; e. (bacon/nitrates); f. (cottage cheese); i. (canned tuna and pickles); j. (commercial soups and some crackers)
27. With a low-salt diet, you do not add salt while preparing food or at the table.
28. c
29. See text and Tables 11-6, 11-7, 11-8,11-10, and 11-11.
30. a. 4; b. 3; c. 2; d. 1
31. a
32. • The older adult may not get thirsty as a sign of dehydration. • Body water is lost more quickly causing dehydration. • Difficulty in assessing skin turgor due to decrease in elasticity of skin.
33. d
34. d
35. c
36. Parathyroid and thyrocalcitonin
37. Fluid intake (amount, types); fluid output (urine, emesis, diaphoresis, conditions leading to increased insensible water loss [IWL]); diarrhea; medications taken (especially diuretics and laxatives); neuromuscular symptoms (heart palpitation, muscle weakness); body weight changes; diet history; thirst sensation; excessive drinking; exposure to environmental heat; history of medical disorders such as renal or endocrine diseases; level of consciousness. (See Chart 11-3 for Gordon's functional health patterns.)
38. Alert; moist eye conjunctiva; moist mucous membranes; volume of urine output with specific gravity of approximately 1.015; resilient skin turgor; skin not excessively dry; body weight; absence of tearing from eyes; pulse volumes; pulse deficit; heart rate; blood pressure; venous filling; peripheral perfusion; body temperature; general sympathetic nervous system arousal; blood chemistry values such as serum sodium hematocrit, and hemoglobin levels; observable degree of client thirst; any fluid loss from wounds, GI tube drainage, fistulas, and blood loss; amount of IWL; neurologic examination; muscle tone, strength, movement, and tremors; cardiac dysrhythmias; bowel sounds. See Chart 11-3 for Gordon's functional health patterns.
39. Psychosocial assessment includes both psychologic and cultural factors that may influence balance. Confusion, anger, hostility, and hypochondriacal tendencies affect the client's reliability as a historian. Psychiatric, social, and cultural behaviors can endanger the client's maintenance of homeostasis.

Case Study

Answers provided on the SIMON website:
http://www.wbsaunders.com/SIMON/Iggy/

STUDY GUIDE NUMBER 3.12

Interventions for Clients with Fluid Imbalances

1. b
2. a. 1; b. 4; c. 2; d. 1; e. 3
3. BUN, creatinine, osmolality, sodium
4. b
5. Increased bounding pulse, presence of crackles, hypertension, peripheral edema, jugular venous distention, increased respiratory rate. (*Answers can be any four of these symptoms.*)
6. a, d, e
7. a. Decreased
   b. Increased (unless the result of SIADH)
   c. Increased
   d. Decreased because of hemodilution
8. a. 4; b. 1; c. 4; d. 5; e. 7; f. 5; g. 6; h. 3; i. 4; j. 1; k. 7
9. a. Decrease in thirst center response in older clients.
   b. Client may be on diuretics, which may induce dehydration if not used appropriately.
   c. Rapid weight loss is an indicator of fluid loss because 1 liter of fluid is equal to 2.2 pounds.
   d. May indicate orthostatic hypotension as a result of fluid volume deficit.
   e. May indicate inability to access fluids.
10. d
11. b, d, a, c

Case Studies

Answers provided on the SIMON website:
http://www.wbsaunders.com/SIMON/Iggy/

STUDY GUIDE NUMBER 3.13

Interventions for Clients with Electrolyte Imbalances

1. See Overview and pathophysiology of hypo- and hyperkalemia.
2. d
3. See text for etiology and Table 13-1. Show your answer to your clinical instructor regarding types of clients.
4. c
5. a
6. See text and Chart 13-2.
7. b
8. b
9. d
10. b
11. See Chart 13-3 on home care assessment and text.
12. d
13. b
14. b
15. d
16. b
17. a
18. See text and Chart 13-5 for interventions related to medications, fluids, and monitoring of clients.
19. a. Tall, peaked T waves. Other ECG changes for hyperkalemia include prolonged PR interval, flat/absent P waves, and widening of QRS complex; cardiac arrest; ECG changes for hypokalemia include ST depression, flat/inverted T waves, prominent U waves, and heart block.
20. Hyperkalemia: a, d, e, f, i, j, l, m. Hypokalemia: b, c, g, h, k, n.
21. *Hypokalemia*: Age; medication use (especially diuretics, steroid, and digitalis); presence of any disease state; any recent illness; diet history; method of food preparation; psychosocial factors including usual mental status, mood, behavior changes, lethargy, and confusion.
    Hyperkalemia: Age; presence of risk factors such as debilitating or chronic illness (renal disease); any recent medical or surgical treatment; urinary output; use of medications; diet history; use of salt substitute; any palpitations or irregular heartbeat; muscle twitching, weak leg muscles; tingling or numbing in extremities or face; explosive diarrhea; decrease in activity level; fatigue; weakness; psychosocial factors including compliance with prescribed dietary restrictions or limitations, knowledge of foods to avoid, use of medications, and details about food preparation.

22. *Hypokalemia*: Shallow, ineffective respirations; diminished breath sounds; cyanotic nail beds and mucosa; thready, weak peripheral pulses; variable heart rate; postural hypotension: ECG change (ST depression, flat/inverted T waves, prominent U waves, heart block); mental status changes (transient irritability or anxiety, lethargy, confusion, coma); decreased sensory perception; muscle weakness including weak hand grasps; hyporeflexia; flaccid paralysis; decreased peristalsis; nausea or vomiting; constipation; abdominal distension; decreased bowel sounds; polyuria; low urine specific gravity.
    Hyperkalemia: Cardiovascular changes including slow, weak peripheral pulses; low blood pressure; ECG changes (tall, peaked T waves, prolonged PR interval, flat/absent P waves, widening of QRS complex), complete heart block, or ventricular dysrhythmias; neuromuscular symptoms including muscle twitching, paresthesia, numbness, progressive ascending muscle weakness, and paralysis in arms and legs; increased respiratory rate; hyperactive bowel sounds; watery, explosive diarrhea.
23. a. 1; b. 2
24. a. Cardiac dysrhythmias. Potassium affects the cardiac conduction of the heart affecting nerve impulses and contraction of the muscle.
25. a
26. d
27. b
28. a
29. b
30. c
31. c
32. a; b; c; e; f; h; i; k; n (See Table 13-3 for common causes of hyponatremia.)
33. a
34. d
35. a. Brain cells are the most sensitive to the osmolality of the blood, which causes the cells to shrink and swell resulting in changes in mental status.
36. c
37. a. 2; b. 1; c. 2; d. 3; e. 2; f. 1; g. 3; h. 2; i. 1 (See Table 13-4 and text.)
38. b
39. d
40. d. Signs and symptoms include short attention span, difficulty recalling recent events, and confusion. Manic or seizure episodes can occur with high levels of serum sodium. In an overload situation, the client may be lethargic, drowsy, stuporous, or comatose. (See Table 13-9 and text.)
41. d
42. a

43. *Hyponatremia*: Age; medication usage; presence of risk factors such as kidney or liver disease or congestive heart failure; recent medical treatment or surgery; vomiting; diarrhea; fever; draining wounds; burn injury; urinary output; fluid intake; height; usual weight and any recent weight changes; diet history; recent engagement in strenuous physical activity and the environmental temperature and humidity at the time; behavior changes; headaches; increased somnolence; decreased alertness and attention span; difficulty awakening; muscle weakness, anorexia; abdominal cramping; increased fatigue; signs of edema.

Hypernatremia: Age; presence of renal disease or conditions promoting excessive water loss (fever, vomiting, diarrhea, heavy diaphoresis); urinary fluid output/intake in past 24 hours; recent weight change; medication use; diet history including use of sodium-containing condiments; recent strenuous physical activity as well as temperature and humidity conditions at the time; insomnia or mental irritability; edema; changes in skin texture or turgor; change in activity level; mental status; weakness; fatigue; psychosocial factors including behavior changes, agitation, and manic excitement.

44. *Hyponatremia*: Presenting behavior; altered mental status including level of consciousness, orientation, attention span, memory, and fund of knowledge; headache; muscle weakness; decreased muscle tone; depressed deep tendon reflexes; increased GI motility; nausea; diarrhea; abdominal cramping; hyperactive bowel sounds; visible peristalsis; explosive, watery stools; rapid, weak, thready pulse; decreased peripheral pulses; flat neck veins at 90 degrees and possibly when supine; decreased blood pressure (especially diastolic); orthostatic hypotension; variable central venous pressure; full, bounding peripheral pulses; shallow respirations; variable respiratory rate; rales or rhonchi; edema; urine specific gravity, urine color; daily weight. *Hypernatremia*: Attention span; recall of recent events; ability to perform cognitive functions; agitation; confusion regarding the sequence of events; lethargy; drowsiness; stupor or coma; convulsions; sporadic muscle twitches; progressive muscle weakness; diminished or absent deep tendon reflexes; variable pulse rate; variable blood pressure; changes in peripheral pulse intensity and quality; changes in skin color and turgor; dry mucous membranes and skin; coated tongue and gums; oral fissures; decreased urine output; concentrated urine.

45. a
46. c
47. b

48. a. 2; b. 4; c. 1; d. 1; e. 3; f. 4; g. 2; h. 1; i. 4; j. 2; k. 1 (See Table 13-5.)
49. b
50. d
51. b
52. d
53. a
54. b
55. a
56. d
57. d
58. c
59. b
60. b
61. c
62. b
63. Immobility and the absence of weight bearing causes bone demineralization and resorption of calcium. This results in brittle, fragile bones.
64. Excessive intake of vitamins can lead to increased absorption of calcium if a large amount of the active form of vitamin D is ingested.
65. a
66. a, e, f, g, h, i
67. b, c, d, f, g, h
68. b, c
69. c
70. b
71. *Hypocalcemia:* Age; sex; race; skin exposure to sunlight; activity level (especially weight bearing); diet history; use of calcium supplements; reports of frequent leg cramps ("charley horses"); recent orthopedic surgery or episodes of bone healing; thyroid surgery; neck radiation, or recent anterior neck injury; abdominal cramping; taking medications such as calcium channel blockers; psychosocial factors including subtle behavior changes (anxiety), increasing sensitivity to extraneous environmental stimuli, progressive irritability, irrational thinking, and frank psychosis; ability to understand medication and diet regimen; ability to afford dietary supplements.

Hypercalcemia: Age; presence of other illnesses including malignancy, renal disease, heart disease, and endocrine disorders; medication use, especially antacids, thiazide diuretics, glucocorticoids, thyroid replacements, calcium supplements, and vitamin D supplements; activity level, diet history; nausea, abdominal pain; anorexia.

72. *Hypocalcemia:* Progressive paresthesia in hands or feet (distal to proximal); tingling; numbness; muscle twitching, cramps, or spasms, tetany; presence of Trousseau's or Chvostek's sign; convulsions; hyperactive deep tendon reflexes; hyperactive bowel sounds, diarrhea; hypotension, diminished pulse quality.

Hypercalcemia: Bradycardia; full peripheral pulses; ECG changes (shortened QT interval, widened T wave); profound muscle weakness; diminished deep tendon reflexes; altered level of consciousness (lethargy, drowsiness, time or place disorientation); decreased or absent bowel sounds; increased abdominal girth; vomiting; constipation; renal stone formation. (See Chart 13-10 and text.)

73. a
74. a. 2; b. 1
75. a
76. Monitor client's cardiovascular status and ECG changes, monitor trends in serum calcium levels, Chvostek's and Trousseau's signs every 15 minutes; administer medication slowly, not to exceed 27 g/min and warmed to body temperature. (See text and Chart 13-12.)
77. Hypocalcemia; hypokalemia; hyponatremia
78. c
79. d
80. c
81. b
82. a. 2; b. 1; c. 1; d. 2; e. 1; f. 1; g. 1; h. 2; i. 1
83. Easily obliterated peripheral pulses; generalized muscle weakness; ineffective respiratory movements; prolonged bleeding after sight trauma; bruising; bleeding gums; increased irritability; seizures; coma; spontaneous fractures; renal calculi.
84. b
85. a
86. b
87. b
88. Malnutrition or starvation; prolonged nasogastric suctioning; diarrhea or steatorrhea; destruction of intestinal villi; alcoholism; liver disease; excess phosphorus in the GI tract. (Table 13-8 and text.)
89. • High doses of loop diuretics or osmotic diuretics • Aminoglycoside therapy • ECF volume expansion • Hypoparathyroidism • Hyperaldosteronism (See Table 13-8 and text.)
90. Hyperactive deep tendon reflexes; painful paresthesia; tetanic muscle contractions; positive Chvostek's and Trousseau's signs; skeletal muscle weakness; increased central nervous system irritability associated with depression or psychosis; decreased GI motility; anorexia; nausea; abdominal distention; paralytic ileus. (See Chart 13-16 and text.)
91. d
92. d
93. d is correct. a. IM MgSO4 is not used because it causes pain and tissue damage; b. Fruits do not have concentrations of magnesium (see Table 11-11); c. Oral magnesium causes diarrhea and increases magnesium loss.
94. a

95. Bradycardia; hypotension; prolonged PR interval; widened QRS complex; widening of pulse pressure; lethargy; coma; diminished or absent deep tendon reflexes; progressive muscle weakness including respiratory insufficiency.
96. Foods that are limited include meat, nuts, legumes, fish, vegetables, and whole-grain cereal products. Medications to avoid are those containing magnesium such as antacids and laxatives. (See Chart 13-15 and text.)

Case Studies

Answers provided on the SIMON website: http://www.wbsaunders.com/SIMON/Iggy/

STUDY GUIDE NUMBER 3.14

Infusion Therapy

1. a. The purpose, in general, is to remove any particles that may be in the solution, such as bacteria, dead cells in blood, or any contaminants, when the solutions are being mixed.
   b. Filters are made with either a membrane that has tiny pores or holes or as a depth filter with a maze-like configuration. Various types of filters are available based on the fluid that is going to be infused. For example, the filter used to infuse total parental nutrition is different than that for blood and blood products so the filter needs to be selected with the intended purpose in mind.
2. a. 2; b. 3; c. 1; d. 4
3. a. 3; b. 1; c. 2; d. 2; e. 1; f. 2
4. Volumetric controllers count drops and electronically convert the drops to milliliters per hour. Because drops vary in size this method of infusion is not as accurate as the volumetric pumps that deliver a specific volume per hour. Pumps actually pump fluids or medications under pressure and therefore are more accurate than controllers. The least accurate method is nonvolumetric controllers because they rely completely on gravity for flow.
5. d
6. a. To receive medications. b. To correct an existing fluid and electrolyte imbalance. c. To prevent a fluid and electrolyte imbalance. d. To provide nutritional support, particularly on a long-term basis.
7. b
8. See Table 14-1 for details.
9. Flow rate, materials used, that is, tubing, equipment function, type of fluid, site condition, and site care. (See Table 14-2 for common maintenance procedures of various venous access devices.)
10. See Chart 14-4 and text.
11. a. 1; b. 2; c. 1; d. 1

12. The catheter of an implanted port is attached to a portal body (port) that is surgically placed in a subcutaneous area of the body. A non-coring device (special needle) is needed to access the port by piercing the skin and puncturing the septum of the port.
13. a
14. c
15. The nurse should monitor the catheter for maintenance or proper placement and provide for safe medication administration including monitoring for side effects.
16. The primary purpose of IPT is to instill medications such as chemotherapy agents directly into the abdominal area and treat the tumor site.
17. Peritonitis, local infection, and catheter problems such as occlusions.
18. Clients who are unable to tolerate oral medication; require subcutaneous injections for greater than 48 hours; require long-term parenteral medication but have poor venous access; need a continuous level of medication to control pain; cannot afford intravenous therapy; and/or are confused or depressed.
19. Yes, because it is the least invasive and safest method for delivering the needed pain medication. Nursing care involves using proper insertion technique and location, slowly infusing the solution (no more than about 80 mL/hr), rotating the site every 5 to 7 days, and monitoring for complications such as site irritation, erythema, heat, swelling, and pooling of the fluid at the site.
20. a. A needle is inserted into the space surrounding the spinal cord. The anesthesiologist inserts the needle. It is an effective method because the pain medication is given slowly and more evenly to block the pain from the site of the needle down to the toes. The anesthesiologist is a physician who usually is responsible for the catheter and medication.
    b. The nurse monitors how well the medication controls the pain, the system, any side effects and complications from the medications, and implements specific policies and protocols for the institution.
    c. (See Table 14-6.)
21. Epidural therapy is administered into the epidural space around the spinal cord. It does not come in contact with the spinal fluid. Intrathecal therapy is administered directly into the ventricular or subarachnoid spaces where cerebrospinal fluid is housed. It is used primarily for administering chemotherapy that does not normally cross the blood tumor barrier. The physician administers the medication and the nurse monitors for side effects and effectiveness of the medication.

22. a. 3 (See Table 14-3.) b. IV would be stopped and restarted at another site if necessary. Warm moist compresses would be applied.
23. a. 4 (See Table 14-3.) b. IV rate would be slowed; the physician notified, oxygen started at 2 L, vital signs checked frequently, diuretics administered as ordered, and client's condition monitored.
24. a
25. c
26. c
27. a
28. b
29. Complete the question and review your answer with your clinical instructor.

Case Study

Answers provided on the SIMON website:
http://www.wbsaunders.com/SIMON/Iggy/

STUDY GUIDE NUMBER 3.15

Acid-Base Balance

1. d
2. • As a result of normal cellular glucose metabolism
   • As a breakdown of fats and proteins
   • Anaerobic metabolism of glucose and fats • As a result of cellular destruction
3. a. 2; b. 1; c. 1; d. 3; e. 4; f. 1; g. 4; h. 2; i. 3
4. d
5. $CO_2 + H_2O \rightarrow H_2CO_3 \rightarrow H^+ + HCO_3^-$
6. a. decrease; b. decrease; c. decrease; d. increase; e. increase
7. • Breakdown of carbonic acid • Intestinal absorption • Pancreatic production • Renal regeneration (reabsorption)
8. a
9. a. 2; b. 3; c. 3; d. 1; e. 4; f. 2
10. a
11. Respiratory
12. c
13. b
14. a. Acid; b. Acid; c. Alkalotic; d. Acid
15. • Less alveolar membrane available for gas exchange • Vascular thickening that impairs gas diffusion • Retention of carbon dioxide that increases hydrogen ion concentration
16. a. Reduced ability to excrete hydrogen ion;
    b. Reduced ability to synthesize bicarbonate
17. c
18. c
19. b
20. c
21. a
22. d

23. c
24. c
25. b
26. d
27. c
28. a
29. b
30. b
31. a. Chemical buffers; b. Lungs; c. Kidneys
32. c
33. Chronic airflow limitation—the kidneys excrete excess hydrogen ions and reabsorb bicarbonate to counter the retained carbon dioxide unable to be released via the lungs.
34. Lactic acidosis resulting from anaerobic metabolism (e.g., running)—excess hydrogen ions in the ECF lead to an increase in the carbon dioxide concentration, which in turn leads to increased depth and rate of respiration in attempts to exhale the excess.
35. *Full compensation* exists when either the lungs or kidneys are able to correct for changes in pH when the other system is unable to mange or is contributing to the cause of the acid-base imbalances. *Partial compensation* exists when the lungs or kidneys are unable to correct completely for pH changes and the pH is not within the normal range.
36. • Structure and function of many proteins are altered • Fluid and electrolyte imbalance • Altered excitable membrane responses • Altered uptake, activity, and distribution of drugs and hormones
37. b

STUDY GUIDE NUMBER 3.16

Interventions for Clients with Acid-Base Imbalances

1. c
2. a
3. a. 1; b. 2; c. 3; d. 1; e. 4
4. b
5. a. 3; b. 2; c. 1; d. 4; e. 3; f. 2; g. 1; h. 2; i. 2; j. 2; k. 4
6. d
7. *May be any of the following*: albuterol, isoproterenol, terbutaline, aminophylline, theophylline, beclomethasone, dexamethasone, flunisolide, triamcinolone
8. c
9. a. Metabolic
   b. Metabolic
   c. Respiratory
   d. Respiratory
   e. Metabolic
10. b
11. c

12. a
13. c
14. d
15. c
16. c
17. a. 3; b. 2; c. 1; d. 4; e. 2; f. 2; g. 4; h. 4; i. 1; j. 2; k. 4
18. *Indirect:* Conditions that increase the concentration of acids or bases at a rate beyond the body's capacity to regulate.
    Direct: Pathologic conditions that directly impair specific regulatory mechanisms.
19. *Acidosis* is the process that causes blood pH to decrease. *Acidemia* is the result of acidosis when there are too many hydrogen ions in the ECF and the arterial pH drops below 7.35.
20. Alkalosis is the process that causes blood pH to increase. Alkalemia is the result of alkalosis when there are too few hydrogen ions in the ECF and the arterial pH rises above 7.45.
21. Respiratory acidosis with complete compensation
22. Metabolic alkalosis without compensation
23. Respiratory alkalosis with partial compensation
24. Metabolic acidosis with partial compensation
25. Metabolic acidosis with complete compensation
26. Metabolic alkalosis with complete compensation
27. • Metabolic disturbances • Respiratory disturbances • Combined metabolic and respiratory disturbances
28. b
29. b
30. c
31. a
32. b
33. d
34. b
35. a
36. b
37. a
38. b
39. c
40. c
41. a
42. c

Case Studies

Answers provided on the SIMON website: http://www.wbsaunders.com/SIMON/Iggy/

STUDY GUIDE NUMBER 4.17

Interventions for Preoperative Clients

1. d
2. b
3. d
4. d

5. True
6. False. The nurse performs a comprehensive head-to-toe physical assessment.
7. True
8. True
9. True
10. False. All lab values should be reported.
11. professional legal responsibility
12. Urinalysis, blood type and crossmatch, CBC, hemoglobin level and hematocrit, coagulation studies, electrolyte levels, serum creatinine level, possible chest x-ray, and ECG
13. b
14. d
15. c

Case Study

Answers provided on the SIMON website:
http://www.wbsaunders.com/SIMON/Iggy/

STUDY GUIDE NUMBER 4.18

Interventions for Intraoperative Clients

1. b
2. a. 2; b. 3; c. 6; d. 1; e. 5; f. 4
3. a, b, c, d
4. Using ECG monitoring, pulse oximetry, end-tidal carbon dioxide monitoring, and arterial blood gases, and hemodynamic monitoring
5. An artificially-induced state of partial or total loss of sensation, occurring with or without loss of consciousness.
6. To block the transmission of nerve impulses, suppress reflexes, promote muscle relaxation, and, at times, to achieve a controlled level of unconsciousness.
7. a. Stage 3; b. Stage 2; c. Stage 4; d. Stage 1
8. Inhalation anesthetics and succinylcholine
9. d
10. d
11. False
12. • If endotracheal tube is not in place, intubate immediately. • Stop all inhalation anesthetic agents and succinylcholine. • Ventilate the client with 100% oxygen, using highest flow rate possible. • Use active cooling techniques. • Assess ABGs, serum chemistries. • Treat any dysrhythmias.
13. a. 4; b. 1; c. 5; d. 3; e. 2

Case Study

Answers provided on the SIMON website:
http://www.wbsaunders.com/SIMON/Iggy/

STUDY GUIDE NUMBER 4.19

Interventions for Postoperative Clients

1. d
2. b
3. a
4. Smoking, older clients, obesity; diseases that decrease immunity; physical condition, age, stress on the surgical wound
5. c
6. b
7. c
8. Type and extent of surgical procedure; type of anesthesia; client's tolerance of procedures; client's allergies; pathologic conditions; vital sign status; type and amount of IV fluids and medications administered; estimated blood loss; complications; preoperative condition; pertinent medical history; intake and output of fluids during surgery.
9. d
10. a
11. c, e
12. d
13. a, d, b
14. g
15. b
16. c
17. d
18. f
19. a
20. e, b, c
21. g
22. c, b, a
23. c, d, f
24. d
25. a
26. f
27. g
28. f, e
29. g, c
30. b, c
31. g
32. f
33. a, c, b
34. d
35. b
36. g
37. a
38. Key points include patent airway; if receiving oxygen, amount and type; pulse oximetry readings; rate, pattern and depth of respirations; breath sounds; inspection of chest wall for accessory muscle use, sternal retraction, and diaphragmatic breathing.
39. a. 7; b. 3; c. 4; d. 5; e. 6; f. 2; g. 1

40. *Impaired Gas Exchange* related to the residual effects of anesthesia, pain, the use of opioid analgesics and immobility. *Impaired Skin Integrity* related to surgical wounds, decreased mobility, inflammatory processes, drains and drainage and tubes. *Acute Pain* related to the surgical incision, positioning during surgery, and endotracheal tube irritation.
41. a. 2; b. 3; c. 4; d. 5; e. 1

STUDY GUIDE NUMBER 5.20

Concepts of Inflammation and the Immune Response

1. c
2. • Individual recognition code • Nonspecific human membrane proteins • Receptors • Tissue-specific membrane proteins • Plasma membrane • Cytoplasm • Nucleus
3. • Nutritional status • Environmental conditions • Medications • Presence of disease • Age
4. True
5. • Antibody-mediated immunity (AMI) • Humoral immunity • Cell-mediated immunity (CMI)
6. • Recognition of self versus self • Phagocytic destruction of foreign invaders and unhealthy or abnormal self cells • Lytic destruction of foreign invaders and unhealthy self cells • Production of antibodies directed against invaders • Activation of complement • Production of hormones that stimulate increased formation of leukocytes in bone marrow • Production of hormones that increase specific leukocyte growth and activity
7. b
8. d
9. b
10. c
11. a. 1; b. 4; c. 3; d. 2; e. 1; f. 1; g. 2; h. 3
12. d
13. c
14. False
15. a
16. d
17. warmth, redness, swelling, pain, loss of function
18. b
19. c
20. c
21. b
22. b
23. Exposure, Invasion, Antigen recognition, Lymphocyte sensitization, Antibody production and release, Antigen-antibody binding, Antibody-binding reactions, Sustained immunity memory
24. a

25. c
26. a
27. a. 2; b. 3; c. 1; d. 4; e. 5
28. d
29. • Active immunity • Passive immunity
30. a. Response to chickenpox virus, b. vaccination, c. mother's breast milk or placenta, d. tetanus or snake bite
31. • Helper/inducer T-cell • Suppressor T-cell • Cytoic/cytolytic T-cell
32. a
33. a. 1; b. 4; c. 3; d. 2; e. 5
34. True
35. True
36. Hyperacute rejection, acute rejection, chronic rejection
37. a. 1; b. 2; c. 1; d. 2; e. 3; f. 2; g. 3; h. 1; i. 3; j. 3; k. 3
38. d
39. a. 2; b. 5; c. 1; d. 4; e. 3; f. 8; g. 6; h. 7
40. a. 8; b. 5; c. 3; d. 7; e. 1; f. 6; g. 4; h. 2; i. 8

STUDY GUIDE NUMBER 5.21

Interventions for Clients with Connective Tissue Disease

1. Connective tissue disease
   Degenerative joint disease
   Osteoarthritis
   Hormone replacement therapy
   Estrogen replacement therapy
   Erythrocyte sedimentation rate
   Total joint replacement
   Total hip replacement
   Deep vein thrombosis
   Total knee replacement
   Rheumatoid arthritis
   Temporomandibular joint
   Progressive systemic sclerosis
   Systemic lupus erythematosis
2. d
3. d
4. arthritis
5. • Progressive degeneration of the joint • Loss of cartilage in the joint
6. d
7. d
8. (Any three of these answers.) Developmental, genetic, metabolic, or traumatic factors
9. obese
10. d
11. c
12. d
13. c
14. b

15. a
16. a, b, c
17. • Chronic Pain • Impaired Physical Mobility • Activity Intolerance • Self-care Deficit • Disturbed Body Image • Impaired Mobility • Ineffective Coping • Imbalanced Nutrition
18. Acetaminophen—reduce inflammation
Topical salicylates—temporary pain relief
Capsaicin products—blocks neurotransmitter for pain
NSAIDs—anti-inflammatory
Cortisone—temporary pain reduction in joint
Hyaluron and Synvisc—synthetic joint fluid
COX-1—produces prostaglandin that helps regulate cell activity
COX-2—produces prostaglandin mainly in sites of inflammation
19. • Local rest • Systemic rest • Psychologic rest • Positioning • Thermal modalities
20. c
21. d
22. True
23. b
24. True
25. c
26. b
27. a
28. True
29. False
30. a
31. d
32. a, c, d
33. True
34. a
35. a
36. Impaired Mobility
37. c
38. a
39. c
40. b
41. Thigh-high stockings, elastic bandages, sequential compression device (SCD)
42. c
43. a
44. Refer to Chart 21-4.
45. Refer to Figure 21-4.
46. True
47. b, c, d
48. • Kneeling • Hyperflexion of knee
49. Articulation, subluxation, dislocation
50. Infection resulting from excessive tissue cutting
51. a, b, d
52. a. Impaired Physical Mobility
    b. Interventions: Therapeutic exercise; Promotion of ADLs; Ambulation with assistive device.

53. c
54. b
55. • Verbalizes pain relief • Ambulates independently • Independently performs ADLs
56. a, b, c
57. b
58. • Fibrous adhesions • Bony ankylosis • Clacification • Loss of bone density
59. osteoporosis
60. d
61. a
62. b
63. See Chart 21-9.
64. a
65. a
66. c
67. a, b, c
68. c
69. b
70. d
71. • Pleurisy • Pneumonitis (Diffuse interstitial fibrosis) • Pulmonary hypotension
72. Pericarditis, myocarditis
73. True
74. a
75. a, b, c, d
76. d
77. a, b, c
78. a. Low; b. Low; c. Low; d. High; e. High
79. b
80. gastrointestinal problems
81. a. 7; b. 3; c. 2; d. 5; e. 9; f. 8; g. 1; h. 4, i. 6
82. d
83. TENS, hypnosis, acupuncture, magnet therapy, imagery, music therapy, stress management, nutrition
84. b, c
85. Increased pain, sleep disorder, weakness
86. CBC, check stool for blood, PT referral, pain relief, energy conservation. (Use Chart 21-8.)
87. Use Charts 21-2, 21-6, 21-8, 21-11, and 21-12.
88. DLE and SLE; SLE affects only the skin.
89. b
90. d
91. Use Chart 21-13.
92. Skin biopsy
93. • Continue medication during remission • Monitor body temperature • Protect skin. (See Chart 21-14.)
94. See Chart 21-13.
95. skin (integumentary); renal
96. • Calcinosis • Raynaud's phenomenon • Esophageal dysmobility • Sclerodactyly • Telangectasias
97. a, b, c
98. a, b, c, d

99. • No smoking • Skin inspection • Bed cradle or foot board • Wear gloves and socks • Small frequent meals • Avoid spicy foods, caffeine, alcohol
100. b, d
101. True
102. • Asymptomatic hyperuricemic • Acute • Intercritical • Chronic
103. c
104. True
105. True
106. Colchicine, NSAIDs
107. Dermatomyositis
108. Neoplasms
109. a, b
110. a
111. Arthritis, conjunctivitis, urethritis
112. d
113. a, b
114. True
115. False
116. • Pain • Muscle stiffness • Spasms • Sensory changes • Exhaustion
117. Hypnotics and antidepressants

STUDY GUIDE NUMBER 5.22

Interventions for Clients with HIV and Other Immunodeficiencies

1. c
2. a. 6; b. 3; c. 1; d. 4; e. 2; f. 5
3. True
4. b, c, c, c, a, b, b, b, c
5. False
6. False
7. A retrovirus only has ribonucleic acid (RNA) as its genetic material. It contains enzymes called *reverse transcriptase* for increasing viral replication.
8. b
9. d
10. c
11. d
12. c
13. c
14. b
15. c
16. True
17. True
18. b
19. a. Clean equipment, fill needle and syringe, and flush with clean water. b. Fill syringe with bleach. c. Shake filled syringe for 30 to 60 seconds and rinse with clean water
20. b
21. a
22. True
23. True
24. c
25. (Any seven of these symptoms.) Cough, night sweats, weight loss, nausea and vomiting, fatigue, diarrhea, fever, lymphadenopathy
26. True
27. True
28. True
29. e
30. a
31. c
32. b
33. c
34. True
35. False
36. False
37. True
38. a
39. b, c, d
40. shingles
41. False
42. False
43. d
44. True
45. False
46. True
47. True
48. True
49. True
50. False
51. True
52. a
53. Risk for Infection, Impaired Gas Exchange, Acute Pain, Imbalanced Nutrition, Diarrhea, Impaired Skin Integrity, Disturbed Thought Processes, Disturbed Self-esteem, Social Isolation
54. False
55. True
56. False
57. True
58. False
59. a, b, c
60. a
61. a, b, c
62. True
63. False
64. True
65. False
66. a, b, c
67. c
68. a, b, d

69. • Anorexia associated with chronic disease, acute infection, or treatment often leads to poor oral intake • Absorption and assimilation of nutrients is sometimes impaired in gastrointestinal disease and with absorption problems. • Host defense mechanisms mobilized in infection result in increased demand for nutrients, met at the expense of the body's store. • Hospitalized clients often receive a semistarvation regimen with many hours of nothing by mouth because of procedures to be performed or because of the lack of essential nutrients in IV fluids.
70. • Leanness and cachexia • Decreased effort tolerance • Lethargy • Intolerance to cold • Ankle edema • Dry, flaking skin and dermatitis • Poor wound healing • Higher than usual incidence of postoperative infections.
71. True
72. False
73. True
74. True
75. True
76. a, c
77. True
78. False
79. True
80. False

STUDY GUIDE NUMBER 5.23

Interventions for Clients with Immune Function Excess: Hypersensitivity (Allergy) and Autoimmunity

1. True
2. a, b, c
3. a
4. b
5. Inhaled, ingested, injected, and contacted
6. anaphylaxis
7. True
8. False
9. a. 7; b. 5; c. 6; d. 3; e. 2; f. 4; g. 1
10. a. 3; b. 2; c. 1; d. 4
11. c
12. a, b, d
13. a. 2; b. 1; c. 3; d. 4; e. 5
14. True
15. True
16. False
17. • Feeling of uneasiness • Apprehension • Weakness • Impending danger • Urticaria • Angioedema
18. a, b
19. b
20. True
21. True

22. False
23. True
24. False
25. True
26. a, b, d
27. Client receiving the wrong blood type
28. Discontinue treatment
29. True
30. True
31. a
32. c
33. True
34. a, b, c, d
35. Benadryl
36. Inappropriate stimulation of normal cell surface receptors by an antibody, resulting in a continuous "turn on" state for the cell. Common form: Graves' disease.
37. b
38. Antibodies or lymphocytes are directed against healthy normal cells and tissue.
39. a, b, c, d, e
40. c
41. b
42. c
43. b
44. d
45. d
46. a, b
47. a. 3; b. 1; c. 2; d. 1; e. 2; f. 1; g. 4
48. c
49. a, e
50. Renal failure
51. High-dose corticosteroids

STUDY GUIDE NUMBER 5.24

Altered Cell Growth and Cancer Development

1. c
2. b
3. True
4. b
5. a, c
6. b, d
7. True
8. True
9. False
10. True
11. True
12. True
13. d
14. True
15. c

16. e
17. d
18. e
19. True
20. a, b, c
21. True
22. False
23. d
24. a, b, c
25. True
26. False
27. a, b, c
28. True
29. a, b, d
30. a, b, c, d
31. True
32. False
33. a, c
34. a, b, c
35. b, c, d
36. d
37. True
38. a, c, d
39. False
40. True
41. True
42. c
43. b, c, d, e
44. True
45. b
46. True
47. d
48. Solar (sun)
49. True
50. a, b, c
51. True
52. a, b, d
53. False
54. False
55. True
56. Aging
57. c
58. See Table 24-14.
59. c
60. b, c
61. b, d
62. True
63. True
64. False
65. False

STUDY GUIDE NUMBER 5.25

Interventions for Clients with Cancer

1. a, c, d
2. a, b, c, d, e
3. a, b, c, d
4. b, c, d
5. c
6. a, b, d
7. a, c
8. d
9. False
10. True
11. False
12. a, c, d
13. True
14. True
15. a, b, c, d
16. False
17. b
18. a, b
19. True
20. a, b, c
21. False
22. b
23. b
24. True
25. c
26. True
27. False
28. b
29. False
30. a, b, c
31. a
32. True
33. d
34. False
35. a, c
36. True
37. True
38. True
39. False
40. a
41. a, b, c
42. True
43. c
44. a. 3; b. 4; c. 5; d. 1; e. 2
45. b
46. b
47. c
48. b, c
49. c
50. a, b, c, d
51. b

52. a
53. True
54. a
55. b, c, d
56. True
57. a, b
58. a, b, d
59. True
60. False
61. a, b, c
62. c
63. a, c
64. b
65. c
66. a, c
67. True
68. a
69. True
70. a. 3; b. 1; c. 2
71. a
72. a, b, c
73. b
74. False
75. True
76. True
77. a

STUDY GUIDE NUMBER 5.26

Interventions for Clients with Infection

1. a. 3; b. 7; c. 4; d. 8; e. 6; f. 9; g. 5; h. 2; i. 1
2. a. People, animal, insects
   b. Soil, water, medical equipment
3. a. 3; b. 2; c. 1
4. True
5. Passive: short-term; placental transfer. Active: years; vaccine. For explanation, see text.
6. False
7. Hormonal (diabetes) and environmental (chemicals).
8. a. 5; b. 4; c. 1; d. 2; e. 1; f. 3; g. 2
9. a. 4; b. 5; c. 1; d. 2; e. 3
10. True
11. Review Table 26-5. Know tissue, action, and defense.
12. True
13. False
14. True
15. Endogeous (normal skin flora) and exogenous (hands of health care personnel)
16. Protect the client, health care personnel, and others. Accomplish this in timely fashion and be cost-effective.

17. True
18. False
19. False
20. a. 3; b. 4; c. 2; d. 1
21. True
22. a, b, c, d
23. True
24. a, b, c, d
25. a, b
26. False
27. True
28. True
29. a. 7; b. 8; c. 6; d. 5; e. 4; f. 3; g. 2; h. 1
30. • Hyperthermia related to increased metabolic state.
    • Social Isolation related to effects of illness.
31. a, b, c, d
32. a, b, c, d
33. True
34. True
35. True

STUDY GUIDE NUMBER 6.27

Assessment of the Respiratory System

1. a. 1; b. 1; c. 2; d. 2; e. 2; f. 1; g. 2; h. 1; i. 1; j. 1; k. 2; l. 2
2. Cleans, warms, and humidifies the air moving into the lungs.
3. a. Surfactant is a protein-rich fluid that forms a lining in the alveoli.
   b. Maintains a moist surface of the alveoli, maintains surface tension of alveoli fluid, and keeps the lung from collapsing.
4. The bronchial system is part of the systemic circulation and is not involved in gas exchange like the pulmonary system.
5. a. 2; b. 3; c. 1
6. Items on the concept map would include age; sex; race; childhood illnesses; adult illnesses; immunizations; operations; injuries; hospitalizations; last chest x-ray; PFTs; environmental data such as home and living conditions; exposure to environmental irritants; smoking habits; travel outside of local area; area of residence; current and past medication use; allergies; family history of genetically transmitted respiratory disorders; diet history, especially for food allergies; occupational history; current health problems; hobbies; leisure activities; current problem with cough; sputum production, chest pain, shortness of breath, dyspnea on exertion, paroxysmal nocturnal dyspnea; orthopnea; recent weight loss; night sweats; psychosocial factors such as effect of stress on respiratory conditions, coping ability, effect of illness on family, financial status,

and support systems; cough (productive, nonproductive); sputum production (color, consistency, amount); hemoptysis; external nose deformity or mass; nostril symmetry; nasal flaring; nasal polyps; deviated septum; color of nasal mucosa; septal perforation; sinus tenderness; decreased sinus transillumination; movement of soft palate and uvula with phonation; color and symmetry of posterior oral cavity; postnasal drainage; tonsilar enlargement; pharyngeal edema or ulceration; neck symmetry; use of neck muscles for respiration; palpable lymph nodes; tracheal deviation from midline; tracheal swelling; abnormal voice; thorax skin color, lesions, and masses; spinal deformities; respiratory rate, rhythm, and depth; symmetry of thoracic movement; inspiratory to expiratory ratio; ratio of anteroposterior to lateral diameter of chest; chest movement with respiration; muscle retraction with respiration; respiratory excursion; crepitus; vocal fremitus (increased, decreased, or absent); diaphragmatic excursion; chest percussion note resonant over lung fields; decreased, diminished, or absent breath sounds; adventitious breath sounds, (crackles, wheezes, pleural friction rubs); bronchophony; whispered pectoriloquy; egophony.

7. b
8. I. Assess the client's knowledge of the procedure as a starting point.
   II. Chose a quiet place to give the client information.
   III. Provide information by answering the following questions:
       A. What is PFT? How well the lung functions
       B. How will results be determined? Results are compared against normal for age.
       C. Where will I go for the test? The test is performed in the respiratory therapy department.
       D. What should I do to prepare for the test? In preparing for tests, the client should be advised to not smoke for 6 to 8 hours before a test for accuracy of results. Advise the client to take no respiratory medication for 4 to 6 hours before the test.
       E. What will happen during and after the test? There will be no pain. Client will breathe in and out of a tube attached to a machine. Respiratory drugs will be available if dyspnea occurs.
       F. What will happen after the test? The client may be tired and will be encouraged to rest. Nurses monitor for respiratory difficulty and notify the physician if it occurs.
9. c
10. a. 4; b. 3; c. 1; d. 5; e. 2; f. 7; g. 6

11. Forced expiratory volume. This test requires effort; the older adult and those with respiratory disorders do not have the strength to maximally force/exhale the air in the first second.
12. c
13. a
14. d
15. d
16. b
17. Refer to Chart 27-1 and discussion in the textbook.
18. b
19. b
20. a. 4; b. 8; c. 5; d. 7; e. 3; f. 1; g. 9; h. 2; i. 4 and 11; j. 10
21. a. 2; b (See Table 27-1.); c (See Chart 27-1 and related chapters such as Postoperative Care to Prevent Complications and Inadequate Gas Exchange.)
22. d
23. b
24. b
25. c
26. b
27. c
28. See Table 27-6.
29. Answer a is correct; b. Intermittent dyspnea during sleep; c. Slow respiration; d. Fast respirations.
30. See 27-9 for illustration and answers.
31. Lungs, chest, and nose
32. a
33. Submit the completed exercise to the clinical instructor.
34. Submit the completed exercise to the clinical instructor.
35. • Symmetry of chest movement • Rate, rhythm, and depth of respiration • Use of accessory muscles for breathing
36. d
37. b
38. d
39. a. Place thumbs on spine at ninth rib.
    b. When client inhales, the thumbs move apart.
    c. On exhalation, the thumbs return to midline.
    d. Watch for symmetry of both sides.
40. c
41. b
42. d
43. c
44. a
45. b
46. a
47. b
48. b
49. Complete assignment and validate findings with your instructor.
50. b

51. False. ICU clients may need hemodynamic monitoring to determine adequate oxygenation.
52. b
53. Answer *c* is correct. a. Dye is given IV; b. No isolation, no radioactivity; substance leaves body within 8 hours; d. Not a screening test.
54. d
55. a. 7; b. 6; c. 5; d. 1; e. 3; f. 2
56. b
57. c
58. a
59. a
60. Examples of assessment findings that indicate a positive response are pulse oximetry should be above 92% to 95%; nail beds and mucous membranes are pink, not pale or cyanotic; ambulation without shortness of breath; respiratory rate even, not labored, and within normal limits; able to speak without shortness of breath; decreased anxiety; improved level of consciousness; improved energy level; no use of accessory muscles with chest movements. (See Signs and Symptoms of Adequate Oxygenation.)
61. c. It is unlikely that oxygen will help this client because the client lacks the Hgb that carries the oxygen and the Hgb that exists is already filled to 99%, which is within normal limits.
62. a. Y. Vasoconstriction.
    b. Y. Low hemoglobin count.
    c. Y. Abnormal shaped red blood cell interferes with blood flow.
    d. N. Hypothermia causes vasoconstriction.
    e. N. Oxygen administration route has no direct affect on the device itself.
    f. Y. Peripheral vasoconstriction occurs when peripheral vascular system shuts down.
    g. N. Can affect respirations but not the pulse ox device directly.
    h. Y. Deeper coloration of the nail bed than those of whites can cause artificially low results by 3% to 5%.
    i. N. Makes no difference in the ability to read the saturation even though women have larger airways than men.
    j. N. The pulse oximetry can be low because of respiratory diseases affecting the ability to oxygenate but not affect the device itself causing an artificially low result.
    k. N. Part of a respiratory assessment and can affect the client's ability to breathe but not cause artificially low results.
63. Answer *d* is correct. a. Mediastinoscopy is performed to obtain samples of lymph nodes; b. Laryngoscopy is performed to visualize the vocal cords to remove lesions or obtain a biopsy; c. A gastroscopy is a type of gastrointestinal test and not related.
64. The throat is anesthetized. A tube is inserted to look into the throat and lungs. Medications are given to relax the client and help him or her forget the procedure. The client will return to the unit after the test. The test is not painful.
65. d
66. b. The nurse would encourage the client to perform vigorous coughing and deep breathing exercises and then reassess the client for effectiveness. The client would not develop pneumonia immediately postoperative. Pneumonia occurs after stagnation of fluids over several days. Rhonchi indicate thick secretions or obstruction; wheezes indicate bronchospasms/narrowing of the airways.
67. b. Is cough productive, nonproductive; dry, hacking; frequency; time of day; length of time had cough; things to relieve it.
68. b. Sputum can also be yellow when there is an infection of the respiratory tract.
69. d
70. a
71. d
72. Subjective feeling of shortness of breath
73. c

Case Study

Answers provided on the SIMON website: http://www.wbsaunders.com/SIMON/Iggy/

STUDY GUIDE NUMBER 6.28

Interventions for Clients with Oxygen or Tracheostomy

1. a. Decreased oxygen blood level; not enough oxygen is being carried in the blood that goes to the cells and tissues.
   b. Not enough tissue oxygen; there is not enough oxygen going inside the tissue, then cells and tissue die.
   c. There is too much carbon dioxide in the blood.
   d. Indicates how saturated the red blood cell is with oxygen; measure in % saturation.
   e. A blood gas measurement to indicate available oxygen in arterial blood.
   f. Amount of oxygen being delivered as supplemental oxygen; reported as liter per minute or %.
2. b
3. a. True
   b. True
   c. True

d. False. The amount of oxygen should be regulated by parameters such as pulse ox/blood gas/respiratory assessment to administer the lowest level possible with least harmful side effects, not just symptom management.

e. True

f. False. Oxygen does not burn itself but is needed for something to burn.

4. c

5. a

6. c. CO_2 necrosis does cause the normal mechanism to turn off but is not the stimulus to breathe in these clients. It is the low oxygen level rather than the high CO_2 level that stimulates these clients to breathe. There is a shift from the brain chemoreceptors sensing the high CO_2 level to the peripheral chemoreceptors in the aortic arch and carotid sinus areas sensing the low oxygen level.

7. c

8. Answer *d* is correct. a. These are signs of ARDS and not related; b. Hypoventilation does occur in the first 30 minutes of administering oxygen to a high-risk client; however, the signs are just the opposite–there is an improvement in color; c. Always be concerned with lack of oxygen because in order for cells to survive, oxygen is necessary.

9. Answer *d* is correct because too much oxygen can override the nitrogen that is needed in the room air to prevent alveolar collapse. Therefore, initially monitor the client every 1 to 2 hours for absorption atelectasis by auscultating for crackles and decreased breath sounds.

10. All statements should be checked.

11. a

12. b

13. d

14. False

15. b

16. True. Knowing about the devices is important in the proper care of the client.

17. d

18. *Low flow* supplements the client to meet the inspiratory demand. The client needs to be able to breathe in and use air from the room. The total oxygen received depends on the client's respiratory rate and tidal volume. *High flow*, by contrast, provides a flow rate that is provided to meet the entire inspiratory demand and tidal volume of the client. Used for critically ill clients.

19. a. 2; b. 2; c. 1; d. 1; e. 1; f. 1; g. 2; h. 2; i. 2

20. See text under "Home Care Management" for details. See Figure 28-10 as an example of a portable oxygen delivery system.

21. The goal is to enable the client to realize that compliance with oxygen therapy is important so that normal activities of daily living (ADLs) and events that bring enjoyment can be continued.

22. The three methods are compressed gas, liquid oxygen, and oxygen concentrator. (See text "Equipment for Home Oxygen Therapy" for details.)

23. a. False

    b. True

24. See text for low-flow and high-flow delivery systems, Tables 28-1 and 28-2, and Figures 28-2, 28-3, 28-4, 28-5, and 28-6.

25. Answer c is correct. a. Maintain reservoir bag to 2/3 full; b. Relates to partial re-breather mask; non-rebreather delivers 80% to 95%; d. If ineffective, the next step is intubation.

26. c

27. Answer *b* is correct. a. This system can deliver oxygen or room air; c. It is not a form of airway intubation; d. There are two methods: BiPAP and nasal continuous positive airway pressure.

28. See "Noninvasive Positive-Pressure Ventilation" in textbook.

29. a (See "Transtracheal Oxygen Therapy" in textbook and Figure 28-9.)

30. *Correct answers:* a, b, d, e, f, g. *Incorrect answers:* c. Use a water base lubricant instead of Vasoline; e. Humidification is used for 4 L/min or more. (See Chart 28-2 for best practices.)

31. b (See Chart 28-1 for further details.)

32. d

33. a

34. a

35. Clients who need prolonged intubation or mechanical ventilation such as with ARDS, shock, postoperative, clients who have acute upper airway obstruction such as with secretions, burns, inflammation, obstructive sleep apnea; retention of secretions; decreased airway dead space from tumors; also those who need airway protection to prevent large aspirations; prophylaxis against airway obstruction during surgery; or as a result of severe injury; laryngectomy—temporary or permanent. (See Table 28-3 for indications for tracheostomy.)

36. c

37. Complications include tube displacement; airway obstruction; aspiration; cuff leak and rupture; tracheomalacia; tracheal stenosis; tracheoesophageal fistula; trachea-innominate artery fistula, bleeding; pneumothorax; infection. (See text under "Postoperative Care, Complications for Assessment Findings, Collaborative Management with Prevention Strategies and Table 28-4.)

38. d

39. c

40. b

41. d

42. a. 4; b. 5; c. 8; d. 9; e. 1; f. 10; g. 2; h. 6; i. 3 (See text and Table 28-5 for further details.)
43. a
44. a. Other measures include coughing and deep breathing, providing inner cannula care, and humidifying the oxygen source.
45. b
46. See text for details.
47. a
48. d
49. a. 4; b. 7; c. 11; d. 5; e. 2; f. 8; g. 3; h. 12; i. 1; j. 10; k. 6; l. 13; m. 9; n. 14 (See Chart 28-3 for "Best Practices for Suctioning Artificial Airways.")
50. One person secures the tube while a second person changes the neckties. If one person is changing the ties alone, the old neck ties are not removed until the new ties are in place and secured.
51. a. 6; b. 2; c. 5; d. 8; e. 12; f. 7; g. 1; h. 14; i. 3; j. 11; k. 9; l. 15; m. 10; n. 4; o. 13; p. 16 (See text and Chart 28-4 for "Best Practices of Tracheostomy Care.")
52. Answer *a* is correct. b. Suction intermittently while rotating catheter for no more than 10 to 15 seconds; c. Do not use glycerin swabs—dries the mucous membranes; d. Clean incision with saline or 50/50 solution; peroxide damages the skin.
53. b
54. d
55. A collar surrounds the entire tracheostomy tube and is used to deliver high humidity and desired oxygen to the client. A T-piece is a special adapter that attaches to the tracheostomy tube to deliver the desired FIO_2 to the client with a tracheostomy or endotracheal tube. (See Figure 28-7, text, and Table 28-2 for nursing interventions and rationales.)
56. d
57. c. A fenestrated tube has a precut opening in the outer cannula for when the inner cannula is removed and a re-decannulation stopper is in place; the client is able to speak. (See text and Table 30-5 for information about other types of tubes.)
58. a. 8; b. 3; c. 4; d. 1; e. 7; f. 6; g. 2; h. 5
59. There is a pilot balloon attached to the outside of the tube that is inflated or deflated. It indicates the absence or presence of air in the actual cuff of the tracheostomy tube.
60. d. The occlusive technique is used with cuffed tracheostomy tubes with pressure relief valves.
61. Client's condition, such as malnutrition, hypotension, dehydration, hypoxia; age: skin of older adults may damage more easily; receiving corticosteroids; suctioning; unstable tube causing friction and movement. Interventions would include maintaining proper cuff pressure, stabilizing the tube, judicious suctioning and preventing or treating malnutrition, hemodynamic stability, adequate oxygenation, and hydration.
62. a (See text and Chart 28-1 for further details.)
63. b
64. Answer *c* is correct. a. The client should "tuck" chin to chest. Hyperextension opens the airway and increases risk; b. Thick liquids are better; d. Have client in most upright position during meals, when receiving tube feedings, and 30 minutes after eating. (See text and Chart 28-6 for further interventions.)
65. Hyperoxygenate with 100% oxygen before suction; avoid prolonged suctioning time, excessive suction pressure, and too frequent suctioning; and use proper catheter size. (See text under "Hypoxia" for details.)
66. c
67. False
68. The client can use a "magic slate," communication board, pen and paper, pictures, letters, hand signals, computer, answer "yes" or "no" questions, and use the call bell system at the nurse's desk. When possible, change the trach tube to a fenestrated tube or a special one-way valve.
69. See text "Continuing Care."

STUDY GUIDE NUMBER 6.29

Interventions for Clients with Noninfectious Upper Respiratory Problems

1. See an anatomy and physiology textbook and Chapter 27.
2. Respiration, swallowing, and speech.
3. c
4. How many times during the night does the wife observe her husband stop breathing and does she notice changes in his personality. Husband complains of waking up tired, awakening several times during the night, sleepiness during the day, and irritability.
5. An overnight sleep study will be performed; all phases of sleep will be observed, along with the type of sleep, respiratory effort, oxygen saturation adequacy, and muscle movement. An EEG (looking at the electrical activity in the brain will be performed. Nurse will explain about the electrodes to the head, that there is no harm to client, and that post test care includes washing the hair to remove all the paste). Nurse explains ECG (heart monitor to see change from lack of oxygen when sleep apnea occurs), pulse oximeter (how much oxygen is being carried in the body by the red cells), and EMG (looking at the electrical activity of muscle movement) used during the test.
6. d

7. a

8. a

9. d

10. c

11. Mustache dressings are used post-surgically after an open reduction due to nasal trauma, as in a rhinoplasty. Antiseptic packing is applied and then dressing. Monitor for respiratory status, obstructions, drainage type and amount, and swallowing ability with postnasal drip for bleeding. A splint or cast may cover the nose for additional alignment and protection. Instruct when to call a physician. (See Figure 29-1.)

12. c

13. b

14. c

15. See "Epistaxis: Collaborative Management" in textbook.

16. a

17. See "Epistaxis" in textbook.

18. a. True
    b. True
    c. False. Usually hospitalized only for posterior because of risks involved.
    d. False. Packing is painful and client must avoid NSAIDs or like products.
    e. True
    f. True
    g. True
    h. False. Relates to posterior packing only.

19. a

20. b

21. a

22. Airway, hemorrhage and extent of trauma to determine patency of airway, any airway obstruction and the interventions services that may be needed such as a specialist in ENT, plastic surgery, trauma team will optimize post-trauma recovery

23. Shortness of breath, dyspnea, anxiety, restlessness, hypoxia, hypercarbia, decreased oxygen saturation, cyanosis, and loss of consciousness. Early recognition is essential to prevent further complications and avoid respiratory arrest.

24. See text, "Facial Trauma–Assessment" for details.

25. (See "Potential Causes of Upper Airway Obstruction to Help with Identifying Types of Clients.") Show your answer to your clinical instructor.

26. c

27. b

28. c

29. a

30. c

31. c

32. b

33. Nodules: People who use their voices a lot, such as teachers, coaches, sports fans, singers. Polyps: People who smoke, people with allergies, people who live in dry climates.

34. d

35. d

36. a

37. c

38. The edema can occlude the airway, leading to respiratory arrest.

39. c

40. d

41. Knife wounds, gunshot wounds, traumatic accidents

42. a, b, c

43. Slate board and chalk, pen or pencil and paper, magic slate, alphabet board, point to the object, yes/no by raising one or two fingers.

44. c

45. d

46. Prolonged use of tobacco and alcohol, exposure to chemicals, infection, voice abuse, chronic laryngitis, and neglect of oral hygiene. Smoking and alcohol are the highest. See Evidence-based Practice for Nursing "Smoking Cessation is Hard." (See Figure 29-6.)

47. a

48. Color changes in mouth or tongue; a sore that does not heal; a lump in mouth or neck; unexplained persistent bleeding; hoarseness; persistent or recurring pain in ears or face; numbness in mouth or lips; difficulty swallowing.

49. c

50. a. The airway is separated from the esophagus, making aspiration impossible.

51. d. Other procedures would be subtotal and vertical laryngectomies.

52. The purpose of the epiglottis is to allow food to go into the esophagus instead of the lung. Supraglottic laryngectomy removes the epiglottis and false vocal cords. Assess the client's ability to perform supraglottic swallowing.

53. See Chart 29-4.

54. a

55. See textbook; the client will need a gastrostomy tube for feeding in order to prevent aspiration.

56. c. All others are diagnostic tests for head and neck cancers.

57. c

58. Mechanical devices, esophageal speech, tracheoesophageal fistula. (See Chart 29-2: "Communication Enhancement: Speech Deficit" and text under "Speech Rehabilitation" for details.)

59. See text for "Esophageal Speech" and "Tracheoesophageal Fistula."

60. d

61. a. True
    b. True
    c. True
    d. False. Erythroplasia; white lesions are leuko-
       plakia.
    e. True
    f. False. Specific locations and small tumors.
    g. True
    h. False. Partial laryngectomy.
    i. True
    j. True
62. b. (For points of emphasis for the teaching plan see
    text "Radiation Therapy.") Include in plan items
    such as location of treatment, length of time, infor-
    mation and interventions related to the side effects
    of hoarseness, sore throat, skin and salivary glands.
    (See text and Chart 29-2.)
63. a
64. c
65. See Table 29-2.
66. d. Flaps are used for head and neck resections.
    Other items to include are coughing and deep-
    breathing exercises, pain control, nutritional sup-
    port, and possibly ventilator support.
67. b
68. See text and Charts 29-5 and 29-6.

STUDY GUIDE NUMBER 6.30

Interventions for Clients with Noninfectious Lower Respiratory Problems

1. a. 10; b. 4; c. 6; d. 1; e. 2; f. 11; g. 5; h. 9; i. 3; j. 7;
    k. 8
2. ventilation; perfusion
3. a
4. c
5. a
6. a. 1, 2; b. 2; c. 3; d. 3; e. 2, 3; f. 2; g. 2, 3; h. 1; i. 2;
    j. 1, 2, 3; k. 1; l. 1; m. 1; n. 3; o. 1; p. 3; q. 1; r. 2, 3;
    s. 1; t. 1; u. 1
7. b
8. a
9. b
10. c
11. The client complains of tightness in the chest and
    inability to "get air," causing an increase in respira-
    tory rate in an attempt to get air. In attempting to
    move the air, the client may use accessory muscles
    so retraction may be noted. The client unable to
    breathe will find it difficult to talk. There will be
    decreased pulse oximetry. Wheezing is more pro-
    nounced on exhalation but can progress to both
    inhalation and exhalation.

12. Since asthma attacks are intermittent, the goals of
    care are to improve airflow, relieve symptoms, and
    prevent episodes. The client is educated in the step
    methods and co-manages the disease with the health
    care provider using peak flow meters twice a day,
    and keeping a diary of signs and symptoms, trigger-
    ing episodes, medications used, and response to
    medications.
13. b
14. b
15. a. 4; b. 6; c. 2; d. 5; e. 1; f. 3
16. Smoking paralyzes the ciliary motion of the lungs;
    mucus secretion cannot be mobilized and removed
    from the lungs effectively during sleep. Upon awak-
    ening and with increased inspiratory effort, the
    smoker has excess mucus, which triggers the cough
    reflex to remove the local irritant.
17. b. By definition, it occurs when the client is lying
    down and is relieved by sitting up.
18. d
19. b
20. c
21. d
22. b
23. c
24. a
25. b
26. a. 1, 2; b. 3, 4; c. 6, 2; d. 2, 3; e. 3, 4; f. 1; g. 2, 7
27. d
28. b
29. The client combines the PEF/FVC values with fre-
    quency of episodes; symptoms such as wheezing,
    shortness of breath, use of accessory muscles, and
    physical limitations to determine the step/severity of
    episode and interventions. Interventions include
    inhalers such as bronchodilators and steroids, sys-
    temic steroids with frequency of use. (See Step Sys-
    tem chart.)
30. Using a hand-held "peak" flow device, the client
    takes as big a breath as possible, then blows out the
    air AS QUICKLY AND AS FAST as possible INTO
    this peak flow device. Do *not* continue to force/push
    air out of the lungs. There is a gauge on the device
    that indicates the peak flow value. The client should
    know the "normal" value for himself or herself. If
    the value drops a certain percentage below the
    client's normal, it indicates there is restriction in
    breathing and intervention is needed.

31. Impaired Gas Exchange; Ineffective Breathing Pattern; Ineffective Airway Clearance, Anxiety; Imbalanced Nutrition (less than body requirements); Activity Intolerance; Risk for Infection; Powerlessness; Ineffective Role Performance; Self-care Deficits related to specific ADLs; Deficient Knowledge related to disease process, treatments, and self-care activities; and Ineffective Coping. Others may be identified. Show your answers to your clinical instructor.

32. b

33. b

34. b (See Figure 30-6.)

35. c. Dyspnea control during meals consists of eating the largest meal when hungry and well rested. Eating six small meals reduces fatigue and dyspnea as opposed to eating three large meals. (See Chart 30-7.)

36. • Bronchodilators • Anticholinergics • Corticosteroids • Cromolyn sodium • Mucolytics (See Chart 30-4.)

37. a. Beta$_2$ agonists—trigger smooth muscle relaxation; there are two kinds of beta agonists. One is short-acting for acute episodes or prevention (Proventil) and the other is long-acting for longer effects only.

    b. Cholinergic antagonists—block the parasympathetic nervous system to bronchodilate and decrease secretions. Example: Atrovent.

    c. Methylxanthines—relax smooth muscles of bronchial tubes. Rarely used today. Example: Theo-Dur.

38. a

39. a

40. c

41. This medication is necessary for treatment of this client to prevent respiratory distress and should have a designated line. A separate line also is needed for safe administration because this medication is incompatible with several medications.

42. c

43. (See pathophysiology section on inflammation.)
    a. Nonsteroidal inhalers—inhibits the release of inflammatory mediators from respiratory epithelial and white cells. Example: Tilade.

    b. Mast cell stabilizers—prevents mast cell from reacting to the allergen that causes the inflammation. Example: cromolyn sodium.

    c. Leukotriene antagonists—blocks leukotriene, a biochemical mediator in the inflammatory process causing lasting effects of inflammation. Example: Singulair.

44. Refer to text Chart 30-5 for details.

45. d

46. b

47. c

48. See charts in text for both asthma and drug therapy: bronchodilators.

49. See charts in text.

50. c. After meals is not recommended because of the risk of gastric reflux and aspiration. a. Is recommended—it eliminates mucus collected during the night; b. Facilitates a more pleasant meal by cleaning the airway; d. At bedtime so the client can rest better.

51. See text under COPD "Controlled Coughing."

52. Chest physiotherapy, postural drainage, positioning, hydration/nutrition, coughing techniques, deep breathing exercises, energy conservation activities, use of medications and inhalers, preventive measures for respiratory infections or triggering "flare ups," signs and symptoms of emergency care, assistive devices such as humidifiers, oxygen therapy, and others.

53. See Chart 30-3: Education Guide: Asthma.

54. c

55. See text and Chart 30-8.

56. See text and dyspnea assessment tool in Figure 30-7.

57. See Charts 30-7 and 30-9.

58. c

59. Items to include are age; sex; ethnic background; family history of asthma and emphysema; smoking history; type of cigarettes smoked; cough pattern and sputum production described; dyspnea episodes; activity intolerance; wheezing; orthopnea; feet swelling; diet history; practice of special breathing maneuvers; current medications; emergency plan; exposure to environmental irritants in home or work setting; psychosocial factors such as isolation; hobbies, pets, coping abilities, anxiety, fear, support systems, and significant others; financial circumstances; ability to answer questions lucidly, with or without breathlessness; weight; respiratory rate; breathing pattern; use of accessory muscles; anteroposterior diameter relative to lateral diameter of chest; presence of cyanosis; capillary refill; clubbing; decreased fremitus; abnormal percussion note; auscultation for breath sounds; chest wall retractions and tenderness; heart rate and rhythm; pedal edema.

60. b

61. c

62. a

63. a. 4; b. 5; c. 1; d. 3; e. 2

64. Answer *d* is correct. a. More deaths than the three combined; b. Survival rate is low, 15% or less; c. No early detection; detection is often made after metastasis has occurred.

65. a. True
    b. True

c. True
d. True
e. False (Small cell)
f. False (15 years)
g. False (All those factors combined.)
h. False (Reverse is true.)
i. False (AF/Am is higher.)
j. True
k. False (There can be a missing gene in women that makes those who smoke at a higher risk.)
l. False (late signs)
m. False (Indicates advance disease; there are no screening tools for lung cancer.)
n. False (Cancer cells are not always in the sputum, various methods are used for diagnostic testing—see text.)
o. True
p. True
66. c
67. a. 1; b. 2, 3, 4; c. 1; d. 2; e. 3; f. 1, 4; g. 2; h. 1; i. 2, 3, 4; j. 3; k. 2, 3; l. 1, 2, 3, 4; m. 2, 3, 4
68. a
69. c
70. b. Answers *a, c,* and *d* are types of surgical interventions done as a result of a thoracotomy. a, The removal of a lobe; c, removal of the entire lung; d, removal of a portion of one section of the lung along with removal of other complete sections of the lung.
71. d. The entire side of lung has been removed and space must fill with fluid.
72. b
73. a. Chamber 1 is used for the collection of drainage and air from chest cavity. Do not empty; frequently monitor the amount, color, etc. Mark amount of drainage from bottle at least every 8 hours, more frequently if needed. Keep connections to client tight; drainage is not emptied. Report excessive amount of drainage. b. Chamber 2 is a water seal—a specific amount of water is used as a water seal. Observe for air leaks: excessive bubbling; observe for the rise of fluid during inspiration and fall during expiration as normal; no fluctuation can mean the lung has re-expanded or there is a problem. When gravity drainage is used, the small tube leading to this section must be left *unclamped*. c. Chamber 3 serves as the suction control—determined by the level of water and not the amount of bubbling. Refill chamber as needed to maintain level of suction ordered by physician. (See Figures 30-14 and 30-15.)
74. a
75. d
76. c
77. a

78. See textbook for "Client Care Plan."
79. d
80. a. Pain
b. Ineffective Airway Clearance
c. Impaired Gas Exchange
81. b
82. a
83. c
84. d
85. d
86. b
87. a
88. c
89. b
90. b
91. a. True
b. True
c. True
92. a
93. c
94. c
95. b
96. d
97. a
98. See Chart 30-1 in text for details.

STUDY GUIDE NUMBER 6.31

Interventions for Clients with Infectious Respiratory Problems

1. c
2. d
3. b
4. d
5. b
6. b
7. Yes, because the client has difficulty breathing and a productive cough may indicate a secondary bacterial infection from the sinusitis.
8. b
9. d (See text and Chart 31-2.)
10. c
11. c
12. a
13. c
14. c
15. a
16. c
17. • Edema of interstitial lung tissue • Extravasation of fluid into alveoli • Hypoxemia and carbon dioxide retention
18. a. 8; b. 5; c. 7; d. 11; e. 2; f. 12; g. 3; h. 6; i. 10; j. 4; k. 9; l. 1
19. b

20. b
21. b
22. d
23. d. The older adult usually does not have leukocytosis.
24. a. Incentive spirometry. (See Chart 31-5 for other NIC nursing interventions.)
25. a. 1; b. 2; c. 2; d. 2; e. 1; f. 1; g. 2; h. 3
26. Dyspnea and respiratory distress, rapid breathing, and dry cough
27. c
28. Answer *c* is correct. a. Smoking damages lungs; b. Immunosuppression; d. Postoperative and decreased mobility
29. d
30. a
31. c
32. a
33. b
34. • Noninfection by aspiration or inhalation. • Infectious invasion by environment. • Invasive devices or equipment.
35. b
36. c
37. c
38. d
39. d
40. a
41. b
42. b
43. c
44. See Continuing Care section under "Pneumonia" heading.
45. a
46. a
47. d
48. b
49. b
50. a (See Table 31-5.)
51. *Clients at risk:* Clients who are receiving tube feedings. Clients who had procedures interfering with swallowing, such as a bronchoscopy. Clients who have difficulty swallowing, such as those who have had a stroke or head injury. Clients with a change in level of consciousness.
Nursing interventions: Head of bed should always be elevated unless feeding is turned off. Assess tube placement and residual and adjust feeding as needed. Assess gag reflex before resuming diet or fluids. Monitor the client's ability to swallow small bites. Drinking thick liquids and eating soft foods. Consult a dietitian and obtain swallowing studies. Administer no thin liquids. Monitor client's ability to swallow saliva; if unable, turn client's head to the side to prevent aspiration. Do not feed client.

52. Inhaling chemicals, cleaning agents, smoke, fumes.
53. Increased respiratory rate, dyspnea, fever, cough, purulent, blood tinged, or rust-colored sputum, pleuritic chest discomfort. (See text and Table 31-6 for pathophysiology of assessment findings.)
54. c. Because of age and community-acquired pneumonia.
55. b
56. b
57. b
58. a. 8; b. 2; c. 6; d. 1; e. 7; f. 5; g. 3; h. 4
59. c
60. d
61. a
62. a
63. d
64. c
65. Multidrug regimens destroy organisms as quickly as possible and minimize the emergence of drug-resistant organisms.
66. d
67. d
68. d
69. b
70. There is a three-drug regimen of isoniazid, rifampin, and pyrazinamide, then ethambutol or streptomycin is added.
71. The medication regimen of 6 months or longer must be strictly adhered to. When adherence to the protocol is in question, the direct observation treatment (DOT) method is implemented. A public health nurse or a responsible family member watches the client swallow the medication.
72. b
73. b
74. a. 5; b. 2; c. 4; d. 1; e. 3; f. 6; g. 1; h. 4; i. 2; j. 4
75. b
76. c
77. c
78. See text for HP 2010 chart under "Tuberculosis" heading.
79. b
80. Past exposure to someone with TB; foreign travel or residence; past skin testing for TB and results; and vaccination with BCG; diffuse anxiety or nervousness.
81. a
82. d

Case Study

Answers provided on the SIMON website:
http://www.wbsaunders.com/SIMON/Iggy/

STUDY GUIDE NUMBER 6.32

Interventions for Critically Ill Clients with Respiratory Problems

1. c
2. a. Y. Postoperative immobility; decreased fluids; usually age >50 years of age.
   b. Y. Hypercoagulability.
   c. N. Out of bed; home; no risk.
   d. Y. Damage to veins; increases risk.
   e. Y. Increase viscosity of blood; >60 years old; hospitalized.
   f. Y. Abnormal red blood cells.
   g. N. No causes.
   h. Y. Obesity: large abdomen causes decreased venous return and increases risk for DVT.
   i. Y. Same as *h*.
   j. Y. Risk for amniotic fluid PE.
   k. N
   l. Y. Decreased mobility; surgical client.
   m. Y. Clot to brain, lung, intestine.
   n. Y. No muscle pumping; stagnation of blood in legs; risk for DVT.
   o. N. Not *all* clients; however, this is a consideration in determining risk.
3. d
4. a
5. b
6. b
7. The majority of clients' signs and symptoms are complaints of sudden onset of shortness of breath; sharp stabbing localized pain in the chest when taking in a breath (inspiration). Client points to the site of pain. Increased breathing rate and increased heart rate. Sometime there is a dry cough; flu-like symptoms—rash on chest and axilla with a low-grade fever or crackles in lungs of 50% of clients. Monitor for more severe dangerous signs of hypoxemia—cyanosis of lips, mucous membranes, conjunctiva, and nail beds; changes in heart sounds; adventitious lung sounds; diaphoresis; fear of impending doom; ECG changes; distended neck vein; changes in blood gases; and changes in oxygen saturation. Severe respiratory distress/ARDS and respiratory/cardiac arrest can occur.
8. b
9. Answer *d* is correct because client was started on heparin therapy. a. Client needs immediate anticoagulant therapy and oral agents take 2 to 3 days to reach therapeutic range. b. Elevate head of bed to facilitate breathing and frequently perform a respiratory assessment for changes in status—notify physician. c. Provide oxygen therapy via nasal cannula or mask.

10. d
11. b
12. a
13. b, c
14. c
15. c
16. c
17. b
18. See Charts 32-7 and 32-8.
19. a. Blowing off CO_2, coughing; the body has not converted to anaerobic.
20. See textbook under DVT and PE headings.
21. See text and Chart 32-4.
22. c
23. d
24. b. After pulmonary contusion develops, flail chest may result; shock is not a problem and aggressive fluids are not used because it is a respiratory issue and prevention of ARDS is the concern; clinical manifestations are insidious and can occur hours later.
25. c
26. c
27. b
28. a
29. b
30. d
31. b
32. d
33. b
34. b
35. a
36. a. 2; b. 1; c .3; d. 2; e. 1; f. 1; g. 2; h. 3; i. 2; j. 1; k. 1; l. 2; m. 1; n. 1; o. 3; p. 2; q. 1; r. 1; s. 2
37. d
38. Severe changes in respiratory pattern leading to Ineffective Breathing Pattern related to inability to effectively cough, poor chest movements, diminished or inaudible breath sounds, and wheezing.
39. a
40. c
41. a
42. c
43. b
44. • Maintain a patent airway. • Reduce the work of breathing. • Provide a way to remove secretions. • Provide ventilation and oxygen. See Table 32-4.
45. a. 3; b. 1; c. 4; d. 2
46. In addition to the correct size tube and insertion supplies, other supplies needed are a resuscitation bag; source for 100% oxygen; suction equipment; oral airway; and a means to secure the tube.
47. c
48. (See text and Chart 32-9.) Listen for bilateral breath sound to detect dislodgment.

49. a
50. a. 1, 2, 3; b. 3; c. 2; d. 1; e. 1, 2, 3; f. 1
51. a. 8; b. 3; c. 2; d. 5; e. 7; f. 10; g. 6; h. 1; i. 9; j. 4; k. 11
52. a. No problem, but low oxygen; give oxygen.
    b. Metabolic acidosis; correct metabolic cause.
    c. Respiratory acidosis; increase ventilations, especially length of expiration with pursed-lip breathing.
    d. Respiratory alkalosis; decrease ventilations or have client re-breathe ventilations.
    e. No problem; no treatment needed.
    f. Respiratory acidosis; give oxygen, increase length of expirations and ventilations.
53. a. Hypotension, fluid retention
    b. Pneumothorax, blood gas abnormalities; subcutaneous emphysema, pneumomediastinum
    c. Fatigue, stress ulcer, malnutrition
    d. Infection
    e. Loss of muscle mass, decreased strength
54. c (See text.)
55. b
56. a
57. a
58. d
59. d. All others indicate respiratory distress and possible re-entubation.
60. a, b, d, g, h, i. All other answers are incorrect. (See text and Chart 32-10 for further details.)
61. c
62. a

STUDY GUIDE NUMBER 7.33

Assessment of the Cardiovascular System

1. a. SA node rate is 60 to 100 beats/min; b. AV node rate is 40 to 60 beats/min; c. Bundle of His is 20 to 40 beats/min.
2. c
3. b
4. c
5. Electrical and mechanical
6. a. 1; b. 6; c. 1; d. 5; e. 2; f. 3
7. a. by cardiac output
   b. Cardiac output (CO) is the amount of blood pumped, in liters, from the left ventricle each minute.
   c. CO = heart rate (HR) • stroke volume (SV)
   d. SV is the amount of blood ejected by the left ventricle during each systole. Variables include preload, afterload, heart rate, and contractility.
   e. Preload refers to the degree of myocardial fiber stretch at the end of diastole and just before contraction of the heart. It is determined by left ventricular end-diastole (LVED) volume.
   f. The more the heart is filled during diastole (within limits), the more forcefully it contacts. However, excessive filling of the ventricles results in excessive LVED volume and pressure and a decreased cardiac output. (See Figure 3-7.)
   g. Afterload is the pressure or resistance that the ventricles must overcome to eject blood through the semilunar valves into the peripheral blood vessels. The amount of resistance directly relates to arterial blood pressure. Aortic compliance and total systemic vascular resistance affect afterload.
   h. Heart rate refers to the number of times the ventricle contracts per minute. It affects cardiac output by increasing the rate as needed via the effect of the autonomic nervous system.
8. (See Figure 33-5.) Electrophysiologic properties of the heart muscle are responsible for regulating heart rate and rhythm. Cardiac muscle cells are unique because they possess the following special characteristics: automatic function, excitability, conductivity, contractility, and refractoriness.
9. The left ventricle is the major workhorse of the heart that pumps oxygenated blood throughout the body; therefore it directly impacts systolic and diastolic values. The blood pressure is determined by the quantity of blood or the cardiac output (CO). The formula for determining blood pressure is BP = CO × PR.
10. The left ventricle increases in size and becomes stiff and diastolic filling is slower, resulting in decreased cardiac output, decreased stroke volume, decreased ejection fraction. This results in decreased compensatory mechanism during increased activity to meet oxygen demand. Chest pain can occur. Changes in blood pressure, which occur in conjunction with other vascular changes of the aorta (i.e., atherosclerosis), can result in hypertension. Other changes in baroreceptor can result in decreased blood pressure with symptoms of dizziness and fainting. Changes in body positioning may be affected by the autonomic nervous system. The respiratory cycle causes paradoxical changes in the systolic blood pressure. Older clients can have a wider pulse pressure.
11. The nervous, renal, and endocrine systems. (See text for details and external factors.)
12. The baroreceptors, chemoreceptors, and stretch receptors. (See text for descriptions.)
13. a. False
    b. False
    c. True
    d. True
    e. False
    f. True

14. d
15. a
16. a
17. See Chart 33-1.
18. See Figures 33-12 and 33-11.
19. a
20. c
21. d
22. c
23. (See Figure 33-10.) In assessing the client's hands, arms, feet, and legs for skin changes, vascular changes, capillary filling, and edema, the nurse also will assess for clubbing of the fingers and toes. Clubbing results from chronic oxygen deprivation in these tissue beds. Clubbing is characteristic in clients with advanced chronic pulmonary disease, congenital heart defects, and cor pulmonale. Clubbing is identified by assessing the angle of the nail bed. The angle of the normal nail bed is 160 degrees. With clubbing, this angle increases to greater than 180 degrees, and the base of the nail becomes spongy.
24. b
25. a. 3; b. 6; c. 4; d. 3; e. 1; f. 1; g. 6; h. 2; i. 5; j. 2; k. 5; l. 3; m. 4
26. Chest pain is not indicative of angina or MI but indicates pericarditis. (See Table 33-1 for more information regarding differentiation of chest pain.)
27. a
28. c
29. c
30. Compare your answer with Chart 33-2.
31. Age; sex; ethnic origin; height; weight; major illness (e.g., diabetes mellitus, kidney disease, anemia, high blood pressure, stroke, bleeding disorders, connective tissue diseases, chronic pulmonary disease, heart disease, thrombophlebitis); history of streptococcal infection or rheumatic fever; congenital heart defects; drug allergies; habits (e.g., alcohol consumption, use of drugs, caffeine intake, smoking activity level and type); family history; diet history (especially intake of sodium, sugar, cholesterol, and fat); household members (spouse, children, others); living environment; occupation; hobbies; history of obesity or weight gain; estrogen intake; emotional stress; details of current health problems such as chest pain, dyspnea, fatigue, palpitations, weight gain, syncope, pain in extremities; psychosocial factors such as support systems, coping abilities, fear about pain, disability, self-esteem, physical dependence, change in family role dynamics.
32. Objective data can include general build and appearance; skin color; distress level; level of consciousness; shortness of breath; position (posture); clubbing; capillary fill delay; edema; paresthesia;

muscle fatigue; loss of hair; blood pressure; pulse pressure; jugular venous pressure; presence of hepatojugular reflux; quality of peripheral arterial pulsations; pulsus alternans; pulsus bisferiens; carotid bruit; tachypnea; use of accessory muscles of breathing; dyspnea; shallow respirations; Cheyne-Stokes respirations/hemoptysis; adventitious breath sounds (crackles or wheezes); precordial vibration or movement except at PMI; heaves; lifts; thrills; auscultation for rate, rhythm, murmurs, extra systolic sounds, and rubs; abnormal splitting of S_2; presence of S_3 or S_4.
33. a
34. One-half pack/day • 2 years = 1 pack-year, one pack/day • 4 years = 4 pack-years, two packs/day • 20 years = 40 pack-years for a total of 45 pack-years
35. Complete the exercise and show your clinical instructor.
36. b
37. b
38. b
39. a. True
    b. False
    c. True
    d. True
    e. True
40. a. False. It begins with inspection.
    b. True
    c. True
    d. False. They are associated with palpation.
    e. True
    f. False. Turn the client to the left.
    g. False. It is for high-frequency sounds.
    h. True
    i. True
41. c
42. d (See Figure 33-19 for placement of precordial ECG leads.)
43. c (See text for details regarding cardiac catheterization and Table 33-6 for complications.)
44. a. 3; b. 2; c. 5; d. 1; e. 4
45. Cholesterol, triglycerides, LDLs
46. HDLs, high HDL-to-LDL ratio
47. a. 2; b. 3; c. 1
48. d
49. d
50. a. Hemodynamic monitoring refers to invasive monitoring that uses a continuous electronic device to monitor the arterial or venous system.
    b. There are three primary types: (1) intra-arterial monitoring (A-line) for BP monitoring and arterial blood access; (2) central venous pressure (CVP line) for measuring pressures in right side of the heart; and (3) pulmonary artery monitoring (PA line/Swan Ganz line). All of these pro-

vide data that are useful in evaluating left and right ventricular function, management of clients with cardiac failure or shock and effectiveness of drugs. These types of monitoring devices can determine pulmonary artery pressure, pulmonary artery wedge pressure, and cardiac output.

c. Postoperative states, circulatory shock, ARDS, ARF, MI, clients on mechanical vents, left ventricular failure, preoperative assessment of high-risk surgical clients, shock unresponsive to fluid therapy.

d. Technical aspects include leveling transducer, no air bubbles in system, maintaining system with heparinized saline at 300 mm Hg, special tubing; written consent is required, adherence to strict milliliter policies and procedures for maintaining lines, prevention of complications such as pulmonary infarction, hemorrhage, accurate readings and interpretations of values.

e. Impedance cardiography (ICG) is noninvasive monitoring. Its main purpose is to measure the resistance to the flow of electricity in the heart.

51. d
52. cardiac catheterization
53. seafood and contrast agents.
54. The client should be informed that he/she may experience palpitations (as the catheter is passed up to the left ventricle), a feeling of heat or a hot flash (as the dye is injected into either side of the heart), and a desire to cough (as the dye is injected into the right side of the heart).
55. Client education regarding purpose of the test, the length of time, sensations the client may experience, and appearance of the room. Obtain any blood work or results and perform an assessment of the vital signs, heart and lung sounds, and all peripheral pulses. If the client does have an allergy to seafood, obtain a physician order for an antihistamine. Assess any medication the client is taking and obtain instruction from the physician regarding administration of these medications before the test. (Often digitalis and diuretics are withheld.) The physician obtains an informed consent and explains the complications.
56. intravascular ultrasonography
57. c, d, e, f, g, h
58. a
59. The purpose is to monitor cardiac activity for an extended period of time (usually 24 hours). This is a type of portable ECG. The client keeps a log in order to correlate assessment findings with the ECG readings. Clients are to avoid heavy machinery, using electric shavers and hair dryers, bathing, or showering.
60. a. True
    b. False
    c. True

d. False
e. False
f. True
g. True
h. True
i. True
j. True
k. True
l. False
m. False

61. It is used to assess myocardial scarring and perfusion, detect the location and extent of an acute or chronic MI, evaluate graft patency after coronary bypass surgery, and evaluate antianginal therapy, thrombolytic therapy, or balloon angioplasty.

Case Study

Answers provided on the SIMON website: http://www.wbsaunders.com/SIMON/Iggy/

STUDY GUIDE NUMBER 7.34

Interventions for Clients with Dysrhythmias

1. a. 9; b. 2; c. 7; d. 8; e. 6; f. 5; g. 1; h. 4; i. 3
2. a. 4; b. 10; c. 1; d. 8; e. 6; f. 3; g. 5; h. 9; i. 2; j. 7; k. 11
3. b
4. Bundle of His, right and left bundle branches, Purkinje fibers
5. a. AV node
   b. Bundle of His
   c. Purkinje fibers
6. The term *arrhythmia* means a complete absence of rhythm, which is the electrical conduction and mechanical contraction that results in a heartbeat. *Dysrhythmia* is a disorder or irregularity in the cardiac cycle. There is still a heartbeat, but it may not be effective in producing a cardiac output sufficient to sustain life.
7. a. True
   b. True
   c. False. The QRS complex is formed.
   d. True
   e. True
   f. False. It is just the ventricles and not the atria.
8. b
9. a. 4; b. 1; c. 3; d. 6; e. 5; f. 2
10. (1) Analyze the P waves; (2) analyze the QRS complexes; (3) determine the atrial rhythm or regularity; (4) determine the ventricular rhythm or regularity; (5) determine the heart rate; (6) measure the PR interval; (7) measure the QRS duration; (8) interpret the rhythm. (See Chart 34-1.)

11. b

12. See Figure 34-3.

13. a

14. d

15. 60—1500 divided by 25

16. 60—bradycardia

17. b

18. b

19. c

20. See Chart 34-2.

21. See text, Table 34-2, and Chart 34-3.

22. a. True
    b. False. There is a delay in the AV node conduction and all impulses reach the ventricles.
    c. True
    d. True
    e. False. P-R interval is constant.
    f. False. First-degree and Mobitz type I may not need interventions.
    g. True

23. a. 7; b. 4; c. 6; d. 6; e. 8; f. 3; g. 1; h. 2; i. 6; j. 5 or 6

24. Ischemia of cardiac tissue; digitalis toxicity, increased catecholamine release; hypoxia; electrolyte imbalances; overuse of stimulants; lack of sleep and anxiety

25. a. Confusion, lightheadedness, seizures; hypotension related to decreased cardiac output. VT, VF, asystole
    b. Ventricular rate, location of block, and cardiac output
    c. (4)
    d. Oxygen and pacemaker
    e. Permanent. It is used for conduction disorders such as CHB.
    f. Interventions include surgical intervention; battery replacement after many years; activity is gradually increased; gentle range-of-motion exercise to affected shoulder; initially, monitoring of ECG occurs at regular intervals via community programs; and site care. Teaching includes information that the use of microwave ovens is safe; avoid MRI scanners; and travel without restrictions.

26. d (See Chart 34-3.)

27. Both types are hooked up to an external generator. *External/noninvasive* is the use of large electrode patches in an emergency situation for profound bradycardia or asystole. It is temporary until client converts or invasive measures are used. *Invasive* is the use of lead wires. Two types of invasive pacing are transvenous and epicardial. Transvenous is pacing wires percutaneously placed through a vein to the right ventricle. Epicardial pacing is done after cardiac surgery and is accomplished by wires on the epicardial surface of the heart.

28. Discomfort, skin irritation, and diaphoresis

29. Demand mode means that a cardiac pacemaker is set so that it produces an electrical impulse to trigger a contraction only if the client's own intrinsic rhythm is less than a targeted range. If the client's heart is capable of producing and conducting its own impulses, the demand pacemaker does not function.

30. d

31. c

32. b

33. c

34. d

35. *Subjective data* include history of cardiac arrest, coronary artery disease, heart failure, congenital defects, and rheumatic fever; cardiac medications including diuretics, supplemental electrolyte therapy; palpitations; shortness of breath; chest pain; weakness; dizziness; confusion; black-outs; diaphoresis; caffeine and alcohol intake; smoking history; and psychosocial factors such as fear of incapacitation or death and fear of recurrence of an MI. *Objective data* include heart rate; rhythm; hypotension; confusion; restlessness or anxiety; dyspnea; oliguria; irregularity of apical or radial pulse; pulse deficit; delayed capillary refill; pale, ashen, or cyanotic skin color; cool, diaphoretic skin; adventitious lung sounds such as crackles; weakness; fatigue.

36. Decreased Cardiac Output

37. • Type of dysrhythmia • What is the cause of the dysrhythmia? • What effect does it have on the cardiac output? • The risk to the client

38. a

39. b

40. c

41. d

42. a

43. b, c, d, e (See text and Chart 34-6 for details on purpose, dosage, and nursing interventions.)

44. c

45. b

46. a. False
    b. True
    c. True
    d. False
    e. True
    f. True

47. b

48. b

49. Stress management, take medications regularly, and stop smoking and avoid caffeine.

50. ROM exercises, follow-up appointment with physician, teach how to take pulse, what signs and symptoms to report, medications, pacemaker battery follow-up, medical alert bracelet, indications of battery

failure, diet, physical activity, do not operate electrical appliances directly over the pacemaker, inform dentist regarding pacemaker. (See Chart 34-9.)

51. See text and Chart 34-10 for details.
52. See Chart 34-8.
53. a
54. c
55. a
56. a
57. d
58. c
59. b
60. b
61. d
62. Atrial flutter
63. Bradycardia with premature atrial contraction (PAC)
64. Atrial tachycardia
65. Atrial flutter
66. Sinus arrest
67. Sinus tachycardia
68. Ventricular fibrillation
69. First-degree heart block
70. Normal sinus rhythm with PVC
71. Ventricular fibrillation
72. Ventricular tachycardia
73. Asystole
74. Atrial fibrillation
75. Atrial flutter
76. First-degree heart block
77. Second-degree heart block (Wenckebach)
78. Normal sinus rhythm with PJC
79. Third-degree heart block/complete heart block
80. Second-degree heart block Type II
81. PVCs (bigeminy)

Case Study

Answers provided on the SIMON website:
http://www.wbsaunders.com/SIMON/Iggy/

STUDY GUIDE NUMBER 7.35

Interventions for Clients with Cardiac Problems

1. a, d, e, f
2. Fever; chills; malaise; night sweats; fatigue; heart murmurs; peripheral edema; weight loss or gain; anorexia; shortness of breath; crackles; sudden abdominal pain radiating to left shoulder and rebound tenderness; flank pain radiating to groin with hematuria or pyuria; transient ischemic attacks; cerebrovascular accident; confusion; aphasia; dysphagia; pleurisy; dyspnea; cough; petechiae; splinter hemorrhages; Osler's nodes; Janeway's lesions; splenomegaly; finger clubbing

3. b
4. c
5. c
6. a
7. b
8. b
9. See text and Chart 37-10.
10. c
11. a. True
    b. False. In the first 48 to 96 hours before steroid therapy.
    c. True
    d. False. Best heard over the left lower sternal border.
    e. True
    f. True
    g. True
    h. False. Includes NSAIDs.
    i. False. Streptococcal infection.
12. b
13. (See Chart 35-12.)
14. b
15. a
16. a. 3; b. 4; c. 7; d. 5; e. 2; f. 1; g. 6; h. 8; i. 9
17. a. True
    b. True
    c. False
    d. False
    e. True
18. See text, "Acute Cardiac Tamponade."
19. a. 2; b. 4; c. 3; d. 7; e. 1; f. 5; g. 7; h. 6
20. c
21. a. True
    b. False
    c. True
    d. True
    e. True
    f. False
    g. True
    h. True
    i. False
22. a
23. See text under "Transplantation" heading.
24. d
25. a. True
    b. True
    c. False. Left side.
    d. False. Mitral valve.
    e. True
    f. True
    g. True
    h. False. Stenosis.
    i. True
    j. False. Left-sided and cardiac output.
26. b and e

27. c
28. a
29. a
30. b
31. c
32. a. 2; b. 4; c. 1; d. 5; e. 1; f. 3; g. 1; h. 5; i. 2; j. 2; k. 2; l. 3; m. 3; n. 4; o. 4
33. See text for details and table on valvular heart disease.
34. b
35. c

36. b
37. a
38. Specifics related to disease process, preventive care, etiology, epidemiology, medications, surgery, self-care measures, and psychosocial support.
39. a
40. c
41. d
42. d
43. b

44.

Compensatory Mechanism	Action to Increase CO with Long-Term Damaging Effect
SNS—Adrenergic receptors	*Action*: Increased heart rate and vasoconstriction. There is also increased venous return to the heart, which stretches the myocardial fibers. This increased stretch is a preload that makes a more forceful contraction, increasing stroke volume and CO. *Long-term effect*: Increase oxygen demand, increase afterload; the resistance against which the heart must pump, too much stretch (preload).
Cardiac dilation	*Action*: The chambers of the cardiac muscle are stretched. The stretching increases the force of contraction. *Long-term effect*: This puts a burden on the muscle and valves.
Cardiac hypertrophy	*Action*: The walls of the heart become thick, increasing muscle mass and increasing the force of contraction. *Long-term effect*: The heart cannot meet the increased oxygen demand that hypertrophied condition requires.
Hormonal response	*Action*: Activates the renin-angiotensin-aldosterone mechanism to raise the blood pressure by increasing fluid retention and vasoconstriction. More blood goes to the left ventricle than out to the system. *Long-term effect*: This eventually increases the stretch (preload) and the resistance (afterload).

45.

Heart Failure Classification	Definition	Effect on System
Systolic dysfunction	LV is unable to eject blood adequately into the circulation.	Left ventricle is unable to relax during diastolic. Hypertrophy can cause this condition
Diastolic dysfunction	Diminished tissue perfusion and blood accumulates in lungs.	Similar to systolic

46. a
47. b
48. d
49. d
50. d
51. a. False. Age is over 70.
    b. True
    c. True
    d. True
    e. True
    f. True
    g. True

52. c
53. See text and Chart 35-6.
54. d
55. See Chart 35-4 and text.
56. b
57. b
58. c
59. b
60. c
61. • Decrease sodium and fat intake • Weight loss • Stop smoking • Exercise • Prompt treatment of infection.

62. b, c, d, e
63. d
64. b
65. a. 3
    b. 2 to 3 days
    c. 3 to 5 days
    d. Several times
    e. At rest
66. a
67. Check vital signs and assess for changes in heart rate and blood pressure; assess for signs and symptoms of poor tissue perfusion—check capillary refill, talk with family members regarding client's memory, interview client regarding activities, rest and sleep pattern, signs and symptoms of cold; meals, amount and type of food; medication, understanding especially the possible side effects and when to call the doctor. Physical assessment of edema in legs, lung sounds, murmurs, skin color, and jugular vein distinction. Interview client regarding urine output—color and amount. Observe client walking and assess any shortness of breath. Assess client and family ability to cope with diagnosis and changes in lifestyle patterns. Contact social worker or aids as needed to help client and family. Encourage client to be as independent as possible.

Case Study

Answers provided on the SIMON website:
http://www.wbsaunders.com/SIMON/Iggy/

STUDY GUIDE NUMBER 7.36

Interventions for Clients with Vascular Problems

1. Atherosclerosis is a thickening or hardening of the arterial wall resulting in a loss of elasticity. Atherosclerosis is a form of arteriosclerosis that involves the formation of plaque within the arterial wall, which leads to eventual interference with blood flow through the artery. Atherosclerosis is the most common cause of vascular disease.
2. b, d, a, c
3. a. Plaque is white and fibrous and partially or completely blocks the flow of blood in an artery.
   b. Mechanical injury: hypertension; chemical injuries: toxins from renal failure, CO from cigarette smoking; natural causes: aging; diseases such as diabetes, hyperlipidemia; others: stress, obesity, and sedentary lifestyle.
   c. Rate of progression depends on factors that cause the injury and the number of risk factors that a client has. For example, if a client is older,

eats a high-fat diet, and has diabetes, the rate of progression is high.
   d. This is a fatty deposit on the inner lining of the arteries but not enough to block blood flow.
4. c
5. d
6. d
7. b
8. a. True
   b. False. 25%.
   c. True
   d. True
   e. True
   f. False. Highest amount.
   g. True
   h. False. Lowers the levels.
   i. True
   j. True
   k. True
9. *Subjective data* would include age; sex; race; weight; height; exercise habits; smoking habits; diet; family diseases; and client's previous health problems (diabetes, hypertension, hyperlipidemia); previous vascular diseases such as cerebrovascular accident, myocardial infarction, and peripheral vascular disease; previous surgical procedures (coronary bypass, carotid endarterectomy, lower extremity revascularization); previous angioplasty or thrombolytic therapy medications; pain and its characteristics; psychosocial factors such as denial of need for assessment or intervention, fear, stressors and stress management, and social support systems. *Objective data* would include areas of dry skin; atrophic changes (hair loss, muscle atrophy, thickened or clubbed nails, circumoral pallor, pale nail beds, reddened skin); cellulitis and distended veins; varicosities; edema; ulcerations of peripheral extremities; shortness of breath; lethargy, irregular heart rate; murmur; pericardial rub; bruits; arterial pulse rates, rhythms, and quality; temperature difference between comparable extremities; nail bed capillary refill delay; pain upon palpation of extremities; positive Homan' test.
10. Review the client's cholesterol level and other lab values—HDL is the good cholesterol and lowers risk and LDL is bad cholesterol and increases risk. Monitor for high triglycerides and homocysteine. Discuss frequency of monitoring. Review normal blood pressure values. Review personal risk factors. Discuss interventions to do before taking medications to minimize risk. It is never too late to decrease risk or slow progression of atherosclerosis and prevent high blood pressure. For atherosclerosis, modify lifestyle: low-fat diet, stop smoking, minimize stress, and begin exercise such as a walking

program. For controlling blood pressure—teach about low salt diet, reducing weight, and importance of exercise, stop/avoid smoking, moderation of alcohol intake, stress control, monitor blood pressure. (See "Hypertension—Deficient Knowledge" in Chapter 36.) Medications that relate to lowering total and LDL cholesterol are available. Provide needed information on drug names, dosages, side effects, and actions. (See Chart 36-1 for drug therapy and related nursing interventions.)

11. c
12. (Also see Chart 36-3, text, and a pharmacology book.)

Antihypertensive Drugs Comparison			
Category and Action	**Common Drugs**	**Unique Side Effects**	**Nursing Implications**
Diuretics—decreases peripheral vascular resistance	Thiazide and Thiazide-like Chlorothiazide (Diuril) Hydrochlorothiazide (Esidrix) Metolazone (Zaroxolyn) Loop Furosemide (Lasix) Ethacrynic acid (Edecrin) Potassium-sparing Spironolactone (Aldactone) Carbonic anhydrase inhibitors Acetazolamide sodium (Diamox)	Loss of potassium	Monitor labs, signs and symptoms for hyper- or hypokalemia. Signs and symptoms of hypokalemia are irregular pulse and muscle weakness. Monitor intake and output. Administer medications early in the day to prevent interruption of sleep. Teach the client regarding potassium supplements either by diet (orange juice or bananas) or medications related to potassium-loosing drugs. Monitor compliance and evaluate for once-a-day dosing. Monitor closely in the older adult.
Beta-adrenergic blocking agents— blocks beta-receptors in the heart and peripheral vessels, reducing cardiac rate and output	Propranolol (Inderal) Atenolol (Tenormin) Nadolol (Corgard) Metoprolol (Lopresor)	Bradycardia Heart failure Shortness of breath and wheezing in clients with history of asthma or bronchospasms Sexual dysfunction Fatigue No usual signs and symptoms of hypoglycemia Weakness Depression—crosses blood brain barrier	Monitor pulse—bradycardia and heart failure Monitor for respiratory difficulty— wheezing and shortness of breath Assess for history of asthma or bronchospasm Hypoglycemic symptoms may be blocked—monitor blood glucose levels Teach to report side effects promptly Monitor closely in the older adult

Antihypertensive Drugs Comparison (continued)			
Category and Action	**Common Drugs**	**Unique Side Effects**	**Nursing Implications**
Calcium channel blockers— inferfere with the transmembrane flux of calcium ions, resulting in reduced vasoconstriction	Nifedipine (Procardia, Adalat) Verapamil (Calan, Isoptin) Diltiazem hydrochloride (Cardizem)	Decreased heart rate Constipation	Monitor pulse with blood pressure Monitor constipation Pedal edema can occur as a result of peripheral vasodilation BP can drop within 30 min of oral dose Monitor for dizziness and orthostatic hypotension; take special precautions with the older adult
Angiotensin-converting enzyme inhibitors: convert angiotensin I to angiotensin II— therefore blocks vasoconstrictors in the body.	Captopril (Capoten) Enalapril (Vasotec) Lisinopril (Prinivil)	Severe hypotension after first dose— postural hypotension Renal function	Monitor renal function tests— creatine and BUN. Monitor for hypotension, especially with first dose. Clients are advised to remain in bed for 2-4 hours to avoid severe hypotension effect; BP is monitored q 15 min. Less effective in older adults and African Americans. More effective in young white adults.
Central alpha agonists—act on the central nervous system, preventing re-uptake of norepinephrine, resulting in a lowering of peripheral vascular resistance and blood pressure	Clonidine hydrochloride (Catapres) Methyldopa (Aldomet)	Hemolytic anemia Sedation, common Postural hypotension, common Impotence, common in males Rash with transdermal patch	Administer at bedtime Instruct client to sit for a few minutes before arising; lie down after first dose and subsequent increases in dosage because of sedation; monitor for other side effects; report any difficulty Monitor closely in the older adult Evaluate client for clonidine patch which provides control up to 7 days
Vasodilators— relax vascular smooth muscle tone; therefore reduces peripheral vascular resistance	Minoxidil (Loniten) Alpha-receptor blockers (Cardura) Terazosin (Hytrin) Nitroglycerin	Postural hypertension	Monitor blood pressure Have client sit or lie down Get up from lying position slowly Seek medical attention if lightheadedness occurs Provide client education regarding how to apply nitroglycerin patch or sublingual form Give first dose at bedtime Monitor closely in the older adult

13. False assumptions that the hypertension is under control because there are no symptoms; false assumptions that the disease has been "cured" because blood pressure is normal; unpleasant side effects from the medications; cost of the medications.
14. d
15. a
16. a, b, c

17. c (See Chart 36-6 for a complete description of stages.) The client may place the leg in a dependent position by lowering the leg down off the side of the bed to facilitate arterial blood flow to the leg and foot. This is a grave sign and an indication of advanced disease that may require intervention or loss of limb.
18. b
19. Arterial: a, b, e, f, g, h, j, k, l, and n. Venous: c, d, i, m, and o.

20. 0.77. The index for normal arterial flow is 1.0. These results indicate a moderate decrease in arterial flow to the extremity. Less than 0.5 indicates a severe decrease in flow.

21. c

22. c

23. a, c, d

24. d

25. Follow plan for atherosclerosis; avoid exposure to cold and constrictive clothing; never apply direct heat to the limb, such as a hot water bottle, heating pad, or hot water; use compression stockings, meticulous foot care (see Chart 36-9); apply dressing to leg ulcers as directed; assess home environment for hazards of injury that may cause infection resulting from poor circulation; report any worsening of symptoms; walking program if appropriate; instructions regarding drug therapy. Meticulous foot care is provided—examine feet daily for any cracks, blisters, wounds because of high incidence of infection; check bathing water with thermometer or elbow, not the hand; avoid going barefoot, wear closed-toed shoes; see podiatrist for trimming of toenails. (Also see Chart 36-8 for more details.)

26. Moisten the dressing until just damp and allow it to dry before changing. Remove dry dressing to debride the wound. Monitor for any signs of infection and report it to the physician immediately. *Do not* use any tape on the skin to secure the dressing or wrap a dressing tightly.

27. b

28. a. False. One or more arteries are dilated with a balloon catheter advanced through a cannula, which is inserted into or above an occluded/stenosed artery.
    b. False. This is not a cure but a local procedure to improve circulation to a given area.
    c. True
    d. True
    e. True

29. a. The six Ps are (1) pain, (2) pallor (changing to cyanosis to black as circulation decreases), (3) paresthesias (numbness and tingling), (4) pulselessness, (5) paralysis, and (6) poikilothermic (changes in temperature from warm to cool to cold) of the legs and feet. Frequent observation, palpation, and interviewing of the client about the symptoms are necessary because changes can occur slowly or quickly as a result of a clot. Compare the assessment findings of the operative leg with the nonoperative leg and preoperative assessment findings. A Doppler device may be necessary to assess the presence of a pulse. Use the back of the hand to assess the temperature of the skin. Perform a pain assessment and do not assume the pain is from the surgical incision site. Document all findings and monitor trends. Notify the physician of any changes that indicate problems of arterial flow.
    b. Pain. Throbbing pain means return of good blood flow. Sharp pain increases as a result of ischemia and is similar to the pain before surgery caused by poor circulation. However, if any of the six P's signs are assessed or the client's condition changes, notify the physician immediately.
    c. Notify the physician immediately and prepare the client for either a thrombectomy to be performed at the bedside or administration of intra-arterial thrombolytic medication.

30. b

31. compartment syndrome.

32. c

33. a. Venous ulcer. (See text and Chart 36-7 for illustrations and explanation of differences and "Physical Assessment/Clinical Manifestations.")
    b. Elevation of legs above the heart versus dependent position of legs facilitates venous return. Avoid crossing the legs and long periods of standing and sitting. Wear elastic stockings to facilitate the blood return when walking. When there is a leg ulcer, take special care to avoid infection.

34. a. False. Changed weekly
    b. False. Moistened with zinc oxide
    c. True
    d. True
    e. False. Toes to knee
    f. True
    g. True

35. Buerger's: a, f, g; Raynaud's: b, c, d, e, h

36. a. 2; b. 1; c. 3

37. Thrombus formation (venous thrombosis) and defective values (venous insufficiency and varicose veins)

38. c

39. Calf or groin tenderness and pain, sudden onset of unilateral swelling of the leg, pain in the calf, may have warmth and edema.

40. d. Heparin SQ is a prophylactic dose for immobilized clients. Heparin IV is fast-acting. Coumadin takes several days to take effect and clients will go home on Coumadin.

41. Coumadin is started after the first dose of LMW heparin. PT and INR values only are monitored. PTT is not monitored.

42. Clients are not hospitalized and receive 1 mg/kg of body weight not to exceed 90 mg every 12 hours. Clients must be instructed in subsequent self-infection technique of this mediation, which includes not massaging the site after the injection. Monitor for improvement in signs and symptoms. Once Coumadin is at a therapeutic range, the LMW heparin is discontinued. Monitor for signs and symptoms of bleeding.
43. protamine sulfate; vitamin K
44. b
45. a. False. May be absent, therefore monitor clients who are known to be at risk.
    b. False. Never advisable because only present in 10% of clients with DVT and may cause PE.
    c. True
    d. True
    e. True
    f. True
    g. True
46. c
47. b
48. c
49. Inform dentist about taking warfarin, follow-up laboratory test, monitor for signs and symptoms of bleeding; use soft bristle toothbrush; avoid traumatic situations as contact sports; when to call physician; carry identification; avoid over-the-counter drugs that affect medication, such as aspirin, antihistamines, large doses of vitamin C, anti-inflammatory agents such as Motrin and Motrin-like products and some antacids; alcohol and wine as advised. (See Chart 36-10 for further details.)
50. b
51. c
52. c
53. • Puncture • Laceration • Transection
54. b
55. c
56. • Establish patent airway • Control bleeding • Restoration of blood flow
57. a. 3; b. 2; c. 1
58. a
59. c
60. a, b, c
61. b
62. a
63. d
64. a
65. c
66. c
67. c. Paralytic ileus.

68. b
69. d
70. b
71. Monitor pulses and signs and symptoms of perfusion. Report any abdominal fullness or pain, and pain in back. Avoid heavy lifting for 6 to 12 weeks as well as straining or pushing/pulling. Avoid driving for several weeks. Comply with taking blood pressure medications, no smoking, and maintain a low-fat, low-cholesterol diet. Control blood glucose levels.
72. b

Case Studies

Answers provided on the SIMON website: http://www.wbsaunders.com/SIMON/Iggy/

STUDY GUIDE NUMBER 7.37

Interventions for Clients in Shock

1. Mean arterial pressure (MAP)
2. b, c, d
3. Cardiac output, total amount of blood
4. Size of the capillary bed
5. c
6. • Lactic acidosis • Fluid and electrolyte imbalances • Myocardial depression
7. b
8. a. 3; b. 1; c. 2; d. 2; e. 1
9. a. True
   b. False. Shock progresses in a predictable, orderly fashion, but death is not inevitable.
   c. False. These are clients who are high risk, but anyone is susceptible to shock if there is lack of oxygen to the cells.
   d. False. In the early stages of shock, the blood pressure is within normal limits or slightly decreased because of adequate compensatory mechanism.
   e. True
   f. True
   g. True
   h. False. Phase I sepsis is easily diagnosed.
   i. True
   j. False. It is hypovolemic, not cardiogenic, shock.
   k. True
   l. True
10. b
11. See text and Chart 37-1.
12. False

13. See text and Table 37-3.

Stage of Shock	General Body Response and Compensation
Initial/early stage	Drop of 5-10 mm Hg in MAP. In this stage, the body compensates by activation of mechanisms to oxygenate vital organs. Compensation by vascular constriction and heart rate to correct MAP. This stage is difficult to detect because of subtle clinical manifestations. It is reversible.
Nonprogressive/compensatory stage	Drop of 10-15 mm Hg in MAP. Cardiac compensation is not enough. Renal (aldosterone, renin, ADH) and chemical (acidosis, hyperkalemia) activated to deliver oxygen to vital organs. Changes in blood pressure systems, pulse pressure; pulse pressure decreases; heart rate increases; urine output decreases because of sodium reabsorption; skin pale, cool because of vasoconstriction; signs and symptoms of hypoxia, e.g., restlessness, increased respiratory rate; increased serum sodium; reversible stage.
Progressive/intermediate stage	Drop of 20 mm Hg in MAP. Compensatory mechanism is failing, leading to anoxia and ischemia of cells. Toxic build-up is life-threatening. Immediate interventions are needed to reestablish MAP. Acidosis significant—signs and symptoms evident; hyperkalemia changes; skin cool, pale. Pulse thready—peripheral system shutting down. Signs and symptoms of anoxia, e.g., altered sensorium, renal failure.
Refractory stage of shock/irreversible	Too much cell death and tissue damage related to tissue hypoxia. Body is unable to respond to interventions. MAP unable to be restored. Build-up of toxic metabolites. Multiple organ dysfunction syndrome (MODS), death.

14. c
15. c
16. a. 3; b. 4; c. 2; d. 1
17. a. 4; b. 6; c. 3; d. 2; e. 1; f. 1; g. 3; h. 1; i. 6; j. 4; k. 1; l. 3; m. 1; n. 1; o. 6; p. 1; q. 6; r. 1
18. d
19. c
20. a (See Table 37-4 for other causes.)
21. d (See Table 37-4 for other causes.)
22. c (See Table 37-4 for other causes.)
23. b (See Table 37-4 for other causes.)
24. b
25. a
26. c
27. b
28. d
29. a. 1; b. 2; c. 2; d. 1; e. 1; f. 2; g. 1
30. c
31. b
32. b
33. d
34. c
35. b
36. b
37. d
38. c
39. a
40. b
41. b

42. a. Control blood loss and monitor for further bleeding.
    b. IV access with large-gauge needle (16-gauge preferred).
    c. Replace intravascular volume with fluids, blood, blood products.
    d. Monitor client, including coagulation studies.
43. a. Triple antibiotic therapy
    b. Crystalloid fluids
    c. Vasopressors
    d. Frequent hemodynamic monitoring
    e. Life support
44. a
45. a
46. c
47. d
48. b
49. d
50. • Deficient Fluid Volume • Decreased Cardiac Output • Disturbed Thought Processes
51. a
52. b
53. See text and Charts 37-2, 37-3, and 37-4.
54. b
55. a
56. Hypernatremia

57. a. True
    b. True
    c. True
    d. True
    e. False. Present in the blood.
    f. True
    g. True
    h. False. Age is very important, particularly in older adults. (See Chart 37-6 for other risk factors of shock.)
    i. False. Increases cardiac output in this phase.
    j. True
58. b
59. Large amounts of toxins and endotoxins produced by the bacteria are secreted into the blood, causing a whole-body inflammatory reaction.
60. Goals: (a) maintain tissue oxygenation, (b) increase body fluid compartment volumes to normal ranges, and (c) support operating compensatory mechanisms. Administer and monitor: (d) oxygen therapy, (e) IV therapy, (f) drug therapies.
61. Hyperdynamic, high-output, or warm shock and hypodynamic, low-output or cold shock.
62. a (See Chart 37-7 for details.)
63. c
64. Yes; see text for discussion of prevention measures.

Case Study

Answers provided on the SIMON website:
http://www.wbsaunders.com/SIMON/Iggy/

STUDY GUIDE NUMBER 7.38

Interventions for Critically Ill Clients with Coronary Artery Disease

1. b
2. a
3. b
4. b
5. Coronary artery spasm, platelet aggregation, and emboli from mural thrombi
6. Fear, anxiety, and anger resulting from inability to do the things they want to do (i.e., limits independence and socialization)
7. c
8. a. Oxygen and nutrients are delivered to the anterior wall and septal wall by the anterior descending coronary artery. Mortality is high because the end result of an MI to this area is decreased cardiac output resulting from pump failure of the left ventricular and/or ventricular dysrhythmias.
9. b
10. a
11. b

12. d
13. b
14. b
15. Ineffective Tissue Perfusion
    b. Administer nitroglycerin as ordered and continue to monitor chest pain. Continue monitoring for signs of an MI. Administer oxygen, nasal cannula at 2 liters. Check pulse oximetry for greater than 92% and increase to 4 liters as needed. Elevate head of bed if not contraindicated to minimize dyspnea. Notify physician. Obtain a 12-lead ECG—check for dysrhythmias; continue to observe the cardiac monitor. Monitor vital signs every 5 minutes. Complete physical assessment including monitoring for an S_3, lungs for wheezes or crackles, and peripheral pulses. Check patency of IV access. Be prepared to administer morphine IV push to relieve chest pain if nitroglycerin is ineffective. Pain increases heart rate, which, in turn, increases oxygen demand. Morphine relieves chest pain, which decreases the heart rate and oxygen demand of the heart. Morphine also reduces circulating catecholamines. Be prepared to draw blood for laboratory tests indicating an MI. Provide comfort care to decrease anxiety. Be prepared to transfer the client to ICU for further treatment of dysrhythmias and monitoring. Prepare for a code situation.
16. See Chart 38-4 and discussion under "Management of Dysrhythmias—Nonsurgical Interventions" in Chapter 34.
17. b
18. d
19. Description of chest discomfort, including pain in upper back, jaw, and arms and type of sensation, location, radiation, and duration; before hospitalization for angina or MI; medications; family history; modifiable risk factors, including eating habits; lifestyle; physical activity levels; nausea during pain episodes; dizziness; weakness; palpitations; psychosocial factors such as denial, fear, anxiety, and anger.
20. Chest pain that lasts longer than 30 minutes; vomiting; diaphoresis; shortness of breath; blood pressure; apical pulse; presence of dysrhythmias; weakened distal peripheral pulses; cool skin temperature; diaphoretic skin; S_3 gallop; increased respiratory rate; breath sounds for crackles or wheezes; S_4; elevated temperature.
21. b
22. See "Class IV Heart Failure: Cardiogenic Shock" in text.
23. Positive inotropic medication to increase cardiac output. (See "Medical Management" in text.)

24. c
25. b
26. The primary reasons for surgery are disease progression is evident or medical management has failed. Candidates for surgery are those with angina with greater than 50% occlusion of the left main coronary artery, unstable angina with severe two-vessel or moderate three-vessel disease, ischemia with heart failure, acute MI, signs of ischemia or impending MI after angiography, or PTCA.
27. (See text.) It is designed to inflate during diastole and deflate before systole.
28. c
29. See text for details and Chart 38-5.
30. a
31. d
32. hemodynamic compromise, increase myocardial oxygen demand, risk of lethal ventricular dysrhythmia
33. d
34. *b, f,* and *g* are correct. a. Take 1 tablet every 5 minutes for the first 15 minutes; if pain is not relieved, then go to the emergency department; the client may be experiencing a heart attack; c. Keep pills with you at all times, but keep them separate from the other pills and within easy reach; d. Nitroglycerin is used only as needed; e. Nitroglycerin under the tongue is fast acting and should relieve the pain quickly. (See Chart 38-11.)
35. b
36. b
37. See Chart 38-2.
38. b
39. b, c, e, f
40. See Table 38-4.
41. Conditions related to decreased cardiac output, pulmonary dysfunction, neurologic dysfunction, acute renal failure, gastrointestinal dysfunction, and infection. (See Table 38-5 for specific problems in these categories.)
42. c
43. b
44. The nurse and physician evaluate the blood pressure, PAWP, right atrial pressure, cardiac output, cardiac index, systemic vascular resistance, and urine output to determine the fluid needs of the client.
45. c. Knowing this is an emergency, the nurse would notify the physician stat, prepare the client for a stat CXR or echo to confirm the diagnosis and interventions by the physician to correct the problem.
46. a. True
    b. False. Infections develop after 4 days.
    c. True
47. See Chart 38-8 and text.

48. Topics include anatomy and physiology of heart, pathophysiology of angina and MI, risk factor modification, activity, exercises, medications, and when to seek medical attention. (See text for details related to these topics and Chart 38-9.)
49. a
50. See Chart 38-1.
51. Review Chart 38-4, "Drug Therapy for Coronary Artery Disease" to familiarize yourself with the drugs, dosage, and nursing interventions. Be ready to use this information in the care of any adult client with cardiac problems.
52. Obtain a complete pain assessment with vital signs and obtain an ECG. Notify the physician, administer nitroglycerin, administer oxygen via nasal cannula starting at 2 to 4 liters or as prescribed. Remain calm and stay with client if possible or have someone stay with the client to monitor his or her condition. Reassess the client 5 minutes after administration of medication. Repeat medications if necessary; notify physician if vital signs deteriorate or if pain is not relieved after three doses of nitroglycerin. If blood pressure is stable, the client can assume position of comfort; however, semi-Fowler's enhances comfort and tissue oxygenation. A quiet, calm environment reduces client's anxiety. Clients may complain of headache caused by the nitroglycerin; administer Tylenol as needed.
53. Begin a walking program. Start by walking the same distance at home as in the hospital three times a day. Gradually increase the walking until the distance total is 2 miles at least three times a week. You may need to walk a short distance several times a day to build up to the total. Carry nitroglycerin with you; monitor your pulse before, during, and after exercise. Stop any activity with an elevation of 20 beats per minute, shortness of breath, angina, or any dizziness. Avoid any straining (i.e., bowel movements, push-ups, pull-ups, weight-lifting). Consult an expert in exercise if necessary.
54. a. True
    b. True
    c. False. Not commonly used.
    d. False. Greater than 30 minutes.
    e. True
55. When the client arrives in the open-heart unit, the nurse cares for the client on mechanical ventilation for up to 6 hours. The nurse connects the mediastinal tubes to drainage containers and monitors closely for the amount and signs of cardiac tamponade; the epicardial pacer wires are grounded and connected to the pacemaker box; pulmonary artery and arterial pressures are monitored as well as heart rate and any dysrhythmias. In addition, fluids and electrolytes, hypothermia, and altered cerebral perfusion are monitored.

56. a
57. Acute pain, Ineffective Tissue Perfusion, Activity Intolerance, Ineffective Individual Coping.
58. Chest pain is caused by ischemia. Pain stimulates the sympathetic nervous system, which increases heart rate and then increases oxygen demand and causes more chest pain. Morphine relieves the MI pain, which decreases myocardial oxygen demand, and reduces circulating catecholamines to reduce heart rate.
59. Respiratory depression, hypotension, and severe vomiting.
60. b
61. a
62. a
63. Heart failure; cardiogenic shock
64. • Blood pressure and pulse in client's acceptable range • Adequate urine output • Mental alertness • Clear lungs on auscultation • Palpable pulses
65. d
66. a
67. The nurse monitors for problems such as acute closure of the vessel, bleeding from insertion site, reaction to the dye, hypotension, hypokalemia, and dysrhythmias. The nurse administers and teaches the client about medications such as calcium channel blockers, aspirin, and beta blockers or ACE inhibitors. Clients with stents need to be instructed about Coumadin, which they will continue to take for 1 to 3 months until endothelial covering is laid over the stent. The nurse also instructs the client in any lifestyle changes relating to coronary artery disease.
68. b
69. All are true.
70. • Fluid and electrolytes • Hypotension • Hypothermia • Hypertension • Bleeding • Pain • Altered levels of consciousness

Case Studies

Answers provided on the SIMON website:
http://www.wbsaunders.com/SIMON/Iggy/

STUDY GUIDE NUMBER 8.39

Assessment of the Hematologic System

1. Blood, blood cells, lymph system, and some organs
2. See textbook under "A+ Preview" heading, especially boldfaced items.
3. Bone marrow
4. RBC, platelets, WBC
5. Fetus develops cells in the liver and spleen until the last month of gestation, at which time the bone marrow begins to form cells. At birth every bone of the neonate is producing blood cells. Flat bones will always produce blood cells. Long bones gradually reduce production until the age of 18 years and then only the ends produce cells.
6. See Figure 39-1.
7. *Albumin:* increases osmotic pressure and prevents leaking of plasma into tissue. *Globulin:* transports substances and protects against infection, a component of antibodies. *Fibrinogen:* activates to form fibrin, an important part of clotting.
8. No nucleus, biconcave disk, able to change shape without breaking
9. See Figures 39-1 and 39-2.
10. b
11. Iron molecule
12. Buffers and helps maintain acid base balance
13. Kidneys control RBCs by producing erythropoietin. Hypoxia increases the flow of erythropoietin, which stimulates bone marrow to produce RBCs. When oxygenation is too high, the kidneys shut down production of erythropoietin.
14. Iron, vitamin B_{12}, folic acid, copper, pyridoxine, cobalt, and nickel.
15. anemia
16. b
17. Sticks to blood vessel walls and forms platelet plugs to stop blood flow to a specific area; produces substances specific to coagulation; maintains blood vessel integrity; performs aggregation
18. thrombopoietin
19. Produced in bone marrow, stored in the spleen, 80% released slowly and 20% stored, life span 1 to 2 weeks, used up or destroyed in normal clotting activities.
20. *White pulp:* filled with lymphocytes and macrophages, filters out old RBCs and bacteria; *red pulp:* has sinuses that store RBCs and platelets; *marginal pulp:* forms ends of arteries and veins.
21. (1) Destroys old RBCs and imperfect ones; (2) assists with iron metabolism; (3) stores platelets; and (4) filters antigens
22. Primary production of blood clotting factors and prothrombin, produces bile salts (critical to vitamin K production in GI tract); stores WBCs and blood cells; converts bilirubin to bile; and stores extra iron within a protein called *ferritin;* produces small amounts of erythropoietin.
23. Localize blood clotting undamaged while circulation is maintained.
24. Platelet aggregation with formation platelet plug; for the three steps of clotting, see text under "Hemostasis/Blood Clotting" heading.
25. aggregate
26. platelet plug
27. False

28. The final result of a platelet plug is a large reaction (compares to a landslide).
29. Anti-antibody reactions, circulating debris, prolonged venous stasis, bacterial endotoxin
30. See Table 39-2.
31. a
32. Calcium and more platelets
33. See Table 39-2.
34. See Figure 39-5.
35. b
36. Refer to textbook.
37. anticoagulant forces
38. (See Figure 39-6.) Digests fibrin, fibrinogen, prothrombin, and factors V, VIII, XII.
39. • Total body water decreased • Lower concentration of plasma proteins • Decreased plasma osmotic pressure • Loss of blood volume into interstitial tissue • Fewer blood cells • Lower RBC and WBC count • Lymphocytes are less reactive to antigens and lose some immune function • Antibody levels and response are lessened • Leukocyte count does not rise as high with infection • Hemoglobin levels are lower.
40. Exert effect by interfering with one or more steps. For categories, see text.
41. Degrade fibrin threads. Common agents: tissue plasminogen activator (TPA), streptokinase, reteplase, anistreplase.
42. CVA, MI, limited arteriole thrombosis, occluded shunts
43. b
44. a, b, c
45. a, b, c, d
46. anemia
47. nutritional deficiencies
48. protein and iron
49. Average number of pads used, recent changes in amount, clot sizes (e.g., compare size to coins)
50. fatigue
51. Vertigo, tinnitus, anorexia, dysphagia, sore tongue
52. Mucous membranes, nailbeds, gums, conjunctiva, palmer creases
53. Petechiae: Pinpoint hemorrhage (best visible on soles of feet and palms of hand); ecchymoses: large bruises.
54. Pernicious anemia and iron deficiency cause a smooth tongue. Nutritional deficiency causes a smooth red tongue and possible fissure.
55. hematuria
56. liver; spleen
57. Cerebral, olfactory, spinal cord, peripheral nerve function, and neurologic damage
58. See Chart 39-3.

59. Elevated macrocytes, abnormally large, megaloblastic anemia. Decreased microcytic, abnormally small, iron deficiency anemia.
60. myelogenous leukemia
61. Demonstrate
62. Coumadin and Warfilone; 1½ to 2 times
63. 2.0 to 3.0
64. 2 times normal
65. Factors II, IX, X, and vitamin K
66. von Willebrand's disease
67. True
68. Biopsy: solid tissue and cells. Aspiration: cells and fluid
69. pressure; pain

STUDY GUIDE NUMBER 8.40

Interventions for Clients with Hematologic Problems

1. d
2. • Number of RBCs • Quantity of hemoglobin or hematocrit
3. See Table 40-1.
4. a. S; b. R; c. S; d. R; e. S; f. S; g. S; h. S; i. R; j. R; k. S
5. Disease has two abnormal genes, trait has only one abnormal gene.
6. b
7. a, b
8. • Hypoxia • Dehydration • Infections • Vascular status • Low body temperature • Acidosis • Strenuous exercise • Anesthesia
9. Pain: treat initially with opioids IV, then give orally as client pain is controlled.
10. a. Heart rate up, blood pressure down
    b. Pale, cyanotic, jaundice
    c. Spleen and liver enlarged
    d. Vascular occlusion
    e. Cerebral hypoxia
11. Warm room causing disorientation, distraction, relaxation, proper positioning, aroma therapy, therapeutic touch, warm compresses, or soaks
12. a, b, c
13. b, c
14. c
15. Review explanation in book.
16. See Chart 40-8.
17. Use text and Table 40-3 and review with instructor.
18. d
19. True
20. a, b, c, d
21. Oral alkylating agents, irradiation, with injection radioactive phosphorus, bone marrow transplant

22. Lymphocytic/lymphoblastic: within the committed lymphoid pathway
    Myelocytic/myelogenous: within committed myeloid pathway
23. Malignant transformation of stem cells; an abnormal proliferation shuts down normal bone marrow production
24. Refer to text under "Etiology of Leukemia" heading.
25. True
26. b
27. a, b, c
28. Immature cells are dividing
29. Use textbook under "Analysis for Leukemia" heading.
30. Client's normal flora overgrows and penetrates the internal environment from another person or thing in the environment.
31. a. 2; b. 1; c. 3; d. 2
32. c
33. d
34. Use textbook under "Collaborative Management for Leukopenia" heading.
35. a
36. True
37. b
38. a. 2; b. 3; c. 1
39. Stem cell procurement, conditioning, transplantation, engraftment, post transplantation
40. False
41. a, b, c
42. a
43. Chemotherapy or hematopoietic growth factor are administered to make stem cells circulate in peripheral blood and increase WBCs.
44. Catheter clotting, hypocalcemia, chills, abdominal and muscle cramps, chest pain, hypotension, paresthesia
45. True
46. False
47. d
48. d
49. Insufficient number of cells transplanted; insufficient attachment or rejection of donor cells; infection in the donor cells, unknown biologic factor
50. See textbook (Graft cells are attacking client cells.); skin, GI tract, liver
51. False
52. c
53. b
54. Greatest point of bone marrow suppression
55. See Charts 40-10 and 40-11.
56. 6 to 12 hours after completion of chemotherapy
57. False
58. See textbook. Increase RBC production.
59. Same as hospital—prevent infection.

60. See textbook under "Overviews for Leukemia" and "Lymphoma" headings.
61. a. 1; b. 1; c. 2; d. 2; e. 1; f. 1; g. 1; h. 2; i. 1; j. 1; k. 2; l. 1
62. See Table 40-14.
63. See textbook under "Continuing Care for Thrombocytopenia" heading.
64. a. ITP; b. TTP; c. ITP; d. TTP; e. ITP; f. ITP; g. TTP; h. TTP; i. ITP
65. b
66. a
67. b
68. b
69. c
70. d
71. True
72. True
73. a, b, c, d
74. a
75. Factor VIII; cryoprecipitate
76. Degenerating joint function caused by bleeds
77. a, b, c
78. Type, volume, special conditions
79. True
80. Testing donor's blood and recipient for compatibility
81. c
82. True
83. b
84. a
85. False
86. False
87. b
88. b
89. True
90. True
91. A, B, AB, O-no antigen
92. See textbook. Rh: cannot receive Rh+.
93. Rh-immune globulin
94. See text discussion of platelet transfusion.
95. d
96. False
97. True
98. See textbook for blood transfusion discussion.
99. True
100. See textbook for blood transfusion discussion.
101. c
102. Same as symptoms for fluid excess, such as increased blood pressure, bounding pulse, crackles in lungs, edema; older adults are most at risk.
103. See textbook for discussion of Blood Transfusion.
104. d
105. True
106. See textbook for discussion under Blood Transfusion heading.

STUDY GUIDE NUMBER 9.41

Assessment of the Nervous System

1. c, d
2. knob; cleft
3. Strength of stimulation, inhibition by another neuron, extracellular fluid changes, anoxia, anesthetics. (See pp. 3-4.)
4. b
5. a. 3; b. 1; c. 1; d. 2; e. 1; f. 2; g. 2
6. a. 3; b. 1; c. 2; d. 4
7. Brain, spinal cord
8. c
9. a and b
10. a. 3; b. 1; c. 2; d. 5; e. 7; f. 4; g. 6
11. a. 3; b. 4; c. 1; d. 4
12. a, c, and d
13. c
14. b
15. b
16. a. 1; b. 2; c. 2; d. 1; e. 1; f. 1; g. 2; h. 1
17. a. 3; b. 1; c. 2; d. 4
18. • Spinal nerves • Cranial nerves • Autonomic nervous system
19. a and b
20. c
21. • Sympathetic nervous system (SNS) • Parasympathetic nervous system (PAS)
22. a. 1; b. 2; c. 1; d. 1; e. 2; f. 2
23. c
24. See Chart 41-2.
25. a
26. a
27. a. 4; b. 3; c. 5; d. 2; e. 1; f. 6
28. c
29. b
30. a. 4; b. 5; c. 1; d. 3; e. 2
31. b
32. c
33. c
34. a. True; b. True; c. False; d. False; e. True
35. a, c, and e
36. d

STUDY GUIDE NUMBER 9.42

Interventions for Clients with Problems of the Central Nervous System: The Brain

1. a. 1; b. 2; c. 2; d. 2; e. 1; f. 2; g. 1; h. 2; i. 2; j. 1
2. a, c
3. a
4. a

5. a. 3; b. 2; c. 1; d. 4
6. a. True; b. True; c. False; d. False; e. True
7. Type of seizure activity; events surrounding onset.
8. a, b, d
9. a, e
10. a, c, d
11. a, b, d
12. All
13. Via the blood stream, penetrating trauma, and subarachnoid space
14. a. 2; b. 3; c. 1; d. 2; e. 1
15. a, c
16. a
17. c
18. b
19. a, b
20. a, b, d, e
21. c
22. d
23. a
24. c
25. Onset; progression; presence of rigid facial expression; other changes
26. b
27. a
28. Decreased brain weight, enlarged ventricles, widening cerebral sulci, narrowing gyri.
29. a, c
30. b
31. a. 3; b. 1; c. 1; d. 3; e. 2; f. 2; g. 1
32. d
33. a
34. b
35. a, b
36. a
37. a, c

STUDY GUIDE NUMBER 9.43

Interventions for Clients with Problems of the Central Nervous System: The Spinal Cord

1. Obesity, smoking, congenital conditions
2. Degenerative joint disease, rheumatoid arthritis
3. a
4. Proper positioning, exercise, anti-inflammatory drugs, analgesics, and heat and ice
5. b
6. c
7. c
8. a
9. a. 2; b. 1; d. 1; d. 2; e. 1; f. 2

10. *Hyperflexion*—forcefully forward; head on collision. *Hyperextension*—head accelerated then decelerated; struck from behind. *Vertical compression*—axial loading; diving accident. *Rotation*—turning beyond normal range.
11. a. 3; b. 1; c. 2
12. d
13. a
14. c
15. a. 4; b. 3; c. 1; d. 5; e. 2
16. a, b, and c
17. Postural hypotension, skin breakdown; DVTs; osteoporosis; constipation; pulmonary emboli
18. d
19. Mobility and activity skills, ADLs, bowel and bladder training, skin care, medication, and sexuality education
20. a, b, c
21. b, d
22. b
23. a, c
24. c
25. a, b, c, d
26. c
27. b

STUDY GUIDE NUMBER 9.44

Interventions for Clients with Problems of the Peripheral Nervous System

1. c
2. Medical and surgical history; antecedent infection in the last 1 to 8 weeks.
3. c
4. b, c, d
5. c
6. c, d
7. c

8. Perform ambulation, transfers, and bed mobility. No experience of pressure ulcers, constipation, or pulmonary emboli.
9. a
10. d
11. Describe symptoms, specifically noting affected muscle groups; difficulty with ADLs, ptosis, diplopia, and choking.
12. c
13. b
14. a
15. c
16. d
17. Weight loss, client's smile, muscle strength, sensation
18. d
19. a
20. a, b, d
21. Vitamin B_{12} deficiency, drug toxicity, infections, trauma, metabolic disturbances, alcohol.
22. d
23. b
24. c
25. Contusion, stretching, constriction, compression
26. b
27. Recent trauma to pelvic area; pain after injection; penetrating injury.
28. c
29. a. 1; b. 2; c. 2; d. 1; e. 2; f. 2; g. 2; h. 1; i. 2; j. 2

STUDY GUIDE NUMBER 9.45

Interventions for Critically Ill Clients with Neurologic Problems

1. b
2. b, d
3. a

4.

	Type of Stroke		
	Thrombotic	**Embolic**	**Hemorrhagic**
Onset	Daytime; gradual	Daytime; sudden	Daytime; sudden or gradual
Evolution	Intermittent Stepwide	Abrupt, steady progression	Usually abrupt
Contributing Factors	Hypertension Atherosclerosis	Cardiac disease	Hypertension Vessel disorders
Duration	Takes weeks to months	Rapid improvement	Variable

5. a, c
6. a
7. a
8. c
9. a, b, d
10. a, c, d
11. a. 2; b. 1; c. 2; d. 2; e. 2; f. 1; g. 2; h. 1; i. 2; j. 2
12. b
13. a. 4; b. 7; c. 5; d. 2; e. 3; f. 6; g. 1
14. b
15. c
16. c
17. b, c
18. d
19. a
20. Prepare for craniotomy; monitor for hydrocephalus (See textbook for additional interventions under "Stroke" heading.)
21. c
22. b, c, d
23. a. 1; b. 2; c. 1; d. 2; e. 1; f. 2; g. 1; h. 2
24. c
25. c
26. Medication schedules, mobility transfer skills, communication skills, safety, self-care skills, dietary needs
27. c
28. a, c, d
29. a. 8; b. 4; c. 1; d. 2; e. 7; f. 5; g. 9; h. 6; i. 3
30. a. Abnormal permeability of vessels
    b. Disturbance in cellular metabolism
    c. Elevated blood pressure or CSF pressure
31. a. 2; b. 3; c. 1
32. d
33. a
34. c
35. a, c, d
36. a. 3; b. 1; c. 5; d. 4; e. 2
37. c

38. (See Chart 45-5.) decreased LOC, restless, irritable; headache, nausea and vomiting, aphasia, slurred speech, pupil changes
39. c
40. b
41. b, c, d
42. See Table 45-5.
43. Breast, lung, GI tract, and kidney
44. d
45. b
46. a. 1; b. 1; c. 2; d. 2; e. 1; f. 1; g. 2; h. 1; i. 2; j. 2
47. c
48. b
49. c
50. d
51. a, b, d
52. a, d
53. b
54. Nose, ears, and mastoid
55. Heart, lung, dental, and peritonsillar abscesses
56. b
57. d
58. a
59. c

STUDY GUIDE NUMBER 10.46

Assessment of the Eye and Vision

1. c
2. Cornea, aqueous humor, lens, vitreous humor
3. a. 4; b. 2; c. 10; d. 5; e. 7; f. 1; g. 3; h. 6; i. 8; j. 9
4. a
5. a. 2; b. 4; c. 1; d. 3
6. astigmatism, myopia, presbyopia, hyperopia, emmetropia
7. a. 4; b. 5; c. 7; d. 1; e. 3; f. 8; g. 2; h. 6
8. • Foreign body sensation • Photophobia • Glaucoma • Diplopia • Pruritus

9.

Health History	Reason for Obtaining Information
Family history	Some eye conditions show a familial tendency.
Current medical systemic diseases	Diseases like diabetes and hypertension can affect the eye and vision.
Types of sports activities they participate in	Some injuries to the eyes are more common in specific sports.
All medications	Some medications have significant ocular effects.

10. d
11. a. Confrontation
    b. Hemianopsia
12. MRI
13. a. 3; b. 4; c. 5; d. 1; e. 2
14. b, d
15. a
16. b
17. a, b
18. b, c
19. red reflex, optic disk, optic blood vessels, fundus, macula
20. c

STUDY GUIDE NUMBER 10.47

Interventions for Clients with Eye and Vision Problems

1. a. 3; b. 6; c. 1; d. 2; e. 4; f. 5
2. a, b, c
3. • Always wash hands before and after administration. • Avoid touching the tip of the tube to the conjunctiva. • Understand that vision may be blurred by the ointment. • Remove the ointment before driving or operating equipment.
4. a. Hordeolum
   b. Warm compresses and antibiotic ointment
5. c
6. Preventing the spread of the disease.
7. a
8. a, c, d
9. • Elevate the head of the bed 30 degrees • Instill antibiotic eye drops • Close the eyes and apply a small ice pack to the closed eyes
10. • Bleeding • Wound leakage • Infection • Graft rejection
11. c
12. Thorough description of eye pain (location, quantity, quality, timing, setting, aggravating and relieving factors, associated signs and symptoms); visual history including surgery or injury, visual environment, concurrent medical conditions, current and past use of medications; psychosocial data, including age,

any loss of vision and accompanying grieving, anxiety, involuntary change of vocation, loss of self esteem or role identity; chance in lifestyle, feelings of isolation. Decrease visual acuity; photophobia; eye secretions; hazy or cloudy cornea, altered corneal reflex; changes in the integrity of cornea.
13. c
14. Age; presence of other factors such as trauma to the eye; exposure to radioactive materials or x-rays; systemic diseases (diabetes mellitus, hypoparathyroidism, Down syndrome, atopic dermatitis); use of medications such as corticosteroids, miotics, chlorpromazine; presence of intraocular disease (recurrent uveitis); description of client's vision; psychosocial factors such as denial of visual loss, fear of losing eyesight, anxiety interference with activities of daily living: slightly blurred vision; decreased color perception; double blurred images; decreased visual acuity, difficulty or inability to visualize retina with the ophthalmoscope, inability to elicit red reflex.
15. • Bending from the waist • Sneezing • Coughing • Blowing the nose • Straining to have a bowel movement • Sexual intercourse • Keeping the head in a dependent position • Vomiting
16. • Sharp, sudden pain • Increased bleeding or discharge • Lid swelling • Decreased vision • Flashes of light or floating shapes
17. b

18.

Open-Angle	Closed-Angle
1. Most common	1. Rare
2. Asymptomatic	2. Severe pain around eyes; may be accompanied with vomiting, headache, or halos around lights
3. Gradual onset	3. Sudden onset
4. The visual fields initially show a small crescent-shaped defect that gradually progresses to a larger defect.	4. Sclera may appear reddened with shallow anterior chamber and moderately dilated nonreactive pupil.
5. Tonometry reading is between 10-21 mm Hg	5. May be 30 mm Hg or higher

19. (1) Physically constricting the pupil so that the ciliary muscle is contracted, which allows better circulation of the aqueous humor to the site of absorption. (2) Inhibiting the production of aqueous humor.
20. 1a: Beta blocker
    1b: Reduce aqueous humor production
    1c: Monitor the client's heart rate and blood pressure
    2a: Miotic
    2b: Constricts the pupil and contracts the ciliary muscle

2c: Use with caution with clients who have urinary tract obstruction; warn the client that visual acuity is decreased in low light environments
21. Trauma, hypertensive retinopathy, and proliferative diabetic retinopathy
22. d
23. a, b
24. c
25. Arteriole narrowing; arteriovenous nicking; soft exudates (cotton wool patches); flame hemorrhages; papilledema; retinal detachment

26. Background and proliferative
27. c
28. Cryotherapy (freezing probe), photocoagulation (laser), or diathermy (high-frequency current)

29. c
30. b
31. Myopia
32. a. 4; b. 2; c. 1; d. 3

33.

Radial keratotomy	Outpatient for treatment of mild-to-moderate myopia. Eight to 16 diagonal incisions are made but the central cornea is not incised.
Photorefractive keratotomy (PRK)	A laser pulses a brief but powerful beam of ultraviolet light on the central superficial cornea and removes small portions of the tissue surface, which reshapes the cornea to properly focus the image on the retina. Use for people with mild-to-moderate myopia and low astigmatism.
Laser-in-situ (LASIK)	Newest procedure that corrects near and farsightedness and astigmatism using the excimer laser. Superficial layers of the cornea are lifted while a laser pulses the deeper layers for reshaping. Superficial layers are placed back in their position.

34. Color fades gradually and disappears in about 10 days.
35. Melanoma
36. d
37. a, b, c, d
38. Have a friend or relative visit once a week to set up medications. Different shapes are helpful for different times of the day. Talking clocks help remind them of the times. Each day's medication can be in a box with raised letters.

STUDY GUIDE NUMBER 10.48

Assessment of the Ear and Hearing

1. a
2. hearing; balance
3. a. 1; b. 2; c. 2; d. 3; e. 1; f. 3; g. 2
4. a. 5; b. 1; c. 2; d. 3; e. 4; f. 6
5. d
6. a. 2; b. 4; c. 1; d. 3; e. 5
7. b
8. a, c
9. b
10. c, d
11. The long and short processes of the malleus and the umbo.
12. Air conduction of sound is more sensitive than bone conduction and is normally heard 2 to 3 times faster than by bone conduction.
13. a, d
14. a. 2; b. 4; c. 5; d. 1; e. 2; f. 3
15. a
16. a, b, c
17. a. 2; b. 4; c. 1; d. 3
18. Explain the procedure and its purpose. Inform the client that he will need to fast for several hours before the test. Instruct him to avoid caffeine-con-

taining beverages for 24 to 48 hours before the test. Explain that fluids need to be carefully introduced after the test to prevent nausea and vomiting.
19. Assesses the ability to discriminate among similar sounds or words
20. a

STUDY GUIDE NUMBER 10.49

Interventions for Clients with Ear and Hearing Problems

1. d
2. b
3. Congenital malformations, allergic response in the ear canal, cysts or growths, hematoma
4. a, c
5. c
6. Located on outer half of external canal, area swollen and red, intense local pain upon light touch, tight skin covering the area.
7. a
8. a
9. a. His left tympanic membrane has perforated. b. A culture of the drainage.
10. b, c
11. a
12. b
13. d
14. b
15. a, b, c, d
16. Meniere's disease, exposure to loud noises, otosclerosis, ototoxic drugs
17. Restrict head motions, move slowly, take medications with antivertiginous effects such as Dramamine, maintain adequate hydration, maintain a safe environment, use a cane or walker to maintain balance during periods of vertigo
18. a, b, c

19.

Characteristics	Pathologic Changes
Tinnitus	Overproduction or decreased reabsorption of endolymphatic fluid, causing a distortion of the entire inner-canal system. This distortion leads to decreased hearing from dilation of the cochlear duct, vertigo because of damage to the vestibular system, and tinnitus from unknown causes.
Fluctuating unilateral sensorineural hearing loss	
Vertigo	

20. a, b, c
21. c
22. Cerumen-blocking ear canal, foreign body obstructing ear canal, edema of ear canal related to infection of external or middle ear, tumors, otosclerosis, scar tissue build-up on ossicles
23. a. Prolonged exposure to loud noise
    b. Presbycusis
    c. Ototoxic substances
    d. Meniere's disease
    e. Acoustic neuroma
    f. Diabetes mellitus
    g. Labyrinthitis
    h. Infection
    i. Metabolic and circulatory disorders
    Exposure to loud noises is preventable.
24. Degeneration or atrophy of the ganglion cells in the cochlea, loss of elasticity of the basilar membrane, and a decreased vascular supply to the inner ear.
25. c
26. b
27. Encourage the client to start using the hearing aid slowly and limit wearing time to short periods at first. Instruct the client to limit the hearing aid at home at first. Encourage listening to the TV and reading aloud to help the client adjust to new sounds. Inform the client that they will need to learn to filter out background noises.
28. d
29. a, b
30. Avoid straining when you have a bowel movement. Avoid air travel for 2 to 3 weeks. Avoid coughing excessively for 2 to 3 weeks. Stay away from people with colds. If you need to blow your nose, blow gently one side at a time with your mouth open. Avoid getting your head wet, washing your hair and showering for 1 week. Keep your ear dry for 6 weeks by placing a ball of cotton coated with petroleum jelly in your ear and change the cotton daily. Change your ear dressing every 24 hours as directed. Report excessive drainage immediately to your physician.
31. b, d
32. Position yourself directly in front of the client. Get the client's attention before you speak. Keep objects away from your mouth when speaking. Speak clearly and slowly. Use appropriate hand motions.

Keep distractions to a minimum. Rephrase sentences and repeat information to aid in understanding. Write messages if client is able to read.

STUDY GUIDE NUMBER 11.50

Assessment of the Musculoskeletal System

1. a. Long bones (femur, humerus)
   b. Short bones (phalanges)
   c. Flat bones (sternum, scapula)
   d. Irregular bones (carpals)
2. a. 6; b. 3; c. 2; d. 5; e. 4; f. 8; g. 11; h. 1; i. 10; j. 9; k. 7
3. *Answers may be in any order.*
   a. Provides body framework
   b. Supports surrounding tissues
   c. Assists movement
   d. Manufactures blood cells
   e. Protects vital organs
   f. Provides storage for mineral salts
4. Completely immovable (cranium)
5. Slightly immovable (pelvis)
6. Synovial, freely movable (elbow and knee)
7. False. Shoulder, hip.
8. True
9. False. Rotation only.
10. True
11. False. And slight rotation.
12. (Nonstriated) contractions of organs and blood vessels
13. Contraction of the heart
14. Movement of the body and its parts
15. a. 2; b. 3; c. 9; d. 8; e. 5; f. 7; g. 1; h. 6; i. 4
16. False. Decreases.
17. False. Degenerates.
18. True
19. Prior fall; surgery; musculoskeletal disease; or current problem
20. Young male, older adult
21. Older adult female
22. Accidents; illnesses; medications; previous or concurrent disease.
23. Inadequate nutrition, particularly inadequate amounts of protein, calcium, and vitamin C; obesity

24. Insufficient exposure to sunlight; inadequate intake of calcium, protein, and vitamin C; homebound or institutionalized
25. Occupation
26. African-Americans
27. Date and time of onset; factors that cause or exacerbate the problem; course of the problem (intermittent or continuous); clinical manifestations and the pattern of their occurrence; measures that improve clinical manifestations.
28. Improper alignment; spinal deformity
29. Limp; any abnormal stance
30. Use of ambulatory device; inadequate ROM
31. Masses; tenderness; pain; crepitus; swelling; inability to flex, extend, or rotate the neck
32. Tenderness; improper alignment
33. Swelling; deformity; mal-alignment; tenderness; pain; improper ROM; unequal size of digits
34. Pain; inadequate degree of mobility or ROM; mal-alignment; deformity
35. Inadequate grip strength; abnormal size, shape, or tone
36. Prolonged absence from job; chronic pain; numerous stressors
37. d
38. c
39. d
40. a
41. b
42. d
43. a. 3; b. 5; c. 6; d. 12; e. 2; f. 4; g. 7; h. 13; i. 8; j. 9; k. 1; l. 11; m. 10

STUDY GUIDE NUMBER 11.51

Interventions for Clients with Musculoskeletal Problems

1. a. A metabolic disease in which bone demineralization results in decreased density and subsequent fractures; osteoporosis is an irreversible osteopenia.
   b. Not associated with an underlying pathologic condition. Type I (post menopausal) occurs in women between the ages of 55 and 65. Type II (senile) occurs in those older than 65 years of age and affects women twice as often as men.
   c. Results from an associated medical condition, such as hyperparathyroidism, long-term drug therapy, or prolonged immobility.
   d. A reversible metabolic disease in which there is a defect in the mineralization of bone.
   e. A metabolic disorder of bone remodeling or turnover, in which increased resorption or loss results in bone deposits that are weak, enlarged, and disorganized.

2. a. 3; b. 1; c. 2
3. • No smoking or alcohol • Increased exposure to sunlight • Decrease caffeine • Increase calcium, vitamin D, milk and dairy products, and green leafy vegetables.
4. a. 3; b. 1; c. 2; d. 1; e. 1; f. 3; g. 2; h. 1; i. 2; j. 1; k. 3; l. 2; m. 1
5. a. 2; b. 3; c. 3; d. 1; e. 2; f. 1; g. 2; h. 1; i. 3
6. Blocks bone resorption by inhibiting cytokines (slows bone loss).
7. Lack of calcium stimulates the parathyroid gland to produce parathyroid hormone (PTH); PTH triggers the release of calcium from the bony matrix.
8. Adequate vitamin D is needed for optimal calcium absorption.
9. Inhibits bone resorption by binding with crystal elements in bone, especially spongy trabecular bone tissue.
10. Mimics estrogen in some parts of the body while blocking its effect elsewhere; increases bone mineral density; reduces bone resorption and lowers serum cholesterol.
11. Inhibits osteoclastic activity, thus reducing bone loss.
12. a. 6; b. 4; c. 3; d. 1; e. 5; f. 2
13. a. anticonvulsants
    b. barbiturates
    c. fluoride
14. An infection lasting less than 4 weeks; infection occurring in another part of the body moves to and invades bone tissue, particularly the long bones and the vertebrae.
15. An infection lasting longer than 4 weeks; may result from any of the acute types.
16. Bone and often the surrounding tissue are invaded by one or more pathogenic microorganisms. The bone and soft tissue become inflamed, leading to increased vascularity and edema. Vessels in the area occlude, resulting in ischemia and eventual bone necrosis. The necrotic bone tissue forms a sequestrum, which delays healing and causes superimposed infection. The cycle of inflammation, thrombosis, and necrosis is repeated.
17. c
18. b
19. d
20. a. 4; b. 5; c. 2; d. 1; e. 6; f. 3
21. a. 4; b. 3; c. 1; d. 2
22. a. 3; b. 4; c. 1; d. 2
23. a. Prostate
    b. Breast
    c. Kidney
    d. Thyroid
    e. Lung

24. a. Vertebra
    b. Pelvis
    c. Femur
    d. Ribs
25. True
26. False. Most malignant.
27. True
28. False. Dull pain.
29. True
30. Has client had previous radiation therapy for cancer; question general health.
31. Pain; local swelling; tender palpable mass; low grade fever; fatigue; pallor and anemia
32. Feeling loss of control; fear of illness; outcome; grieving; anxiety
33. Nursing diagnoses: Grieving; Impaired Mobility. (Refer to textbook for further discussion, common nursing diagnoses and collaborative problems, and Chart 51-6.)
34. a. 2; b. 1; c. 2; d. 2; e. 1; f. 2; g. 1
35. • Analgesics
    • NSAIDs
    • Chemotherapy
    • Radiation therapy
    • Surgical excision or resection
    • Bracing and immobilization
36. c
37. a, b, d
38. a. State the pain is reduced or alleviated
    b. Perform ADLs and ambulation activities independently
    c. Seek health care resources as needed, including cancer support group
    d. State the body image perception is improved
    e. Return to a functional lifestyle (or accept impending death in the case of advanced metastasis)
    f. State the anxiety regarding medical diagnosis and treatment is decreased
39. a. The median nerve in the wrist becomes compressed, causing pain and numbness. A group of nine tendons, enveloped by synovium, share space with the median nerve in the carpal tunnel. When the synovium becomes thickened or swollen, the nerve is compressed.
    b. Excessive hand exercise; jobs that require repetitive hand activities involving pinch or grasp during wrist flexion.
40. Client is asked to relax the wrist into flexion or place the backs of the hands together and flex both wrists simultaneously. A positive test produces paresthesia in the median nerve distribution within 60 seconds.

41. A test for CTS; tapping lightly over the area of the median nerve in the wrist to elicit a tingling sensation.
42. a. Drug therapy: aspirin, NSAIDs, injection of corticosteroids directly into the carpal tunnel.
    b. Immobilization: splint
43. a. Open carpal tunnel release (OCTR): incision is made and a synovectomy is performed or the removal of a space occupying lesion (if present) is removed. Whatever the cause of nerve compression, the physician removes it either by cutting or with laser.
    b. Endoscopic release: very small incision is made, endoscope inserted, and surgical instruments are used to free the trapped nerve.
44. a. 1; b. 3; c. 1; d. 2; e. 3; f. 1; g. 2; h. 1; i. 2; j. 1; k. 1
45. a. 2; b. 3; c. 1; d. 3; e. 4; f. 5; g. 1; h. 2; i. 1; j. 4; k. 5; l. 5; m. 2
46. True
47. True
48. False. Women are affected more than men.
49. False. During their middle school years.
50. False. Most common.
51. True
52. a. 2; b. 1; c. 2; d. 1; e. 1
53. Make the client as comfortable as possible; reinforce technique and exercise taught in the physical therapy program. The nurse's role in caring for a client with cardiac or other organ involvement is the same as for any client with dysfunction of these areas.

Case Study

Answers provided on the SIMON website: http://www.wbsaunders.com/SIMON/Iggy/

STUDY GUIDE NUMBER 11.52

Interventions for Clients with Musculoskeletal Trauma

1. Refer to textbook, "Classification of Fractures," and Figure 52-1.
2. a. 3; b. 2; c. 1
3. a. 4; b. 3; c. 1; d. 2
4. a. 3; b. 5; c. 1; d. 4; e. 2
5. • Acute compartment syndrome • Shock • Fat embolism syndrome • Thromboembolitic complications • Infection • Avascular necrosis • Fracture blisters • Delayed union or nonunion
6. Increased pressure within one or more muscle compartments of an extremity causes reduced circulation to the area. This may lead to the ischemia-edema cycle, which if left untreated, can cause

irreversible neuromuscular damage and permanent loss of function in the extremity.

7. *Answers may be in any order.*
   a. Pallor of the extremity
   b. Weakened peripheral pulses
   c. Swollen and tense skin surface
   d. Numbness
   e. Tingling
   f. Cyanosis
   g. Paresthesia
   h. Severe pain unrelieved by analgesics

8. *Answers may be in any order.*
   a. Infection
   b. Persistent motor weakness
   c. Contractures
   d. Myoglobinuric renal failure

9. An incision through the skin and subcutaneous tissues, into the fascia of the affected compartment, to relieve pressure, to restore circulation to the affected area

10. Hypovolemic shock related to hemorrhage

11. • Long bones (hip) • Multiple fractures • Pelvis

12. Altered mental status

13. Respiratory distress; tachycardia; tachypnea; fever; petechiae

14. • Smokers • Obese clients • Clients with history of heart disease • Clients with a history of thromboembolitic complications

15. a. 4; b. 3; c. 2; d. 5; e. 3; f. 1

16. a continuous grating sound created by bone fragments

17. Refer to textbook: common and additional nursing diagnoses and collaborative problems for additional discussion.

18. Assess and treat first: respiratory distress, bleeding and head injury; remove any clothing over suspected fracture site; control bleeding from fracture site with applied pressure; assess vital signs; position in supine; keep warm; assess fracture site using inspection and palpation; assess distal pulses and motor function; immobilize fracture by splinting.

19. • Bandages and splints • Casts • Traction • Internal fixation • External fixation

20. Neurovascular status including color, temperature, presence of sensation, motor ability, peripheral pulses, skin blanching, swelling, and snugness of device.

21. Promote air drying of wet cast (leave uncovered); handle wet cast with palms of hand; use a firm mattress under cast; use cloth-covered pillow for extremity elevation if cast is wet; inspect cast for drainage, cracking, crumbling, alignment and fit; prevent cast contamination from urine or feces; petal cast edges when dry.

22. So that the wound can be observed and cared for properly

23. Infection; circulation impairment; peripheral nerve damage; joint contracture; degenerative arthritis in joint(s); muscle atrophy; other complications of prolonged immobility (e.g., skin breakdown, thromboembolism, constipation, pneumonia, atelectasis).

24. a. 3; b. 5; c. 1; d. 2; e. 4

25. Never remove weights, lift weights, or let them rest on the floor; weights must hang freely. Instruct other caregivers and colleagues regarding the weights. Inspect skin integrity and condition at least every 8 hours, especially at pin sites. Perform pin care according to agency's policy. Maintain body alignment and countertraction. Check all equipment for proper functioning.

26. Injury to the skin

27. Inflammation; infection of pin tract may result in osteomyelitis

28. • Opioid analgesics • Anti-inflammatory agents • Muscle relaxants

29. • Hot or cold therapy applications (depending on source of pain) • Warm bath • Back rub • Therapeutic touch • Distraction and imagery • Deep breathing • Music therapy and other forms of relaxation therapy

30. It permits early mobilization, therefore decreasing the susceptibility to the complications of immobility.

31. Advantages: Minimal blood loss; allows for early ambulation and exercise of the affected body part while relieving pain; maintains alignment in closed fractures that will not maintain position in a cast; stabilizes comminuted fractures that require bone grafting; permits easy access to the wound and promotes healing
    Disadvantage: Pin tract infection

32. Risk for Infection; Impaired Physical Mobility. (Refer to textbook: ORIF postoperative care for further discussion.)

33. • Thromboembolitic complications • Respiratory complications (pneumonia, atelectasis) • Contractures or muscle atrophy • Skin breakdown • Elimination problems (constipation, urinary retention) • Cerebral dysfunction

34. c

35. Used for clients who have or are likely to develop an infection. Wound remains open, and drains allow exudate to escape from the site until infection resolves; skin flaps may be sutured over the wound at a later date.

36. The surgeon pulls the skin flaps over the bone end and sutures them in place at the time of the amputation.

37. This happens when a body part is severed unexpectedly (chain saw, knife, automobile accident).

38. • Hemorrhage • Infection • Phantom limb pain
    • Problems of immobility • Neuroma formation
    • Flexion contractures
39. • Middle-aged or older men with diabetes, with a lengthy history of smoking, and failure to care for feet properly
    • Young men who experience motorcycle or other vehicle accidents or are injured at work by industrial equipment
40. a. Expect the client to go through a grieving process, client is faced with altered self-concept; may be bitter, angry, hostile, or uncooperative.
    b. May verbalize and feel that an intimate relationship with a mate is no longer possible.
41. • Stage I: lasts 1 to 3 months, client complains of locally severe, burning pain, edema; vaso- and muscle spasm.
    • Stage II: more severe, diffuse pain and edema; muscle atrophy; spotty osteoporosis.
    • Stage III: marked muscle atrophy; intractable (unrelenting) pain; severely limited mobility of the affected area; contractures, and marked profuse osteoporosis.
42. pain relief
43. • Physical therapist • Occupational therapist • Pharmacist, physician, and possibly a psychotherapist
44. • Torn meniscus • Ligament strain or tear • Dislocation • Subluxation
45. A diagnostic technique to determine a torn meniscus. The knee is flexed and rotated by the examiner; then the examiner presses on the medial aspect while slowly extending the leg. The test is positive if "clicking" is heard or palpated.
46. False. Medial meniscus is more likely to tear.
47. True
48. False. Six to 9 months or longer.
49. False. Athletes.
50. True
51. False. Sprain.
52. True
53. True
54. False. Cannot maintain abduction.
55. a. 4; b. 2; c. 1; d. 3

Case Study

Answers provided on the SIMON website: http://www.wbsaunders.com/SIMON/Iggy/

STUDY GUIDE NUMBER 12.53

Assessment of the Gastrointestinal System

1. a. Mucosa: a thin layer of smooth muscle and some exocrine glands

b. Submucosa: made up of connective tissue
   c. Outermost layer: both circular and longitudinal smooth muscles
2. • Secretion • Digestion • Absorption • Motility
3. A mechanical and chemical process, whereby complex foodstuffs are broken down into simpler forms that can be used by the body. During digestion, the stomach secretes hydrochloric acid, the liver secretes bile, and the digestive enzymes are released, aiding in food breakdown.
4. a. Intrinsic contractile stimulation: to maintain the tone of the smooth muscle, and to stimulate movements
   b. Autonomic nervous system: slows movement, inhibits secretions, and contracts sphincters
5. aorta
6. portal vein of the liver
7. liver; hepatic vein; heart; inferior vena cava
8. buccal mucosa; lips; tongue; hard palate; soft palate; teeth; salivary glands
9. Chewing
10. • Parotid glands • Submandibular glands • Sublingual glands
    Purpose: To assist in digestion by moistening food, thus enabling it to be formed into a bolus for swallowing
11. a. 14; b. 7; c. 20; d. 16; e. 2; f. 18; g. 17; h. 13; i. 4; j. 8; k. 9; l. 5; m. 3; n. 10; o. 11; p. 1; q. 10; r. 6; s. 15; t. 12
12. *Subjective*: age; sex; culture; occupation; previous GI disorders or surgeries in self or family members; medications; travel history; diet history including religious or cultural influences; socioeconomic status; in-depth exploration of diarrhea, constipation, flatus, bloating, bowel habits, and any changes; melena; urine changes; weight gain or loss; smoking history; complete description of pain; skin changes (itching, jaundice, bruising, bleeding); heartburn; hematemesis; nausea or vomiting; psychosocial factors such as effect of current health problem on lifestyle, interference with job or leisure activities, job related stress, financial status.
    Objective: height; weight; triceps skinfold thickness; midarm circumference; midarm muscle circumference; inspect and palpate mouth (lips, oral mucosa, gums, teeth or dentures, tongue, odors, tonsils, uvula movement); inspect, auscultate, percuss, and palpate abdomen (skin, contour and symmetry, movement, edema, bowel sounds, bruits, friction rub, venous hum, percussion notes elicited, liver span, spleen size, masses, tenderness); spider telangiectases on upper torso and neck; presence of leg edema and peripheral pulses; asterixis.
13. The correct sequence is inspection, auscultation, percussion, and then palpation. This sequence is

preferred so that palpation and percussion do not increase intestinal activity and hence increase bowel sounds.

14. Uncontrolled diabetes mellitus
15. Tumor; pancreatic cyst; or gastric dilation
16. Ovarian tumors, fibroid tumors, pregnancy, or bladder distention
17. Intraperitoneal hemorrhage
18. Presence of an aneurysm
19. After abdominal surgery; peritonitis or paralytic ileus
20. Diarrhea or gastroenteritis, or above a complete intestinal obstruction
21. b
22. a
23. Presence of blood in the stool from GI bleeding, such as with colorectal cancer
24. a. 9; b. 7; c. 1; d. 8; e. 4; f. 6; g. 5; h. 2; i. 3
25. a. 4; b. 3; c. 2; d. 1

STUDY GUIDE NUMBER 12.54

Interventions for Clients with Oral Cavity Problems

1. • Infection • Allergy • Vitamin deficiency • Systemic disease • Radiation
2. *Primary*: usually a result of systemic disorders *Secondary*: generally the result of infection by opportunistic viral or bacterial organisms in clients who already have lowered host resistance.
3. a. 4; b. 2; c. 1; d. 3
4. True
5. False. Symmetric white oral lesions.
6. True
7. False. White plaquelike lesions.
8. False. Fungal infection resulting from an overgrowth of normal flora.
9. True
10. c
11. b
12. Swish the solution around in the mouth before swallowing (swish and swallow)
13. *Subjective*: onset of disease process; location and duration of symptoms; history of a similar problem; presence and location of pain and its nature; presence of systemic symptoms (fever, malaise, nausea, vomiting); disability resulting from condition; routine oral hygiene regimen; dentures or orthodontic appliances; effectiveness of any current treatment; nutritional habits; ability to chew and swallow; nutritional status; stress level; medications; psychosocial factors such as perception of current stressors, changes in lifestyle, emotional trauma, situational crises, coping patterns, perceived impact of

oral lesions on self-concept.
Objective: oral cavity lesions; coating, cracking, fissures, odors, location, size, shape, color, drainage, anterior lymphadenopathy; uvula displacement from midline; airway obstruction.

14. • Avoidance of contact with the causative agent • Mental health practices that reduce stress levels and emotional tension • Maintenance of proper nutritional status • Routine oral hygiene
15. Oral hygiene; drug therapy (Refer to textbook Chapter 54 and Charts 54-1 and 54-2 for further discussion.)
16. a. 5; b. 3; c. 1; d. 4; e. 2
17. • Increasing age • Tobacco use • Alcohol ingestion • Occupations (textile workers, plumbers, coal and metal workers) • Overexposure to the sun • Poor dietary habits • Poor oral hygiene • Infection with the human papillomavirus (HPV)
18. *Subjective:* occupation; exposure to known oral carcinogens or irritants (sunlight, heat, mechanical, alcohol, tobacco); family history of cancer or oral cancer; routine oral hygiene regimen; dentures or oral appliances; hemoptysis; nutritional status; appetite; problems with chewing or swallowing; weight loss; medications; psychosocial factors, including fear of cancer, support systems, coping mechanisms, impact on self-concept, comfort level, limitations to education or therapy.
Objective: lip color, texture, symmetry; pain; color of buccal mucosa, texture, presence of lesions; tongue movement; floor of mouth; speech; cervical nodes for enlargement or tenderness.
19. Ineffective Airway Clearance; Impaired Oral Mucosa Membrane (Refer to textbook and Chart 54-3 for further interventions.)
20. • Placement of a temporary tracheostomy for approximately 10 days and the concomitant nursing care (oxygen and suctioning) • Temporary loss of speech because of the tracheostomy • Need for vitals to be taken frequently postoperatively • Need to take nothing by mouth for 10 to 14 days (approx.) or until intraoral suture lines are healed • Need to have IV lines in place for medication delivery and hydration • Postoperative medications and activity • Surgical drains
21. Removal of the tongue (total or partial)
22. Airway management is a priority; use sterile technique (See textbook for postoperative care discussion.)
23. suctioning
24. 30
25. throbbing; pounding
26. IV morphine
27. • Ability to swallow without difficulty • Any aspiration • Leakage of saliva or fluid from the suture line

28. Nutritional management, medications, resources available (Refer to textbook on community-based care for further discussion.)
29. • Maintains a patent airway through removal of oral secretions • Maintains nutritional status by eating foods that are well tolerated and nutritious • Communicates thoughts and feelings to family members, friends, and health care personnel • Maintains the integrity of the oral mucous membrane
30. • Acute sialadenitis • Postirradiation sialadenitis • Salivary gland tumors
31. • Infectious agents • Irradiation • Immunologic disorders
32. • Hydration • Application of warm compresses • Massage of the gland • Use of saliva substitute • Use of sialagogues
33. Very dry mouth caused by severe reduction in the flow of saliva
34. facial weakness or paralysis (partial or total) on the affected side
35. Client's ability to:
• Wrinkle the brow • Raise the eyebrows • Squeeze the eyes shut • Wrinkle the nose • Pucker the lips • Puff out the cheeks • Grimace or smile
36. Surgical removal of the parotid glands

STUDY GUIDE NUMBER 12.55

Interventions for Clients with Esophageal Problems

1. the backward flow of gastrointestinal contents into the esophagus
2. • Incompetent lower esophageal sphincter • Irritation from the refluxate • Abnormal esophageal clearance • Delayed gastric emptying
3. a. Location in the abdomen where the intra-abdominal pressure is higher than the intrathoracic pressure
   b. The acute angle of His formed where the lower portion of the esophagus enters the stomach
4. During the normal process of healing, the body may substitute a columnar epithelium (Barrett's epithelium) for the normal squamous cell epithelium of the lower esophagus. This new tissue is more resistant to acid, but it is considered premalignant and is associated with an increased risk of cancer. The fibrosis and scarring that accompanies the healing process can produce esophageal stricture, resulting in the narrowing of the esophageal lumen.
5. c
6. Nighttime reflux tends to result in prolonged exposure of the esophagus to acid because being recumbent tends to impair peristalsis and gravity clearance mechanisms.

7. a. 1; b. 3; c. 5; d. 2; e. 4
8. *Subjective*: pain pattern (heartburn), including onset, frequency, duration, intensity, associated environmental or physical aggravating factors; regurgitation; water brash; dysphagia; odynophagia; dietary patterns; use of medications to relieve pain and their effect; work and leisure activities; psychosocial factors, including disruption of lifestyle and daily activities, knowledge about disorder, coping mechanisms used, resources available, support systems.
   Objective: general physical appearance, nutritional status, especially unplanned weight loss; ability to swallow smoothly and smoothness of laryngeal movement; auscultation for aspiration if regurgitation occurs; dysphagia; belching; flatulence; nausea or vomiting.
9. An acidic solution is infused via a tube inserted into the distal esophagus. Clients with normal esophageal mucosa experience no symptoms when the acid is infused, clients with esophagitis experience immediate heartburn.
10. d
11. b
12. 1; 2 to 3
13. gastric acid secretions
14. increase the rate of gastric emptying
15. *Sliding hernia:* Occurs as a result of weakened hiatal muscle support structures and increases in intra-abdominal pressure. The esophagogastric junction and a portion of the stomach fundus move through the diaphragm into the thorax.
    Rolling hernia: Results from an anatomic defect whereby the stomach is not securely anchored below the diaphragm. The gastroesophageal junction remains below the diaphragm, whereas portions of the stomach roll into the thorax.
16. *Subjective*: age; sex; weight; body build; daily work and leisure activities; dietary patterns; heartburn; regurgitation pattern; pain; dysphagia; belching; feeling of fullness after eating; breathlessness; feeling of suffocation; chest pain; psychosocial factors such as changes in lifestyle (work and leisure activities), knowledge of the disease and its treatment, self-care measures, ability to learn, coping mechanisms, support systems. *Objective:* general physical appearance; nutritional status; location of any pain; auscultation of chest for signs of aspiration or decreased lung sounds.
17. The surgeon wraps a portion of the stomach fundus around the distal esophagus to anchor it and reinforce the LES.
18. False; at least 30 degrees
19. True
20. False; first 8 hours

21. False; meals need to be both smaller and more frequent
22. True
23. False; notify physician
24. An esophageal motility disorder in which the LES fails to relax properly with swallowing and in which the normal peristalsis of the esophagus is replaced with abnormal contractions.
25. • Esophageal candidiasis • Lower esophageal diverticula • Airway obstruction • Aspiration pneumonia
26. a
27. c
28. • Tobacco use • Alcohol ingestion • Long-term exposure to gastric contents • High levels of nitrosamines (found in pickled and fermented foods) and foods high in nitrate • Diets that are chronically deficient in fresh fruits and vegetables • Genetic factors
29. white males of middle to upper socioeconomic status
30. African Americans
31. areas of northwest China
32. • Dysphagia (most common) • Weight loss
33. *Subjective:* race; culture; age; sex; alcohol consumption; tobacco use; history of esophageal problems (stricture, reflux); extreme weight loss; anorexia; dysphagia; pain pattern; dietary pattern; psychosocial factors, including fear of choking, reactions to the diagnosis of cancer, financial concerns.
    Objective: general physical appearance; weight; nutritional status; skin turgor; condition of mucous membranes; auscultation for signs of aspiration; palpation of cervical, neck, and axillary nodes; dysphagia; odynophagia; regurgitation; vomiting; foul breath; chronic hiccups; chronic cough; increased secretions; hoarseness.
34. Imbalanced Nutrition: Less than Body Requirements related to impaired swallowing.
35. Refer to textbook for further discussion, additional nursing diagnoses, and collaborative problems.
36. • Nutritional support • Radiotherapy • Photodynamic therapy • Dilation of strictures • Prosthesis insertion • Chemotherapy • Surgical removal of the tumor
37. True
38. False; forward flexion, back of the mouth
39. True
40. False; avoid exposure to sunlight for 1 month, and wear sunglasses and protective clothing to cover all exposed body areas
41. False; temporary relief
42. True
43. False; with no evidence of advanced disease
44. esophagogastrostomy
45. Respiratory care
46. atelectasis; pneumonia
47. deep; turning; coughing
48. 1; 2
49. semi-Fowler's; high Fowler's; reflux
50. chest tubes; volume; color
51. overload; lymph node
52. edema; jugular venous pressure
53. does not
54. Client should be knowledgeable about symptom management, wound management. (Refer to "Community-Based Care" in textbook for further discussion.)
55. Sacs resulting from the herniation of esophageal mucosa and submucosa into surrounding tissue.
56. By x-ray examination and barium swallow.
57. • Diet therapy • Positioning
58. • Blunt injuries • Chemical burns • Surgery • Endoscopy • Stress of protracted severe vomiting
59. • Presence of airway • Chest pain • Dysphagia • Vomiting • Bleeding
60. a, b, c, d

STUDY GUIDE NUMBER 12.56

Interventions for Clients with Stomach Disorders

1. Inflammation of the gastric mucosa (stomach lining).
2. Prevents the stomach from digesting itself by a process called *acid autodigestion.*
3. A thickened, reddened mucous membrane with prominent rugae, or folds.
4. *Acute:* Inflammation of the gastric mucosa or submucosa after exposure to local irritants, with complete regeneration and healing usually occurring within a few days.
   Chronic: Appears as a patchy, diffuse inflammation of the mucosal lining of the stomach, and usually heals without scarring but can progress to hemorrhage and the formation of an ulcer.
5. a. 2; b. 1; c. 1; d. 2; e. 1; f. 2; g. 1
6. • Epigastric discomfort • Anorexia • Cramping • Nausea • Vomiting • Gastric hemorrhage
7. • Nausea • Vomiting • Upper abdominal discomfort • Epigastric pain that simulates ulcer-like distress • Anorexia • Pain exacerbated by eating spicy or fatty foods
8. Esophagogastroduodenoscopy (EGD)
9. relieving the symptoms; removing the cause
10. a. 1; b. 2; c. 3; d. 4
11. d
12. PUD: results when gastric mucosal defenses become impaired and no longer protect the epithelium from the effects of acid and pepsin.

13. a. Gastric ulcers—usually occur on the lesser curvature of the stomach, near the pylorus
    b. Duodenal ulcers—usually occur in the first portion of the duodenum
    c. Stress ulcers—usually occur at the proximal portion of the stomach and duodenum
14. • Hemorrhage • Perforation • Pyloric obstruction • Intractable disease
15. a. 1; b. 3; c. 2; d. 4; e. 2; f. 3; g. 1; h. 2; i. 1; j. 4; k. 3
16. *Subjective:* age; sex; occupation; use of medications (especially corticosteroids, salicylates, endomethacin, phenylbutazone); diet history; eating patterns; daily stressors; smoking and alcohol use; caffeine consumption; any history of GI upset or symptoms; history of radiation treatment; occurrence and pattern of pain and its relationship to food ingestion, aggravating and relieving factors; early satiety; anorexia; nausea; heartburn; psychologic factors, particularly impact on lifestyle, stressors, income, educational levels, leisure activities.
    Objective: Nutritional status; pain location; posture; facial expression; dress; grooming; hygiene; abdominal tenderness, fullness or guarding to palpation; vomiting; melena; orthostatic change in vital signs and dizziness.
17. Pain; Risk for Fluid Volume Deficit. (Refer to common nursing diagnoses and collaborative problems in textbook for further discussion.)
18. Esophagogastroduodenoscopy (EGD)
19. • Provide pain relief • Eradicate *H. pylori* infection • Heal ulcerations • Prevent recurrence
20. Suppress the enzyme system of gastric acid production, available as sustained-release tablets; therefore they must not be crushed before administration
21. Used for indigestion and heartburn; inhibits gastric acid secretions. Administered in a single dose at bedtime and are used for 4 to 6 weeks in combination with triple therapy.
22. Reduces gastric acid secretion and enhances gastric mucosal resistance to tissue injury. This drug is contraindicated in pregnant women.
23. Buffer gastric acid and prevent the formation of pepsin; give about 2 hours after meals; can interact with certain drugs (administer other medications 1 to 2 hours before or after the antacid); clients with past or present heart failure should avoid antacids containing a high sodium content
24. Forms a protective coating; given on an empty stomach 1 hour before each meal and at bedtime
25. loss; upper; lower; complications
26. a. Slight feelings of weakness and mild perspiration may be present
    b. Signs and symptoms of shock may be manifested, such as hypotension, chills, palpitations, diaphoresis, and a weak, thready pulse

27. Transfusion therapy
28. • Cessation of the acute bleeding episode • Prevention of recurrent bleeding
29. • Endoscopic therapy • Acid suppression • NG tube placement • Saline lavage
30. • Thermal contact using a heater probe or electrocoagulation • Injection of the bleeding site with diluted epinephrine or a sclerosing agent (alcohol) • Laser therapy
31. This allows surgery to take place without contamination of the peritoneal cavity by gastric secretions.
32. To prevent the accumulation of secretions, which may lead to vomiting or gastrointestinal distention and pressure on the suture line.
33. Gastroenterostomy, vagotomy, pyloroplasty. (Refer to textbook and Chart 56-2 for further discussion.)
34. True
35. False; not done unless specifically ordered by the surgeon
36. False; epigastric pain and a feeling of fullness, hiccups, tachycardia, and hypotension
37. d
38. b
39. Teach to recognize and report complications; diet; identify situations that cause stress. (Refer to "Community-Based Care" in textbook for further discussion.)
40. • Maintains hemodynamic stability; free of disease or surgical complications • States that pain is reduced or alleviated by prescribed interventions • Identifies potential causes and risks of disease recurrence • Avoids the intake of irritating foods and beverages • Avoids smoking • Avoids over-the-counter medications containing aspirin or ibuprofen • Identifies early symptoms of recurrence or complications • Identifies and copes successfully with stressful situations • Adheres to long-term medication regimen and appropriate follow-up with the health care provider
41. ZES is manifested by upper GI tract ulceration, increased gastric acid secretion, and the presence of a non–beta cell islet tumor of the pancreas (gastrinoma). Diarrhea may be a manifestation of this disorder.
42. An excessive amount of fat in the feces
43. To suppress acid secretion to control symptoms
44. a. Spread within the gastric wall and into regional lymphatics; b. direct invasion of adjacent structures (liver, pancreas); c. hematogenous spread via the portal vein to the liver; d. systemic circulation to the lungs and bones; e. peritoneal seeding via the gastric serosa to the omentum, peritoneum, and ovary.
45. • Infection with *H. pylori* • Pernicious anemia • Gastric polyps • Chronic atrophic gastritis • Achlorhydria • Ingestion of pickled foods (over long period of

time) • Ingestion of salted fish (over long period of time) • Ingestion of salted meats (over long period of time) • Ingestion of nitrates from processed foods (over long period of time) • High consumption of salt (over long period of time) • Cigarette smoking (controversial) and alcohol consumption (controversial) • Genetic factors • Gastric surgery

46. • Native Americans • African Americans • Hispanics

47. • Indigestion (heartburn) • Abdominal discomfort

48. c

49. b

50. • Pneumonia • Anastomotic leak • Hemorrhage • Reflux aspiration • Sepsis • Reflux gastritis • Paralytic ileus • Bowel obstruction • Wound infection • Dumping syndrome

51. c

52. folate; iron; vitamin B_{12}

53. TPN may be needed as a supplement to oral intake or for complete dietary management if a client cannot maintain adequate nutritional status.

54. Fear of returning home related to inability to care for themselves. (Refer to "Community-Based Care" in textbook for further discussion.)

STUDY GUIDE NUMBER 12.57

Interventions for Clients with Noninflammatory Intestinal Disorders

1. IBS is a functional GI disorder, characterized by the presence of chronic or recurrent diarrhea, constipation, and/or abdominal pain and bloating (most common digestive disorder seen in clinical practice).

2. There is no inflammation present causing alteration in the bowel mucosa or intestinal wall.

3. • Diverticular disease • Ingestion of coffee or other gastric stimulants • Lactose intolerance

4. c

5. b

6. *Subjective:* sex; age; race; occupation; habits (cigarettes, alcohol, caffeine consumption); current stressors; dietary patterns; bowel patterns; past health problems; weight loss; nausea; belching; flatulence; anorexia; bloating; fatigue; anxiety; headaches; difficulty concentrating; psychosocial factors, including impact of the illness on individual and recent period of stress or emotional tension.
Objective: repeated episodes of diarrhea or constipation; abdominal cramps or pain; LLQ pain; fatigued appearance; normal bowel sounds; diffuse tenderness over abdomen.

7. True

8. False; limit caffeine and avoid alcohol

9. False; usually recommended

10. False; drink 8 to 10 cups of liquid each day

11. True

12. d

13. • Pregnancy • Obesity • Abdominal distention • Ascites • Heavy lifting • Coughing

14. a. 4; b. 1; c. 6; d. 3; e. 2; f. 5; g. 7

15. c

16. *Subjective:* sex; age; body build; weight; height; past or concurrent medical problems; medications; exercise patterns: occupation (any lifting); past herniation or symptoms; psychosocial factors including developmental stage, home situation, support systems.
Objective: abdominal bulging at rest or with straining; presence of bowel sounds; changes in inguinal ring with increased intra-abdominal pressure.

17. d

18. a. *Herniorrhaphy*—surgeon makes an abdominal incision and places the contents of the hernial sac back into the abdominal cavity before closing the opening.
   b. *Hernioplasty*—surgeon reinforces the weakened muscle wall with mesh, fascia, or wire.

19. coughing

20. b

21. a. 4; b. 2; c. 6; d. 1; e. 3; f. 5

22. • Liver (most frequent site) • Lungs • Brain • Bones • Adrenal glands

23. • Bowel perforation and peritonitis (gradual intestinal obstruction, pressure on nearby organs) • Abscess formation • Fistula formation to the urinary bladder or vagina • Frank bleeding

24. *Subjective:* age; sex; diet history; geographic location of residence; presence of risk factors, including family history of ulcerative colitis, polyposis, adenomas; recent weight loss; malaise; reports of abdominal pain or discomfort, fullness; change in bowel habits such as diarrhea or constipation; nausea; psychosocial factors, including fear, denial, guilt, loss of control, anger.
Objective: overall appearance (energy level, listlessness, weakness); cachexia; loose skin; muscle wasting; abdominal distention; abdominal guarding; palpable abdominal mass; rectal bleeding; vomiting; ascites.

25. False; decreased

26. False; positive

27. True

28. False; used to locate distant sites of metastasis

29. • Clients must cope with a diagnosis that inspires fear and anxiety about treatment • Pain • Possible disfigurement • Shortened life span

30. It involves the excision of the involved area of the colon, leaving an area of clean margins.

31. It is the surgical creation of an opening of the colon onto the surface of the abdomen.

32. To advise on the optimal placement of the ostomy and ET will instruct the client about the rationale and general principles of ostomy care
33. An ET is a registered nurse with specialized training and is certified in ostomy care.
34. Elective surgery, hemicolectomy, bowel prep (Refer to textbook for further discussion.)
35. b
36. a
37. c
38. b
39. Social worker, ET, Ostomy associations (Refer to health care resources in textbook for further discussion.)
40. a. 3; b. 5; c. 4; d. 2; e. 6; f. 1
41. *Small intestine:* adhesions and hernias. *Large bowel:* tumors, diverticulitis, and volvulus.
42. a. 3; b. 1; c. 2
43. Peristaltic waves across abdomen; borborygmi; absent bowel sounds; abdominal distention, vomiting (may contain bile and mucus; orange-brown and foul smelling); hiccups; absence of stool or gas per rectum or ribbon-like stools; guarding; tenderness; low-grade fever; possible elevated pulse rate. (Refer to textbook and Chart 57-6 for more discussion.)
44. c
45. b
46. 4; proper placement; patency; output
47. Abdominal; same
48. nausea; increased; placement
49. d
50. c
51. a
52. a. Blunt abdominal trauma: motor vehicle accidents, falls, aggravated assaults, contact sports
    b. Penetrating abdominal trauma: gunshot wounds, stabbing, impalement with an object
53. • Risks of hemorrhage • Shock • Peritonitis
54. • Mental status of client • Skin perfusion
55. d
56. Internal bleeding
57. a. During percussion: resonance over the right flank with the client lying on his left side
    b. Ruptured spleen
58. Fluid volume replacement needs are extensive. Blood replacement products, crystalloids, and isotonic saline are given, as well as intravenous antibiotics. All these interventions require multiple infusion ports and large-bore catheters to ensure a means of quick access. An upper extremity or central line is used to prevent fluid pooling in the abdominal cavity.
59. Serial blood work helps to identify true blood loss, whereas single samples may reflect hemoconcentration and volume loss.
60. sterile dry dressing

61. • To identify bleeding • To minimize the risk of vomiting and aspiration
62. Hemorrhage related to the trauma can occur weeks after blunt abdominal trauma. A client who is alerted about what to watch for can seek medical intervention immediately and possibly avoid further complications.
63. a. True; b. True; c. True; d. False; e. False; f. True; g. False; h. True; i. False; j. True
64. c
65. Bleeding and prolapse
66. a
67. • Pain • Urinary retention • Hemorrhage
68. • Bile salt deficiency (fats, fat-soluble minerals) • Enzyme deficiency (lactase, vitamin B_{12}) • Bacteria overgrowth (fats, vitamin B_{12}) • Disrupted small bowel mucosa (most nutrients) • Altered lymphatic or vascular circulation (protein, minerals, vitamin B_{12}, folic acid, lipids) • Decreased absorptive surface area (vitamin B_{12}, bile salts, and other nutrients)
69. Diarrhea
70. • Steatorrhea • Weight loss • Bloating and flatus • Decreased libido • Purpura • Anemia • Bone pain • Edema
71. Avoidance of dietary substances that aggravate malabsorption and supplementation of nutrients
72. d

Case Study

Answers provided on the SIMON website:
http://www.wbsaunders.com/SIMON/Iggy/

STUDY GUIDE NUMBER 12.58

Interventions for Clients with Inflammatory Intestinal Disorders

1. The appendix has no known function.
2. a. 6; b. 9; c. 5; d. 8; e. 3; f. 1; g. 7; h. 2; i. 4
3. A fecalith is a stone-like (calculi) mass of feces. Such "stones" are a common cause of obstruction in the appendix.
4. a
5. *Subjective*: age; sex; history of abdominal surgery (especially appendectomy); other medical conditions; recent barium intake; diet history including fiber intake; complete pain description (location, sequence related to other symptoms); pain localizing to RLQ; pain relief with flexion of right hip or knees; nausea or vomiting; anorexia; urge to defecate; urge to pass flatus; psychosocial factors, including ability to cope with an abrupt onset of illness and surgery.
   Objective: vomiting following pain onset; tender-

ness on palpation (varies with time related to symptom onset); tenderness or rebound tenderness over McBurney's point; muscle rigidity; elevated temperature, tachycardia.

6. • Perforation • Abscess formation • Peritonitis
7. a. Heat may increase circulation to the appendix and result in increased inflammation and perforation.
   b. This position will allow any abdominal drainage to be contained in the lower abdomen.
   c. To prepare for the possibility of emergency surgery and to avoid aggravating the inflammatory process.
   d. To prevent fluid and electrolyte imbalance and to replenish fluid volume.
   e. These could cause perforation of the appendix.
8. d
9. a. *Primary peritonitis* is an acute bacterial infection unassociated with perforation of an abdominal organ. It may result from an infection located elsewhere within the body that travels to the peritoneum via the vascular system.
   b. *Secondary peritonitis* is a result of bacterial invasion after perforation or rupture of an abdominal organ or direct contamination by foreign bodies, surgical instruments, peritoneal catheters, or ascending reproductive tract infections
10. c
11. a
12. *Subjective:* history of abdominal pain (including whether localized or generalized); aggravating factors such as respiration or movement; reports of pain relief with knee flexion; abdominal distention; anorexia, nausea, vomiting, fever and chills, inability to pass flatus or feces; recent surgery; current or past medical conditions; last menstrual period (women); psychosocial factors, including fear, concerns related to the illness, coping ability, support systems.
   Objective: lying still with knees flexed; abdominal guarding with cough or movement; location of pain; abdomen either rigid and distended (generalized) or localized tenderness and rebound tenderness (localized); high fever; tachycardia; dry mucous membranes; decreased turgor; decreased urinary output; hiccups; dry mouth; possible difficulty with respirations.
13. b
14. c
15. d
16. Gastroenteritis is an inflammation of the mucous membranes of the stomach and intestinal tract. It primarily affects the small bowel.
17. Viral and bacterial

18. a. Noninflammatory—organism releases an enterotoxin
    b. Inflammatory—organism attaches itself to mucosal epithelium
    c. Penetrating—organism penetrates the intestine
    All of these can result in alteration in normal intestinal flora allowing increased capability of invading organisms to attach to the intestinal mucosa (client receiving antibiotics, malnourished, debilitated).
19. • *E. coli* • *Campylobacter* species • *Shigella* species
20. The primary route of transmission of the infecting organism is the fecal-oral route via contaminated food, water, fomites, or contact with infected animals or infants.
21. • Avoid all water and food identified as possibly being contaminated. • Limit exposure to other people who have symptoms of gastroenteritis throughout the period of communicability. • Wash hands meticulously before and after eating, after contact with animals, after each defecation. • Symptomatic individuals should limit (or avoid) contact with others, restrict the use of glasses, utensils, dishes, tubes of toothpaste etc. to themselves.
22. Ulcerative colitis is characterized by diffuse inflammation of the intestinal mucosa; the result is a loss of surface epithelium, which allows for ulceration and possible abscess formation. These changes result in an inability of the bowel to absorb nutrients and water, contributing to malnutrition, anemia, and dehydration.
23. • Intestinal perforation with resultant peritonitis and fistula formation • Toxic megacolon • Hemorrhage • Increased risk for colon cancer • Abscess formation • Malabsorption • Bowel obstruction • Extraintestinal clinical manifestations such as arthritis
24. *Subjective:* sex; age; race; family history of IBD; previous or current therapy for illness, including surgery; dietary history, including relationship of elimination patterns to intolerance of milk and milk products, greasy fried foods, spicy or hot foods; frequency, number, and characteristics of stools; medication history; recent travel; allergies; occupation; stressors; nausea or vomiting; psychosocial factors, including impact of the disease on lifestyle, events related to exacerbations, job-related stressors and symptoms, smoking or alcohol use and effect on bowels, sleep patterns, support systems, weight loss, and change in body image; restrictions on activities, especially outside the home; stage of development.
    Objective: presence or absence of bowel sounds and their characteristics; presence of abdominal scars; skin turgor; areas of increased or localized abdominal tenderness; rebound tenderness; localized pain or cramping; rectal fissures or hemorrhoids; characteristics of stools, including presence of blood, pus, or mucus; presence of tachycardia or fever.

25. occult; ova (eggs); parasites; culture; viral and bacterial dysenteries
26. b
27. Diarrhea, pain. (Refer to nursing diagnoses and collaborative problems in textbook for further discussion.)
28. a. 3; b. 1; c. 2; d. 1; e. 4; f. 3; g. 2
29. In the right lower quadrant of the abdomen, below the belt line
30. Intra-abdominally
31. The client would feel a sense of fullness, the pouch would be drained several times a day by inserting a urinary catheter into the pouch, and client would wear a small dressing over the stoma to keep it moist.
32. salt; water; loss
33. Prevention of skin problems, ostomy care, drug therapy. (Refer to postoperative care in textbook and Chart 58-4 for further discussion.)
34. • Be free of diarrhea, rectal bleeding, and cramping. • Maintain adequate hydration. • Understand the factors that can influence exacerbations of the disease. • Maintain ideal body weight. • Understand and adhere to the prescribed drug regimen. • Remain free of complications of the disease. • Identify and seek care for extraintestinal manifestations of the disease.
35. A chronic inflammatory bowel disease that can affect any part of the GI tract, from the mouth to the anus (terminal ileum is the site most affected).
36. • Severe malabsorption by the small intestine • Fistula formation
37. Nutritional status is at risk; GI secretions are composed of fluids, electrolytes, and digestive enzymes. Malnutrition, dehydration, and hypokalemia are common complications. Skin excoriation can occur, as well as abscesses and sepsis.
38. d
39. a
40. *Subjective:* data are similar to those with ulcerative colitis. Also include any current or past history of fistulas. *Objective:* initial discomfort in the RLQ; diarrhea; low-grade fever; tenderness; guarding; palpable mass in RLQ; periumbilical pain before or after bowel movements; steatorrhea; weight loss; anorexia.
41. a. 3; b. 2; c. 3; d. 1; e. 2; f. 3; g. 2; h. 1
42. Glucocorticoids
43. nutrition; electrolyte; skin; infection
44. Skin care, infection, and psychosocial. (Refer to Crohn's disease in textbook for further discussion.)
45. Impaired Skin Integrity related to fistula formation.
46. Refer to textbook under "Community-Based Care" heading for Crohn's disease.

47. Diverticula are congenital or acquired pouchlike herniations of the mucosa through the muscular wall of the small intestine or colon.
48. d
49. c
50. The risk of perforation of an inflamed diverticulum or a localized abscess is high.
51. Rupture of the diverticulum with subsequent peritonitis • Pelvic abscess • Bowel obstruction • Fistula • Persistent fever • Pain after 4 days of medical treatment • Uncontrolled bleeding
52. c
53. high-fiber
54. Dietary fiber, add gradually; avoid foods containing seeds. (Refer to health teaching in textbook for further discussion.)
55. a. 3; b. 1; c. 2
56. • Sitz baths • Analgesics • Bulk-producing agents • Stool softeners
57. Sitz baths help promote circulation to the perianal area, are soothing, and help relax the anal sphincter, thereby decreasing spasm. The soaks also assist in cleaning the perianal skin area. These actions help to decrease pain and reduce risk of infection.
58. Fecal-oral transmission via contaminated food or water is the most common mode; also fecal-oral transmission from oral-anal sexual practices or contact with feces from a contaminated person.
59. Close, intimate contact increases the risk of exposure to and transmission of parasites, particularly if bathroom facilities are shared and food is prepared without careful handwashing.
60. Botulism; it causes severe illness and can be life-threatening if paralysis and respiratory failure occur.
61. *Food poisoning:* not directly communicable person to person; has a relatively short incubation period (1 hour to 4 days depending on organism); does not result in acquired immunity because reinfection can occur; symptoms include diarrhea, nausea, and vomiting.
    Gastroenteritis: readily transmitted person to person; period of communicability can range from days to weeks; can result in acquired immunity; symptoms include diarrhea, nausea, and vomiting.
62. Discard cans of food that are punctured or swollen or have defective seals. Sterilize containers for home canned-foods by boiling for at least 20 minutes. Never slow cool food after it is cooked. Thoroughly cook all foods, including beef, pork, and fish. Have drinking water tested. Check all stored foods thoroughly for roaches, arthropods, and droppings. Meticulous handwashing before and after meals and defecation. Keep toilet areas clean, maintain personal hygiene, and avoid contact with stool from animals or people.

Case Study

Answers provided on the SIMON website:
http://www.wbsaunders.com/SIMON/Iggy/

STUDY GUIDE NUMBER 12.59

Interventions for Clients with Liver Problems

1. a. 2; b. 4; c. 1; d. 3; e. 1; f. 1; g. 1; h. 4; i. 2; j. 3; k. 4; l. 3
2. a. 5; b. 3; c. 1; d. 6; e. 2; f. 7; g. 4
3. Laënnec's cirrhosis—it is preventable with complete abstinence from alcohol.
4. Chronic infection with the hepatitis B virus.
5. *Subjective*: age; sex; race; employment history (chemical toxin exposure); history of alcoholism in client or family; pattern of alcohol intake; past health problems related to the hepatobiliary system, viral infection, blood transfusion, heart failure, respiratory disorders; weight loss; generalized weakness; loss of appetite; early morning nausea or vomiting; dyspepsia; flatulence; bowel habit changes; psychosocial problems such as personality and behavior changes, emotional lability, sleep pattern disturbance, interruptions in work or family life, financial difficulties.
   Objective: gastrointestinal bleeding; jaundice; ascites; spontaneous bruising; dry skin; rashes; purpuric lesions; palmar erythema; spider angiomas; hepatomegaly; peripheral edema; distended abdomen or bulging flanks; protruding umbilicus; orthopnea; dyspnea; problems with maintaining balance; inguinal hernia; increases in abdominal girth; presence of blood in emesis or stool; fetor hepaticus; amenorrhea or testicular atrophy; gynecomastia; impotence; mentation or personality changes; asterixis.
6. Excessive fluid volume most common; potential for hemorrhage. (Refer to nursing diagnoses and collaborative problems in textbook for further discussion.)
7. a. 1; b. 4; c. 3; d. 5; e. 1; f. 3; g. 2; h. 3; i. 1; j. 2
8. a. Initial means of controlling fluid accumulation in the abdominal cavity
   b. If sodium serum levels fall, and in an effort to reverse the fluid overload and raise the serum sodium level
   c. Clients are usually malnourished, and these are typically added because of the liver's inability to store vitamins
   d. To reduce fluid accumulation and to prevent cardiac and respiratory impairment
   e. To monitor the effect of diuretic therapy
   f. To monitor the effect of diuretic therapy
   g. To monitor the effect of diuretic therapy
   h. To screen for electrolyte imbalances that may accompany diuretic therapy
   i. For hypokalemia
   j. Controlling fluid (i.e., sodium levels) the kidneys retain sodium
   k. To minimize shortness of breath
9. d
10. These clients are susceptible to infection, disseminated intravascular coagulation (DIC), bleeding varices, and anesthesia reactions.
11. The shunt drains ascitic fluid from the peritoneal cavity to the superior vena cava, thereby reducing fluid accumulation. The client is expected to improve by losing weight, decreasing abdominal girth, increasing urinary output, and excreting renal sodium.
12. imbalances; frozen plasma; K; red blood; bleeding
13. • Gastric intubation • Balloon tamponade • Drug therapy • Replacement of blood products • Injection sclerotherapy • Transjugular intrahepatic portal-systemic shunt (TIPS)
14. c
15. • Large crystalloid solutions • Colloids (plasma) • Packed red blood cells • Fresh frozen plasma
16. d
17. Portal systemic shunts
18. • Increased blood pressure • Decreased heart rate • Increased urinary output
19. Proteins
20. b
21. Diet therapy—dietician, alcohol abstinence —counseling (Refer to health teaching and home care in textbook for further discussion.)
22. AA, spiritual support (Refer to "Community-Based Care" section in textbook for further discussion.)
23. • Experience a decrease in or no ascites • Have electrolytes within normal limits • Have blood pressure within normal limits • Not experience hemorrhage, or be managed immediately if bleeding occurs • Not experience PSE, or be managed immediately if PSE occurs • Have the optimal quality of life possible
24. Hepatitis is the widespread inflammation of liver cells; can be either acute or chronic.
25. a. 5; b. 2; c. 4; d. 7; e. 3; f. 1; g. 6
26. • Hepatitis A virus (HAV) • Hepatitis B virus (HBV) • Hepatitis C virus (HCV) • Hepatitis D virus (HDV) • Hepatitis E virus (HEV)
27. Hepatitis B virus (and most recently hepatitis C virus)
28. a. 4; b. 1; c. 5; d. 1; e. 1; f. 2; g. 3; h. 2; i. 3; j. 2; k. 3
29. a. Drink water treated by a purification system or bottled water; wash hands before eating and after using toilet. Avoid oral-anal sexual practices.

b. Use standard precautions, take hepatitis B vaccine.

c. Avoid sharing razors, nail clippers, and toothbrushes. Do not share needles for injection or tattooing.

30. Leading cause of cirrhosis; increased incidence (Refer to textbook for cost of care and legal-ethical issues and further discussion.)

31. a. 2; b. 1; c. 3

32. obstruction; edema; bile channels

33. b

34. c

35. a. 2; b. 1; c. 3; d. 2; e. 3; f. 1; g. 1; h. 3; i. 1; j. 2; k. 3

36. • Primary cancers of the esophagus, stomach, colon, rectum, breasts, and lungs • Malignant melanoma

37. • Cirrhosis • Viral hepatitis • Trauma • Nutritional deficiencies • Carcinogen exposure • Hepatotoxin exposure • Metastatic process

38. • Liver lobe resection (surgical excision) • Cryosurgical ablation of the liver • High-dose chemotherapy • Hepatic artery ligation • Liver transplantation

39. The client with end-stage liver disease who has not responded to conventional medical or surgical intervention

40. The client with severe end-stage liver disease with life-threatening complications and possibly the client with malignant neoplasms

41. Head trauma victims in the United States

42. • Acute graft rejection • Infection • Hemorrhage • Hepatic artery thrombosis • Fluid and electrolyte imbalances • Pulmonary atelectasis • Acute renal failure • Chronic graft rejection • Psychologic maladjustment

43. Usually beginning 4 days to 2 weeks after surgery

44. • Tachycardia • Fever • Right upper quadrant or flank pain • Increasing jaundice

45. • Cyclosporine (Cyclosporine A) • Azathioprine (Imuran) • Prednisone (Deltasone) • Most recently tacrolimus (FK 506) and mycophenolate mofetil (CellCept)

Case Study

Answers provided on the SIMON website: http://www.wbsaunders.com/SIMON/Iggy/

STUDY GUIDE NUMBER 12.60

Interventions for Clients with Problems of the Gallbladder and Pancreas

1. *Acute cholecystitis* is usually a result of obstructed bile flow from a gallstone, or less commonly, bacterial invasion. This condition leads to edema, vascular congestion, and inflammation. The trapped bile is reabsorbed by the gallbladder and causes chemi-cal irritation. This irritation, coupled with the edema, leads to tissue ischemia, sloughing, necrosis, and gangrene.
Chronic cholecystitis results from prolonged inefficient bile emptying and diseased muscle wall tissue. This condition may or may not be associated with gallstones.

2. • Trauma • Inadequate blood supply • Prolonged anesthesia and surgery • Adhesions • Edema • Neoplasms • Long-term fasting • Prolonged dehydration • Gallbladder trauma • Prolonged immobility • Excessive opioid use

3. c

4. Decreased blood flow to the gallbladder, which causes "gallbladder shock"

5. b

6. *Subjective:* sex; age; race; ethnic group; if female, obstetric history, menopausal state, use of birth control pills, estrogen, other hormones; food preferences and intolerances (include gastrointestinal symptoms); daily activity and exercise level; client or family history of gallbladder disease and its treatment; abdominal pain and its associated characteristics; anxiety; fears.
Objective: height; weight; tenderness with palpation; muscle guarding or rigidity; rebound tenderness; palpable mass in right upper quadrant below liver border; jaundice; clay-colored stools; dark urine; steatorrhea; possible fever, tachycardia, dehydration, pallor and diaphoresis.

7. A differential diagnosis must rule out other diseases that may cause similar symptoms such as PUD and GERD.

8. Ultrasonography

9. a

10. Cholecystectomy

11. splinting; pillow; blanket; jarring; deep breathing; turning

12. incision; drain; T-tube

13. Six weeks or longer

14. c

15. b

16. ambulatory; same day

17. early; absorption; dioxide

18. within 1 day

19. Within 1 to 3 weeks

20. Bile stasis resulting from impaction of the cystic duct by gallstones

21. a. 4; b. 3; c. 1; d. 2

22. • Cholesterol • Bilirubin • Bile salts • Calcium • Various proteins

23. ERCP

24. a

25. a. 5; b. 3; c. 1; d. 4; e. 2

26. Teach regarding postcholecystectomy syndrome; report symptoms of biliary tract disease. (Refer to community based care in textbook and Chart 60-2 and 60-4 for further discussion.)

27. a. *Lipolytic process*: Lipase acts on pancreatic endocrine and exocrine cells, causing fatty acids to be released. These acids combine with calcium and result in a rapid decrease in serum calcium.
   b. *Proteolysis*: Trypsin activates proteolytic enzymes, which attack pancreatic parenchyma. Damage may be localized or involve the entire organ.
   c. *Necrosis of blood vessels*: Elastase is activated and acts on the elastic fibers of pancreatic blood vessels and ducts leading to bleeding. Kallikrein causes release of peptides, which contributes to increased vascular permeability, vessel destruction, and hemorrhage.
   d. *Inflammatory stage*: This last stage results when leukocytes converge around the hemorrhage and necrotic pancreatic tissue. Lesions may become infected by bacteria, producing suppuration, or may become walled off and lead to an abscess.

28. Autodigestion is a process in which the pancreas lyses its own cells with the digestive enzymes it normally produces.

29. • Bile reflux • Hypersecretion-obstruction • Alcohol-induced • Reflux of duodenal contents

30. a. 5; b. 3; c. 6; d. 2; e. 1; f. 4

31. • Alcoholism • Biliary tract disease with gallstones

32. *Subjective*: reason for seeking treatment; presence of abdominal pain, characteristics and related details; alcohol intake and related details; family history of alcoholism, pancreatitis, or biliary tract disease; prior abdominal surgery or procedures; presence of other medical problems causative of pancreatitis; recent viral infections; recent drug consumption; stated weight loss; nausea; psychosocial factors such as excessive alcohol intake, recent traumatic loss.
   Objective: weight loss; vomiting; jaundice; Cullen's sign; Turner's sign; absent or decreased bowel sounds; abdominal tenderness, rigidity, muscle guarding; palpable mass; dullness on percussion (ascites); possible fever, tachycardia, hypotension, adventitious breath sounds, dyspnea, orthopnea, changes in behavior and sensorium.

33. • Elevated serum amylase levels • Elevated serum lipase levels

34. True

35. False; decrease vagal, decrease GI

36. False; titration of opioids

37. False; fetal position

38. True

39. True

40. False; elevated blood glucose levels

41. Meticulous skin care, nutrition, pain (Refer to textbook and Chart 60-5 for further discussion.)

42. A progressive, destructive disease of the pancreas, characterized by remissions and recurrence

43. *Chronic calcifying pancreatitis*: is alcohol induced and characterized by protein precipitates that plug the ducts, leading to obstruction, inflammation, and fibrosis of pancreatic tissue. Cysts may form, and the organ becomes hard and firm.
   Chronic obstructive pancreatitis: is a result of obstruction of the sphincter of Oddi by gallstones, causing spasm and inflammation and leading to ductal erosion, inflammation, and autodigestion in the head of the pancreas.

44. a. 2; b. 2; c. 1; d. 2; e. 1

45. calcification; tissue; biopsy

46. • Serum bilirubin • Serum alkaline phosphatase level • Amylase level • Lipase level (and transient glucose levels)

47. *Subjective*: data are similar to those for acute pancreatitis. Ask specifically about alcohol intake, time and amount consumed, and its relationship to pain development; abdominal pain characteristics; psychosocial factors, especially the use of opioid analgesics, use of street drugs, economic hardship on family.
   Objective: abdominal tenderness; palpable mass in the left upper quadrant; dullness on abdominal percussion; adventitious breath sounds, dyspnea, orthopnea; steatorrhea; weight loss; muscle wasting; jaundice; dark urine; associated signs of diabetes mellitus.

48. The client may become or already be dependent on opioids. This problem complicates accurate assessment of pain episodes because the client may use manipulative behavior to obtain needed opioids. When the client is hospitalized, opioid or alcohol withdrawal may result, especially if the client is misleading about the quantity of either depressant substance he or she is accustomed to taking.

49. True

50. False; given with meals or snacks

51. False; fruit juice or applesauce

52. False; not mixed with proteins

53. False; wet towel or washcloth

54. False; every 2 to 4 hours

55. False; decrease

56. a

57. Pain and nutritional intake. (Refer to textbook and Charts 60-7 and 60-8 for further discussion.)

58. • Lung • Breast • Thyroid • Kidney • Skin melanoma

59. Tumors are usually not found until in the last stages of development. They grow rapidly and metastasize easily via the lymphatic and vascular systems.

60. b
61. c
62. ERCP
63. head; pancreas
64. The development of a fistula
65. a. Checking for undue stress or kinking and maintain them in a dependent position, monitoring drainage—color, amount, etc.
    b. So it does not become obstructed
    c. Secretions are corrosive and irritating to the skin, internal leakage causes chemical peritonitis
    d. To reduce stress on the suture line and anastomosis site and to optimize lung expansion
    e. Observing for signs of decreased blood pressure and increased heart rate to detect early signs of shock; temperature may be indicative of infection
    f. Procedure is long and evaporation of fluids and loss of blood, fluids, and electrolytes occurs making client susceptible to third spacing and shock; client is usually malnourished; adequate hydration, nutritional replacement, and electrolyte replacement is essential
    g. Decreased urine output is early indicator for hypovolemia, precursor to shock
    h. Hyperglycemia or hypoglycemia as result of stress and surgical management of the pancreas; insulin may need to be administered
    i. Decreased vascular pressure changes are early signs of hypovolemia; intervention to prevent shock
66. Biopsychosocial needs need to be met. (Refer to textbook, community based care, and Box 60-b for further discussion.)
67. palliative; symptoms; pain
68. diagnosis; cancer; few months; death
69. client and family; done; death
70. will; family members; friends
71. requests; funeral; service; significant others
72. dignified
73. Biopsychosocial needs; need to be met (Refer to textbook and Box 60-b for further discussion.)

STUDY GUIDE NUMBER 12.61

Interventions for Clients with Malnutrition and Obesity

1. • Energy intake • Protein • Vitamins • Minerals
2. d
3. Milk, cheese, and dairy foods but no meats, fish, poultry, or eggs
4. B_{12}
5. • Disease • Infection • Psychologic stress

6. • Disease • Eating behavior • Economic factors • Emotional stability • Medication • Cultural factors
7. • Review of diet history • Food and fluid intake record • Laboratory data • Food-medication interactions • Physical examination and health history • Anthropometric measurements • Psychosocial assessment
8. Measurements that are noninvasive methods of evaluating nutritional status
9. Height, weight, and assessment of body fat
10. False; overestimate height, underestimate weight
11. False; no shoes
12. False; heels together, arms at the sides
13. False; ambulatory
14. False; conditions such as heart failure and renal disease affect fluid balance and, therefore, weight
15. True
16. False; does not
17. True
18. False; and subcutaneous fat
19. energy; stored
20. a. Marasmus—body fat and protein are wasted
    b. Kwashiorkor—lack of protein quantity and quality in the presence of adequate calories
    c. Marasmic-Kwashiorkor—combined protein and energy malnutrition
21. protein; intake; synthesis; negative; weight; decreased; weakness
22. • Functional ability of liver, heart, lungs, GI tract, and immune system diminishes • Hypoproteinemia • Leanness and cachexia • Decreased effort tolerance • Lethargy • Intolerance to cold • Edema • Dry, flaking skin and various types of dermatitis • Poor wound healing and a higher than usual number of infections, particularly postoperative infection
23. • Poverty • Lack of education • Substance abuse • Decreased appetite • Decline in functional ability to eat independently • Infectious diseases • Diseases that produce diarrhea, respiratory, and other infections • Vomiting • Medical treatments • Catabolic processes • Admission to hospital or nursing home • Dysphagia • Anorexia nervosa • Bulimia nervosa
24. starvation; catabolic; infection; injury
25. *Subjective*: usual daily food intake; eating patterns; appetite change; recent weight changes; times of meals and snacks; types of foods usually consumed; change in eating habits or appetite; involuntary weight loss; change in taste; dysphagia; types of food avoided; nausea; vomiting; heartburn; discomfort with eating; dental problems; dentures worn; psychosocial factors such as economic status, educational level, living and cooking facilities; mental status; resources to buy and prepare food.
    Objective: condition of hair, eyes, oral cavity, nails, musculoskeletal, and neurologic systems; height;

weight; skinfold thickness; noted difficulty chewing or swallowing; food and fluid intake.

26. • Dysphagia • Cognitive impairment • Admission to hospital or long term care • Poverty • Unable to eat independently • Multiple medications

27. a. 5; b. 7; c. 1; d. 6; e. 2; f. 4; g. 3

28. Imbalanced Nutrition: Less than Body Requirements related to inadequate food intake or increased nutrient requirements

29. Risk for Infection; Impaired Skin; Anemia (Refer to textbook, additional nursing diagnoses and collaborative problems and Chart 61-4 for further discussion.)

30. • Demonstrate an adequate nutrient intake. • Maintain body mass and weight within normal limits. • Maintain laboratory values within normal limits.

31. c

32. d

33. Nasoenteric tube (NET)

34. A stoma is created from the abdominal wall into the stomach through which a short feeding tube is inserted.

35. a. 3; b. 1; c. 2

36. Development of a clogged tube

37. X-ray study

38. increased; imbalances

39. Circulatory overload and the formation of pulmonary edema

40. Excessive diarrhea

41. Hyperkalemia and hypernatremia

42. PPN

43. PPN

44. TPN

45. PPN

46. TPN

47. TPN

48. PPN

49. The extreme hyperosmolarity of the solutions stimulates fluid shifts between body fluid components

50. Weights; intake; output

51. • Potassium • Sodium • Calcium

52. a. 2; b. 3; c. 1

53. • Diabetes mellitus • Hypertension • Hyperlipidemia • Cardiac disease • Sleep apnea • Cholelithiasis • Chronic back pain • Early degenerative arthritis • Certain types of cancer

54. a. Neuroendocrine causes: injury to hypothalamus, Cushing's disease, polycystic ovary failure, hypogonadism
    b. Dietary obesity associated with high fats such as potato chips, cakes, and pies
    c. Genetic factors: family history
    d. Drug treatment: corticosteroids, estrogens, and others
    e. Physical inactivity: couch potato, no exercise.

55. Higher; women

56. • Coronary heart disease and hypertension • Diabetes • Dyslipidemia • Gallstone formation • Cancer of the reproductive organs

57. • Participate in a structured weight loss program • Approach ideal body weight • Establish a lasting, healthful dietary pattern that will result in permanent, sustained weight loss

58. a

59. appetite

60. lipase; triglycerides

61. • Dry mouth • Constipation • Insomnia • Loose stools • Abdominal cramps • Nausea

62. • Maxillomandibular fixation: jaw wiring • Esophageal banding: encircling the esophagus • Gastroplasty: banding or stapling the stomach • Intestinal bypass: the stomach and jejunum are connected

63. repositioning; suture

64. bowel sounds; flatus

65. health

66. Behavioral management, Weight Watchers or other safe weight-loss programs, exercise. (Refer to textbook, postoperative care, health teaching, resources for further discussion.)

STUDY GUIDE NUMBER 13.62

Assessment of the Endocrine System

1. • Anterior and posterior pituitary • Adrenal cortex and medulla • Thyroid • Alpha, beta, delta islets of Langerhans • Parathyroid • Male (testes) and female (ovaries) gonads

2. hormones

3. Hormones are considered to be biochemicals that affect specific areas of the body known as the *target tissues*. In order to reach the target tissue, the hormones have to travel by way of the circulatory system instead of actual ducts because the target tissue is not in close proximity to the gland that secreted the hormone.

4. Hypothalamus is nervous tissue. The pituitary gland (see Figures 62-1 and 62-4) is divided in anterior and posterior sections. Hypothalamus secretes hormones directly to the posterior pituitary where they are stored until needed. Hypothalamus also stimulates or inhibits the release of various hormones from the anterior pituitary.

5. a. 8; b. 5; c. 3; d. 4; e.1; f. 6; g. 9; h. 3; i. 5; j. 10; k. 7 ; l. 6; m. 2; n. 2; o. 5; p. 1; q.1
   (See Table 62-1.)

6. There is a certain level of any given hormone in the body. The body measures the level and the need for more or less hormone to be secreted. A signal is then sent to increase or decrease the hormone. It forms a loop around from the target site to the gland

that secretes the hormone. The hormone that is secreted causes the opposite action of change that occurred in the body. When this system malfunctions, secreting too much or not enough hormone in response to the need, pathologic conditions result.

7. True

8. a. True
   b. False; short
   c. False; must be free to bind
   d. False; except for two hormones that are not stored and must be continuously produced
   e. True
   f. True
   g. True
   h. True
   i. True
   j. True
   k. True
   l. False; the pituitary gland also has releasing and inhibiting factors that affect specific hormone production. (See textbook and Table 62-2 and Figure 62-3.)

9. c

10. pituitary gland

11. b

12. c

13. See textbook and Table 62-1.

14. b

15. a

16. b

17. a

18. a

19. c

20. b

21. a

22. a. False; affects carbohydrate, protein and fat metabolism
    b. True
    c. False; ACTH from anterior pituitary
    d. False; peaks in morning (See text and Table 62-6 for details.)

23. a. This is because cortisol has a direct effect on the immune system. Stress decreases the body's ability to fight infections.

24. a

25. • Changes in blood pressure and increased heart rate due to vasoconstriction or dilation • Elevated blood glucose as result of gluconeogenesis or glycogenolysis • Increased perspiration • Dilation of pupils • Increased urination related to increased renin release • Diarrhea related to increased GI motility

26. a. False; located anteriorly
    b. True
    c. False; two lobes
    d. False; increase

27. a

28. d

29. a, b, c, d

30. Bone, kidney, gastrointestinal

31. d

32. d

33. c

34. b

35. d

36. b

37. • Reason for seeking health care • Nature of onset • Previous treatment • Any interference with activities of daily living • Age • Sex • Family history of endocrine-related disorders • Change in energy levels • Change in elimination patterns • Change in nutritional status or gastrointestinal disturbances • Sexual and reproductive function such as menstrual cycle changes, male impotence, change in libido, or change in secondary sexual characteristics • Change in hair texture or distribution • Change in facial contour or body proportions • Psychosocial factors such as coping skills, support systems, health beliefs, self-perception, ability to learn and manage self-care, socioeconomic status

38. • Height • Weight • Body fat distribution • Muscle mass • Skin color • Areas of hyperpigmentation • Edema of extremities or at base of spine • Body hair distribution • Nail thickness and strength • Facial structure • Features and expression • Visible thyroid enlargement • Jugular vein distention • Chest size and symmetry • Truncal obesity • Supraclavicular fat pads • Buffalo hump • Breast size, shape, symmetry, pigmentation and any discharge • Reddish striae on breasts or abdomen • Size of external genitalia • Distribution and quantity of pubic hair • Irregular cardiac rate or rhythm • Orthostatic change in pulse or blood pressure • Bruit over thyroid • Thyroid size, symmetry, shape, and nodularity

39. b

40. a. Osteoporosis: decreased ovarian production of estrogen
    b. Decreased glucose tolerance: decreased sensitivity of peripheral tissues to the effects of insulin
    c. Impaired water excretion: decreased concentrating ability of the kidneys
    d. Degenerative cellular metabolism: decreased overall metabolic rate

41. a

42. b

43. b (The only other gland that can be palpated is the testes. See Chapters 69 and 73 for a discussion of palpation of the testes.)

44. b

45. Suppression/stimulation testing challenges the endocrine system to see if it is capable of normal

hormone production. It is use in times when the simple measurement of hormonal levels is inadequate for revealing variations in normal or abnormal levels.

46. c
47. b
48. c, d, e, f
49. Skull films • CT scan • MRI • Vascular studies • Ultrasonography
50. b
51. c
52. d
53. a. • Changes in weight • Difficulty swallowing or chewing • Heat-cold changes • Appetite and food intake • Hair changes in color • Distribution and texture • Fluid intake
    b. Changes in urinary and bowel patterns such as constipation or urinary frequency • Excessive perspiration • Increased thirst
    c. Changes in sleep patterns such as difficulty waking, nightmares, waking up at night
    d. Changes in sexual activity • Questions related to menstrual cycle
    e. Changes in energy level • Changes in ability to perform ADLs
       (See also Chart 62-2, text, or Gordon's textbook for more answers.)
54. b
55. d
56. a
57. c
58. b
59. c (All other answer options are related to specific endocrine problems.)
60. Hair texture or distribution • Facial contours • Heat and cold intolerance • Voice quality • Body proportions • Secondary sexual characteristics • Facial expressions

STUDY GUIDE NUMBER 13.63

Interventions for Clients with Pituitary and Adrenal Gland Problems

1. a. Primary pituitary dysfunction is the result of a problem in the pituitary gland itself, such as a benign or malignant tumor.
   b. Secondary pituitary dysfunction is the result of a dysfunction of the hypothalamus. In either case, one or more hormones are underproduced (hypofunction) or overproduced (hyperfunction).
2. Prolactinomas are the most common. Gonadotropin- and TSH-secreting tumors are the least common.
3. • Growth hormone (GH; somatotropin) • Prolactin (PRL) • Thyrotropin (thyroid-stimulating hormone

[TSH]) • Corticotropin (adrenocorticotropic hormone [ACTH]) • Gonadotropins (follicle-stimulating hormone [FSH] and luteinizing hormone [LH]) • Melanocyte-stimulating hormone
4. Antidiuretic hormone (ADH) • Oxytocin
5. c
6. c; *Nursing diagnosis:* Ineffective Sexuality Patterns
7. a
8. a
9. a
10. b
11. Acromegaly (see Figure 63-1 and Chart 63-2) is more common than gigantism (see Figure 63-2). Acromegaly occurs as a result of excessive GH production after puberty (adults in third or fourth decade). Gigantism occurs before puberty (children before closure of epiphyses). Gigantism causes rapid proportional growth in the length of all bones, resulting in extremely tall children. Acromegaly produces hypertrophy of the skin, increased skeletal (bone) thickness, and enlarged organs and soft tissue. Bone changes include arrowhead-shaped fingertips and degeneration of joint cartilage. Early detection and treatment can reverse symptoms except for skeletal changes, which are permanent. *Nursing diagnosis:* Disturbed Body Image
12. a; GH is an insulin antagonist.
13. Arthralgias or backaches
14. The client would have decreased bone density resulting in pathologic fractures with decreased muscle strength. Increased serum cholesterol levels are noted. *Nursing diagnosis:* Risk for Injury or Risk for Falls.
15. *Thyroid disorder:* hypothyroidism; *a, c, e,* and *g* are correct. Others listed are related to hyperthyroidism. *Nursing diagnoses:* Activity Intolerance; Impaired Memory; Disturbed Body Image; Sexual Dysfunction; and others
16. T3, T4, testosterone, and estradiol are easily measured.
17. d
18. b
19. c
20. d
21. a
22. a. Body changes, visceral enlargement, and visual changes are not reversible. Other characteristics may be altered.
    b. Nasal packing stays for 2 to 3 days with a mustache dressing.
    c. To prevent increase pressure inside the head and improper healing, do not brush teeth for 2 weeks after surgery. Cough, sneeze, blow the nose and bend forward after surgery—bend at the knees, avoid constipation.

d. Nasal and oral specimens are taken preoperatively.

e. Bladder drainage tube, neurologic exams, instruction to report any postnasal drip.

f. Hormone replacement may be necessary. See text and Chart 63-4 for further details.

23. a, b, c, d
24. c, d, e, f, g
25. b
26. CSF leak.
27. d
28. a
29. c
30. b (*a* is an overproduction of ADH.)
31. a. True
    b. False; excessive output of dilute urine even with decreased intake and thirst.
    c. True (See Chart 63-5 for dehydration.)
    d. False; less than 1.005.
    e. True
    f. True; if not taking adequate fluids, there is an increase in plasma osmolarity.
32. b
33. a, b
34. Correct answers are *a, c,* and *d. b* is used for hypertonic saline test. (See Table 63-2.)
35. *c* is incorrect because lithium is a potential cause of DI. (See Chart 63-6 for details regarding medications and nursing interventions.)
36. b
37. DI is associated with ADH deficiency, or inability of the kidney to respond to ADH, resulting in excretion of large volumes of dilute urine. SIADH is associated with ADH excess, resulting in water retention, increased ECF volume, and hyponatremia.
38. b
39. b
40. c
41. a, c, d; *b* is incorrect because it is *hypo-* not *hyper-*natremia.
42. a
43. c; a low percentage of normal saline is needed to replace serum sodium and increase osmolality without adding too much fluid back into the intravascular space and worsening the fluid overload.
44. a. Decreases
    b. Increases
    c. Increases
45. b
46. b
47. d
48. b
49. d
50. d

51. a. Laboratory test results showing decreased serum potassium, elevated serum sodium, low renin levels, and elevated aldosterone levels.
    b. CT scan reveals presence and location of adrenal adenomas.
52. d
53. d (See Table 63-6.)
54. a
55. See Chart 63-2. Changes in fat distribution may result in a buffalo hump, truncal obesity, and fat pads on the shoulders. The trunk is enlarged with thin legs and arms with generalized muscle wasting, and weakness. Skin changes resulting in blood vessel fragility, such as bruises, thin or translucent skin, and wounds that have not healed properly. Reddish-purple striae ("stretch marks") are often present on the abdomen, upper thighs, and upper arms because of cortisol's degradative effect on collagen. Client may have fine facial hair with acne and hyperglycemia.
56. c
57. Cortisol levels vary throughout the day.
58. Points of emphasis would include: save *all* urine for 24 hours; do not take medications, especially phenytoin and phenobarbital for at least 2 days before the test; no stressful procedures such as other diagnostic tests or intense physical therapy during the test; baseline urine is collected on day 1; a medication called dexamethasone will be administered.
59. elevated free cortisol and androgens levels
60. See text "Pathologic fractures."
61. a
62. a. 2; b. 4; c. 1; d. 3
63. Hypophysectomy, adrenalectomy
64. b; glucocorticoid preparations
65. Due to excess cortisol levels, the client is at risk for infection.
66. d
67. In case of client injury or episodes of unconsciousness, confusion, or inability to communicate, health care providers should be made aware of the client's lack of endogenous cortisol and need for exogenous steroid replacement. Otherwise death may result.
68. b
69. • Inadequate secretion of ACTH • Dysfunction of the hypothalamic-pituitary control mechanism • Complete or partial destruction of the adrenal glands
70. a
71. a. Cortisol promotes glyconeogenesis in the liver and muscle tissues, and maintains the glomerular filtration rate and gastric acid production. It helps maintain a normal range for serum glucose levels, serum urea nitrogen level, and gastric acid production.
    b. Aldosterone promotes renal clearance of potassium, sodium, and water. It helps prevent hyper-

kalemia, hyponatremia, hypovolemia, and metabolic acidosis.

c. Androgens crisis is an acute adrenal insufficiency and an emergency. The body's demand for glucocorticoids and mineral corticoids exceeds supplies. Sodium levels fall, potassium levels rise rapidly, and intravascular volume depletion (collapse) occurs. Severe hypotension results.

72. Addisonian crisis is an acute adrenal insufficiency and an emergency. The body's demand for glucocorticoids and mineralocorticoids exceed supplies. Sodium levels fall, potassium levels rise rapidly, and intravascular volume depletion (collapse) occurs. Severe hypotension results.

73. b
74. d
75. *Addison's:* b and f increase; a, c, d, e, and g decrease, i and j are normal. *Cushing's:* a, c, d, e, g, and i increase; b, f, and j decrease.
76. b
77. c
78. c
79. d
80. a
81. b
82. c
83. b
84. See textbook under each endocrine disorder for discussion.

STUDY GUIDE NUMBER 13.64

Interventions for Clients with Problems of the Thyroid and Parathyroid Glands

1. d
2. Increased hormone production causes a hypermetabolic state with increased sympathetic nervous system activity and increased number of beta-adrenergic receptors causing hyperthyroidism. Decreased hormone production results in a hypometabolic state or hypothyroidism.
3. a. 1; b. 2; c. 1; d. 1; e. 1; f. 2; g. 1; h. 1; i. 2; j. 1; k. 1; l. 2; m. 1; n. 2; o. 1; p. 2; q. 1; r. 1; s. 2; t. 2; u. 1; v. 1
4. c
5. b
6. b
7. d
8. b
9. a
10. b
11. • Exophthalmos • Pretibial edema • Eyelid lag • Globe lag • Wide-eyed (startled) appearance
12. a. Abnormal protrusion of the eyes

b. Dry, waxy swelling of the front surfaces of the lower legs
c. Upper eyelid fails to descend when client gazes slowly downward
d. Upper eyelid pulls back faster than the eyeball when the client gazes upward

13. In Graves' disease, antibodies called thyroid-stimulating immunoglobulins (TSIs) attach to the TSH receptor sites on the thyroid tissue, causing the gland to increase in size and overproduce thyroid hormone. Graves' disease creates hyperthyroidism. In Hashimoto's disease, the antibodies and lymphocytes destroy thyroid tissue, causing underproduction of thyroid hormone and increased secretion of TSH. Hashimoto's disease creates hypothyroidism.

14. a. True
b. False; it is not hereditary; however there is a genetic susceptibility to the antibodies.
c. True
d. True
e. True
f. True
g. True
h. True
i. False; hyperthyroidism, particularly Graves' disease, cause these cardiac problems.
j. True
k. True
l. False; one dose is given as outpatient and no radiation precautions are necessary.
m. True

15. *Goiter* is a general term that refers to a noncancerous *enlargement* of the thyroid gland that can occur in either hypo- or hyperthyroidism. It can be cystic or fibrous, containing nodules. *Thyroid nodule* refers to a cancerous or noncancerous lump of the thyroid gland that is usually firm and has a knotty feel. Clients can have more than one nodule; these cases are called *multinodular*.

16. d
17. a. Deficiency of iodine in local soil or water resulting in inadequate iodine in the diet
b. Genetic defects preventing iodine metabolism
c. Diets consisting mainly of goiter-forming foods
d. Medications that contain large amounts of iodine (See textbook for further details.)
18. For the constipation, drink plenty of fluids and eat a well-balanced diet with adequate fiber. Too much fiber can interfere with absorption of thyroid hormone. For the skin, use plenty of lotion with emollients.
19. a
20. b
21. c

22. Thyroid storm is an *extreme case of hyperthyroidism* that is life-threatening. Mortality rate is 25%. Stress, trauma, infection, vigorous palpation of the goiter, exposure to iodine, RAI, and thyroidectomy often trigger thyroid storm. Assessment findings include fever, tachycardia, systolic hypertension, signs and symptoms of heart failure, agitation, tremors, and complaints of feeling anxious. Depending on the severity of the crisis, manifestations may include abdominal pain, nausea, vomiting, diarrhea, confusion, seizures, psychosis, and coma.

23. a

24. b

25. See Chart 64-4 for best practices for management of thyroid storm.

26. a, b, c

27. a. 1; b. 1 and 2; c. 1, 2, 3, and 7; d. 5; e. 6 and 8; f. 4; g. 3, 4, and 5; h. 6; i. 6; j. 2; k. 6; l. 3; m. 6; n. 8; o. 6; p. 6 and 8

28. Correct answers are *b, c, d, e, g,* and *h.* Incorrect answers are *a,* Coughing and deep breathing exercises are encouraged with manual head support; *f,* When awake, the client will be placed in semi-Fowler's position.

29. *a* and *c.* One or both of these may be needed due to swelling around the trachea, tetany, or laryngeal nerve damage resulting in respiratory distress. Observe for signs and symptoms of respiratory obstruction that include changes in respirations, stridor, and vocal cord paralysis. b. Hypocalcemia as result of damage to the parathyroid glands may result.

30. d (See text for details and explanations on other complications.)

31. Hoarseness and a weak voice; reassure the client the hoarseness is usually temporary

32. 1) Ineffective Breathing Pattern related to decreased energy, obesity, fatigue and inactivity—A priority because the airway must be maintained to prevent acidosis, and respiratory failure. Perform complete respiratory assessment. Prepare for ventilatory support and avoid sedation. (See Chart 64-6.)

    2) Decreased Cardiac Output related to decreased stroke volume as a result of electrical or mechanical malfunction from bradycardia and arteriosclerotic coronary artery disease—A priority to treat or prevent cardiovascular collapse from hypovolemia, hyponatremia, and dysrhythmias. Monitor for decreased blood pressure, bradycardia, dysrhythmias, and signs of shock. (See Chart 64-6 for more interventions.)

    3) Disturbed Thought Processes related to increased interstitial edema and water retention—This is a priority because interventions are needed to prevent further cerebral edema, acidosis, and hypoglycemia. Monitor for lethargy, drowsiness, memory deficit, inattentiveness, and difficulty communicating. Provide written information and repeat information when providing client education.

33. Monitor for the following:
    • Cardiac status because medication can exacerbate existing cardiac problems related to hypothyroidism, specifically for chest pain and dyspnea
    • T$_3$, T$_4$, TSH lab values
    • Signs and symptoms of hypothyroidism and hyperthyroidism
    Teach about the following:
    • Medications—dosage is gradually increased over a period of weeks; taken daily for lifetime; preferably similar time each day
    • Signs and symptoms of hypo- and hyperthyroidism
    • Signs and symptoms should improve about 2 weeks after onset of taking medication
    • Safety measures until mental status improves
    • Blood work, return physician visits, wearing medic alert, and when to seek medical advice
    • No over-the-counter medications should be taken
    • Well-balanced diet with no excess fiber
    • Adequate rest
    • Interventions to keep warm. (See Chart 64-6.)
    Provide written information, repeat important points, and educate family because of client's altered mental status. (See Chart 64-9 on home care.)

34. b

35. a.1; b. 2; c. 2; d. 4; e. 3; f. 2; g. 3 and 4; h. 2; i. 2; j. 3

36. *b* and *d*

37. Parathyroid hormone is secreted by parathyroid gland. It maintains serum calcium levels increasing resorption/breakdown from the bone and kidneys, and absorption from the intestines. Calcitonin is secreted by the thyroid gland and has the opposite effect on the body.

38. a. 1; b. 2

39. a

40. c

41. Parathyroid hormone acts directly on the kidney to increase phosphate excretion and *lower* serum phosphate levels. Calcitonin works in the opposite direction.

42. b

43. b

44. c

45. a. 2; b. 2; c. 1; d. 2; e. 2; f. 1

46. *Hyperparathyroidism:* a. +; b. −; c. +; d. +; *Hypoparathyroidism:* a. −; b. +; c. −; d. −

47. a (All the other answers are correct but not the number one priority. See text for rationale on administering other medications.)
48. b
49. Signs and symptoms depend on the severity of low serum calcium. The nurse monitors for tingling and numbness around the mouth, hands, and feet; seizures, mental status change, irritability, inappropriate muscle contractions causing finger, hand, and elbow flexion, Chvostek's and Trousseau's sign.
50. • IV calcium (calcium chloride, calcium gluconate) • Oral elemental calcium • Vitamin D • Magnesium sulfate (See text and pharmacology book for details on these medications.)
51. a
52. a
53. See textbook under each endocrine disorder for discussion.
54. See textbook under each endocrine emergency for discussion.

STUDY GUIDE NUMBER 13.65

Interventions for Clients with Diabetes Mellitus

1. Diabetes mellitus is a complex disease process characterized by a deficiency or lack of insulin. The lack of insulin affects metabolism of carbohydrates, proteins, and fat and leads to long-term complications throughout the body.
2. • Type 1 (or IDDM) • Type 2 (or NIDDM) • Other specific types • Gestational diabetes mellitus
3. c
4. b
5. • Glucagon • Epinephrine • Norepinephrine • Growth hormone • Cortisol
6. b. The increased urination (polyuria) causes the increase thirst.
7. c. There is glucose in the blood but it is not getting into the cells and used for fuel. This causes cellular starvation from lack of glucose going inside the cell, and the body then uses protein and fat for fuel (energy).
8. a. High glucose in the blood causes high glucose in the urine. High glucose in the urine causes an osmotic diuresis which causes increased urination.
9. c
10. d
11. See textbook in Chapter 65 under "Type 1 and Type 2 Diabetes Mellitus" and Table 65-4 under "Differentiation of Type 1 and Type 2 Diabetes."
12. b
13. c
14. c

15. • Diabetic ketoacidosis (not enough insulin) • Hypoglycemia (too much insulin) • Hyperglycemic hyperosmolar nonketotic coma (inadequate amount of insulin but enough to suppress ketosis)
16. d
17. b
18. a
19. c
20. d
21. b
22. c
23. a
24. b
25. b
26. a
27. a
28. b
29. b
30. a
31. b
32. d
33. a
34. c
35. BUN level and serum creatinine levels are indicators of renal function, specifically glomerular filtration. In diabetic nephropathy, nephrons are damaged, glomerular filtration decreases, and BUN and serum creatinine levels rise.
36. Renal threshold is the point at which blood glucose is filtered out of the blood into the urine. It varies among individuals and rises with the aging process and with kidney damage. Consequently, measurements of urine glucose levels are inaccurate and underestimate the true levels of blood glucose, resulting in periods of untreated hyperglycemia.
37. Urine test results can be altered by the amount of fluid ingested; the client may make errors in timing when reading results; a number of medications that the client may be taking interfere with accurate results; some tests are more accurate than others; and there is controversy about whether a first or second voided urine specimen should be used for testing.
38. d
39. b
40. a
41. c
42. • Hypoglycemia • Gastrointestinal effects
43. • Kidney disease • Liver disease • Cardiopulmonary disease • Gastrointestinal disease
44. b
45. c
46. b

47. See textbook under "Insulin Therapy" in Chapter 65, Tables 65-10 and 65-17, and Charts 65-4 and 65-13.

48. • Lack of insulin during the night, resulting in hyperglycemia • Dawn phenomenon, in which blood glucose levels rise between 5:00 a.m. and 6:00 a.m. due to nocturnal hormone secretions • Somogyi effect, in which blood glucose levels rapidly drops between 2:00 a.m. and 3:00 a.m., triggering a release of counter-regulatory hormones to produce a rebound hyperglycemia

49. d

50. c

51. d

52. d

53. a. Call the doctor with blood glucose level, assessment findings and obtain orders.
    b. Draw a *venous* blood glucose as ordered.
    c. Administer Dextrose 50% IVP as ordered and repeat AccuCheck blood glucose test in 10 to 20 minutes. When client awakens, orange juice followed by protein food.

54. a

55. d

56. c

57. a

58. b

59. a

60. c

61. b

62. c

63. c

64. • Infection • Gangrene • Amputation

65. The DCCT study and UKPDS findings showed that lowering blood glucose levels with intensive therapy reduces risk of retinopathy (eye), nephropathy (kidney) and neuropathy (nerve) disease; critical for prevention of cardiovascular (heart) disease (DCCT study), there is a strong relationship between risks for microvascular complications and glucose control (UKPDS).

66. Data include: age; sex; race; usual weight, height, dietary intake for 3 days; previous diagnosis of diabetes and which type; how long symptoms have been present; taking any diabetes medications (name, dose, strength, last dose); sites used for insulin injections; history of hypoglycemia, symptoms, and treatment; current stressors; presence of concurrent illness; use of other medications; type of glucose monitoring used; past illnesses, surgery, immunizations; family history of diabetes mellitus, heart disease, stroke, obesity, level of exercise; fatigue or lethargy; visual changes; intermittent claudication; extremity coolness, tingling, or pain, delayed wound healing; itchy skin; diarrhea with

incontinence; urinary retention or urinary tract infections; postparandial fullness or bloating; history of stillbirth, miscarriage or large babies in women; psychosocial factors such as depression and impaired self-perception or self-concept, ability to function and interact with others, ability to understand and perform self-care techniques, support systems; periodontal disease; cavities; dental extractions; skin turgor; dry skin; level of consciousness; vital signs; fruity breath odor; signs of retinopathy (tortuous vessels or pinpoint hemorrhages or exudates); neuropathy (depressed tendon reflexes, vibratory sense, and perception of sharp versus dull); decreased vascular flow (decreased peripheral pulses and cool skin).

67. • Usual dietary intake • Weight-to-height ratio • Cultural norms • Daily schedule

68. d

69. • Bread • Vegetable • Fruit • Meat • Fat • Milk

70. b

71. b

72. c

73. d

74. • Anorexia nervosa • Bulimia nervosa

75. a

76. Exercise increases the body's ability to utilize calories and decreases the need for insulin. The combined effect of these two actions is that the diabetic client may have a hypoglycemic episode due to having too much exogenous insulin or insufficient glycogen stores. Simple sugars provide a ready supply of useable glucose to meet the body's needs during these episodes.

77. c

78. d

79. a

80. d

81. d

82. • Fear of loss • Fear of having a severe hypoglycemic reaction • Fear of being different • Fear of losing control

83. b

84. c

85. 140; 200 mg/dL

86. c

87. A snack before exercise helps to prevent hypoglycemia. Adequate insulin is needed because of the counter-regulatory hormones that are secreted during exercise, which can cause hyperglycemia.

88. Sometimes this is a better method to achieve tight control (as opposed to frequent injections) and to reduce the risk of complications.

89. b

90. The first priority is the injecting of insulin. Assess the client's ability to self-administer or determine

whether someone else needs to administer the medication. The second priority is the drawing up of the insulin. Assess client's ability or determine whether someone else is needed to do this step and leave it for the client to self-administer. Assess the client's vision to see whether visual aids are necessary to draw up the insulin in the syringe. Does the client need premixed insulin of 70/30? Depending on the client, educating the client regarding types of insulin, action times, and signs and symptoms of hypoglycemia may be necessary. Education should be done in steps. Do not overload the client. Schedule a return appoint to reassess, reinforce the information, and add new information as needed. See text for client education regarding insulin and insulin injections for more information. The nurse plays a very important role in educating clients about insulin. If a client has had diabetes and has been self-administering the insulin for a number of years, do not assume the client can accurately draw up and self-administer. This is particularly true of older clients in whom there can be changes in vision and mental status.

91. This client with two shots of mixed insulin requires a set meal regimen, which includes a bedtime snack to prevent hypoglycemia at night. There needs to be enough glucose to balance the insulin doses.

92. The client should continue taking the medication and have an intake of food with a focus on liquid carbohydrates if necessary. The client should monitor the blood glucose more frequently. Extra insulin is sometimes necessary during this illness due to the normal stress response causing elevated blood glucose level. Notify the physician if glucose is above 250 or if illness continues.

93. Decreasing urine output/oliguria because dehydration is a cause of hypovolemic shock.

94. Slurred speech, irritability, headache, numbness of fingers, sweating, shakiness, inability to concentrate, unawareness of surroundings. The initial signs and symptoms are a result of the sympathetic nervous system response to low blood sugar. If the central nervous system is involved, changes in level of consciousness can occur. Monitor for signs and symptoms of hypoglycemia at peak times of the insulin action. Some medications mask the early warning signs of hypoglycemia such as the beta-blocker Inderal.

95. Different parameters are used for the older adult in that tight control is not implemented because it takes 10 years or more to develop complications and hypoglycemia with risk of falls is a bigger problem. Prevention of hypoglycemia is the priority. The client's medication is often adjusted by symptom management.

96. Part A: 4; Part B: 4.
97. Part A: 2; Part B: 4.
98. Read and study the information related to onset, peak, and duration of the various types of insulin. Apply this information in the care of your clients.
99. See textbook in Chapter 62 under each endocrine emergency. See Chapter 65 under each "Diabetic Emergency" for discussion. See also Tables 65-16, 65-17, and 65-18 and Charts 65-4 and 65-13.

Case Studies

Answers provided on the SIMON website:
http://www.wbsaunders.com/SIMON/Iggy/

STUDY GUIDE NUMBER 14.66

Assessment of the Skin, Hair, and Nails

1. a. 2; b. 1; c. 2; d. 2; e. 3; f. 1; g. 1; h. 3; i. 3; j. 3
2. d
3. c
4. b
5. a, e
6. a. Elevated, marble-like lesions more than 1 cm wide and deep
   b. Small firm lesions less than 1 cm in diameter
   c. Elevated, irregularly shaped, transient areas of dermal edema
7. a. 4; b. 5; c. 2; d. 1; e. 3
8. a
9. d
10. *A:* Asymmetry of shape; *B:* Border irregularity; *C:* Color variation within one lesion; *D:* Diameter greater than 5 mm
11. c
12. a. Hormone imbalance
    b. Prolonged hypoxia or lung cancer
    c. Dehydration, sudden severe weight loss, or normal aging
    d. Fungal infection
13. Explain that the most uncomfortable time is during the injection of the local anesthesia but that the discomfort will subside as anesthesia takes effect. In addition, the nurse can talk with the client during the process in a quiet voice, combined with a gentle touch, to calm the client.

STUDY GUIDE NUMBER 14.67

Interventions for Clients with Problems of the Skin and Nails

1. b
2. a
3. a

4. a, b, e

5. a, b, c, d

6. The discomfort will increase for 1 to 2 days before subsiding. Cool baths and soothing lotions will help with the symptoms. Antibiotic ointments are used only if there are blisters.

7. c

8. depth; tissue

9. b

10. a, b

11. • Progressive flattening of the dermal-epidermal junction predisposes them to skin tears • Skin moisture and irritation from incontinence • Friction over bony prominences places them at risk.

12. Turning 1 to 2 hours, as appropriate. Turn with care to prevent injury to fragile skin. Position with pillows to elevate pressure points off the bed or use a pressure relieving or reduction device. Moisturize dry, unbroken skin. Avoid massaging over bony prominences. Keep client free from fecal or urinary incontinence and use topical barrier protection.

13. II

14. Acute Pain related to skin trauma

15. a. hydrophobic; b. hydrophilic

16. a, b, c

17. a

18. a. 4; b. 2; c. 6; d. 1; e. 3; f. 5

19. a

20. b

21. a. Candidiasis
    b. Cellulitis
    c. Herpes zoster

22. b

23. a

24. a, b, c

25. c

26. a, b, c

27. • Avoid sun exposure between 11 a.m. and 3 p.m. • Use sunscreens with the appropriate skin protection factor for your skin type. • Examine your body monthly for possibly cancerous or precancerous lesions. • Wear a hat, opaque clothing, and sunglasses when you are out in the sun.

28. Postnasal bleeding

29. a, c

30. a, b

31. b

32. degree; resistance

STUDY GUIDE NUMBER 14.68

Interventions for Clients with Burns

1. • Fluid and protein losses • Sepsis • Disturbances of the metabolic system • Disturbances of the endo-crine system • Disturbances of the respiratory system • Disturbances of the cardiac system • Disturbances of the hematologic system • Disturbances of the immune system

2. a. 4; b. 9; c. 7; d. 5; e. 2; f. 8; g. 3; h. 6; i. 1; j. 11; k. 1

3. d

4. b, c, f

5. See Table 68-1 in the text.

6. b

7. b

8. b

9. a

10. a

11. c

12. d

13. a, c, d

14. a, c

15. • Sympathetic nervous system stress response • The inflammatory response

16. • Dry heat • Moist heat • Contact burns • Chemical injury • Electrical injury • Radiation injury

17. d

18. See Chart 68-2.

19. • Time of injury •Source of injurious agent • Whether alcohol or drugs may have been a factor • Physical surroundings in the immediate area where the burn was sustained • Events occurring from the time of the burn to admission in the health care facility

20. a, b, c, d

21. a

22. a, c, d

23. a, b, c, d

24. a

25. It is important for diagnosis and prognosis but also for calculating specific interventions such as drug dose, fluid replacement volumes, and caloric requirements.

26. Sickle cell preparation. Trauma often triggers a sickle cell crisis in clients who have the disease and in those who carry the trait. African Americans are at significant risk for sickle cell disease.

27. d

28. 7000 mL in the first 8 hours

29. Ends at 5 p.m.

30. 1400 mL

31. 0.5 mL/kg (30 mL/hr)

32. b, c, d

33. a

34. c

35. a, b, c, d

36. b

37. a, b, c, d

38. c

39. c
40. a
41. • Pervasive odor • Color changes • Change in texture
    • Purulent drainage exudates • Sloughing grafts •
    Redness at the wound edges extending into non-
    burned skin
42. d
43. a
44. a, b, c
45. a
46. a
47. See Table 68-9 in the text.

STUDY GUIDE NUMBER 15.69

Assessment of Renal/Urinary System

1. Refer to introduction of chapter.
2. Refer to introduction of chapter.
3. See Figure 69-1.
4. d
5. b
6. e
7. a
8. See Table 69-1.
9. 20 to 30
10. True
11. True
12. c
13. a, b, c
14. True
15. a
16. a. R; b. H; c. H; d. R; e. R; f. H
17. c
18. b
19. c
20. b
21. a
22. a, c
23. True
24. True
25. b
26. See Table 69-3.
27. See Figure 69-5.
28. a, b, c, d
29. b
30. True
31. True
32. See Figure 69-9.
33. See Figure 68-6.
34. b
35. a, b, d
36. a
37. d
38. d

39. d
40. See Chart 69-1.
41. a
42. b
43. 1) b; 2) b
44. b
45. 1) b; 2) d
46. See textbook.
47. a, b, c, d
48. a, b
49. b, c, d, e, f
50. d
51. a, c
52. c
53. d
54. See Figure 69-10.
55. a
56. b
57. a
58. a
59. d
60. b
61. a. 6; b. 14; c. 13; d. 7; e. 1; f. 12; g. 2; h. 8; i. 3; j. 9;
    k. 11; l. 4; m. 10; n. 5

STUDY GUIDE NUMBER 15.70

Interventions for Clients with Urinary Problems

1. See textbook.
2. d
3. a, b
4. a, b
5. b
6. b
7. a, b, c, d
8. Treat for the organism that is in the vagina
9. a, b, c, d
10. b
11. c
12. Voiding cystoureterography
13. • Bladder calculi • Bladder diverticula • Urethral
    stricture • Foreign bodies • Travculation (abnormal
    thickening of bladder wall related to urinary reten-
    tion and obstruction)
14. c
15. a
16. a, b, d
17. preterm labor; affect the fetus
18. a
19. a, c
20. a, b, c, d, e
21. A cystocele is a herniation of the bladder into the
    vagina.

22. a, b
23. • Excretory urography • Voiding cystogram • Cystourethroscopy • Cystometrogram • Urethral pressure • Profilometry • Uroflowmetry • Electromyography of pelvic muscles
24. b
25. d
26. See textbook, charts, and tables.
27. • Cause and options • Medication effect • Dietary adjustments • Protective supplies • Self-catheterization teaching • Controlling and managing anxieties and fears • Home care education • Referral to home care • Support group referrals
28. a. Stones in the urinary tract
    b. Stones in the kidney
    c. Stones in the ureters
29. a, b, c, d
30. b
31. True
32. a, b, d
33. See text.
34. See text, Table 70-2, and Chart 70-12.
35. a
36. b
37. c
38. a, b, c
39. d
40. a
41. self image, body image, sexual functioning, self-esteem
42. a, b, c, d, e
43. blunt trauma, fractured pelvis, penetrating wound, sexual assault

STUDY GUIDE NUMBER 15.71

Interventions for Clients with Renal Disorders

1. a, b, c, d
2. b
3. True
4. a, b, c
5. c
6. a
7. True
8. b
9. True
10. a. 1; b. 2; c. 1; d. 2; e. 1 and 2; f. 1; g. 1 and 2; h. 2
11. a, c, d
12. b
13. a
14. c
15. d
16. b

17. c
18. c
19. d
20. b, c
21. a, c, d
22. a
23. a
24. See text and Tables 71-1, 71-2, and 71-3.
25. b
26. b
27. d
28. b, c, d
29. b
30. See textbook under "Etiology for Pyelonephritis" heading.
31. b
32. a, c
33. a, b, c, d, e
34. a
35. d
36. a, b, c, d
37. b, c, d
38. c
39. b
40. a
41. c
42. d
43. a, b, c
44. a, c
45. a, b, c
46. c, d
47. a, b, c
48. d
49. b, c
50. a
51. a, b, c, e, g, h, i
52. b
53. a, b, c, d
54. d
55. a
56. c
57. c
58. d
59. d
60. d
61. a
62. c
63. b
64. False
65. b, c, d, e, g, h
66. True
67. a, b
68. a
69. b
70. True

71. b
72. b
73. c
74. c
75. b
76. b
77. True

STUDY GUIDE NUMBER 15.72

Interventions for Clients with Chronic and Acute Renal Failure

1. True
2. d
3. b
4. False
5. Use Tables 72-2, 72-6, and 72-7.
6. See Etiology for Acute Renal Failure (ARF).
7. See Prevention under Collaborative Management for ARF and Table 72-4.
8. True
9. False
10. a
11. a. 3; b. 1; c. 1; d. 1; e. 2; f. 2; g. 3; h. 2; i. 1
12. c
13. True
14. a
15. b
16. d
17. a, b, c, d
18. True
19. • Hypotension • Tachycardia • Decreased urine output • Decreased cardiac output • Decreased central venous pressure • Lethargy
20. • Oliguria/anuria • Hypertension • Shortness of breath • Jugular vein distention • Elevated central pressure • Weight gain • Rales and crackles • Anorexia • Nausea
21. a, b, c
22. True
23. See "Collaborative Management for ARF" heading in textbook.
24. d
25. True
26. c
27. d
28. a
29. d
30. See textbook discussion under "Dialysis Therapies" heading.
31. True
32. False
33. a, b, c
34. False

35. a. 1; b. 2 and 3; c. 3; d. 1; e. 1; f. 3; g. 2
36. See textbook discussion under CAPD.
37. See textbook under "Chronic Renal Failure."
38. a. 3; b. 2; c. 3; d. 1; e. 1; f. 1, 2, 3; g. 1; h. 2; i. 3; j. 3, k. 3
39. b
40. b
41. b
42. True
43. True
44. False
45. a
46. b
47. True
48. c
49. Diabetes and HTN
50. See textbook.
51. Review Chart 72-7.
52. Fatigue, Excess Fluid Volume, Decreased Cardiac Output
53. True
54. True
55. a, b, c
56. b, c, d
57. Review Chart 72-3.
58. a, b, c
59. a, b, d
60. d
61. True
62. c
63. True
64. See textbook. Use Table 72-8.
65. See textbook for discussion of renal replacement therapies.
66. See textbook for CAPD discussion.
67. True
68. True
69. a, b, c, d
70. See textbook for discussion of dialysis therapies.
71. a, b, c, d
72. • Thrombosis • Stenosis • Infection • Aneurysm • Ischemia • Heart failure
73. True
74. c
75. b
76. True
77. True
78. False
79. See textbook for discussion of PD and Figure 72-8.
80. a, b, d
81. False
82. a, b, c
83. a, b, c
84. See textbook under "Kidney Transplantation."
85. True

86. See textbook under "Kidney Transplantation."
87. Indepth tissue testing, ABO blood group typing, human leukocyte antigen testing
88. True
89. a, b
90. See textbook discussion of postoperative care.
91. Kidney is not working.
92. True
93. True
94. b
95. True
96. Refer to textbook for post-transplantation care.
97. Refer to Table 72-12.
98. a, b, c, d
99. a, c, d

STUDY GUIDE NUMBER 16.73

Assessment of the Reproductive System

1. c
2. b
3. d
4. b
5. c
6. b
7. c
8. d
9. b
10. c
11. a, b, d
12. b
13. d
14. b
15. d
16. c
17. a
18. b
19. a
20. b
21. d
22. c
23. b
24. d
25. d
26. a. 10; b. 4; c. 8; d. 5; e. 1; f. 3; g. 6; h. 9; i. 2; j. 7
27. a. 4; b. 6; c. 5; d. 1; e. 9; f. 2; g. 8; h. 3; i. 7
28. a. Irregular menstrual and ovarian cycles. The levels of estrogen and progesterone gradually decrease until the levels are no longer able to affect the endometrial lining of the uterus. Until menstruation ceases, the menstrual flow may be lighter or heavier and ovulation may fail to occur.
    b. The uterus, cervix, ovaries, vagina, and external female reproductive organs shrink in size as a

direct result of low estrogen levels. Vaginal mucosa becomes thin and dry, making coitus uncomfortable.
   c. Bone density decreases with resulting osteoporosis because the low levels of estrogen decrease calcium uptake by the bone tissue. Low estrogen levels indirectly decrease the absorption of calcium from the intestine by decreasing the amount of vitamin D metabolized in the body.
   d. Bladder support decreases as the pelvic musculature becomes more relaxed from the loss of estrogen.
   e. Hot flashes are very common and result from vasomotor instability. The surges of FSH and LH on the hypothalamus are thought to produce vasodilation and increased heat production.
   f. Risk of cardiovascular disease increases because of secondary effects of decreased estrogen levels.
29. a. Menopause is the biologic end of the woman's ability to reproduce and refers only to the last menstrual period. It is one symptom of the climacteric.
    b. Climacteric is the overall phase of the woman's life that starts with the initial decrease in estrogen production by the ovaries to the cessation of symptoms resulting from the decreasing estrogen level. Also referred to as "The Change of Life."
30. • Radiation • Chemotherapeutic agents • Prolonged use of corticosteroids • Exogenous sources of estrogen or testosterone • Chronic disorders such as diabetes, MS, and CAD • Medications used to treat other diseases, such as antihypertensives or antidepressants • Substance abuse
31. • Menstrual history • Menopausal history or symptoms • Obstetric history • Sexual history • Family history • Self-care practices
32. • Anxiety • Fear • Deficient Knowledge • Acute Pain • Altered Sexuality

STUDY GUIDE NUMBER 16.74

Interventions for Clients with Breast Disorders

1. d
2. b
3. b
4. a
5. b
6. a
7. b
8. d
9. b
10. b
11. b

12. d
13. d
14. c
15. c
16. a, b, c
17. c
18. a
19. d
20. a, b, c, d
21. d
22. a
23. c
24. Most closely related to *age*
25. *Decreases* the woman's risk
26. Are *less* compliant with the performance
27. Any day would be fine, but needs to be done monthly.
28. *Fibrocystic breast disease* is the most common problem
29. Between the ages of *35 and 54*
30. Another name for *prophylactically*, using chemotherapeutic agents to reduce a woman's risk for getting breast cancer. It is for those women at high risk.
31. *Large-breasted* women are at increased risk.
32. Palpable mass with a greenish-brown discharge.
33. Does *not* involve the use of implants
34. Benign nodules can be single or multiple in number and are usually well-circumscribed, movable, and tender. They also do not result in skin retraction or edema of the breast tissue. Malignant nodules are usually singular in number, nontender, nonmoveable, and can be hard to differentiate from surrounding tissue. There are skin changes from dimpling to retraction or gross deformity. The breast tissue can be shiny and edematous.
35. a. Identify the location by the face-of-the-clock method.
    b. Describe the size, shape, and consistency.
    c. Assess whether the mass is fixed or movable and whether the client has pain or soreness around the mass.
    d. Note any skin changes around the mass.
    e. Assess the adjacent lymph nodes, axillary, and supraclavicular.
36. a. The client must know measures to prevent irritation or infection of the incision site. These include wearing light, loose-fitting clothing; not using lotions or creams on the affected area; not using deodorant under the affected arm; recognizing signs and symptoms of infections as redness, swelling, increased heat, and tenderness around the site; and wearing a loose-fitting, nonwired bra with a soft-filled form for the first 6 to 8 weeks.

b. The client should be taught exercises to help her gain full range of motion of the affected arm. These include hospital exercises to continue at home and active ROM exercises to start 1 week after surgery or when drains and stitches are removed; exercises to be done only to the point of pain or pulling; give information on Encore; and teach any specific limitations specified by the physician.
c. Measures to avoid injury, infection, or swelling of the affected arm. These include no blood pressures taken from, infections acquired in, or blood drawn from the affected arm; take precautions to avoid burns in the kitchen, cuts or scrapes with cleaning or gardening; avoid sunburn and insect bites; elevate the arm whenever possible; prevent lymphedema.
d. The home does not have to be modified, but the client will need help with drain care, dressing changes, ADLs, or any type of house work that involves stretching or reaching or lifting heavy objects because of the pain and limited range of motion in the affected arm.
37. The nurse teaches the client: the different types of findings, especially those that can be identified as abnormal; how to identify normal inframammary ridge, rib areas, and breast masses; how to assume the proper position of standing in front of the mirror with arms above the head and then hands on the hip to draw attention to any breast asymmetry or shape changes; the method of examining the breasts while bathing and while lying down with the arms over the head one arm at a time, and the amount of pressure to use; the correct position of the hands for effective assessment; and how to inspect the nipple and areas for symmetrical size, shape, color, and discharge.

STUDY GUIDE NUMBER 16.75

Interventions for Clients with Gynecologic Problems

1. c
2. d
3. a
4. a
5. d
6. c
7. b
8. d
9. c
10. b
11. Children of women who took DES throughout pregnancy, cigarette smoking, multiple sexual partners
12. a, b, c

13. a
14. c
15. b
16. d
17. c
18. c
19. c
20. c
21. c
22. d
23. ...increased production of *prostaglandins.*
24. ...decrease in the hormonal levels of *estrogen.*
25. ...most serious cause of postmenopausal bleeding is *endometrial hyperplasia.*
26. Endometriosis *rarely becomes malignant...*
27. ...is *not always* treated with a hysterectomy. (*usually a last resort*)
28. *Follicular cysts* occur in young menstruating women
29. *Ovarian cancer*
30. The rarest of all gynecologic cancers...is *fallopian cancer.*
31. Depression...*occurs at anytime.*
32. *Cryosurgery* is another treatment for CIN...
33. a. 8; b. 9; c. 2; d. 10; e. 3; f. 6; g. 11; h. 5; i. 4; j. 12; k. 1; l. 7
34. Primary dysmenorrhea is one of the most common gynecologic problems in women in their teens to early 20s. Primary dysmenorrhea is usually not debilitating and is not associated with pelvic pathologic changes. Secondary dysmenorrhea usually begins with an underlying disease condition. Primary dysmenorrhea usually occurs once ovulation is established. Dysmenorrhea refers to painful uterine cramping with characteristic lower abdominal spasmodic pain. It begins with the onset of the menstrual flow and lasts for 12 to 48 hours. The pain causes nausea, vomiting, fatigue, nervousness, and the less common symptoms of headache, syncope, diarrhea, bloating, and breast tenderness. These symptoms arise from prostaglandins produced by the endometrium during the luteal phase, and levels peak at the onset of menses. The elevated levels stimulate the myometrium to spasm, which decreases uterine blood flow and yields ischemia and pain.
35. a. Application of heat or cold; b. Aerobic exercise, swimming; c. Dietary methods, including decrease sodium intake to decrease fluid retention and increase intake of vitamin B$_6$, calcium, magnesium, and protein; d. Biofeedback, relaxation, meditation, yoga, acupressure, and massage
36. *Emotional symptoms:* anxiety, low self-esteem, depression, crying spells, and irritability. *Cognitive symptoms:* short-term memory problems, unclear thinking, and difficulty concentrating. *Physical symptoms:* bloating, fatigue, fluid retention, hot flashes, appetite increases, headaches, food cravings, muscle aches and pains, and insomnia.
37. Primary amenorrhea is the absence of menstruation in that it has never occurred in a woman at least 16 years of age. This dysfunction is associated with anomalies of the reproductive tract, and the prognosis for fertility is poor. Secondary amenorrhea is the absence of menstruation, once it has started, for at least 3 months. It is usually the result of a functional disorder, and the fertility prognosis is better.
38. • Laser therapy • Radiation, internal intracavity • Radiation, externally to involved areas • Chemotherapy • Surgical excision, from the removal of only the involved area (such as vaginectomy or vulvectomy) to TAH with BSO or pelvic exenteration
39. Nursing diagnoses and collaborative problems include: • Risk for Infection • Acute Pain • Potential for Hemorrhage • Disturbed Body Image • Sexual Dysfunction • Anxiety • Fear • Impaired Urinary Elimination • Activity Intolerance • Deficient Knowledge Related to Medications, Treatment Plan, and Plan of Care • Ineffective Coping • Grieving (Any of the above that are present must be addressed for the woman to regain optimal control of her life and functioning.)

Case Studies

Answers provided on the SIMON website:
http://www.wbsaunders.com/SIMON/Iggy/

STUDY GUIDE NUMBER 16.76

Interventions for Male Clients with Reproductive Problems

1. d
2. d
3. d
4. a
5. c
6. c
7. b
8. a
9. d
10. c
11. d
12. c
13. a
14. d
15. c
16. systemic; aging
17. TURP—transurethral
18. Testicular
19. nocturnal

20. perineal
21. Organic erectile
22. Ditropan or Lomine
23. 2
24. a. 9; b. 3; c. 1; d. 12; e. 8; f. 11; g. 4; h. 6; i. 7; j. 10; k. 2; l. 5
25. • Digital rectal exam to reveal a stony hard mass • Prostate-specific antigen (PSA) level greater than 4 mg/mL
26. • Surgical radical prostatectomy • Cryosurgical ablation of the prostate • Radiation therapy • Hormonal therapy with estrogen • Chemotherapy
27. • Surgical procedures • Vascular diseases • Endocrine disorders • Medications • Smoking and/or alcohol abuse • Pelvic fractures or injuries
28. • Sickle cell disease • Diabetes • Malignancies • Trauma
29. • Sexual Dysfunction • Body Image Alteration • Pain • Fear or Anxiety
30. • Hydroureter • Hydronephrosis • Urinary retention or stasis • Urinary overflow or dribbling • Frequency • Urgency • Nocturia • Increased number of UTIs

STUDY GUIDE NUMBER 16.77

Interventions for Clients with Sexually Transmitted Diseases

1. d
2. c
3. a
4. d
5. b
6. c
7. c
8. a
9. d
10. d
11. c
12. b
13. a
14. a, b, c
15. d
16. d
17. c
18. b
19. c
20. b
21. d
22. d
23. c
24. c

25. The use of douches *increases* the risk of PID.
26. ...usually has a *yellow, green, or cheesy* discharge, *if one is present.*
27. Pain is *increased* with ambulation and *relieved by antibiotics.*
28. PID is primarily a secondary infection from an STD. The risks are the same for both STDs and PID.
29. Diagnosis of PID is made on the basis of *elevated WBC, and ESR along with cultures to evaluate the presence of Chlamydia or Neisseria.*
30. PID *may present as asymptomatic* in some women and is *very hard to diagnose.*
31. a. 3; b. 8; c. 5; d. 12; e. 7; f. 1; g. 9; h. 4; i. 11; j. 10; k. 6; l. 2
32. • Intimate sexual contact • Parental exposure to infected blood • Fecal-oral route • Intrauterine transmission to a fetus
33. • Differences in the physiology of the reproductive structures allow for increased transmission of STDs. • Adolescents and postmenopausal women are at a greater risk for STDs because of unprotected sexual intercourse. • Women have more asymptomatic infections, which delay diagnosis and treatment. • Social embarrassment, denial, or fear may further delay diagnosis and treatment.
34. • Syphilis • Gonorrhea • *Chlamydia* infection • Genital herpes
35. a. Drug therapy includes a combination of several oral and IM antibiotics, which can be administered on an outpatient basis. b. Treatment failure is rare, but if symptoms are present after treatment is finished a return visit is necessary because of the chance of reinfection. c. All sexual partners must be treated before resuming sexual relations in order to resolve the infection. d. Systemic infections can develop abruptly and require inpatient treatment with IV and IM antibiotic combinations. Symptoms to watch for include fever, chills, skin lesions on distal parts of the extremities, joint swelling, heat, and erythema.
36. • To decrease pain or discomfort from the ulcerations • To promote healing without secondary infection • To decrease viral shedding • To prevent transmission of the infection
37. a. Collect history of genital lesions or any encounters with partners that had genital lesions. b. Explain cultures, biopsies, or other diagnostic tests. c. Teach about the diagnosis, treatment regimen, and risk for relapse or complications. d. Provide comfort measures. e. Provide emotional support. f. Encourage client to discuss fears, concerns, or other needs.